HEALTH
SCIENCES
INFORMATION
SOURCES

CHING-CHIH CHEN

HEALTH SCIENCES INFORMATION SOURCES

The MIT Press
Cambridge, Massachusetts,
and London, England

This project was sponsored by the National Library of Medicine Publication Grant No. 1-RO1-LM03117-01.

© 1981 by
The Massachusetts Institute of Technology

All rights reserved. No part of this book may be reproduced in any form or by any means, electronic or mechanical, including photocopying, recording, or by any information storage and retrieval system, without permission in writing from the publisher.

This book was set in VIP Baskerville by DEKR Corporation
and printed and bound by The Murray Printing Company
in the United States of America.

Library of Congress Cataloging in Publication Data
Chen, Ching-chih, 1937–
   Health sciences information sources.

   Includes bibliographies and indexes.
   1. Medicine—Bibliography.   2. Reference books—Medicine—Bibliography.   3. Medicine—Information services.   I. Title.
Z6658.C44   [R129]   016.616   80-20557
ISBN 0-262-03074-8

To Anne and Cathy
May their interests in health sciences flourish.

CONTENTS

PREFACE	xxv
ACKNOWLEDGMENTS	xxvii
REVIEW SOURCES	xxix
SUBJECT GUIDE	xxxv

1 SELECTION TOOLS — 1
Indexes to Book Reviews — 1
Basic Tools — 2
Booklists and Serial Union Lists — 3
    Other Subject Booklists — 5
Subject and Library Catalogs for Both Current and
    Retrospective Selection — 6
    General — 6
    Subject — 7

2 GUIDES TO THE LITERATURE — 9
General — 9
General—Medicine — 11
Dentistry — 13
Genetics — 13
Gerontology — 14
Health Services Administration — 14
Infectious Diseases — 14
Nursing — 15
Pharmacy and Pharmacology — 15
Psychiatry and Psychology — 15
Public Health — 16
Urogenital System — 17
Veterinary Medicine — 17

3 BIBLIOGRAPHIES — 18
Reference Tools — 18
General — 19
Allergy and Immunology — 22
Anesthesiology and General Surgery — 22
Brain and Nervous System — 23
Cardiovascular System — 25
Dentistry — 25
Genetics — 26
Gerontology — 26
Health Services Administration — 27

Hematology	28
Infectious Diseases	29
Internal Medicine	30
Nursing	32
Nutrition	33
Oncology and Nuclear Medicine	35
Orthopedics	36
Pediatrics	36
Pharmacy and Pharmacology	37
Physical Medicine and Rehabilitation	40
Psychiatry and Psychology	41
Public Health	46
Radiology	50
Urogenital System	50
Veterinary Medicine	51

4 ENCYCLOPEDIAS 52

General	52
Anesthesiology and General Surgery	55
Internal Medicine	55
Nutrition	56
Ophthalmology	56
Pathology	56
Pediatrics	57
Pharmacy and Pharmacology	57
Physical Medicine and Rehabilitation	59
Psychiatry and Psychology	59
Public Health	60
Radiology	61
Respiratory System	61
Urogenital System	61
Veterinary Medicine	61

5 DICTIONARIES 63

Abbreviations and Acronyms	63
Subject	63
Thesauri and Nomenclatures	65
General	65
Subject	66
Drug Names	68
Multilingual	68
Bibliographies	68
English-French	69
English-German	69
English-Hebrew	70

English-Japanese	70
English-Russian	70
English-Spanish	71
More than Two Languages	71
Spelling Dictionaries	73
Subject Dictionaries	74
General	74
General—Medicine	77
Allergy and Immunology	83
Anatomy	83
Anesthesiology and General Surgery	83
Brain and Nervous System	83
Dentistry	84
Dermatology	84
Genetics	84
Health Services Administration	85
Infectious Diseases	85
Nursing	86
Nutrition	87
Ophthalmology	88
Otorhinolaryngology	88
Pathology	89
Pharmacy and Pharmacology	89
Psychiatry and Psychology	90
Public Health	91
Radiology	92
Respiratory System	92
Urogenital System	92
Veterinary Medicine	93
6 HANDBOOKS	**94**
Index	94
General	94
Allergy and Immunology	97
Anatomy	97
Anesthesiology and General Surgery	98
Brain and Nervous System	99
Cardiovascular System	102
Dentistry	103
Dermatology	104
Endocrinology	104
Gastrointestinal System	105
Genetics	105
Gerontology	106
Health Services Administration	107
Hematology	109

Infectious Diseases 109
Internal Medicine 111
Nursing 115
Nutrition 116
Oncology and Nuclear Medicine 118
Ophthalmology 119
Orthopedics 120
Otorhinolaryngology 120
Pathology 120
Pediatrics 121
Pharmacy and Pharmacology 123
Physical Medicine and Rehabilitation 127
Psychiatry and Psychology 128
Public Health 132
Radiology 136
Respiratory System 137
Urogenital System 138
Veterinary Medicine 138

7 TABLES, ALMANACS, DATABOOKS, STATISTICAL SOURCES 140

Tables 140
  SI Units 140
  Other Tables 140
Almanacs, Databooks 141
  General 141
  Nursing 143
  Nutrition 144
  Pharmacy and Pharmacology 145
  Radiology 146
  Other Subjects 147
Statistical Sources 148
  Guide to Sources of Statistical Information 148
  Governmental Statistical Sources 148
  Nongovernmental Statistical Sources 151
  Commercial Medical Market Research Services 153

8 MANUALS, LABORATORY MANUALS AND WORKBOOKS, AND SOURCE BOOKS 154

Manuals 154
  Style Manuals 154
  General 156
  Allergy and Immunology 157
  Anatomy 157
  Anesthesiology and General Surgery 158

Brain and Nervous System	160
Cardiovascular System	161
Dentistry	163
Dermatology	163
Endocrinology	164
Gastrointestinal System	165
Genetics	165
Gerontology	165
Health Services Administration	165
Hematology	166
Infectious Diseases	167
Internal Medicine	168
Nursing	172
Nutrition	174
Oncology and Nuclear Medicine	175
Ophthalmology	176
Orthopedics	176
Pathology	177
Pediatrics	178
Pharmacy and Pharmacology	179
Physical Medicine and Rehabilitation	180
Psychiatry and Psychology	181
Public Health	182
Radiology	183
Respiratory System	184
Urogenital System	185
Veterinary Medicine	186
Laboratory Manuals and Workbooks	186
General	186
Allergy and Immunology	187
Anatomy	188
Brain and Nervous System	188
Cardiovascular System	188
Dentistry	188
Genetics	188
Hematology	189
Infectious Diseases	190
Internal Medicine	192
Nursing	194
Nutrition	196
Oncology and Nuclear Medicine	196
Orthopedics	196
Pathology	197
Pharmacy and Pharmacology	197
Physical Medicine and Rehabilitation	197
Psychiatry and Psychology	198

Public Health	198
Radiology	198
Rheumatology	198
Urogenital System	199
Veterinary Medicine	199
Source Books	199
General	199
Anesthesiology and General Surgery	199
Cardiovascular System	200
Genetics	200
Gerontology	200
Health Services Administration	200
Nursing	201
Nutrition	201
Oncology and Nuclear Medicine	202
Otorhinolaryngology	202
Pharmacy and Pharmacology	202
Psychiatry and Psychology	203
Public Health	203
Rheumatology	203
9 GUIDES	**205**
General	205
Allergy and Immunology	207
Anatomy	207
Anesthesiology and General Surgery	208
Brain and Nervous System	209
Cardiovascular System	210
Dentistry	211
Dermatology	212
Endocrinology	212
Gastrointestinal System	213
Genetics	213
Gerontology	214
Health Services Administration	214
Hematology	217
Infectious Diseases	217
Internal Medicine	218
Nursing	221
Nutrition	224
Oncology and Nuclear Medicine	225
Ophthalmology	226
Orthopedics	227
Otorhinolaryngology	228
Pathology	228
Pediatrics	228

Pharmacy and Pharmacology	229
Physical Medicine and Rehabilitation	231
Psychiatry and Psychology	232
Public Health	235
Radiology	237
Respiratory System	238
Rheumatology	239
Urogenital System	239
Veterinary Medicine	241

10 ATLASES — 242

Anatomy	242
Anesthesiology and General Surgery	246
Brain and Nervous System	248
Cardiovascular System	251
Dentistry	253
Dermatology	254
Gastrointestinal System	255
Genetics	258
Hematology	260
Infectious Diseases	262
Internal Medicine	263
Oncology and Nuclear Medicine	264
Ophthalmology	265
Orthopedics	266
Otorhinolaryngology	268
Pathology	268
Pediatrics	272
Physical Medicine and Rehabilitation	273
Public Health	274
Radiology	274
Rheumatology	278
Urogenital System	278
Veterinary Medicine	280

11 DIRECTORIES, YEARBOOKS, BIOGRAPHICAL SOURCES — 281

Directories	281
Biographical Sources	281
General	281
General—Medicine	288
General—Medical Education and Care	291
Anatomy	294
Brain and Nervous System	294
Dentistry	294

Genetics	295
Gerontology	295
Health Services Administration	295
Hematology	297
Infectious Diseases	297
Internal Medicine	297
Nursing	298
Nutrition	299
Oncology and Nuclear Medicine	299
Ophthalmology	299
Pathology	300
Pediatrics	300
Pharmacy and Pharmacology	300
Physical Medicine and Rehabilitation	302
Psychiatry and Psychology	303
Public Health	304
Radiology	307
Urogenital System	307
Veterinary Medicine	308
Yearbooks	308
General	308
Anesthesiology and General Surgery	309
Brain and Nervous System	310
Cardiovascular System	310
Dentistry	310
Dermatology	310
Endocrinology	311
Health Services Administration	311
Hematology	311
Infectious Diseases	311
Internal Medicine	311
Nursing	312
Oncology and Nuclear Medicine	312
Ophthalmology	313
Orthopedics	313
Otorhinolaryngology	313
Pathology	313
Pediatrics	314
Pharmacy and Pharmacology	314
Psychiatry and Psychology	314
Public Health	314
Radiology	315
Urogenital System	315
Veterinary Medicine	315
Biographical Sources	315
General	315

Anesthesiology and General Surgery	319
Dentistry	319
Internal Medicine	319
Physical Medicine and Rehabilitation	320
Psychiatry and Psychology	320
Public Health	321
Veterinary Medicine	321

12 HISTORY — 322

General	322
Allergy and Immunology	329
Anesthesiology and General Surgery	329
Brain and Nervous System	330
Cardiovascular System	331
Dentistry	331
Genetics	332
Health Services Administration	332
Infectious Diseases	333
Internal Medicine	334
Nursing	335
Nutrition	336
Ophthalmology	337
Pathology	337
Pediatrics	337
Pharmacy and Pharmacology	337
Psychiatry and Psychology	338
Public Health	341
Radiology	342
Respiratory System	342
Urogenital System	343
Veterinary Medicine	343

13 IMPORTANT SERIES AND OTHER REVIEWS OF PROGRESS — 344

Guide to Series Publications	344
Important Series	344
General	344
Allergy and Immunology	346
Anatomy	347
Anesthesiology and General Surgery	348
Brain and Nervous System	349
Cardiovascular System	352
Dentistry	353
Dermatology	353
Endocrinology	353

Gastrointestinal System	355
Genetics	355
Gerontology	356
Hematology	356
Infectious Diseases	357
Internal Medicine	358
Nursing	359
Nutrition	359
Oncology and Nuclear Medicine	360
Ophthalmology	361
Orthopedics	362
Otorhinolaryngology	362
Pathology	363
Pediatrics	364
Pharmacy and Pharmacology	365
Psychiatry and Psychology	367
Public Health	368
Radiology	370
Respiratory System	371
Rheumatology	371
Urogenital System	371
Veterinary Medicine	372
Other Reviews of Progress	372
Tools to Medical Reviews	372
Reviews	373

14 TREATISES 374

General	374
Allergy and Immunology	375
Anatomy	376
Anesthesiology and General Surgery	377
Brain and Nervous System	378
Cardiovascular System	380
Dentistry	380
Dermatology	381
Endocrinology	382
Gastrointestinal System	382
Genetics	382
Gerontology	383
Hematology	383
Infectious Diseases	383
Nursing	384
Nutrition	385
Oncology and Nuclear Medicine	386
Ophthalmology	387

Orthopedics	388
Otorhinolaryngology	388
Pathology	388
Pediatrics	389
Pharmacy and Pharmacology	390
Psychiatry and Psychology	390
Public Health	391
Radiology	392
Rheumatology	392
Urogenital System	392
Veterinary Medicine	393
15 MONOGRAPHS	**394**
General	394
Allergy and Immunology	398
Anatomy	400
Anesthesiology and General Surgery	401
Brain and Nervous System	403
Cardiovascular System	408
Dentistry	414
Dermatology	416
Endocrinology	418
Gastrointestinal System	420
Genetics	423
Gerontology	426
Health Services Administration	427
Hematology	429
Infectious Diseases	432
Internal Medicine	436
Nursing	439
Nutrition	449
Oncology and Nuclear Medicine	451
Ophthalmology	455
Orthopedics	459
Otorhinolaryngology	461
Pathology	462
Pediatrics	465
Pharmacy and Pharmacology	473
Physical Medicine and Rehabilitation	476
Psychiatry and Psychology	478
Public Health	482
Radiology	485
Respiratory System	488
Rheumatology	491
Urogenital System	492
Veterinary Medicine	497

16 ABSTRACTS AND INDEXES, AND CURRENT-AWARENESS SERVICES 499

Abstracts and Indexes 499
  Guides to Abstracts and Indexes 499
  General 500
  Subject Tools 504
    National Library of Medicine Recurring Bibliographies 504
    General—Medicine 507
    Allergy and Immunology 508
    Brain and Nervous System 509
    Dentistry 509
    Dermatology 510
    Endocrinology 510
    Gastrointestinal System 511
    Genetics 511
    Health Services Administration 511
    Infectious Diseases 512
    Internal Medicine 513
    Nursing 513
    Nutrition 514
    Oncology and Nuclear Medicine 515
    Ophthalmology 515
    Orthopedics 516
    Pharmacy and Pharmacology 516
    Physical Medicine and Rehabilitation 517
    Psychiatry and Psychology 517
    Public Health 519
    Rheumatology 521
    Urogenital System 522
    Veterinary Medicine 522
Current-Awareness Services 522
  General 522
  Subject 522
  Information Services 523

17 PERIODICALS 524

Reference Sources 524
Abbreviations 525
Selective Titles 526
  General 526
  Allergy and Immunology 527
  Anatomy 527
  Anesthesiology and General Surgery 527
  Brain and Nervous System 528
  Cardiovascular System 528

Dentistry	528
Dermatology	529
Endocrinology	529
Gastrointestinal System	529
Genetics	529
Gerontology	529
Health Services Administration	529
Hematology	529
History	530
Infectious Diseases	530
Internal Medicine	530
Nursing	531
Nutrition	531
Oncology and Nuclear Medicine	531
Ophthalmology	531
Orthopedics	532
Otorhinolaryngology	532
Pathology	532
Pediatrics	532
Pharmacy and Pharmacology	532
Physical Medicine and Rehabilitation	533
Psychiatry and Psychology	534
Public Health	534
Radiology	534
Respiratory System	534
Rheumatology	534
Urogenital System	534
Veterinary Medicine	535

18 TECHNICAL REPORTS AND GOVERNMENT DOCUMENTS 536

Technical Reports	536
General Reference Tools	537
Subject Reference Tools	538
Government Documents	539
General Major Bibliographical Sources	539
Subject Bibliographical Sources	542
National Library of Medicine (NLM) Publications	543

19 CONFERENCE PROCEEDINGS, TRANSLATIONS, DISSERTATIONS, AND RESEARCH IN PROGRESS, PREPRINTS, AND REPRINTS 544

Conference Proceedings	544
Calendars and Forthcoming Meetings	544
General	544
Subject	545

Published Proceedings	545
Major Bibliographical Tools	545
Conference Publications	547
General	547
Allergy and Immunology	549
Anesthesiology and General Surgery	549
Brain and Nervous System	549
Endocrinology	549
Gastrointestinal System	550
Genetics	550
Infectious Diseases	550
Nursing	551
Nutrition	551
Oncology and Nuclear Medicine	551
Orthopedics	552
Pathology	552
Pediatrics	552
Pharmacy and Pharmacology	553
Psychiatry and Psychology	553
Translations	553
General Sources	553
Abstracting and Indexing Sources	555
Cover-to-Cover Translations	555
Dissertations and Research in Progress	556
Dissertations	556
General Tools	556
Subject Guides	557
Research in Progress	558
General	558
Subject	561
Preprints	562
Reprints	563
Reference Tools	563
Subject Tools	563
20 CLASSIFICATIONS, STANDARDS, AND PATENTS	**565**
Classifications	565
General	565
Dentistry	566
Health Services Administration	566
Oncology and Nuclear Medicine	566
Psychiatry and Psychology	567
Veterinary Medicine	567
Standards	567
Guides to Standards	568

Major Bibliographical Tools—General	569
Medical Standards	570
General	571
Anatomy	571
Cardiovascular System	572
Gastrointestinal System	572
Health Services Administration	572
Nursing	573
Nutrition	574
Pharmacy and Pharmacology	574
Physical Medicine and Rehabilitation	576
Public Health	576
Radiology	577
Patents	578
Indexes to US and International Patents	579
Sources about Patents	579
US Patents	580
International Patents	581

21 TRADE LITERATURE 583

Guide to Trade Literature	583
Trade Reference Tools	584
Sample Trade Periodicals	585
Monographs	586

22 NONPRINT MATERIALS 587

General Reference Sources	588
AV Equipment	591
Microform Information Services	592
Subject Sources	592
General	592
Anatomy	595
Anesthesiology and General Surgery	595
Brain and Nervous System	596
Dentistry	596
Health Services Administration	596
Infectious Diseases	596
Nursing	596
Oncology and Nuclear Medicine	597
Ophthalmology	597
Orthopedics	598
Pediatrics	598
Pharmacy and Pharmacology	598
Psychiatry and Psychology	598
Public Health	599
Urogenital System	600

23 PROFESSIONAL SOCIETIES AND THEIR PUBLICATIONS 601

Directories 601
Society Publications 603
   Guides 603
Selective List of Professional Organizations 603
   General 603
   Allergy and Immunology 605
   Anesthesiology and General Surgery 605
   Brain and Nervous System 606
   Cardiovascular System 606
   Dentistry 606
   Dermatology 606
   Endocrinology 606
   Gastrointestinal System 607
   Gerontology 607
   Health Services Administration 607
   Hematology 608
   Infectious Diseases 608
   Internal Medicine 608
   Nursing 608
   Nutrition 609
   Oncology and Nuclear Medicine 609
   Ophthalmology 610
   Orthopedics 610
   Otorhinolaryngology 610
   Pathology 610
   Pediatrics 610
   Pharmacy and Pharmacology 610
   Physical Medicine and Rehabilitation 611
   Psychiatry and Psychology 611
   Public Health 612
   Radiology 612
   Respiratory System 612
   Rheumatology 612
   Urogenital System 613
   Veterinary Medicine 613
   Other Organizations 613

24 DATA BASES 614

Directory Sources 614
Evaluation of Data Bases 614
National Library of Medicine 614
   Brief Introduction of the National Library of Medicine 615
   Computerized Literature Retrieval Services of the National Library of Medicine 615

Regional Medical Libraries   616
　　NLM Online Services Program Policy Statement   619
　　Data Bases Available on the Online Network   620
　　　Tools for the Use of NLM Data Bases   623
Selective Data Bases   623

REFERENCE LIST   633

TITLE INDEX   653

AUTHOR INDEX   725

AUTHOR INDEX TO REFERENCE LIST   765

PREFACE

This book is intended primarily as a reference guide for health sciences librarians and their assistants and as a textbook for library school students engaged in the study of the structure, properties, and output of biomedical and clinical literature. It is also my hope that the work will serve as a handy reference manual for physicians, allied health professionals, students in all fields of the health sciences, and others who rely on health sciences library resources.

Given the vast amount of published material in the fields of health sciences, the titles included are necessarily selective, although in most categories no obvious attempt has been made to present only the "best" of the sources available. While the user may find a surprising variety of information suitable for a general library—consumer guides, medical folklore dictionaries—the vast majority of the information sources included are in all likelihood more suited to an academic or special health sciences collection. Since health sciences information must be current, the primary criterion for inclusion in this volume is that the reference be a current source of information. Few titles published prior to 1970 will be evident; the majority of titles have imprint dates after 1975. The last date for inclusion is April 1980.

Most books of this type tend to include only secondary sources, and yet active health professionals in the field rely more heavily on informal and primary channels of communications. This pattern has been substantiated by a significant number of use studies of the information needs of medical scientists, professionals, and students. For this reason, *Health Sciences Information Sources* provides a substantial coverage of primary sources.

Each type of subject literature is useful and sought after in distinctive and separate situations. Thus, the sources are grouped first by types of material and then by subject within each category. Altogether, more than four thousand sources are grouped under twenty-four categories. It is intended that by this arrangement the users of health sciences libraries may have easier access to available information sources. I also hope that health sciences librarians and library school students may be made more keenly aware of the varied uses of each type of information as well as the characteristics and properties of health sciences literature. The necessary discussion of a few types of information has been kept extremely brief. Many useful bibliographical sources for each type of information are provided in the Reference List. Additional discussions of the structure of medical subject literature and other pertinent topics can be located in several sources included in chapter 2, Guides to the Literature. The material incorporates primarily the clinical and biomedical sciences. Few other scientific and technical titles are covered in this book unless they have general applications for health science professionals, since a companion volume, *Scientific and Technical Information Sources*, was published in 1977. Under each type of information sources (each chapter in this book), materials are subgrouped by subject categories, and details on the scope of each subject category are provided in the Subject Guide following this Preface. The subject approach using Medical Subject Headings, adopted in the *Medical Reference Works*, was rejected because I feel that the minute headings hinder the effective use of tools of this type, fragment the listing of sources, and, in effect, make it impossible to browse. Although certain foreign titles are included, this book heavily emphasizes American works.

All entries have been arranged by title rather than by the more conventional main-entry approach. There are several justifications for such a treatment. First, most users, including librarians unfamiliar with health sciences information sources, cannot usually remember the names of authors. Second, many sources are more commonly known by their titles, while many secondary sources frequently change editorship. Finally, many key primary sources (such as *JAMA* and *New England Journal of Medicine*) used by health professionals list reviewed books by title, consequently these individuals are probably more comfortable with such an approach. Those readers seeking to locate a source by author approach can easily do so through the use of an author index.

Most entries are annotated. These generally brief annotations have been designed, whenever possible, to include critical as well as descriptive information, with emphasis on the former. It should be pointed out that while I am familiar with many of the sources, some, particularly more current ones, have been included without personal inspection. These annotations are generally brief abstracts from various review sources.

A major feature of this book is that review sources, when available, are provided at the end of the annotations, introduced by the letter R. The review information is presented with scientific and medical journal sources by alphabetical order first, then nonscience and nonhealth sciences journal sources, and finally book sources. A list of these sources is included following the table of contents. For purposes of comparison, the review citations also include, whenever possible, those for the earlier editions of the titles listed. Another feature of this book is a subject-classified reference list of pertinent sources (Reference List). The list will supply interested readers with starting key references for a specific topic. An author index to this reference list is also provided.

To facilitate the use of this book, a detailed table of contents is included for easy subject approach. There is a complete author index, including personal as well as corporate names, and a comprehensive title index.

A book of this size and scope is necessarily imperfect. I would be most grateful to receive any suggestions, corrections, and additions that readers may be inclined to offer.

ACKNOWLEDGMENTS

I wish to express my deep appreciation to those who have made this book possible. First of all, this project would not have been feasible without a generous Publication Grant from the National Library of Medicine. A project of this scope and complexity could not possibly have been completed without the long involvement of numerous research assistants whose help is deeply appreciated. While it is impossible to thank each one of them individually, I do want to single out two of my assistants, Nina Green and Nancy Padykula, who stayed with the entire project from the very beginning and whose excellent work and tireless devotion to this project made its completion possible. This book has benefited from the wisdom of several consultants. Among them, I want to thank Barbara Hill, Librarian of the Massachusetts College of Pharmacy and Allied Health Sciences, and Mary L. Pekarski, Librarian of the School of Nursing Library of Boston College, for agreeing to work on the project under impossible time pressures and for their critical comments and suggestions. As usual with all my books, I am deeply indebted to every member of my family for their unfailing and unselfish support, love, understanding, and encouragement. Last, but certainly not least, my two daughters, Anne and Cathy, who played major roles in the production of the *Scientific and Technical Information Sources,* the companion volume of this book, deserve again the greatest credit and thanks for their long, active, and most devoted participation in most aspects of the project activities and for their perfect typing of most of this large manuscript.

REVIEW SOURCES

Abbreviations will be given only when they are used in the review information following the annotations, introduced by the letter R.

MEDICAL AND SCIENTIFIC JOURNALS

AAAS Science Books & Films
Abstracts of Hygiene
American Family Physician
American Heart Journal
American Journal of Cardiology
American Journal of Clinical Nutrition
American Journal of Digestive Diseases
American Journal of Diseases of Children
American Journal of Human Genetics
American Journal of Nursing
American Journal of Occupational Therapy
American Journal of Ophthalmology
American Journal of Proctology
American Journal of Psychiatry
American Journal of Psychology
American Journal of Public Health
American Journal of Roentgenology
American Journal of Tropical Medicine and Hygiene
American Journal of Veterinary Research
American Review of Respiratory Diseases
American Scientist
Anaesthesia
Analytical Chemistry
Anesthesiology
Annals of Allergy
Annals of Human Genetics
Annals of Internal Medicine
Annals of Otology, Rhinology and Laryngology
Annals of Thoracic Surgery
Archives of Dermatology
Archives of Environmental Health
Archives of Internal Medicine
Archives of Neurology
Archives of Ophthalmology
Archives of Otolaryngology
Archives of Pathology & Laboratory Medicine
Archives of Physical Medicine and Rehabilitation
Archives of Surgery
Arthritis and Rheumatism
Biology of the Neonate
Biomaterials, Medical Devices and Artificial Organs
Biomedical Engineering
Biomedical Instrumentation and Measurements
Bioscience
Blood
Brain
British Dental Journal
British Journal of Medicine (BMJ)

British Journal of Obstetrics & Gynaecology
British Journal of Ophthalmology
British Journal of Radiology
British Journal of Surgery
British Medical Bulletin
British Medical Journal
Canadian Family Physician
Canadian Journal of Genetics and Cytology
Canadian Medical Association Journal
Canadian Nurse
Cardiac Mechanics
Chemical Marketing Reporter
Chemistry and Industry
Chest
Clinical Chemistry
Clinical Immunology and Immunopathology
Clinical Notes on Respiratory Diseases
Clinical Pediatrics
Clinical Pharmacology and Therapeutics
Comparative Psychology
Computers and Medicine
Contemporary Psychology
Data Processing Digest
Dermatologica
Diabetes
Digestion
Digestive Diseases & Science
Electroencephalography & Clinical Neurophysiology
European Journal of Obstetrics,
Gynecology & Reproductive Biology
Food Engineering
Food Science and Technology Abstracts
Food Technology
Gastroenterology
Geriatrics
Group Practice
Growth
Health Laboratory Science
Health Physics
Heredity
Hospital Administration
Hospital and Health Services Administration
Hospitals
Human Pathology
Immunogenetics
Immunological Communications
Immunology
International Archives of Allergy & Applied Immunology
International Journal of Nursing Studies
International Journal of Radiation Biology
International Nursing Review
Johns Hopkins Medical Journal
Journal of Allied Health
Journal of Anatomy
Journal of Bone and Joint Surgery
Journal of Chemical Education
Journal of Chronic Diseases
Journal of Clinical Pathology

Journal of Community Health
Journal of Dentistry
Journal of Experimental Physiology
Journal of Food Technology
Journal of Gerontology
Journal of Histochemistry and Cytochemistry
Journal of Human Nutrition
Journal of Investigative Dermatology
Journal of Medical Education
Journal of Nervous and Mental Disease
Journal of Neurosurgery
Journal of Nursing Administration
Journal of Nursing Education
Journal of Obstetrics and Gynaecology of the British Commonwealth
Journal of Oral Pathology
Journal of Oral Surgery
Journal of Parasitology
Journal of Pathology
Journal of Pediatrics
Journal of Pharmaceutical Sciences
Journal of Psychiatric Nursing and Mental Health Services
Journal of School Health
Journal of the American Chemical Society
Journal of the American Dental Association
Journal of the American Dietetic Association
Journal of the American Geriatrics Society
Journal of the American Medical Association (JAMA)
Journal of the American Medical Women's Association (JAMWA)
Journal of the American Osteopathic Association
Journal of the American Veterinary Medical Association
Journal of the Kansas Medical Society
Journal of the Medical Society of New Jersey
Journal of the Royal Society of Health
Journal of the Royal Statistical Society
Journal of Veterinary Research
Laboratory Animal Science
Laboratory Practice
Lahey Clinic Foundation Bulletin
Lancet
Mayo Clinic Proceedings
Medical Care
Medical Journal of Australia
Medical Meetings
Microchemical Journal
Military Medicine
Military Review
Modern Healthcare
Nation's Health
Nature
Neurology
Neuropsychology
Neuroscience
New England Journal of Medicine (NEJM)

New Physician
New Scientists
New Zealand Medical Journal
Nurse Educator
Nurse Practitioner
Nursing
Nursing Clinics of North America
Nursing Digest
Nursing Forum
Nursing Research
Nutrition
Nutrition Reviews
Obstetrics and Gynecology
Occupational Health Nursing
Pediatrics
Pharmaceutical Journal
Physical Therapy
Physics in Medicine & Biology
Plastic and Reconstructive Surgery
Postgraduate Medicine
The Practitioners
Proceedings of the Royal Society of Medicine
Psychological Medicine
Quarterly Review of Biology
Radiology
Rheumatology and Rehabilitation
Social Biology
Society of Motion Picture and Television Engineers
South African Medical Journal
Supervisor Nurse
Surgery, Gynecology and Obstetrics
Teratology
Transfusion
Unlisted Drugs
Veterinary Medicine & Small Animal Clinician
Yale Journal of Biology and Medicine

NONMEDICAL AND NONSCIENTIFIC JOURNALS

American Libraries
Aslib Book List (ABL)
Aslib Proceedings
Assistant Librarian
Australian Library Journal
Bibliographical Society of American Papers
Bibliography, Documentation, Terminology
Book Review Digest
Booklist (BL)
British Book Notes
Bulletin of the Medical Library Association (BMLA)
Business Journal
Business Literature
Canadian Library Journal
Catholic Library World
Choice
College & Research Libraries (CRL)
Consultant News
Grant Magazine
Herald of Library Science
Industrial Bookshelf
Inquiry
International Bibliography,

Information, Documentation (IBID)
John Wiley & Sons Librarians' Newsletter
Journal of Academic Librarianship
Journal of Documentation
Journal of the American Society for Information Science (JASIS)
Kemixon Reporter (Spain)
Library Association Record
Library Journal (LJ)
Library of Congress Information Bulletin (LCIB)
Library Quarterly (LQ)
Management Review
Mass Media Booknotes
New Library World
New Technical Books (NTB)
Quarterly Bulletin of the International Association of Argicultural Librarians and Documentalists
Reference and Subscription Book Review
Reference Services Review (RSR)
RQ
Saturday Review
Sci-Tech Book News
Sci-Tech News
Special Libraries (SL)
Technical Book Review Index (TBRI)
UNESCO Bulletin for Libraries (UBL)
Wilson Library Bulletin (WLS)

BOOK SOURCES

Abbreviation Used	Title
ARBA	*American Reference Book Annual.* Vols. 1–. Littleton, CT: Libraries Unlimited, 1970–.
Chen	Chen, Ching-chih, *Scientific and Technical Information Sources.* Cambridge, MA: MIT Press, 1978.
Jenkins	Jenkins, Frances Briggs. *Science Reference Sources.* 5th ed. Cambridge, MA: MIT Press, 1969. (Replaced by Chen)
Katz	Katz, William. *Magazines for Libraries.* 2d ed. New York: Bowker, 1972. Also, suppl. 1, 1974.
Mal	Malinowsky, H. Robert; Gray, Richard A.; and Gray, Dorothy A. *Science and Engineering Literature.* 2d ed. Littleton, CT: Libraries Unlimited, 1976.
MRW	*Medical Reference Works, 1679–1976: A Selected Bibliography.* **John B. Blake and Charles Roos.** Chicago, IL: Medical Library Association, 1967.
MRW, S1	———. Supplement 1, 1967–1968, (1970).
MRW, S2	———. Supplement 2, 1969–1972, (1973).

MRW, S3	_____. Supplement 3, 1973–1974, (1975).
Sheehy	Sheehy, Eugene P. *Guide to Reference Books.* 9th ed. Chicago, IL: American Library Association, 1977. (Eighth edition under Winchell)
Wal	Walford, A. J., ed. *Guide to Reference Material.* 3d ed. Vol. 1: *Science and Technology.* London: Library Association, 1973.
Win	Winchell, Constance M. *Guide to Reference Books.* 8th ed. Chicago, IL: American Library Association, 1967. Also, supps. 1, 1965–1966, (1968); 2, 1967–1968, (1970); 3, 1969–1970, (1972).

CORE LISTS
(See Reference List for further information.)

Allyn	Allyn, Richard. "A Library for Internists Recommended by the American College of Physicians," *Annals of Internal Medicine* 84: 346–373 (1976).
Brandon	Brandon, Alfred N. "Selected List of Books and Journals for the Small Medical Library," *Bulletin of the Medical Library Association* (April issue of the odd year).
Brandon (NO)	Brandon, Alfred N. "Selected List of Nursing Books and Journals," *Nursing Outlook* 27: 672–680 (Oct. 1979).
Stearns & Ratcliff (AJN)	Stearns, Norman S.; Ratcliff, Wendy W.; et al. "A Core Nursing Library for Practitioners," *American Journal of Nursing* 70: 818–823 (1970).
Stearns & Ratcliff (NEJM, 1969)	Stearns, Norman S., and Ratcliff, Wendy W. "A Core Medical Library for Practitioners in Community Hospitals," *New England Journal of Medicine* 280: 474–480 (Feb. 27, 1969).
Stearns & Ratcliff (NEJM, 1970)	Stearns, Norman S., and Ratcliff, Wendy W. "An Integrated Health Science Core Library for Physicians, Nurses and Allied Health Practitioners in Community Hospitals," *New England Journal of Medicine* 283: 1489–1498 (Dec. 31, 1970).

SUBJECT GUIDE

Under each type of information source (each chapter in this book), materials are subgrouped by subject categories. I have considered the approach used by the *Medical Reference Works* arranged by Medical Subject Headings (MeSH), but decided against it because it will fragment the listing and prevent effective use of this book by health sciences professionals who are not familiar with MeSH.

In this work, like in its companion volume *Scientific and Technical Information Sources,* all sources are grouped in broad subjects. The following is a guide to these categories:

Subject Category	Scope
GENERAL	Chemistry, biology, medicolegal ethics, medical education
ALLERGY AND IMMUNOLOGY	Allergy, asthma, immune disorders, all aspects of immunobiology
ANATOMY	Normal growth and structure of the human body, including embryology and physiology
ANESTHESIOLOGY AND GENERAL SURGERY	Anesthesia and analgesic drugs. General surgical techniques, plastic and reconstructive surgery, surgical equipment. Surgery of specific organs is with the organ system
BRAIN AND NERVOUS SYSTEM	Brain, CNS, Spinal cord, tumors of brain, etc. Neurology in general
CARDIOVASCULAR SYSTEM	Heart, blood vessels, circulation, thoracic surgery
DENTISTRY	Oral pathology, oral surgery, teeth, palate, gums, jaw, public health dentistry
DERMATOLOGY	Skin, hair, nails, in both their normal and pathological conditions. Includes skin cancer
ENDOCRINOLOGY	Endocrine glands and their secretions, hormones and hormone chemistry, metabolic diseases, digestive enzymes

GASTROINTESTINAL SYSTEM	Stomach, intestine, colon, liver, pancreas, digestive disorders
GENETICS	Genes, chromosomes, birth defects, genetically inherited diseases, teratology
GERONTOLOGY	All geriatric diseases, studies of aging
HEALTH SERVICES ADMINISTRATION	Hospital administration, including purchasing of equipment; regional, state, and national health planning, health maintenance organizations, office practice, administration of health and special facilities such as geriatric and mental health clinics
HEMATOLOGY	Blood, bone marrow, blood chemistry
INFECTIOUS DISEASES	Microbiology, bacteria and fungi, epidemiology, mycology, communicable diseases, viruses and virology
INTERNAL MEDICINE	General medicine, family practice, trauma, burn, critical care, bedside diagnosis, laboratory medicine
NURSING	All medical literature that relates to the nursing profession, including critical care, anesthesiology, pediatrics, etc.
NUTRITION	Diet, food, nutritional requirements
ONCOLOGY AND NUCLEAR MEDICINE	All forms of cancer treatment and therapy
OPHTHALMOLOGY	Eye diseases and surgery, optometry, mechanisms of vision
ORTHOPEDICS	Bone diseases, orthopedic surgery
OTORHINOLARYNGOLOGY	Ear, nose, throat and their anatomy, pathology, and surgery
PATHOLOGY	Cell biology, histology, microscopy, studies of diseased tissues and organs

PEDIATRICS	All medical literature related to newborns, children, and diseases of newborns, children, adolescents
	Also prenatal care of mother and child
PHARMACY AND PHARMACOLOGY	Composition, chemistry, and interactions of drugs
	Toxicity, adverse reactions, biology of drug reactions, herbal medicine
PHYSICAL MEDICINE AND REHABILITATION	Speech pathology, physical therapy, occupational therapy, aids for blindness, hearing
PSYCHIATRY AND PSYCHOLOGY	Mental health, social work, psychotropic drugs, crisis intervention, biopsychology
PUBLIC HEALTH	Disease vectors, environmental health, contamination and pollution of air, water, land
	Occupational safety, sanitation, health hazards of radiation, toxic chemicals, preventive medicine
RADIOLOGY	Methods of diagnosis, such as ultrasound, computerized axial tomography, X-rays
	Radiology of diseases, bone growth, etc.
RESPIRATORY SYSTEM	Lungs, lung cancer, pulmonary/respiratory disease (i.e. emphysema), metastasis
RHEUMATOLOGY	Arthritis, rheumatic diseases, muscle diseases, diseases of joints and connective tissue
UROGENITAL SYSTEM	Kidney, reproductive organs and diseases (both male and female), urology, infertility
VETERINARY MEDICINE	All animal medical science

Subject Classification Examples

While such categories as Nursing and Dentistry are straightforward, other categories here should be briefly explained as to their content. For example, Internal Medicine would cover a manual of bedside diagnosis, as it would one on clinical laboratory medicine; however, books which are less specifically related to medicine, such as handbooks of biology and chemistry, would be classed in the General category. Another example is the Brain and Nervous System subject section, which would contain a discussion of the medical repercussions of spinal cord injury; however, a book which focuses on the rehabilitative process resulting from this injury would be found in Physical Medicine. Likewise, a book which covers digestive enzymes would be found under Endocrinology, while one which discusses digestive diseases would be located under the Gastrointestinal System.

HEALTH SCIENCES INFORMATION SOURCES

CHAPTER 1   SELECTION TOOLS

Publishers' blurbs and catalogs are usually the most up-to-date information sources of newly available scientific and medical books. But journals are probably the most important sources for critical evaluative information on new medical books. For better understanding and easy identification of the major reviewing journals in the fields of health sciences, the following book should be consulted:

Biomedical, Scientific, and Technical Book Reviewing. **Ching-chih Chen.** Metuchen, NJ: Scarecrow Press, 1976.

Comprehensive, detailed analysis of book reviewing in biomedicine, science, and technology. Approximately 500 journals in field were examined. Among topics explored are identification of major biomedical, scientific, and technical journals that contain book reviews, analysis of reviews, and identification of major publishers of biomedical, scientific, and technical books. Important volume for technical librarians involved in monographic selection and collection development.
R: *Computers and Medicine* 6: 7 (May/June 1977); *BMLA* 65: 487 (Oct. 1977); *CRL* 38: 260 (May 1977); *Journal of Academic Librarianship* 3: 159 (July 1977); 3: 234 (Sept. 1977); *LJ* 102: 210 (Jan. 15, 1977); *LQ* 48: 555 (Oct. 1978); *UBL* 31: 304 (Nov.–Dec. 1977); *ARBA* (1978, p. 704); Chen (p. 1).

INDEXES TO BOOK REVIEWS

Current Book Review Citations. New York: H. W. Wilson. Monthly.

Monthly index to book reviews, 50,000 entries a year that appeared in more than 1,200 periodicals in all major areas of study, including medicine. With no research emphasis.

Index to Book Reviews in the Sciences. Vols. 1–. Philadelphia, PA: Institute for Scientific Information, 1980–. Monthly.

A multidisciplinary index to some 35,000 current book reviews in the life sciences, clinical medicine, physical sciences, agriculture, and engineering. Arranged by author or editor, and subject. Valuable tool for librarians, researchers, professors, and students.

Science Fiction Book Review Index, 1923–1973. **H. W. Hall, ed.** Detroit: Gale Research, 1975.

A complete record of all books, including non-science-fiction books, reviewed in the science-fiction magazines from 1923 to 1973, and a record of all science-fiction and fantasy books reviewed from 1970 to 1973 in selected general magazines. Citations to about 14,000 reviews are included. Indexed.
R: *LJ* (Sept. 1, 1975).

Technical Book Review Index. Vols. 43–. **Carnegie Library of Pittsburgh and Maurice and Laura Falk Library of the Health Professions, University of Pittsburgh.** Pittsburgh, PA: JAAD Publishing Co., 1977–. Monthly except July and August.

Continues the *Technical Book Review Index*, Volume 1–42, 1935–1976, published by the Special Library Association. Same format.
R: Chen (p. 2); Katz (p. 27); Mal (3-7); Wal (p. 10); Win (EA68; EA69).

BASIC TOOLS

Besides the following listed tools, readers are referred to the general section of the chapter on guides to the literature for other major sources for collection development.

Aslib Book List: List of Recommended Scientific and Technical Books, with Annotations. London: Aslib, 1935–. Monthly.

All entries have evaluative annotations by specialists and are graded into categories for users of general, intermediate, highly technical, and reference books. Of special interest to librarians for acquisition purposes. Arranged by universal decimal system categories.
R: Chen (p. 2); Mal (3-4); Wal (p. 5).

British Books in Print 1978. New York: Bowker, 1978.

Medical Books and Serials in Print 1979: An Index to Literature in the Health Sciences. 8th ed. New York: Bowker, 1979.

Early editions under the title *Bowker's Medical Books in Print: Subject Index, Author Index, Title Index,* 1972–78.
An index to author, title, and subject of medical books in print. Also lists serials, publishers. A comprehensive reference for bibliographical information. Contains over 35,000 titles in medicine and allied fields currently available in the United States. Some 5,000 subject areas from psychiatry to veterinary medicine; format is like that of *Books in Print*. Entries are indexed alphabetically by author, title, and subject and provide author, title, price, imprint, publisher, series, ISBN, etc. Provides direct access to monographic medical literature in print.
R: *BL* 70: 451 (Jan. 1973); 73: 1068 (Mar. 1976); *LJ* 97: 72 (Sept. 15, 1972); *RSR* 2: 118 (July–Sept. 1974); 3: 71 (July–Dec. 1975); *ARBA* (1973, p. 605); 1975, p. 732; 1976, p. 725; 1977, p. 705); *MRW* S3, pp. 5, 9, 13, 37, 54; Sheehy (EK4); Win (EK26).

Medical Books '79. A Preferred List. **Major Scientific Books, Inc.** Flemington, NJ: Medical Media Corp., 1979.

A selected catalog of books, encompassing the medical, dental, nursing, veterinary, and related health professions. Includes list of participating publishers. Available free.

New Technical Books: A Selective List With Descriptive Annotations. Vols. 1–. New York: New York Public Library, 1915–. 10 nos./yr.

Provides a selected list of tables of contents from noteworthy publications. Covers pure and applied sciences, mathematics, engineering, industrial technology. Dewey classification, annual author and subject index.
R: Jenkins (p. 28); Mal (3-3); Sheehy (EA36).

NLL Announcement Bulletin. Vols. 1–. Boston Spa, England: National Lending Library for Science and Technology, 1971–.
R: Chen (p. 1).

Science Books: A Quarterly Review. Vols. 1–. Washington, DC: American Association for the Advancement of Science, 1965–. Quarterly.
Annotated, classified list of new books in the pure and applied sciences.
R: *LJ* 92: 1577 (Apr. 1967); Chen (p. 1); Jenkins (A228); Wal (p. 9); Win (1EA6).

Science Books and Films. Washington, DC: American Association for the Advancement of Science, 1965–. Quarterly.
A classified listing. Critical reviews.
R: Chen (p. 1); Mal (3-5).

Scientific and Technical Books in Print. New York: Bowker, 1972–. Annual.
An outgrowth of *Books in Print* and *Subject Guide to Books in Print.* Lists titles available from 1,200 publishers, providing subject, author, and title approach.
R: *ARBA* (1973, p. 533; 1974, p. 542); Chen (p. 1); Mal (3-1).

Technical Books in Print: A Reference Catalogue of Books in Print and on Sale in Great Britain. London: Whitaker, 1964–.
R: Chen (p. 2); Win (1EA7).

BOOKLISTS AND SERIAL UNION LISTS

See also the core lists in the Reference List of this book.

The AAAS Science Book List: A Selected and Annotated List of Science and Mathematics Books for Secondary School Students, College Undergraduates, and Nonspecialists. 3d ed. **Hilary J. Deason, comp.** Washington, DC: American Association for the Advancement of Science, 1970.
Titles numbering 2,441 are arranged under Dewey decimal classification categories. Descriptive annotations and evaluative critiques.
R: Chen (p. 2); Mal (3-6).

Basic Book and Periodical List, Nursing School and Small Medical Library. 4th ed. **Sister Mary Concordia, OSF.** Peru, IL: St. Bede Abbey Press, 1967.

Basic List of Books and Journals for Veterans Administration Medical Libraries. **Central Office Library, US Veterans Administration.** Washington, DC: US Veterans Administration, 1972.

Basic List of Guides and Information Sources for Professional and Patients' Libraries in Hospitals. 8th ed. **Joint Committee on Library Service in Hospitals, Council of National Library Associations.** Chicago, IL: American Hospital Association, 1973.
Seventh edition, 1971.

Annotated bibliography of guides, lists, information sources, and publication facts for hospital libraries. No index.
R: *MRW* S2, p. 62.

Basic Texts of the Food and Agriculture Organization of the United Nations. 2 vols. New York: Unipub, 1971.
Updated to 1974, 2 volumes, 1975.
R: Chen (p. 2).

Books and Periodicals for Medical Libraries in Hospitals. 5th ed. **Jenny Wade, Howard Hague, and Leslie Morton, comps. and eds.** Medical Section, Library Association. London: Library Association, 1978.
Lists some 700 books and periodicals with heavy application in the medical field. Concentrates on clinical practice. Alphabetical arrangement of citations by author's names. Provides complete bibliographic information. No index.
R: *MRW* S3, pp. 5, 31.

A Guide to the Use of the Excerpta Medica Abstract Journals: A List of 4,000 Biomedical Terms Most Commonly Used in Search Formulation of Secondary Publications. **Excerpta Medica Foundation.** Amsterdam: Excerpta Medica Foundation, 1969–. Irregular.
Helpful terminology guide to various sections of *Excerpta Medica*. Alphabetical arrangement of terms with appropriate section accompanying each entry.
R: *MRW* S2, p. 20.

Index of NLM Serial Titles: A Keyword Listing of Serial Titles Currently Received by the National Library of Medicine, DHEW Pub. no. (NIH) 79-267. 2d ed. 2 vols. **US National Library of Medicine.** Washington, DC: US Government Printing Office, 1979.
First edition, 1973.
Designed to assist librarians in identification of biomedical serials and to provide necessary information for requesting interlibrary loans. It is a key word-out-of-context index with some 31,000 entries arranged alphabetically. Citations include key word, journal title and NLM call number. Includes statistical analyses of titles by geographic origin and language.
R: *MRW* S3, pp. 6, 32; Win (EK37).

Library Resources for Nurses: A Basic Collection for Supporting the Nursing Curriculum. **Dale E. Shaffer.** Salem, OH: Dale E. Shaffer (437 Jennings Ave., Salem, Ohio), 1974.
Outdated but still helpful in identifying older but still valid books.

List of Journals in Abridged Index Medicus. Vols. 1–. **US National Library of Medicine.** Washington, DC: US Government Printing Office, 1970–. Monthly.
List of 100 journals included in the *Abridged Index Medicus.* On the cover of each issue.
R: Stearns & Ratcliff (*AJN*); (*NEJM*, 1970).

Medbooks: A Bibliography of New and Forthcoming Books in Human and Dental Medicine. Basel: S. Karger, 1968–. Semiannually.

An international bibliography of medical literature; includes Congress reports, monographs, journals, handbooks. Divided into subject groups. Includes full bibliographic data.

Scientific, Medical, and Technical Books Published in the United States of America: A Selected List of Titles in Print with Annotations. 2d ed. **Reginald Robert Hawkins.** Prepared under the direction of the National Academy of Sciences–National Research Council's Committee on Bibliography of American Scientific and Technical Books. Washington, DC: 1958. Distr. New York: Bowker, 1958.

Useful for books published up to 1956. About 8,000 titles were chosen. Annotated.
R: *Subscription Books Bulletin* 55: 397 (1959); Chen (p. 3); Jenkins (A4); Mal (3-10); Wal (p. 15); Win (EA11).

Sources of Serials: An International Publisher and Corporate Author Directory. New York: Bowker, 1977.

A directory of 90,000 serial titles found in *Ulrich's International Periodicals Directory, Irregular Serials & Annuals,* and *Ulrich's Quarterly.* Arranged by country, then by publisher or corporate author. Current address is provided. Cross referenced and indexed.

Union List of Scientific Serials in Canadian Libraries. Catalogue collectif des publications scientifiques dans les bibliothèques canadiennes. 3d ed. **Canada, National Science Library, Ottawa.** Ottawa: National Science Library, 1969.

First edition, 1957; second edition, 1967.
A computer-generated publication listing more than 40,753 titles in 208 cooperating libraries.
R: Chen (p. 3); Win (3EA10, EA54).

OTHER SUBJECT BOOKLISTS

Braille Book Review. Vols. 1–. Washington, DC: Division for the Blind and Physically Handicapped, US Library of Congress, 1932–. Bimonthly.

Available in Braille and Inkprint editions.
R: *LCIB* 35: 70 (Jan. 30, 1976); 37: 456 (Aug. 4, 1978).

The Harvard List of Books in Psychology. 4th ed. **Harvard University.** Cambridge, MA: Harvard University Press, 1971.

Compiled and annotated by the psychologists at Harvard. Includes psychotherapy and behavior disorders.

SUBJECT AND LIBRARY CATALOGS FOR BOTH CURRENT AND RETROSPECTIVE SELECTION

Besides the tools listed under this section, readers are reminded of the significance of publication catalogs of various governmental and professional organizations, such as the publication catalogs of the National Library of Medicine, National Institutes of Health, World Health Organization, American Medical Association, American Hospital Association, etc. See chapters 18 and 23 for further information.

GENERAL

Author Catalog of the Library of the New York Academy of Medicine. 43 vols. **New York Academy of Medicine.** Boston, MA: G. K. Hall, 1969.

Catalog describes over 370,000 volumes and over 169,000 pamphlets.
R: *ARBA* (1970, p. 133); Win (3EJ6).

Catalog of the Library of the American Hospital Association. 5 vols. **American Hospital Association Library.** Boston, MA: G. K. Hall, 1976.

This dictionary catalog contains approximately 75,000 author, title, and subject entries from the library of the American Hospital Association. Includes all print, nonprint, government documents, theses. Considered a comprehensive collection.
R: *ARBA* (1977, p. 706).

Catalog of the National Library of Medicine. 1948–1965. 18 vols. **US National Library of Medicine.** Washington, DC: US Government Printing Office, 1949–1966. Annual, with quinquennial cumulations beginning 1950/1954–1960/1965.

Title varies: 1948, *Catalog Cards*; 1949–1950, *Author Catalog.*
Library name varies: 1948–1951, US Army Medical Library; 1952–1955, US Armed Forces Medical Library.
Reproductions of cards cataloged by the National Library of Medicine from 1948–1965.
R: Win (EK23).

Current Catalog Proof Sheets. **US National Library of Medicine.** Chicago, IL: Medical Library Association. Weekly.

Illustration Catalog of the Library of the New York Academy of Medicine. 2d ed., enlarged. **New York Academy of Medicine.** Boston, MA: G. K. Hall, 1965.

First edition, 1960.
A photographically reproduced index to over 21,000 illustrations in medical works.
R: Win (EK14).

National Library of Medicine Current Catalog. **US National Library of Med-**

icine. Washington, DC: US Government Printing Office, 1966–. Biweekly, cumulating quarterly, with fourth quarterly annual cumulation.

Supersedes the National Library of Medicine *Catalog*.
Biweekly computer-produced catalog includes citations for works catalogued by the NLM which have an imprint date of current or two preceding years. Cumulations give citations for all publications cataloged except pre-1801 and Americana titles. Entries are listed by subject and by name of persons, corporate bodies, and titles.
R: *CRL* 28: 63 (Jan. 1967); Win (EJ14; 1EJ2).

Portrait Catalog of the Library of the New York Academy of Medicine. 5 vols. **New York Academy of Medicine.** Boston, MA: G. K. Hall, 1960.

First Supplement, 1959–1965, 1965; *Second Supplement, 1965–1971,* 1971.
With supplements, contains over 12,000 separate portraits (paintings, woodcuts, engravings, photographs, etc.) and over 187,000 portraits appearing in books and journals in the Academy's catalog.
R: Win (EK15).

Subject Catalog of the Department Library. 20 vols. **US Department of Health, Education, and Welfare.** Boston, MA: G. K. Hall, 1965.

Subject Catalog of the Library of the New York Academy of Medicine. 34 vols. **New York Academy of Medicine.** Boston, MA: G. K. Hall, 1969.

Reproductions of catalog cards for over 370,000 volumes and over 169,000 pamphlets.
R: Win (EK13).

SUBJECT

Catalogs of the F. B. Power Pharmaceutical Library, School of Pharmacy, University of Wisconsin, Madison. Boston, MA: G. K. Hall, 1976.

Contains complete catalog entries of this pharmacy library which was founded in 1883. Divided into author, title, and subject sections.

Catalog of the Sophia F. Palmer Memorial Library. 2 vols. **American Journal of Nursing Company, New York City.** Boston, MA: G. K. Hall, 1973.

Photographic reproduction of the dictionary style catalog of the important American Journal of Nursing Company Library and its holdings, from the early 1900s through 1972.

Catalog of Works in the Neurological Sciences Collected by Cyril Brian Courville, M.D. **M. L. Manson Thomas and W. Conrad Cooper.** Irvine, CA: Regents of the University of California, 1978.

The catalog of C. B. Courville's collection of works in the neurological sciences. Contains many historical books, though most of the collection is from the twentieth century. Arranged alphabetically by author and then title, the catalog can be used both as a bibliographic reference tool and a record of Courville's achievements in the neurosciences.
R: *BMLA* 67: 342 (July 1979).

Dictionary Catalog on Deafness and the Deaf. 2 vols. **Gallaudet College.** Boston, MA: G. K. Hall, 1970.

A dictionary arrangement of over 35,000 card catalog entries which pertain to deafness from the Edward Miner Gallaudet Memorial Library. Titles date from 1546, and include the Charles Baker collection from the sixteenth century to the Civil War.
R: *MRW* S2, pp. 16, 25.

The Evan Bedford Library of Cardiology: Catalogue of Books, Pamphlets and Journals. **Royal College of Surgeons.** London: Royal College of Surgeons, 1977.

The catalog of this prominent British cardiologist contains over 1,000 citations, many of rare books. Classification and description are extremely well done. A useful publication.
R: *American Heart Journal* 95: 815 (1978).

Shelf List Catalog. **Western Reserve University, Frances Payne Bolton School of Nursing Library.** Cleveland, OH: Bell & Howell, 1966.

CHAPTER 2   GUIDES TO THE LITERATURE

The following are examples of sources that analyze the structure and availability of medical, scientific, and technical literature:

On Documentation of Scientific Literature. **T. P. Loosjes.** London: Butterworths. Distr. Hamden, CT: Archon Books, 1973.

Concentrates on theoretical problems of bibliographic control and information retrieval.
R: Chen (p. 9); Mal (3-12).

Understanding Scientific Literature: A Bibliometric Approach. **Joseph Donohue.** Cambridge, MA: MIT Press, 1972.
R: Chen (p. 9).

Pilot Study on the Use of Scientific Literature by Scientists. **Ralph R. Shaw.** Metuchen, NJ: Scarecrow Press, 1971.
R: *LJ* 96: 2747 (Sept. 15, 1971); *ARBA* (1972, p. 543); Chen (p. 9).

GENERAL

Guide to Reference Books. 9th ed. **Eugene P. Sheehy.** Chicago, IL: American Library Association, 1977.

____. 8th ed. **Constance M. Winchell.** Chicago, IL: American Library Association, 1967.

____, 1st Supplement, 1965–1966, 1968.
____, 2nd Supplement, 1967–1968, 1970.
____, 3rd Supplement, 1969–1970, 1972.

Guide to Reference Material. 3d ed. 3 vols. **Albert J. Walford.** London: Library Association, 1973.

Second edition, 1969.
Volume 1, *Science and Technology*; volume 2, *Philosophy and Psychology, Religion, Social Science, Geography, Biography and History*; volume 3, *Generalities, Language, The Arts, and Literature*.
A standard reference of some 4,300 main entries and 700 subsumed entries. Largely expanded from the earlier edition. Annotations are generally descriptive rather than critical.
R: *BL* 70: 393 (Dec. 15, 1973); *Choice* 10: 1536 (Dec. 1973); *LJ* 91: 3687 (1966); *ARBA* (1974, p. 542); Chen (p. 9); Jenkins (A9); Mal (1-6).

Guide to Russian Reference Books. Vol 5. **Karol Maichel.** Stanford, CA: Hoover Institution Press, 1967.

Volume 1, 1962.
Volume 5 devoted to science, technology, and medicine. Lists almost 2,000 reference sources dealing with Russian sciences from earliest times to 1965. Includes

books and journal articles written in Russian and Western languages. Emphasis on post-World War II period.
R: *BMLA* 56: 347 (1968); *LJ* 93: 2846 (1968); Chen (p. 10); Jenkins (A5); *MRW* S1, p. 3; Wal (p. 14); Win (AA300; AA390; EK3; 2EAI).

Guide to the Literature of the Life Sciences. 8th ed. **Roger C. Smith and W. Malcolm Reid.** Minneapolis, MN: Burgess, 1972.
First edition, 1942; seventh edition, 1967.
Latest edition of this guide has been increased to include plant diseases, with the title accordingly changed from *Guide to the Literature of the Zoological Sciences.* Manual includes eight chapters devoted to various sources, and a ninth deals with preparation of papers and their publication. A valuable source, useful in familiarizing one with the main branches of the sciences.
R: *Journal of Parasitology* 59: 146 (Feb. 1973); *ARBA* (1973, p. 549); Mal (9-3); *MRW* S2, pp. 13, 14, 110.

How to Find Out: A Guide to Sources of Information Arranged by the Dewey Decimal Classification. 4th ed. **G. Chandler.** New York: Pergamon Press, 1974.
R: Chen (p. 10).

Improving the Dissemination of Scientific and Technical Information: A Practitioner's Guide to Information. **Prepared by Capital Systems Group for the Office of Science Information Service.** National Science Foundation, 1975.
Focus is on the primary dissemination of information—the technical journal or its equivalent.
R: Chen (p. 10).

Information Sources in Science and Technology. **C. C. Parker and R. V. Turley.** Boston: Butterworths, 1975.
R: Chen (p. 10).

LC Science Tracer Bullet. **US Library of Congress. Science and Technology Division. Reference Section.** Washington, DC: US Library of Congress, 1974–. Irregular.
An irregular series of reference aids provides guide to systematically searching the literature of specific topic areas. Intended to aid those who seek a clearer understanding of a specific topic. Some of the sample reference aids include: *Diabetes Mellitus* (11 pages); *The History of Psychology* (14 pages); *Nuclear Safety* (10 pages); *Science Education in America* (13 pages); *Recombinant DNA Controversy* (16 pages).
R: *LCIB* 34: 92 (Mar. 7, 1975); 34: 472 (Nov. 28, 1975); 34: 488 (Dec. 12, 1975); 35: 592 (Sept. 24, 1976).

The Literature of Science and Technology Approached Historically: A Brief Guide for Reference. **Raymond V. Turley.** Southampton, England: University of Southampton, 1973.
Bibliographical guide groups annotated entries under headings commonly em-

ployed in guides to current literature such as encyclopedias, patents, etc. In addition contains categories of manuscripts and microforms. A hundred or so titles listed, two-thirds are more general sources.
R: *Library Association Record* 75: 123 (June 1973).

Scientific and Technical Information Sources. **Ching-chih Chen.** Cambridge, MA: MIT Press, 1978.

A comprehensive and up-to-date guide to the literature of science and technology. Over 3,600 sources are included together with both critical and descriptive annotations. Author index and subject arrangement by types of literature. A major tool for scientific and technical libraries. Replaces Jenkins's *Science Reference Sources*.
R: *AAAS Science Books & Films* 15: 1 (May 1979); *Unlisted Drugs* 30 (July 1978); *Engineering Societies Library Book Review* (Mar. 1978); *BL* 74: 405 (Aug. 1978); 75: 81 (Sept. 1978); *Book Review Digest* (Nov. 1978); *Choice* 15: 836 (Sept. 1978); *CRL* 39: 324 (July 1978); *Grant Magazine* 1: 79 (Mar. 1978); *Journal of Academic Librarianship* (1979); *Kemixon Reporter* (Spain) No. 287 (1979); *Library Association Record* 80: 105 (Mar. 1978); *LJ* 103: 1034 (May 15, 1978); *Mass Media Booknotes* 9: 157 (June 1978); *New Library World* 79: 935 (May 1978); *Sci-Tech Book News* 2: 2 (Feb. 1978); *SL* 69: 236 (May/June 1978).

The Use of Biological Literature. 2d ed. **R. T. Bottle and H. V. Wyatt, eds.** Hamden, CT: Archon Books, 1971.

First edition, 1966.
A comprehensive survey of biological literature divided into subfields. Ample coverage of government publications, bibliographies, patents, and abstracts, though primary emphasis is on British sources. Includes chapters on library use and research methods.
R: *Assistant Librarian* 65: 68 (Apr. 1972); *Bibliographical Society of America Papers* 61: 290 (July/Sept. 1967); *WLB* 42: 220 (1967); *ARBA* (1973, p. 549); Chen (p. 14); Jenkins (G1); Mal (9-1); *MRW* S1, p. 7; Wal (p. 191); Win (2EC1).

GENERAL—MEDICINE

Biological and Biomedical Resource Literature. **Ann E. Kerker and Henry T. Murphy.** Lafayette, IN: Purdue University, 1968.

A two-part bibliographical guide based in part on *Literature Sources in the Biological Sciences* by Ann E. Kerker and Esther M. Schlundt, 1961. Materials are presented in more than 50 categories and subdivisions. Author and title index.
R: Chen (p. 14); Jenkins (G3); Mal (9-2); *MRW* S1, p. 2. Wal (p. 192); Win (2EC2).

Biomedical Subject Headings: A Reconciliation of National Library of Medicine and Library of Congress Subject Headings. 2d ed. **Eugene V. Muench.** Hamden, CT: Shoe String Press, 1979.

First edition, 1971.
A standard reference of medical subject headings of the National Library of Medicine and the Library of Congress. Both are cross referenced. Extremely helpful for controlled vocabulary in computer interface. Also helpful for librarians and catalogers.

Classics and Other Selected Readings in Medical Librarianship. **Jack D. Key and Thomas E. Keys, eds.** Huntington, NY: Krieger, 1980.

A handy and concise anthology of significant writings in the field of medical librarianship. Includes both historical and current topics. A must for practicing medical librarians and library school students.

Consumer Health Information: A Guide to Sources. **Alan M. Rees.** Littleton, CO: Libraries Unlimited, 1980.

Selectively annotated compilation of informative and accurate health care information sources available for the lay public. Emphasis on major health concerns: cancer, heart disease, drugs and drug abuse, health concerns of women, etc. Invaluable reference tool for collections in consumer health.

Current Medical References. 6th ed. **Paul J. Sanazaro and Milton J. Chatton, eds.** Los Altos, CA: Lange Medical Publications, 1970.

First edition, 1959; third edition, 1963; fourth edition, 1965.
Some 15,000 items representing English-language medical literature. Entries arranged under 35 sections, dealing with various aspects of medicine. Consists mainly of books, journal articles, and reviews. Many items annotated. Includes subject index.
R: *MRW* S2, p. 11; Win (EK18; 1EJ1); Stearns & Ratcliff (*NEJM*, 1970).

A Guide to Canadian Health Science: Information Service and Sources. **Phyllis J. Russell.** Ottawa, Canada: Canadian Library Association, 1974.

Handbook on Canadian information services and sources for health science libraries. Covers national library services, professional organizations, computerized information retrieval, and audiovisual services. Selection and reference sources are listed. Includes a directory of Canadian publishers, book dealers, and library suppliers.
R: *UBL* 29: 226 (July–Aug. 1975).

Health Sciences Librarianship: A Guide to Information Sources. **Beatrice K. Basler and Thomas G. Basler, eds.** Detroit, MI: Gale Research, 1977.

Annotated bibliography covers recent publications on theory and practice of health science librarianship. Includes microforms, computer technology, manpower, and education. Approximately 550 nonjournal sources are cited.
R: *SL* 68: 424 (Nov. 1977).

An Introduction to the Literature of the Medical Sciences. 3d ed. **Myrl Ebert.** Chapel Hill, NC: University of North Carolina Press, 1970.

Medical Reference Works, 1679–1966: A Selected Bibliography. **John B. Blake and Charles Roos, eds.** Chicago, IL: Medical Library Association, 1967.

———. Supplement 1, 1967–1968, 1970.
———. Supplement 2, 1969–1972, 1973.
———. Supplement 3, 1973–1974, 1975.

Collection of annotated citations arranged by subject, author, and title. Titles selected for usefulness in answering questions in bioscience libraries. Informative

annotations are contained in this publication which is important for public, college, and special library collections.
R: *RSR* 4: 90 (Apr.–June 1976); *MRW* S1, p. 2; Win (EK1; EK24; 2EJ2; 3EJ3); Sheehy (EK1).

Sourcebook on Health Sciences Librarianship. **Ching-chih Chen.** Metuchen, NJ: Scarecrow, 1977.

A source book for medical librarians. The book consists of two parts. Part I is a systematic study of the articles of the *Bulletin of the Medical Library Association,* 1966–1975. Part II is a citation bibliography of over 3,000 citations, arranged by broad subjects. Indexed.
R: *BMLA* 65: 488 (Oct. 1977); *Canadian Library Journal* 34: 459 (Dec. 1977); *CRL* 38: 362 (July 1977); *LJ* 102: 889 (April 15, 1977); *RQ* 17: 184 (Winter 1977); *Reference and Subscription Books Reviews 1977–1978*: 132; *ARBA* (1978, p. 107).

Use of Medical Literature: Information Sources for Research and Development. 2d ed. **Leslie T. Morton, ed.** London: Butterworths, 1978.

First edition, 1978.
Comprehensive guide to major information sources in medical sciences and clinical specialties. First five chapters relate to general aspects of the literature such as libraries, standard reference sources, and mechanized information retrieval. These are followed by thirteen expertly written chapters, each devoted to a specific medical area. Literature available in each area is organized under journals, abstracts and indexes, reviews, monographs, dictionaries, etc. Listings include informed comments. Intended for use by clinicians, medical scientists, and librarians.
R: *British Medical Bulletin* 31: 98 (1975); *BMJ* 4: 539 (Nov. 30, 1974); *Journal of Medical Education* 50: 307 (Mar. 1975); *Lancet* 2: 324 (Aug. 10, 1974); *BMLA* 63: 71 (Jan. 1975); *Journal of Documentation* 31: 55 (Mar. 1975); *ARBA* (1975, p. 732); *MRW* S3, p. 6.

DENTISTRY

Basic Dental Reference Works. **Aletha Kowitz, comp.** American Dental Association, Bureau of Library Services. Chicago, IL: American Dental Association, 1975.

Lists 104 annotated entries to dental reference literature. Includes dictionaries, indexes, directories, bibliographies, histories, etc.
R: Sheehy (EK25).

GENETICS

Teratology and Congenital Malformations: A Comprehensive Guide to the Literature. 3 vols. **Lois Weinstein, ed.** New York: Plenum, 1976.

Three-volume set containing references of retrospective searches on congenital malformations caused by agents in "Teratogenicity, Mutagenicity, and Carcinogenicity Current Awareness Bulletin," published between 1963 and 1974. Volume 1 lists references in chronological sequence; volume 2 and parts of volume 3 classify literature by key words; and volume 3 ends with author index. Quick source of reference up to 1974.

R: *American Journal of Human Genetics* 29: 413 (July 1977); *Annals of Human Genetics* 41: 270 (Oct. 1977); *Quarterly Review of Biology* 52: 334 (1977).

GERONTOLOGY

Current Literature on Aging. New York: National Council on the Aging, 1963–.

Subject guide to selected publications relating to aging in such fields as housing, employment, health, recreation.

HEALTH SERVICES ADMINISTRATION

Health and Medical Economics: A Guide to Information Sources. **Ted J. Ackroyd, ed.** Detroit, MI: Gale Research, 1977.

Guide to information sources in the economic aspects of health care delivery. Covers general hospitals, physicians' practices, health insurance, public health.

Health Care Administration: A Guide to Information Sources. **Dwight A. Morris and Lynne D. Morris, eds.** Detroit, MI: Gale Research, 1978.

A bibliographic guide to health care administration. Contains over 1,000 entries which are annotated and classified by subject. Contains subject and author index. Nonbibliographic sources (i.e. directories) are listed in appendixes.
R: *BMLA* 67: 342 (July 1979).

Health Sciences and Services; a Guide to Information Sources. **Lois F. Lunin.** Detroit, MI: Gale Research, 1978.

Hospital Literature Subject Headings. 2d ed. **Alice Dunlap, ed.** Chicago, IL: American Hospital Association, 1977.

First edition, 1965.
List of subject headings used by American Hospital Association library provides guide to *Hospital Literature Index* prior to 1978 and *Cumulative Index of Hospital Literature* series. Useful reference for administrators, librarians, and other health care professionals.
R: *SL* 68: 374 (Sept. 1977); *MRW* S1, p. 14.

Hospital Literature Subject Headings Transition Guide to Medical Subject Headings. **Alice Dunlap et al., eds.** Chicago, IL: American Hospital Association, 1978.

Shows correlation between hospital literature subject headings used in *Hospital Literature Index* and the Medical Subject Headings. Useful research tool in establishing appropriate headings for locating health care articles.

INFECTIOUS DISEASES

Guide to the Literature for the Industrial Microbiologist. **Peter A. Hahn.** New York: Plenum, 1973.

Covers 1960–1973 literature period. Outlines citations to textbooks, journals, meetings, courses, and review articles in four sections. Includes complete biblio-

graphic data and applicable specific information such as price and journal contents.
R: *MRW* S3, p. 34.

NURSING

Nursing Staffing Methodology: A Review and Critique of Selected Literature. **Myrtle K. Aydelotte.** Washington, DC: US Government Printing Office, 1973.

Presents critical assessments of approximately 200 nurse staffing studies and a bibliography of over 1,000 items. Staffing methods are explored, along with the identification of problems and issues, with ensuring recommendations and hypotheses.
R: *American Journal of Nursing* 74: 92 (Jan. 1974).

PHARMACY AND PHARMACOLOGY

Comprehensive Guide to the Cannabis Literature. **Ernest L. Abel, comp.** Westport, CT: Greenwood, 1979.

Guide to Drug Information. **Winifred Sewell.** Hamilton, IL: Drug Intelligence Publications, 1976.

A bibliographical essay as well as a useful ready reference tool. In four parts: drug supplier and information sources; primary reference sources; index and abstracting sources, microfiche, etc.; suggestions for future use of information technology in the drug field. For pharmacists, health professionals, and librarians.
R: *ABL* 41: entry 363 (Sept. 1976); *ARBA* (1978, p. 733); Sheehy (EK34).

PSYCHIATRY AND PSYCHOLOGY

Child Care Issues for Parents & Society: A Guide to Information Sources. **Andrew Garoogian and Rhoda Garoogian, eds.** Detroit, MI: Gale Research, 1977.

Covers 45 subject areas related to child care, including child abuse, learning, health, day care.

A Guide to Psychiatric Books in English. 3d ed. **Karl A. Menninger.** New York: Grune & Stratton, 1972.

First edition, 1950; second edition, 1956.
Classified arrangement of approximately 3,600 entries to books in psychiatry. Source listings include author, title, publisher, and year. There is an appendix of publishers and addresses as well as a name index.
R: *RSR* 1: 19 (June 1973); *MRW* S2, p. 81.

Guide to the Literature in Psychiatry. **Bernice Ennis.** Los Angeles, CA: Partridge Press, 1971.

Source book of psychiatric literature. Sources include: journals; information sources (abstracts, indexes, bibliographies, etc.); psychiatric monographs; pamphlets, brochures, and exhibit literature; government documents; controlled cir-

culation publications; translations; psychiatric libraries; and list of publishers. Yields valuable source descriptions. Not an exhaustive list of reference books. Lacks annotations. Geared toward clinical and academic psychiatrists.
R: *LJ* 97: 862 (Mar. 1, 1972); *ARBA* (1973, p. 606); *MRW* S2, p. 81.

How to Find Out in Psychiatry: A Guide to Sources of Mental Health Information. **Bette Greenberg.** New York: Pergamon, 1978.

Complete coverage of sources of mental health information. Divided into twelve chapters (drug therapy, directories, statistical sources, etc.). Each page of text lists from eight to twelve titles of books and journals with emphasis on English-language material. Nonprint not included. Includes an appendix, labeled "classics in psychiatric literature," listing 79 annotated books. Highly recommended to libraries serving departments of psychiatry, medicine, nursing, social work, and allied areas of psychiatry.
R: *Choice* 16: 648 (July–Aug. 1979).

PUBLIC HEALTH

Chemical Mutagenesis: A Survey of the Literature. **Environmental Mutagen Information Center.** Oak Ridge, TN: US Energy Research and Development Administration, Oak Ridge National Laboratory, 1971.

Extensive review of the international literature; 2,500 citations arranged numerically. All titles in English. Includes KWIC index, author index, chemical registry.
R: *MRW* S3, pp. 35, 36, 54.

Environmental Toxicology: A Guide to Information Sources. **Robert L. Rudd.** Detroit, MI: Gale Research, 1977.

Annotated bibliographic descriptions of 1,000 books and articles. Information sources covering general material, consequences of pollution, and special aspects of environmental toxicology.

Findings of Drug Abuse Research, DHEW Pub. no. (ADM) 75-0255, National IDA Research Monograph Series 1. 2 vols. **US Department of Health, Education, and Welfare. National Institute on Drug Abuse. National Clearinghouse for Drug Abuse Literature.** Washington, DC: US Government Printing Office, 1975.

An annotated bibliography of over 3,500 titles and abstracts of drug abuse literature resulting from NIDA and NIMH grants from 1967–1974. Volume 1 contains three sections pertaining to methodology and findings of drug abuse research. Volume 2 has entries on behavioral and clinical aspects of drug abuse research. Each volume has indexes by author/editor and subject/drugs.
R: *RSR* 4: 108 (Oct.–Dec. 1976).

Occupational Safety and Health; A Guide to Information Sources. **T. P. Peck.** Detroit, MI: Gale Research, 1974.

Primary Prevention in Drug Abuse: An Annotated Guide to the Literature, DHEW Pub. no. (ADM) 76-350. **Prevention Branch, US National Insti-**

tute on Drug Abuse. Washington, DC: US Government Printing Office, 1977.

Organizes literature and resources available to workers in field of drug abuse prevention. For the most part, the materials were produced within the last five years. Major sections are drug abuse prevention, education, community action; multimedia, information sources, evaluation; and additional readings. Citations are complete, and annotations are informative. Appendixes list state and federal agencies.
R: *ARBA* (1978, p. 734).

UROGENITAL SYSTEM

Guide to the 1968–1972 International Abortion Research Literature. **International Reference Center for Abortion Research.** Silver Spring, MD: International Reference Center for Abortion Research, 1973.

Monographs, journal articles, and conference proceedings dealing with induced abortion compose the nearly 1,800 citations. Includes foreign language references but no ephemeral, anonymous, or popular literature. Includes three indexes: author, subject, and geographical.
R: *MRW* S3, p. 1.

VETERINARY MEDICINE

Comparative & Veterinary Medicine, A Guide to the Resource Literature. **A. E. Kerker.** Madison, WI: University of Wisconsin Press, 1973.

CHAPTER 3 BIBLIOGRAPHIES

REFERENCE TOOLS

Bibliographic Guide to Technology: 1978. **The Research Libraries of the New York Public Library and the Library of Congress.** Boston, MA: G. K. Hall, 1979.

Bibliography of Medical Bibliographies. **US National Library of Medicine.** Washington, DC: US Government Printing Office, 1970.

Includes published and unpublished bibliographies, NLM Literature Searches, bibliographies from specialized research centers. Entries, arranged alphanumerically. Includes description and source information.
R: *MRW* S2, p. 12.

Biological Sciences: A Bibliography of Bibliographies. **Theodore Besterman.** Totowa, NJ: Rowman & Littlefield, 1972.

Bibliography of bibliographies. Citations in original language.
R: *ARBA* (1973, p. 549); Chen (p. 27); *MRW* S2, pp. 10, 12.

Computext Book Guides: Medicine. Vols. 1–. Boston, MA: G. K. Hall, 1974–. Monthly.
R: *ARBA* (1976, p. 725).

Handbook of International Documentation and Information. 6th rev. ed. 15 vols. New York: K. G. Saur, 1978.

Volume 1, *International Scientific Documentation and Information*, 4th rev. ed., 1969; volume 3, *International Bibliography and Bibliographies in Technology, Science and Economics*, 2d ed., 1969; volume 4, *International Bibliography of Special Dictionaries*, 6th ed., 1979; volume 13, *World Guide to Scientific Associations and Learned Societies*, 2d ed., 1978; volume 14, *Anglo-American and German Abbreviations in Science and Technology*, 3 parts, Peter Wennrich, 1976/1978.

Medical Books for the Layperson: An Annotated Bibliography. **Marilyn M. Philbrook, comp.** Boston, MA: Boston Public Library, 1976.

Concentrates on 300 in-print medical books published between 1969 and 1975. Culled from vast holdings of the Boston Public Library. Author arrangement with subject index. Topics covered: specific illnesses, staying healthy, quality of health care, and personal narratives. Aid to general public and library collection development.
R: *WLB* 51: 442 (Jan. 1977); *ARBA* (1977, p. 708).

Medicine: A Bibliography of Bibliographies. **Theodore Besterman.** Totowa, NJ: Rowman & Littlefield, 1971.

A retrospective bibliography. Includes sources on anatomy, medicine, pharmacology. Citations are from international sources and in original language. Includes number of references for each citation.
R: *ARBA* (1973, p. 605); *MRW* S2, p. 12.

National Library of Medicine Classification: A Scheme for the Shelf Arrangement of Books in the Field of Medicine and Its Related Sciences, Public Health Service Pub. no. 1108. 3d ed. **US National Library of Medicine.** Washington, DC: US Government Printing Office, 1969.

First edition, 1951; second edition, 1964.
R: *MRW* S2, p. 14.

National Library of Medicine Literature Search. **US National Library of Medicine.** Bethesda, MD: National Library of Medicine, 1965–.

Individually produced bibliographies generated from the MEDLARS computer file which cover a variety of health science topics. Available from the National Library of Medicine upon request.
R: *MRW* S1, p. 1.

GENERAL

Bibliography of Bioethics. 5 vols. **LeRoy Walters, ed.** Detroit, MI: Gale Research, 1975–1979.

Considered an important source of bioethical literature, providing bibliographic control of pertinent print and nonprint publications. Covers English-language journals, newspapers, monographs, court decisions. Volumes 1–5 cite over 7,000 documents published from 1973 through 1978. Available on-line through BIOETHICSLINE.
R: *Annals of Internal Medicine* 85: 696 (Nov. 1976); 91: 344 (Aug. 1979); *BL* 74: 632 (Dec. 1, 1977); *LJ* 100: 2316 (Dec. 15, 1975); *RSR* 3: 71 (July–Dec. 1975); 4: 86 (Apr.–June, 1976); *WLB* 52: 92 (Sept. 1977); *ARBA* (1976, p. 727; 1978, p. 706; 1978, p. 707).

Bibliography of Society, Ethics and the Life Sciences. 1979–1980 edition. **Sharmon Sollitto and Robert Veatch, comps.** Hastings-on-Hudson, NY: Institute of Society, Ethics, and the Life Sciences, 1978.

First edition, 1973.
Approximately 1,000 references from all primary sources, topically arranged. Includes full bibliographic citations and occasional annotations. Out-of-date citations are replaced in succeeding editions by newer ones; classic works are retained. Author index.
R: *MRW* S3, pp. 24, 49.

Bibliography on Medical Education. Vols. 1–. **Association of American Medical Colleges.** Washington, DC: Association of American Medical Colleges, 1966–. Monthly.

Included in the *Journal of Medical Education.*

British Medicine. Vols. 1–. London: Medical Department, British Council, 1972–. Monthly.

Monthly publication which lists new books, pamphlets, official publications, brochures, reports, and journal articles in medicine and allied fields. No index.
R: *MRW* S2, pp. 11, 65, 77.

Clinical Education in the Health Professions: An Annotated Bibliography. **M. L. Moore, J. F. Perry, and A. W. Clark, eds.** Washington, DC: Section for Education, American Physical Therapy Association, 1976.

An aid in the assessment of clinical education programs and guide for clinical staff development. Includes 573 references, carefully cross-indexed. Most citations reflect recent literature but valuable older sources also included. Highly recommended reference for those involved in the education of health professionals.
R: *Physical Therapy* 56: 1315 (1976).

The Euthanasia Controversy 1812–1974: A Bibliography with Select Annotations. **Charles W. Triche, III, and Diane S. Triche.** Troy, NY: Whitston Publishing, 1975.

Selected, annotated bibliography covering all angles of this issue. Divided into three main sections: a list of books and essays with specific chapters analyzed; a section on periodicals, alphabetically arranged by article title within nineteen subject categories; and an author index. Contains no abbreviations. Described as a "near complete" bibliography.
R: *RSR* 4: 86 (Jan–Mar. 1976); *ARBA* (1977, p. 709).

Family Therapy and Research: An Annotated Bibliography of Articles and Books Published 1950–1970. **Ira D. Glick and Jay Haley.** New York: Grune & Stratton, 1971.

Includes nearly 2,100 references. Concentrates on family research studies dealing with psychiatry, psychology, and social work. Subject arrangement. Contains author index.
R: *MRW* S2, p. 45.

Index of Legal Medicine, 1940–1970: Annotated Bibliography. **William V. Nick.** Columbus, OH: Legal Medicine Press, 1970.

_____. Supplement 1–, 1970/1971–. Quarterly.
Cites over 15,000 references to monographs, books, reviews, symposium proceedings, and journal articles from legal and medical publications. Comprehensive coverage of international literature on this topic in English. Not all citations are fully annotated. Specific subject arrangement of entries. Includes a subject heading index and a list of indexed journals. No author index.
R: *MRW* S2, p. 47; Win (EK160).

McGraw-Hill Basic Bibliography of Science and Technology. Rev. ed. New York: McGraw-Hill, 1966.

Intended as a supplement to the *McGraw-Hill Encyclopedia of Science and Technology.* Lists books under subject headings.
R: *LJ* 91: 969 (Mar. 1, 1966); Chen (p. 23); Wal (p. 7); Win (1EA5).

Minority Groups in Medicine: Selected Bibliography, DHEW Pub. no. (NIH) 72-331.**US Division of Physician and Health Professions Education.** Washington, DC: US Government Printing Office, 1972.

The 146 citations date mainly from 1969–1972. Deals with health-related prob-

lems of minority groups. Monographs and journal articles provide most of the references.
R: *MRW* S2, pp. 52, 69.

Museum Publications. 2 vols. **Jane Clapp.** New York: Scarecrow Press, 1962.

Part 2. *Publications in Biological and Earth Sciences.*
Books, pamphlets, and serial reprints of 276 American museums are included in this classified bibliography. Indexed by author and subject.
R: Chen (p. 33); Mal (9-9); Wal (p. 143, 182, 191); Win (EE14).

NASA Continuing Bibliography Series. Washington, DC: National Aeronautics and Space Administration.
Aerospace Medicine and Biology, NASA-SP-7011, monthly; *Aeronautical Engineering,* NASA-SP-7037, monthly; *Patent Abstracts Bibliography,* NASA-SP-7039, semiannually; *Earth Resources,* NASA-SP-7041, quarterly; *Energy,* NASA-SP-7043, quarterly; *Management,* NASA-SP-7500, annually.
Annotated bibliographies of unclassified reports and articles. Most include accession numbers, price, and ordering information.
R: Chen (p. 35).

NOVA; Science Adventures on Television: A Series of Reading Lists. Boston: Boston Public Library, 1975.
R: *RQ* 15: 358 (Summer 1975); *ARBA* (1976, p. 632); Chen (p. 23).

New Titles in Bioethics. Vol. 1–. Washington, DC: Kennedy Institute of Ethics, Georgetown University, 1975–. Monthly.
Includes the classified lists of the Institute's weekly acquisitions of books, reports, hearings, special issues of journals, and audiovisuals.

Recurring Bibliography on Education in the Allied Health Professions. Vols. 1–. **Ohio State University. School of Allied Medical Professions.** Columbus, OH: Ohio State University, School of Allied Medical Professions, 1969–. Annual.

Science, Technology, and Public Policy: A Selected and Annotated Bibliography. 2 vols. **Lynton K. Caldwell, ed.** Prepared for the National Science Foundation by the Program in Public Policy for Science and Technology. Bloomington, IN: Indiana University, Department of Government, 1968–1969.
Volume 1: books, monographs, documents, and whole issues of journals; volume 2: articles in journals.
Covers the years 1945–1967.
R: Chen (p. 23); Win (2EA4, 3EA5).

Scientific American Resource Library. 15 vols. San Francisco: W. H. Freeman, 1969.
Readings in the Earth Sciences, 2 volumes; *Readings in the Life Sciences,* 7 volumes;

Readings in the Social Sciences, 1 volume; *Readings in Psychology*, 2 volumes; *Readings in the Physical Sciences and Technology*, 3 volumes.
Authoritative scientific articles in a uniquely clear and informative style for a large and varied audience of educated laity and scientists.
R: *ARBA* (1971, p. 472); Chen (p. 23).

Selected Abstracts on Animal Models for Biomedical Research. **Charles B. Frank and Marilyn J. Anderson, comps. and eds.** Washington, DC: Institute of Laboratory Animal Resources, National Research Council, National Academy of Sciences, 1971.
Over 100 citations from primary reference sources of medical research on animal models. Topically arranged, includes author directory.
R: *MRW* S2, p. 32.

Traditional Medicine. **Ira E. Harrison and Sheila Cosminsky.** New York: Garland Publishing, 1976.
Annotations describe the use of traditional healers in "modern" systems, illnesses which they treat, training and rationale behind traditional systems. Three primary divisions are general: African, Latin American, and Caribbean. Within those divisions, items are divided into seven subcategories, i.e. ethnomedicine, maternal and child health. Each section has author index, and country index appears at end of volume.
R: *LJ* 101: 2162 (Oct. 15, 1976); *ARBA* (1977, p. 707).

ALLERGY AND IMMUNOLOGY

Interferon and Antiviral Substances Bibliography. **US National Institute of Allergy and Infectious Diseases.** Springfield, VA: National Technical Information Service. Annual.

Interferon Bibliography from MEDLARS, September 1973–August 1974. **National Institute of Allergy and Infectious Diseases, US Department of Health, Education, and Welfare.** Washington, DC: US Government Printing Office, 1974.
National Library of Medicine MEDLARS generated bibliography.
R: *RSR* 4: 110 (Oct.–Dec. 1976).

Rapid Methods & Automation in Microbiology & Immunology: A Bibliography. **Wendy J. Palmer and Suzanne E. LeQueene, comps. and eds.** Washington, DC: Information Retrieval, 1976.
Contains 2,500 references with complete bibliographic citations to international journal literature published between 1967–1975. Author and subject index.

ANESTHESIOLOGY AND GENERAL SURGERY

Anesthesiology Bibliography. **American Society of Anesthesiologists.** Park Ridge, IL: Wood Library-Museum of Anesthesiology, 1968–. Quarterly.

Quarterly citations obtained from MEDLARS. Sponsored by the American Society of Anesthesiologists.
R: *MRW* S1, p. 33.

Bibliography of Surgery of the Hand. Vols. 1–. **American Society for Surgery of the Hand.** Denver, CO: American Society for Surgery of the Hand, 1967–. Annual.

Current Bibliography of Plastic and Reconstructive Surgery. **American Society of Plastic and Reconstructive Surgeons.** Chicago, IL: American Society of Plastic and Reconstructive Surgeons. Bimonthly.

BRAIN AND NERVOUS SYSTEM

The Alpha Syllabus: A Handbook of Human EEG Alpha Activity. **Barbara B. Brown and Jay W. Klug, eds.** Springfield, IL: Charles C. Thomas, 1974.

Approximately 650 abstracts relating to alpha activity of the brain are extracted from world medical literature from 1960–1972. Comprehensive bibliographic citations are arranged by major topics. Bibliography of earlier papers. Descriptor index. Useful for researcher, student, teacher, and clinician.
R: *Archives of Neurology* 31: 282 (Oct. 1974); *Brain* 98: 186 (Mar. 1975); *Journal of Neurosurgery* 43: 114 (July 1975); *MRW* S3, p. 21.

Bibliography of Translations in the Neural Sciences 1950–1966, US Public Health Service Pub. no. 1635. **Richard T. Louttit and Michael J. Hanik.** US National Institute of Mental Health. Washington, DC: US Government Printing Office, 1967.

Lists more than 1,000 translation sources. Over 90 percent were originally published in Russian.
R: *MRW* S1, p. 18.

A Centennial Bibliography of Huntington's Chorea, 1872–1972. **G. W. Bruyn, F. Baro, and N. C. Myrianthopoulos.** The Hague, The Netherlands: Martinus Nijhoff, 1974.

Inspired by the Centennial Symposium on Huntington's Chorea held in Columbus, Ohio, in April 1972. Analyzes every paper on Huntington's Chorea published in the scientific press over a period of a century. Includes references to over 200 articles. Includes a geographical index for those who analyze migration patterns. Billed as the first exhaustive literature search on a specific disease.
R: *Neurology* 25: 300 (Mar. 1975).

The CNS Depressant Withdrawal Syndrome and Its Management: An Annotated Bibliography: 1950–1973, DHEW Pub. no. (ADM) 75-206. Special Bibliographies no. 2. **National Clearinghouse for Drug Abuse Literature, National Institute on Drug Abuse, US Department of Health, Education, and Welfare.** Washington, DC: US Government Printing Office, 1975.

Contains 182 abstracts dealing with withdrawal problems and syndromes of drug abuses, manifesting adverse effects on the CNS. Special emphasis on neonatal

and adult withdrawal from barbiturates, benzodiazepine, methaqualone, peperidinedione. Includes author index.
R: *RSR* 4: 108 (Oct.–Dec. 1976).

The Collaborative Study on Cerebral Palsy, Mental Retardation, and Other Neurological and Sensory Disorders of Infancy and Childhood, Bibliography no. 8, July 1974–June 1975, DHEW Pub. no. (NIH) 76-1050. **National Institute of Neurological and Communicative Disorders and Stroke, US Department of Health, Education, and Welfare.** Washington, DC: US Government Printing Office, 1975.

Annual publication covering 30 manuscripts. Emphasis on approved sampling methods presented at national and international conferences and published in the professional literature.
R: *RSR* 4: 107 (Oct.–Dec. 1976).

Epilepsy Bibliography, 1900–1950. **US National Institute of Neurological Disease and Stroke.** Washington, DC: US Government Printing Office, 1973.

Consists of 11,825 citations arranged under nine major headings. Includes subject and author index.
R: *ARBA* (1974, p. 625).

Hearing, Speech, and Communication Disorders: Cumulated Citations 1973. **Information Center for Hearing, Speech, and Disorders of Human Communication.** New York: Plenum, 1974.

Contains 13,000 citations of over 1,700 books, journal articles, and technical reports received during 1973 by the Information Center at the Johns Hopkins Medical Institutions. Multidisciplinary in coverage and international in scope Entries arranged alphabetically by author under specific subjects. No annotations. Includes author index. Monumental work geared toward therapists, special education personnel, and researchers in the field of hearing, language, and speech and communication disorders.
R: *Neurology* 25: 694 (July 1975); *ARBA* (1976, p. 726); *MRW* S3, pp. 28, 51.

Literature Relating to Neurosurgery and the Neurologic Sciences: A Bibliography From 1945 Through 1968 With a Few Earlier Classics in this Field. **John L. Fox, comp.** Washington, DC: US Government Printing Office, 1969.

Consists of some 601 references. Alphabetical arrangement by author under three sections: journals, yearbooks, and conference proceedings; books; and publishers and distributors, with appropriate abbreviations. No indexes. Although somewhat dated, the bibliography serves as a building block for future compilations on this topic. Geared toward residents in the field of neurosurgery.
R: *MRW* S1, p. 17; *MRW* S2, pp. 70, 71.

Neuronal Activity in Sleep: An Annotated Bibliography, NINDS Neurological Information Network, NIH 70-2063. **J. Allan Hobson and Robert W. McCarley.** Los Angeles, CA: Brain Research Institute Publications Office, 1971.

Abstracts from journals, theses, book chapters concerning electrode recording cells in sleep. Over 100 references in loose-leaf format. Author and subject indexes.
R: *MRW* S2, pp. 71, 95.

Parkinson's Disease and Related Disorders: Cumulative Bibliography: 1800–1970. 3 vols. **Parkinson Information Center, US National Institute of Neurological Diseases and Stroke.** Washington, DC: US Government Printing Office, 1971.

This is a bibliography of over 8,000 references on Parkinson's Disease cumulated over the past 170 years. Citations from primary sources are arranged in chronological order. Subject descriptors and scope of studies are included.
R: *MRW* S2, pp. 20, 76.

CARDIOVASCULAR SYSTEM

Cardiovascular Disease: Epidemiology, Prevention, and Rehabilitation: A Guide to Literature. Vols. 1–. **Senta S. Rogers and Irvin C. Mohler, comps.** New York: Plenum, 1974–.

Volume 1, 1960–1973.
Contains over 5,000 references from 756 international journals on the topics of physical activity/exercise in rehabilitation of heart disease patients. Alphabetical arrangement by authors; provides author and subject indexes. Foreign-language titles are translated into English.
R: *MRW* S3, p. 8.

International Bibliography of Cardiovascular Ausculation and Phonocardiography: Journal Articles: 1820–1966; Books, Theses, Dissertations, Phonodiscs, 1819–1968. **Abe Ravin and Florence K. Frame, comps.** New York: American Heart Association, 1971.

Comprehensive bibliography of over 6,000 references to international literature. Emphasis on ausculation and phonocardiography. Volume divided into five sections: journal articles and book chapters covering 1820–1966; books, theses, dissertations, and phonodiscs for the time span 1819–1968; abbreviations, complete titles, and origin of journals; author index; and subject index.
R: *ARBA* (1972, p. 611); *MRW* S2, pp. 53, 78.

DENTISTRY

Cranio-Facial–Cleft Palate Bibliography. **American Cleft Palate Association.** Chapel Hill, NC: University of North Carolina, Dental Research Center. Quarterly.

Research in Dental Education: Selected Abstracts, 1933–1968. **John G. Shrock and Virginia G. Sturwold.** San Francisco, CA: Dental Health Center, Education Research Branch, 1969.

A selective abstract focusing on dental education studies published as journal

articles. Citation includes description, problem, methods, procedures, and findings. Author and subject indexes.
R: *MRW* S2, p. 39.

GENETICS

Bibliographica Genetica Medica, 1930–1970 with Technical Assistance of Martine De Boel. **Luc Goeminne.** Ghent, Belgium: E. Story-Scientia, 1971.

Over 600 references to human genetics in English, French, Flemish. Covers a wide range of interests; abstracts from reference books, handbooks, proceedings, monographs.
R: *MRW* S2, pp. 48, 53.

Bibliography on Speech, Hearing, and Language in Relation to Mental Retardation, 1900–1968. **Maryann Peins.** US Maternal and Child Health Service. Washington, DC: US Government Printing Office, 1969.

Close to 2,000 references from English-language books, theses, dissertations. No index.
R: *MRW* S2, pp. 40, 53, 61, 98.

Down-Syndrome: Mongolismus. **Gerhard Koch.** Erlangen: In Kommission bei Palm & Enke, 1973.

Over 3,000 citations on the physiological and genetic aspects of Down's Syndrome. Covers all primary sources and languages. Alphabetically arranged by author. Separates citations pre- and post-1960.
R: *MRW* S3, p. 35.

Down's Syndrome (Mongolism): A Reference Bibliography. **Rudolf F. Vollman.** US National Institutes of Health. Washington, DC: US Government Printing Office, 1969.

A bibliography of close to 700 citations from international sources related to Down's Syndrome. Includes the full text of six classic papers. Subject index.
R: *MRW* S2, p. 69.

Social and Psychological Aspects of Applied Human Genetics: A Bibliography, DHEW Pub. no. (NIH) 73-412. **James R. Sorenson.** Fogarty International Center. Washington, DC: US Government Printing Office, 1973.

International coverage of books and articles about social and psychological issues of applied human genetics. About 1,400 references from 1960–1972 in a subject arrangement.
R: *ARBA* (1974, p. 564); Chen (p. 27); *MRW* S3, pp. 25, 28.

GERONTOLOGY

Words on Aging: A Bibliography of Selected Annotated References Compiled for the Administration on Aging by the Department Library. **US Administration on Aging, US Department of Health, Education, and Welfare Library.** Washington, DC: US Government Printing Office, 1970.

More Words on Aging, Supplement, 1971.

An annotated bibliography on aging; citations are from books (1900–1968) and articles (1963–1967). Entries arranged topically. Includes government documents. Indexes: author, subject.
R: *MRW* S2, pp. 3, 49.

HEALTH SERVICES ADMINISTRATION

Administrator's Collection. 1978 ed. Chicago, IL: American Hospital Association, 1978.
A bibliography for health care administrators.

American Hospital Association Resource Catalog. Chicago, IL: American Hospital Association, 1979.
A free publication; lists all AHA available resources.

A Bibliography of the Socioeconomic Aspects of Medicine. **Theodora Andrews.** Littleton, CO: Libraries Unlimited, 1975.
Very useful collection building tool in the field of health care. Emphasizes socioeconomic aspects of health.
R: Sheehy (EK2).

Comprehensive Bibliography on Health Maintenance Organizations: 1970–1973. **Health Services Administration, US Department of Health, Education, and Welfare.** Washington, DC: US Government Printing Office, 1974.
Entries are listed under the following main categories: Health Care Systems; Legislation and Laws; Medical Services and Staff; Administration; Organizational Structure. Includes an additional bibliography by author. Lists serials, journals, annuals, abstracts, indexes, and newspaper indexes which deal with HMO. Aimed at those involved in HMO management.
R: *RSR* 3: 100 (July–Dec. 1975).

Health Manpower: An Annotated Bibliography. Rev. ed. **Barbara I. Bloom.** Chicago, IL: American Hospital Association, 1976.
Lists over 400 references in the sections "Manpower" and "Employment of Minorities and Women" alone. Emphasis on health manpower in journal articles, books, and pamphlets. Includes a useful list of publishers and addresses.
R: *Modern Healthcare* 6: 81 (Sept. 1976).

Methodology in Evaluating the Quality of Medical Care: An Annotated Selected Bibliography, 1955–1968. Rev. ed. **Isidore Altman, Alice J. Anderson, and Kathleen Barker.** Pittsburgh, PA: University of Pittsburgh Press, 1969.
First edition, 1962.
Cumulates close to 400 references which detail newer methods for improving the quality of medical care.

Selected Studies in Building Research, Applicable to the Design and Construction of Health Facilities, Public Health Service Pub. no. 930-D-26. **US Health**

Facilities Planning and Construction Service. Washington, DC: US Government Printing Office, 1970.

Annotated citations concerning health care architecture design and planning. Over 600 citations numerically arranged. Key word index.
R: *MRW* S2, pp. 54, 89.

The Sociology of Medicine and Health Care: A Research Bibliography. **Theodor J. Litman.** San Francisco, CA: Boyd & Fraser, 1976.

Listing of material available in field of medical sociology through 1971 with the exclusion of the topics of drug addiction, family problems, social gerontology, sexual deviancy, and mental health. Journal, book, government, and pamphlet literature is divided into thirteen broad categories. Indexed by author and subject. Valuable for reference collections in medical, university, and large public libraries.
R: *ARBA* (1978, p. 708).

A Technology of Health Manpower Utilization: Uniform Measurement and Evaluation, DHEW Pub. no. (NIH) 73-429. **National Center for Health Services Research and Development, Bureau of Health Manpower Education, US National Institutes of Health.** Washington, DC: US Government Printing Office, 1973.

Studies of utilization and distribution of health manpower from 1960–1971 are covered in this bibliography containing over 250 annotated references. Material is indexed by subject, author, and organization. Chronological list.
R: *MRW* S3, pp. 26, 27, 45.

The Utilization of Health Services: Indices and Correlates: A Research Bibliography, 1972, DHEW Pub. no. (HSM) 73-3003. **Lu Ann Aday and Robert Eichhorn.** US Health Services and Mental Health Administration. Washington, DC: US Government Printing Office, 1973.

Utilization Review: A Selected Bibliography, 1933–1967. **Donald C. Reidel.** Arlington, VA: US Division of Medical Care Administration, 1968.

Entries are arranged under three subjects in an alphabetical listing by author. Contains no indexes.
R: *MRW* S1, p. 26.

HEMATOLOGY

Frozen Blood: A Review of the Literature 1949–1968. **Arthur R. Turner.** New York: Gordon & Breach, 1970.

The Sickle Cell Hemoglobinopathies: A Comprehensive Bibliography 1910–1972. **Charles W. Triche, III, and Diane Samson Triche.** Troy, NY: Whitston, 1974.

Supplemented by an update, 1973–1975, published in 1976.
Comprehensive collection of literature on the subject. The volumes are divided in three sections: books and scientific essays, scientific journal literature subdivided into 44 subjects, and popular periodical literature and newspaper articles.

Arrangement is alphabetical by title. Both English- and foreign-language material is covered, and an author index is included.
R: *ARBA* (1975, p. 735; 1977, p. 709); *MRW* S3, p. 3.

INFECTIOUS DISEASES

Chagas's Disease: (South American Trypanosomiasis): A Bibliography Compiled From Sleeping Sickness Bureau Bulletin, 1908–1912, and Tropical Diseases Bulletin, 1912–1970. **M. A. Miles and Jean E. Rouse.** London: Bureau of Hygiene and Tropical Diseases, 1970.

A compilation of 2,035 entries to significant publications on Chagas's disease. Consists mostly of journal articles. Alphabetical arrangement of entries by author under specific topics. Titles listed in original language and in English. Author index included.
R: *MRW* S2, p. 105.

Hepatitis Bibliography. **US National Institute of Allergy and Infectious Diseases.** Springfield, VA: National Technical Information Service. Annual.

Schistosomiasis: A Bibliography of the World's Literature From 1852 to 1962. **2 vols. Kenneth S. Warren and Vaun A. Newill.** Cleveland, OH: Press of Western Reserve University, 1967.

Two-volume work contains 10,286 citations. The first book is a key word index with complete entries arranged chronologically under key word. Volume 2 is the author index with complete entry under each author. Foreign-language titles are in English only.
R: *MRW* S1, p. 11.

Schistosomiasis: The Evolution of a Medical Literature: Selected Abstracts and Citations, 1852–1972. **Kenneth S. Warren.** Cambridge, MA: MIT Press, 1973.

Close to 400 core references from the medical literature on schistosomiasis spanning 120 years. Abstracts from international journals, topically arranged. Includes bibliography, illustrations, author and subject indexes.
R: *Lancet* 2: 384 (Aug. 17, 1974); *MRW* S3, p. 46.

Schistosomiasis III: Abstracts of the Complete Literature 1963–1974. 2 vols. **Kenneth S. Warren and Donald B. Hoffman, Jr.** Washington, D.C. Hemisphere Publishing, 1976.

Condenses the literature on schistosomiasis from 1963 to 1974. Consists of over 8,000 citations alphanumerically arranged. Abstracts in English contain much useful information. Key word index. The third in a chronological series; considered an important addition to the literature of the field.
R: *ARBA* (1978, p. 709).

Venereal Disease Bibliography, 1966–1970. **Stephen H. Goode.** Troy, NY: Whitston, 1972.

Supplemented by *Venereal Disease Bibliography for 1972,* published in 1974, and

Venereal Disease Bibliography for 1973, published in 1975 by the same author, as well as annual updates.

Each bibliographical entry is given once in alphabetical title listing and once in a subject listing. Author and subject indexes. Includes both book and periodical materials. Of interest to medical scientists, students, nurses, and psychologists.
R: *BL* 70: 431 (Dec. 15, 1974); *RSR* 1: 45 (Dec. 1973); 2: 118 (July–Sept. 1974); *ARBA* (1973, p. 624; 1975, p. 733; 1976, p. 725).

Work Done in India on Viral and Rickettsial Infections of Vertebrates: A Bibliography. **Surendar Mohan and T. R. Srinivasan, comps.** Delhi, India: Indian National Scientific Documentation Centre, 1967.

Includes 3,267 entries from 84 journals from 1900–1964.
R: *MRW* S1, p. 10.

INTERNAL MEDICINE

Acupuncture: A Research Bibliography. **Allen Y. Liao.** New York: New York University Medical Center Library, 1975.

This bibliography covers materials published from 1960 to 1975. It assists health professionals and others interested in acupuncture research; citations are from scientific journals, books, audiovisual materials.
R: *ARBA* (1977, p. 708).

Acupuncture: An International Bibliography. **Billy K. S. Tam and Miriam S. L. Tam.** Metuchen, NJ: Scarecrow Press, 1973.

A bibliography with over 900 entries covering developments in acupuncture from A.D. 282 to 1972. Abstracted from a variety of source materials; also includes a directory of acupuncture research institutions.
R: *ARBA* (1974, p. 624), *MRW* S3, p. 1.

An Annotated Bibliography on Diving and Submarine Medicine. **Charles W. Shilling and Margaret F. Werts.** New York: Gordon & Breach, 1971.

Prepared under the auspices of the Office of Naval Research, this bibliography covers literature on deep sea diving medicine from 1962–1969. Approximately 2,000 abstracts from all primary sources. Alphabetically arranged by author; permuted subject index.
R: *ARBA* (1972, p. 612); *MRW* S2, pp. 33, 100.

Chiropractic: An International Bibliography. **Lawrence Klein and Sharon Meyer.** Des Moines, IA: Foundation for Chiropractic Education and Research, 1976.

A compilation of over 1,600 items dealing with chiropractic and manipulative therapy. Arranged by kind of material. Introductory section presents an historical outline of manipulative therapeutics, and lists of sources searched and abbreviations used. Book and journal citations comprise the bulk of bibliography.
Useful appendix provides a list of chiropractic associations, directory information on accredited chiropractic colleges and chiropractic periodicals. Includes author and subject indexes.
R: *ARBA* (1978, p. 723).

Emergency Medical Services: Selected Bibliography. **John H. Noble, Jr., et al., eds.** New York: Behavioral Publications, 1974.

Based on the references to the companion book, *Emergency Medical Services: Behavioral and Planning Perspectives.* Consists of 1,000 entries to monographs, articles, and unpublished literature. Topical arrangement of entries according to chapters in the companion volume. Most recent references are from early 1972. No subject or author index. Adequate tool for a beginning literature search. Rapid changes in the field requires additional current material.
R: *RSR* 2: 122 (Apr.–June 1974); *ARBA* (1975, p. 734); *MRW* S3, p. 22.

Health Physics Research Abstracts. No. 6. **International Atomic Energy Agency.** Vienna: International Atomic Energy Agency, 1976.
No. 5, 1974. Irregularly published.
Summary of research reports on health physics from member states of the agency. Titles and abstracts are in original languages in which they were submitted. Includes information on current research and environmental protection.
R: *IBID* 4: 242 (Sept. 1976).

International Bibliography on Burns: Thermal, Electrical, Chemical, Radiation, Cold Injuries, for Better Patient Care, Research, and Teaching. **Irving Feller.** Ann Arbor, MI: American Burn Research Corporation, 1969.
_____. Supplement, 1970–. Annual.
Covers some 9,000 references collected from 4,000 medical publications issued since 1950. Represents 27 languages; however, all titles given in English. Entries arranged in classified manner under twelve major categories. Includes author and subject heading indexes. First supplement appeared in 1970.
R: *MRW* S2, p. 15; Win (EK9; 3EJ4).

Physical Fitness/Sports Medicine. Vols. 1–. **US President's Council on Physical Fitness and Sports.** Washington DC: US Government Printing Office, 1978–. Quarterly.

The Physiology of Physical Stress: A Selective Bibliography, 1500–1964. **Carleton B. Chapman and Elinor C. Reinmiller.** Cambridge, MA: Harvard University Press, 1975.

An historical bibliography on exercise physiology; articles subsequent to 1964 are in MEDLARS file. Topically arranged citations in original language with translation provided for oriental languages. Of interest to physiologists. Author and subject index.
R: *LJ* 100: 1810 (Oct. 1, 1975); *RSR* 3: 34 (July–Dec. 1975); *ARBA* (1976, p. 725).

Quality of Care Assessment and Assurance: An Annotated Bibliography With a Point of View. **Norbert Hirschhorn et al.** Boston, MA: G. K. Hall, 1978.
A selective overview of the literature on the assessment and assurance of quality care in ambulatory medicine. Includes books, articles, and monographs. Valuable resource for health planners, teachers, researchers in public health, and health center providers.

Recurring Bibliography of Hypertension. Vols. 1–. **American Heart Association.** New York: American Heart Association, 1969–. Bimonthly.

Bimonthly compilation of articles obtained from MEDLARS data base. References are listed in format used by *Index Medicus* and divided into subject and author sections.
R: *MRW* S2, p. 55.

Underwater Medicine and Related Sciences: A Guide to the Literature: An Annotated Bibliography, Key Word Index, and Microthesaurus. Vol. 2. **Charles W. Shilling and Margaret F. Werts.** New York: Plenum, 1976.

Volume 1, 1973.
Updates *An Annotated Bibliography on Diving and Submarine Medicine.* Includes nearly 1,800 citations, primarily from 1970 and 1971, each carrying an abstract. Other features include permuted subject index, author index, and microthesaurus (seven pages of relevant terms). References arranged alphabetically by author from government and scientific reports, proceedings, books, and articles from 298 journals.
R: *Neurology* 27: 104 (Jan. 1977); *ABL* 38: entry 634 (Nov. 1973); *ARBA* (1975, p. 734); *MRW* S3, pp. 17, 51.

NURSING

A Bibliography of Nursing Literature, 1859–1960. **Alice M. C. Thompson, ed.** London: Library Association, 1968.

____, *1961–1970.* **Alice M. C. Thompson, comp. and ed.** London: Library Association, 1974.

An historical bibliography of nursing articles and monographs. In five sections: history of nursing, biography, nursing as a profession, specialties of knowledge, and hospitals. Supplemental volume contains index to both bibliographies. For all nursing and medical libraries.
R: *ARBA* (1975, p. 735); *MRW* S1, p. 20; Win (EK165; 3EJ20).

Bibliography of Nursing Monographs. **The Dahlgren Memorial Library, Georgetown University, comp.** Washington, DC: The Dahlgren Memorial Library, Georgetown University, 1979.

Lists works published since 1970 on nursing practices as well as basic health sciences prepared by Georgetown University faculty and medical librarians.

Canadian Nurses' Association Bibliographies. Ottawa, Ontario K2P IE2.

List of bibliographies on specific topics available on request.

Ethics in Nursing: References and Resources, ANA Pub. no. G137. Kansas City, MO: American Nurses Association, 1979.

A selective, nonevaluative list of books, periodical articles, and audiovisuals which will assist nurses in locating additional references in ethics literature.

Instruments for Measuring Nursing Practice and Other Health Care Variables,

DHEW Pub. no. 78-53, 54. Vols. 1–2. Washington, DC: US Government Printing Office, 1978.

Instruments For Use in Nursing Education Research. **Mary Jane Ward and Mark E. Fetler.** Boulder, CO: Western Interstate Commission for Higher Education, 1979.

Nursing Care of the Aged: An Annotated Bibliography for Nurses, Public Health Service Pub. no. 1603. **Myrtle I. Brown.** US Adult Health Protection and Aging Branch. Washington, DC: US Government Printing Office, 1967.
Entries cover years 1954–1965.
R: *MRW* S1, p. 20.

NUTRITION

Annotated Bibliography on Maternal Nutrition, Public Health Service Pub. no. 2055. **Committee on Maternal Nutrition, US Maternal and Child Health Service, National Research Council.** Washington, DC: US Government Printing Office, 1970.

An annotated bibliography of almost 800 references of material published from 1958 to 1968 in English. Physicians and nutritionists concerned with maternal nutrition will find it most useful. Alphabetically arranged by author, with divisions by topics such as diabetes and birth weight.
R: *ARBA* (1971, p. 528); *MRW* S2, p. 73.

An Annotated International Bibliography of Nutrition Education: Materials, Resource Personnel, and Agencies. **Clara Mae Taylor.** New York: Teacher's College Press, 1971.
R: Chen (p. 29).

Beverage Literature: A Bibliography. **A. W. Noling, comp.** Metuchen, NJ: Scarecrow Press, 1971.

About 5,000, mostly unannotated, titles covering all aspects of beverages and related topics.
R: *LJ* 96: 2071 (June 15, 1971); *ARBA* (1972, p. 640); Chen (p. 29).

The Diet Food Finder. **Joan T. Casale,** New York: Bowker, 1975.
Contents of over 200 books and pamphlets are arranged in relation to 25 special diets. An annotated bibliography of books and pamphlets about specific diets also provided. A useful guide to students in nutrition courses.
R: *ARBA* (1976, p. 747); Chen (p. 29).

Food and Nutrition/Alimentation et nutrition/Alimentacion y nutricion: Annotated Bibliography, Author, and Subject Index. **Food and Agriculture Organization of the United Nations.** Distr. New York: Unipub, 1974.
A selected list of publications and documents issued between 1945 and 1972.
R: *ARBA* (1975, p. 763); Chen (p. 29).

Food and Nutrition Information and Educational Materials Center Catalog. **Food and Nutrition Information and Educational Materials Center, US National Agricultural Library.** Beltsville, MD: National Agricultural Library, 1973.

Topical arrangement of over 2,000 references to articles on nutrition education and related subjects. Of interest to food service and nutrition education professionals. Indexes: subject, author, title.
R: *MRW* S3, pp. 8, 25, 38, 52.

Food Composition Tables: Updated Annotated Bibliography, Nutrition Information Document Series, 1. **Food and Agriculture Organization of the United Nations.** Rome, Italy: Food and Agriculture Organization, 1975.

A publication of the FAO Food Policy and Nutrition Division. Updates *Food Composition Tables: Annotated Bibliography.* Emphasis on data relating to food consumption by populations. International coverage. Entries list the following: reference, background, portion analyzed, nutrients, presentation and grouping, and additional information. An aid for food planners, nutritionists, food policy makers, and clinicians.
R: *IBID* 4: 36 (Mar. 1976); Sheehy (EK28).

Index of Nutrition Education Materials. 2d ed. **The Nutrition Foundation.** Washington, DC: The Nutrition Foundation, 1977.

Cites more than 2,000 booklets, pamphlets, audiovisual aids that pertain to nutrition and are government publications. Color-coded format; includes directory of nutrition agencies and associations. A valuable ready reference.
R: *American Journal of Clinical Nutrition* 31: 1713 (Sept. 1978); *Journal of the American Dietetic Association* 72: 459 (Apr. 1978).

Lists of Volatile Compounds in Foods. A Bibliography. **S. van Straten and F. deVryer,** New York: Plenum, 1973.
R: Chen (p. 29).

Nutrition and Aging: A Selected Annotated Bibliography, 1964–1972, DHEW Pub. no (SRS) 73-20237. **Margaret D. Simko and Karen Colitz, comps.** US Administration on Aging. Washington, DC: US Government Printing Office, 1973.

Over 250 references to books, pamphlets, and journal articles on nutritional problems of aging. Intended for both students and professionals. Author arrangement under broad topics. Does not include an index.
R: *MRW* S3, p. 38.

Nutrition Education Materials. **The Nutrition Foundation.** Washington, DC: The Nutrition Foundation, 1974.

Describes sources of nutrition. Publications annotated according to user group, subject matter. Includes audiovisual materials, listing of pertinent associations and societies. An invaluable tool for nutrition educators.
R: *Journal of School Health* 46: 490 (Oct. 1976).

Nutrition, Nutricion: Index, Indice, 1945–1966. **Documentation Center,**

Food and Agriculture Organization of the United Nations. Rome, Italy: Food and Agriculture Organization, 1968.

A bibliography of 1,400 entries covering documents of the FAO from 1945 to 1966. Analytical and author index.
R: *MRW* S1, p. 21.

Obesity: A Bibliography, 1964–1973. **Hilary Whelan and Trevor Silverstone, comps.** Washington, DC: Information Retrieval, 1974.

Contains over 2,000 references to publications dealing with obesity; divided into major areas such as general reviews, descriptive material, and management. Entries give title, clinical subject, author, citation, type of publication, numbers of references. Bibliography will be useful in university and medical libraries. Includes complete author and subject indexes.
R: *Nutrition Reviews* 35: 160 (June 1977); *RSR* 3: 33 (Apr.–June 1975).

Obesity: A Bibliography 1964–1973. **Hilary Whelan and Trevor Silverstone.** London: Information Retrieval Ltd., 1974.

Deals with all aspects of obesity and related topics. Subject and author index. Contains over 2,000 references.

Selected Bibliography of Nutrition Materials. **Doris Flax Kaplan, ed.** Orono, ME: Folger Library, University of Maine, 1973.
R: *Choice* 10: 1700 (Jan. 1974); *TBRI* 40: 281 (Sept. 1974); Chen (p. 30).

Selected References on Cereal Grains in Protein Nutrition: Human and Experimental Animal Studies of Major and Minor Cereals, 1910–1966, US Agricultural Research Service (ARS) 61-5. **Callie M. Coons.** Agricultural Research Service, US Department of Agriculture. Washington, DC: US Government Printing Office, 1968.

Arranged by type of grain, 1,512 entries to journal articles and monographs are included. No indexes.
R: *MRW* S1, p. 21.

ONCOLOGY AND NUCLEAR MEDICINE

Bibliographic Control of the Literature of Oncology, 1800–1960. **Pauline M. Vaillancourt.** Metuchen, NJ: Scarecrow Press, 1969.

A bibliographic handbook which describes tools pertinent to cancer research. Arranged by subjects such as history of oncology, medical bibliography. Emphasizes retrospective searching; indexed.
R: *WLB* 44: 567 (1970); *ARBA* (1970, p. 131); *MRW* S2, pp. 12, 70.

Bibliography on Nuclear Medicine, TID 3319-S6. **US Energy Research and Development Administration.** Springfield, VA: National Technical Information Service, 1975.
R: *RSR* 4: 109 (Oct.–Dec. 1976).

Reading Guide to the Cancer-Virology Literature. Vols. 1–. **Alerting Service,**

Viral Oncology Branch, US National Cancer Institute. Bethesda, MD: National Cancer Institute, 1964–. Monthly.
Entries are arranged alphabetically by journal title. Information on author's addresses, number of references, and abstracts are included in entry. No indexes.
R: *MRW* S1, p. 16.

Readings on Cancer: An Annotated Bibliography, DHEW Pub. no. (NIH) 75-678. Rev. ed. **National Cancer Institute, US Department of Health, Education, and Welfare.** Washington, DC: US Government Printing Office, 1975.
Original edition, Public Health Services Pub. no. 457, 1969.
Designed to meet the literature needs of cancer patients, students, and educators. Arrangement by form: books, articles, pamphlets, etc. Annotations accompany the more than 180 items. Sources are graded. Features valuable listing of major medical libraries in each state.
R: *RSR* 4: 109 (Oct.–Dec. 1976); *ARBA* (1970, p. 133).

ORTHOPEDICS

Annual Bibliography of Orthopaedic Surgery. Vols. 1–. **Journal of Bone and Joint Surgery.** Boston, MA: Journal of Bone and Joint Surgery, 1960–. Annual.

PEDIATRICS

Adolescence: A Select Bibliography. **D. R. Boorer and S. J. Murgatroyd.** Caerphilly, Wales, England: MTM Publishing House, 1972.
A listing of monographs on adolescence published since 1955. Alphabetical by author; divided into six subject categories.
R: *MRW* S2, p. 3.

Bibliography on Early Childhood. **Project Head Start, US Office of Child Development.** Washington, DC: US Government Printing Office, 1970.
Lists over 140 references to books, pamphlets, and government documents. Alphabetically arranged by author; includes directory of publishers.
R: *MRW* S2, pp. 19, 76.

The Child With a Chronic Medical Problem—Cardiac Disorders, Diabetes, Haemophilia: Social, Emotional and Educational Adjustment: An Annotated Bibliography. **Doria Pilling.** New York: Humanities Press, 1973.
A National Children's Bureau report. Consists of 107 citations, all published between 1958–1972. Includes journal articles, society reports, British government publications, and WHO documents. Chronological arrangement under three sections: emotional and social adjustment, family adjustment, and educational attainments. Author index.
R: *MRW* S3, pp. 10, 49.

Normal Child Development: An Annotated Bibliography of Articles and Books

Published 1950–1969. **Janice B. Schulman and Robert C. Prall.** New York: Grune & Stratton, 1971.
Over 700 references alphabetically arranged by author under topical divisions. Author index.
R: *MRW* S2, p. 19.

Sudden Infant Death Syndrome: An Annotated Bibliography for the Layman. **Michael J. Archuleta and Alyce J. Archuleta.** San Diego, CA: Current Bibliography Series, 1975.
Focuses on sudden infant death syndromes. Arrangement of references is by type of media. Attempts a critical evaluation of references. Features a useful list of organizations concerned with SIDS. Handy reference tool for professionals and laymen.
R: *ARBA* (1976, p. 724).

Sudden Infant Death Syndrome: Selected Annotated Bibliography, 1960–1971, DHEW Pub. no. (NIH) 73-237. **Scientific Publications Section, National Institute of Child Health and Human Development, US Department of Health, Education, and Welfare.** Washington, DC: US Government Printing Office, 1972.

_____, DHEW Pub. no. (NIH) 76-237, 1972–1974, 1975.
Includes 205 annotated entries for period 1972–1974 from journal and monographic literature. Arranged alphabetically by authors under year of publication and indexed by author and subject.
R: *RSR* 4: 107 (Oct.–Dec. 1976); *MRW* S3, p. 13.

PHARMACY AND PHARMACOLOGY

Bibliography of Pharmaceutical Reference Literature. **Magda Pasztor and Jenny Hopkins.** London: Pharmaceutical Press, 1968.
Incorporates post-1960 works in pharmaceutics, pharmacology, pharmacognosy, pharmaceutical chemistry, and biological sciences. Arranged by type: handbooks, dictionaries, directories, etc. Includes annotations; well indexed.
R: Win (EK183, 3EJ22).

Cannabis '71. **Paul D'Encarnacao and Pat D'Encarnacao, comps.** Memphis, TN: Psychopharmacology Researchers, 1972.
Marijuana bibliography of 1,400 entries for books, journal articles, and government documents. Covers the period from 1825 through 1971. Entries arranged alphabetically by author. No annotations or index.
R: *ARBA* (1973, p. 621).

A Cocaine Bibliography-Nonannotated, Research Issues no. 8. **Joel L. Phillips and Ronald D. Wynne.** National Institute on Drug Abuse, US Department of Health, Education, and Welfare. Washington, DC: US Government Printing Office, 1975.
Some 1,800 nonannotated references dating from 1585 to the present. Emphasis

on scientific and popular literature. Reflects on the sociopsychological, biomedical, political, and economic aspects of cocaine.
R: *RSR* 3: 101 (July–Dec. 1975).

A Comprehensive Guide to the Cannabis Literature. **Ernest L. Abel, comp.** Westport, CT: Greenwood Press, 1979.

Drug Information Sources. A World-wide Annotated Survey. **J. P. Revill, ed. and comp.** Oxon, England: Gothard House Publications, 1978.

Listing of some 500 professional geographical and trade pharmaceutical organizations. Includes company codes, price lists, handbooks, journals, and other prescription pharmaceutical publications. Basic reference tool for pharmacists, librarians, or market research executives.

Drugs: An Annotated Bibliography and Guide to the Literature. **Alfred M. Ajami, Jr.** Boston, MA: G. K. Hall, 1973.

Over 500 entries which cover a wide range of topics. Divided into four sections: physiological psychology, pharmacology, drugs in society, cultural and philosophical overviews. Entries are from scholarly and popular journals. For medical and university libraries.
R: *Journal of Pharmaceutical Sciences* 62: 1909 (Nov. 1973); *ARBA* (1974, p. 641); *MRW* S3, pp. 17, 18, 40.

Drugs of Addiction and Non-addiction; Their Use and Abuse: A Comprehensive Bibliography, 1960–1969. **Joseph Menditto.** Troy, NY: Whitston Publishing, 1970.

International coverage of drug abuse literature in monographs and periodicals. Lists over 6,000 entries arranged under broad subject areas: amphetamines, narcotics, marijuana, etc.
R: *Choice* 10: 1354 (Nov. 1973); *RQ* 10: 173 (Winter 1970); 14: 161 (Winter 1974); *RSR* 2: 122 (Apr.–June 1974); 2: 38 (July–Sept. 1974); 4: 86 (Jan.–Mar. 1976); *ARBA* (1974, p. 641; 1975, p. 749; 1976, p. 737); *MRW* S2, pp. 33, 34; Win (3EJ25).

The Fate of Drugs in the Organism: A Bibliographic Survey. Vols. 1–. **J. Hirtz, ed.** Societe Francaise des Sciences et Techniques Pharmaceutiques Working Group, comp. New York: Marcel Dekker, 1974–.

Volume 4, 1977.
A bibliographic series tracing the fate of drugs in man and animals. Deals with the processes of absorption, distribution, metabolism, and excretion. Includes citations to significant papers in pharmacology, biochemistry, and clinical medicine. General format of each bibliography: references arranged numerically; an analytical table of references arranged by drug name; an empirical formula table.
R: *Journal of Pharmaceutical Sciences* 65: 633 (Apr. 1976); *ARBA* (1978, p. 730).

Interaction of Alcohol and Other Drugs: An Annotated Bibliography of the Scientific Literature on the Interaction of Ethanol and Other Chemical Compounds

Normally Absent in Vivo. 2d rev. ed. **E. Polacsek et al., comps.** Toronto, Canada: Addiction Research Foundation, 1972.

Research reports, clinical studies, review articles, and papers comprise most of the 1,500 citations. Stresses medicolegal aspects and commentaries. Multilingual coverage. Each entry lists full bibliographic information. Includes key word, author, and drug indexes.
R: *MRW* S3, pp. 1, 19.

LSD Research: An Annotated Bibliography: 1972–1975, DHEW Pub. no. (ADM) 76-293. **National Clearinghouse for Drug Abuse Literature, National Institute on Drug Abuse, US Department of Health, Education, and Welfare.** Washington, DC: US Government Printing Office, 1975.

Annotated references to 315 selected reports and articles from 1972 through April 1975. Follows the following types of LSD studies: human studies in clinical and nonclinical studies, pharmacological and behavioral studies on animals, the synthetic manufacture and analysis of the drug. Includes author index.
R: *RSR* 4: 108 (Oct.–Dec. 1976).

Medical Readings on Heroin. San Francisco, CA: Boyd & Fraser, 1972.

Heroin addiction in the United States forms the basis for the 161 abstracts of journal articles and reports. Arranged by topic. Includes subject index.
R: *MRW* S3, pp. 13, 18.

Medicinal Chemistry Reviews: A Select Bibliography. **Gwynn P. Ellis.** Hamden, CT: Archon Books, 1972.

Guide to important review literature arranged by 60 subject classifications includes about 4,000 entries. Covers January 1950 to late 1971. Primarily in English, but some in French or German. Well-selected bibliography; detailed subject index. Recommended to research workers, information scientists, and librarians in biochemistry, pharmacy, etc.
R: *Aslib Proceedings* 25: 228 (June 1973); *ARBA* (1974, p. 624); *MRW* S3, pp. 6, 9, 20.

Psychopharmacology Bibliography. **US National Institute of Mental Health. International Reference Center for Psychotropic Drugs.** Rockville, MD: National Institute of Mental Health. Quarterly.

Published in the *Psychopharmacology Bulletin.*

Recent Surveys of Nonmedical Drug Use: A Compendium of Abstracts. **William A. Glenn and Louise G. Richards.** National Institute on Drug Abuse, US Department of Health, Education, and Welfare. Washington, DC: US Government Printing Office, 1974.

Bibliographical and statistical abstracts of the nonmedical uses of drugs, grouped accordingly: nationwide survey, high school populations, university populations, other populations. Indexed.
R: *RSR* 3: 101 (July–Dec. 1975).

Selected Bibliography on Detection of Dependence-Producing Drugs in Body

Fluids, WHO Offset Pub. no. 17. **T. L. Chrusciel and M. Chrusciel, comps.** Geneva: World Health Organization, 1975.

Contains list of analytical methods that can be used to detect dependence-producing drugs in the body. Scientific literature published between 1969 and October 1974 is arranged under eleven headings: methods of detection, opiates and synthetic narcotic drugs, hallucinogens, etc. Multilingual volume; when language of publication is other than English or French, the titles are translated into both.
R: *Pharmaceutical Journal* 219: 200 (1977); *IBID* 3: 243 (Dec. 1975); *RSR* 4: 43 (Jan–Mar. 1976).

Toxicity Bibliography: A Bibliography Covering Reports on Toxicity Studies, Adverse Drug Reactions, and Poisoning in Man and Animals. **US National Library of Medicine.** Washington, DC: US Government Printing Office, 1968–1978. Quarterly.

Quarterly publication prepared from MEDLARS file which covers about 2,300 biomedical journals. Part 1 covers drugs and chemicals and includes subject and author indexes. Part 2 covers adverse reactions to drugs and chemicals. Contains 18 subject subsections, but no indexes.
R: *MRW* S1, p. 24; Win (EK221).

PHYSICAL MEDICINE AND REHABILITATION

Cerebral Palsy and Related Developmental Disabilities Prevention and Early Care: An Annotated Bibliography. 3 vols. **Raymond R. Rembolt and Beth Roth.** Columbus, OH: Ohio State University Press, 1975.

Published under the auspices of the United Cerebral Palsy Association. Annotated bibliography mainly concerned with prevention and early care of cerebral palsy. Consists of three volumes: items published before 1964 through 1971, items published 1968 to 1972, and items published in 1972 and 1973. Not intended to be exhaustive. Excellent reference source for therapists. Free publication.
R: *Archives of Physical Medicine and Rehabilitation* 57: 45 (Jan. 1976).

Disability and Rehabilitation: A Selected Bibliography. **Lawrence E. Riley, Elmer A. Spreitzer, and Saad Z. Nagi, eds.** Columbus, OH: Forum Associates, 1971.

A collection of 2,500 references to English-language monographs and journal articles, dating from before 1940 through 1970. Entries arranged by topic. Covers various aspects of physical disability except for medical and mental illness topics. Author index.
R: *MRW* S3, pp. 17, 26, 44.

The Handicapped Child: Research Review. **Rosemary Dinnage.** London: Longman, 1970.

References to literature published from 1958 to 1968 about neurologically handicapped children. Lists English, American, French, and German publications. Emphasizes research methods and materials. Includes subject index. Study funded by grant of the National Fund for Research into Crippling Diseases.
R: *MRW* S2, pp. 15, 61.

Sex and the Handicapped: A Selected Bibliography (1927–1975). **US Veterans Administration Hospital.** Cleveland, OH: US Veterans Administration Hospital, 1975.

Focuses on some twenty disabling conditions with various effects on sexual activity. Printed sources comprise most of the citations. Includes an annotated bibliography of eight rental films. Reference aid for afflicted individuals and counselors.
R: *ARBA* (1978, p. 708).

PSYCHIATRY AND PSYCHOLOGY

Alcohol Education Materials: An Annotated Bibliography. **Gail G. Milgram, ed.** New Brunswick, NJ: Rutgers Center of Alcohol Studies, 1975.

Citations from trade publications, state boards of education.
R: *LJ* 101: 604 (Feb. 15, 1976); *ARBA* (1977, p. 708).

A Bibliography of Books on Death, Bereavement, Loss, and Grief, 1935–1968. **Austin H. Kutscher, Jr., and Austin H. Kutscher, comps.** New York: Health Science Publishing Corp., 1969.

Approximately 1,200 English-language citations from books on death. Intended for the lay person and the professional; arranged alphabetically by subject.
R: *MRW* S3, pp. 4, 12, 26.

Bibliography of Child Psychiatry and Child Mental Health with a Selected List of Films. **Irving N. Berlin, ed.** New York: Human Sciences Press, 1976.

For mental health professionals. Citations from all aspects of the literature. Chronologically arranged. Good format. A valuable tool for professionals working with children.
R: *ARBA* (1977, p. 705).

A Bibliography of Drug Abuse, Including Alcohol and Tobacco. **Theodora Andrews.** Littleton, CO: Libraries Unlimited, 1977.

An extensive compilation of over 700 titles covering aspects of drug abuse. In two parts: general reference sources and material by subject area, such as history, hallucinogens, stimulants. Complete citations include summary of contents, evaluation of appropriate level.
R: *Choice* 15: 369 (May 1978); *WLB* 52: 585 (Mar. 1978); *ARBA* (1978, p. 729).

Bibliography of Drug Dependence and Abuse, 1928–1966. **US National Clearinghouse for Mental Health.** Chevy Chase, MD: US National Clearinghouse for Mental Health, 1969.

Contains 3,000 citations from books, articles, legal documents arranged by topic. No annotations. Compiled for use by specialists and research workers.
R: *ARBA* (1970, p. 132).

Bibliography on Suicide and Suicide Prevention: 1897–1957, 1958–1970, DHEW Pub. no. (HSM) 72-9080. **Norman L. Farberow.** US National Institute of Mental Health. Washington, DC: US Government Printing Office, 1972.

Intended as a single reference source for those concerned with suicide prevention. Consists of two chronologically divided lists, totaling about 3,500 citations. Alphabetically arranged; provides full citations, author and subject indexes. Tends to exclude medical aspects of the literature.
R: *ARBA* (1970, p. 137); *MRW* S2, p. 100; *MRW* S3, p. 52.

Conceptual Index to Psychoanalytic Technique and Training. 5 vols. **Henry H. Hart.** Croton-on-Hudson, NY: North River Press, 1972.

Abstracts from the psychoanalytic literature from 1949 to 1969. Topically arranged by approximately 300 concepts. Includes full bibliographic citation and brief annotation. Cross-referenced.
R: *MRW* S2, p. 82.

Cooperative Studies in Mental Health and Behavioral Sciences: An Annotated Bibliography Summarizing Two Decades of Cooperation in Mental Health and Behavioral Sciences 1956–1975. **Susan Abrams and Sandra Ciufo.** Department of Medicine and Surgery, US Veterans Administration, 1975.

Deals with published Veterans Administration reports. Emphasis on drug therapy, psychological studies, methodological studies, and psychopathological studies performed on mental health patients. Arranged by subject; no indexes.
R: *RSR* 4: 110 (Oct.–Dec. 1976).

Death: A Bibliographical Guide. **Albert J. Miller and Michael J. Acri.** Metuchen, NJ: Scarecrow Press, 1977.

Partially annotated bibliographical guide to literature of death and dying. Its 3,848 entries include periodical articles, books, essays, and audiovisual material written through 1974. Focuses on material in English and provides an author and extensive subject index.
R: *LJ* 102: 2149 (Oct. 15, 1977); *WLB* 52: 425 (Jan. 1978); *ARBA* (1978, p. 724).

Death, Grief and Bereavement: A Bibliography 1845–1975. **Robert Fulton, comp.** New York: Arno, 1977.

Compiled by the Center for Education and Research. Lists over 3,800 items which are alphabetically arranged by author. Focuses only on references that approach the subject from an empirical viewpoint. Topic of suicide omitted from bibliography; however, contains numerous references to euthanasia, sudden infant death syndrome, organ transplantation, terminal care, and abortion. Generally excludes foreign material.
R: *Choice* 14: 830 (Sept. 1977); *ARBA* (1978, p. 724).

Drug Use and Abuse Among U.S. Minorities: An Annotated Bibliography. New York: Praeger, 1976.

Emphasis on American minority groups: Blacks, Chicanos, Puerto Ricans, American Indians, and Asian Americans. Bibliography consists of scholarly literature. Includes timely critical essay on the topic. Indexes enhance the bibliography's reference usefulness.
R: *ARBA* (1977, p. 724): *Choice* 13: 958 (Oct. 1976).

Dying and Death: An Annotated Bibliography. **Irene L. Sell.** New York: Tiresias Press, 1977.

Some 506 annotated items to articles, books, and audiovisual materials. Emphasis on practical works. Audiovisual section is outstanding. Complements the 3,848-item *Death: A Bibliographical Guide* by A. J. Miller and M. J. Acri. Designed primarily for nurses and health professionals who are faced with the emotional problems of dying patients and their families.
R: *ARBA* (1978, p. 725).

Early Childhood Psychosis: Infantile Autism, Childhood Schizophrenia and Related Disorders: An Annotated Bibliography, 1964 to 1969, DHEW Pub. no. (HSM) 71-9062. **Carolyn Q. Bryson and Joseph N. Hingtgen.** National Clearinghouse for Mental Health Information, US National Institute of Mental Health. Washington, DC: US Government Printing Office, 1971.

Consists of 424 annotations of articles, books, and papers. Topical arrangement of entries. Includes author index.
R: *MRW* S2, pp. 9, 84, 93.

Emotions and Bodily Changes: A Survey of Literature on Psychosomatic Interrelationships, 1910–1953. **Helen F. Dunbar.** New York: Columbia University Press, 1954. Reprint New York: Arno, 1976.

Fills the literature gaps between psychiatric and physiological research. Consists of three segments: Part 1 deals with methodology and orientation; Part 2 concentrates on organs and organ systems; and Part 3 considers therapeutic concerns and conclusion. Includes a fold-out chart of "Personality Profiles of Eight Psychosomatic Diagnostic Groups." Length of abstracts varies; some include commentaries. Worthwhile addition to libraries without original editions.
R: *ARBA* (1977, p. 707).

Homosexuality: A Selective Bibliography of Over Three Thousand Items. **William Parker.** Metuchen, NJ: Scarecrow Press, 1971.

Homosexuality Bibliography: Supplement, 1970–1975. **William Parker.** Metuchen, NJ: Scarecrow Press, 1977.

Homosexuality: An Annotated Bibliography. **Martin S. Weinberg and Alan P. Bell, eds.** New York: Harper & Row, 1972.

Lists 1,265 citations on homosexuality from literature published during 1940–1968 in the English language. References include journal articles, books, dissertations, theses, and unpublished papers. Entries arranged under three sections: physiological, psychological, and sociological aspects. Principle emphasis on fields of psychiatry, psychology, and sociology with scattered interest in related topics. Includes author and subject indexes. Excludes popular magazines and newspaper articles. Useful reference tool for the serious student.
R: *ARBA* (1974, p. 626); *MRW* S2, p. 54.

Human Sexuality in Physical and Mental Illness and Disabilities: An Annotated Bibliography. **Ami Sha'ked.** Bloomington, IN: Indiana University Press, 1979.

Very specialized bibliography. Contains no pre-1940 references. Annotations are explicit.
R: *LJ* 104: 474 (Feb. 15, 1979).

Latino Mental Health: Bibliography and Abstracts, DHEW Pub. no. (HSM) 73-9144. **Amado M. Padilla and Paul Aranda.** US Alcohol, Drug Abuse, and Mental Health Administration. Washington, DC: US Government Printing Office, 1974.

Supplements *Latino Mental Health: A Review of the Literature* (1973). Contains 497 abstracts to predominantly English-language literature dealing with the mental health of the Latin population in the United States. Attempts to be an exhaustive survey of the many mental health related disciplines of the Spanish speaking, Spanish surnamed, and people of Spanish origin. Arrangement by author. Includes subject index.
R: *RSR* 3: 102 (July–Dec. 1975); *MRW* S3, pp. 33, 35.

Mental Health Book Review Index: An Annual Bibliography of Book Reviews in the Behavioral Sciences: Cumulative Author-Title Index of Volumes 1–12, 1956–1967. **Council on Research and Bibliography.** New York: Council on Research and Bibliography, 1969.
R: *ARBA* (1970, p. 137).

Mental Health Emergencies Alert!: An Annotated Bibliography, no. 1. **National Institute of Mental Health, US Department of Health, Education, and Welfare.** Washington, DC: US Government Printing Office, 1974.

Annotated references to recent mental health literature, focusing on emergencies. Emphasizes suicide, drug overdose, alcoholism, child abuse, and rape.
R: *RSR* 4: 110 (Oct.–Dec. 1976).

The Mental Health of the Black Community: An Exploratory Bibliography. **Lenwood G. Davis.** Monticello, IL: Council of Planning Librarians, 1975.
R: *RSR* 3: 71 (July–Dec. 1975).

PsychoSources: A Psychology Resource Catalog. **Editors of Communications Research Machines, Inc.** New York: Bantam Books, 1973.

In a format similar to the *Whole Earth Catalog,* this volume provides bibliography and reviews of books, films, journal articles, and other sources that deal with psychology. Broad topical arrangement, illustrations, lists of publishers, film access information, etc.
R: *MRW* S3, pp. 43, 49.

Publications Resulting from National Institute of Mental Health Research Grants, 1947–1961, Public Health Service Pub. no. 1647. **US National Institute of Mental Health.** Washington, DC: US Government Printing Office, 1968.

Lists 12,325 publications by grant number. Includes investigators, title, sponsoring institution and its location, and duration of project.
R: *MRW* S1, p. 18.

A Selective Guide to Materials for Mental Health and Family Life Education. **Mental Health Materials Center.** Northfield, IL: Perennial Education, 1972.

Alphabetically arranged by subject. Describes over 500 publications in the field of education. Also covers audiovisuals, plays. Provides bibliographic data and evaluation according to audience.
R: *CRL* 38: 106 (Apr. 1977); *MRW* S3, pp. 4, 33.

Urban Environments and Human Behavior: An Annotated Bibliography. **Gwen Bell, Edwina Randall, and Judith E. R. Roeder.** Stroudsburg, PA: Dowden, Hutchinson & Ross, 1973.

Over 500 references from books and journal articles dated 1889–1972 covering relationship between social behavior of humans and urban environments. Topical arrangement, bibliography, author and subject indexes. For those in design and building fields as well as social and behavioral scientists.
R: *MRW* S3, pp. 10, 23, 49.

Volunteer Services in Mental Health: An Annotated Bibliography, 1955–1969, National Clearinghouse for Mental Health Information Pub. no. 1002. **Francine Sobey, prep.** US National Institute of Mental Health. Washington DC: US Government Printing Office, 1969.

Arranged by settings in which volunteers work, over 400 entries about mental health volunteer services in the United States are included. Listing gives bibliographic details and annotations. Volume contains research and statistical studies, list of bibliographies and directories, author index.
R: *ARBA* (1970, p. 138); *MRW* S2, pp. 67, 97, 108.

We Call It Bibliotherapy: An Annotated Bibliography on Bibliotherapy and the Adult Hospitalized Patient, 1900–1966, US Veterans Administration Bibliography, 10-1. **Rosemary Dolan, comp.** Medical and General Reference Library, US Veterans Administration. Washington, DC: US Veterans Administration, 1967.

Contains 403 citations to journal articles and books.
R: *MRW* S1, p. 18.

Women and Drugs: An Annotated Bibliography. **National Clearinghouse for Drug Abuse Literature, National Institute on Drug Abuse, US Department of Health, Education, and Welfare.** Washington, DC: US Government Printing Office, 1975.

Some 180 abstracts explore the psychological, social, and cultural reasons to heavy drug use especially prevalent in middle-aged women. Three main categories are women and narcotics, women and psychotherapeutic drugs, and women and alcohol. Includes author index.
R: *RSR* 4: 109 (Oct.–Dec. 1976).

Women and Mental Health: Selected Annotated References 1970–1973. **Phyllis E. Cromwell.** National Institute of Mental Health, US Department of

Health, Education, and Welfare. Washington, DC: US Government Printing Office, 1974.

Arranged by author under topic, some of which are contraception, motherhood, rape, widowhood. Author index.
R: *RSR* 3: 102 (July–Dec. 1975).

PUBLIC HEALTH

Air Pollution Publications: A Selected Bibliography, 1963–1966, Public Health Service Pub. no. 979. **Division of Air Pollution, US Public Health Service.** Washington, DC: US Government Printing Office, 1966.

Contains approximately 900 entries.
R: *MRW* S1, p. 27.

Asbestosis: A Bibliography of the World's Literature Abstracted and Indexed 1960–1968. **Sylvia Williams.** Johannesburg, South Africa: Pneumoconiosis Research Unit, Council for Scientific and Industrial Research, 1969.

Contains 600 English-language abstracts on asbestosis. Includes full bibliographical citation and evaluation of sources consulted. Author index.
R: *MRW* S2, p. 8.

A Bibliography of Chinese Sources on Medicine and Public Health in the People's Republic of China, 1960–1970, DHEW Pub. no. (NIH) 73-439. **US John E. Fogarty International Center for Advanced Study in the Health Sciences, National Institutes of Health.** Washington, DC: US Government Printing Office, 1973.

Contains over 15,000 entries. In two parts: abstracts from Chinese medical journals, magazines, and newspapers and abstracts from monographs and books. Complete citation includes translation and transliteration. Index of abbreviations and periodicals.
R: *ARBA* (1974, p. 624); *MRW* S3, pp. 6, 44.

A Bibliography of Noise, 1965–1970. **Mary K. Floyd.** Troy, NY: Whitston Publishing, 1973.

Over 4,500 international citations that deal with physiological, psychological, and sociological effects of noise on people. Alphabetically arranged by title and author. Articles and books listed separately.
R: *MRW* S3, p. 36.

Bibliography on Smoking and Health, Public Health Service Pub. no. 1124, Bibliography Series no. 45. **Donald R. Shopland, ed.** Atlanta, GA: Technical Information Center, US National Clearinghouse for Smoking and Health, 1967–. Annual.

An annual which supersedes the *Bibliography on Smoking and Health, 1958–63.* Includes index by author, subject, and corporate author.
R: *MRW* S1, p. 23; Win (EK19).

Biological Aspects of Lead: An Annotated Bibliography. 2 vols. **US Environ-**

mental Protection Agency. Washington, DC: US Government Printing Office, 1972.

Citations concerning the biological aspects of lead from all primary sources, including historical publications. Includes information on water, soil, air pollution, legal regulations, and recommendations.
R: *ARBA* (1973, p. 607).

Biological Effects of Microwaves. **Stanislaw Baranski and Przemyslaw Czerski.** Stroudsburg, PA: Dowden, Hutchinson & Ross, 1976.

Reviews literature from 1973 on the effects of microwaves. Cites numerous studies. Emphasizes biological effects. Comprises a critical survey.
R: *Nature* 266: vii (Apr. 28, 1977); *Quarterly Review of Biology* 53: 207 (1978).

Comprehensive Bibliography of Existing Literature on Tobacco: 1969–1974. **Robert S. Gold, William H. Zimmerli, and Winnifred K. Austin.** Dubuque, IA: Kendall/Hunt Publishing, 1975.

Some 4,000 items devoted to a considerable amount of diverse source material on the tobacco plant, the effects of smoking, experiments, and recent research. Bibliography divided into three separate sections: bibliographic listings by topic outline, alphabetical author index, and subject index with topical arrangement. Represents primarily English-language texts. Compiled for research workers and laymen.
R: *ARBA* (1977, p. 724).

Current Bibliography of Epidemiology: A Guide to the Literature of Epidemiology, Preventive Medicine, and Public Health. Vols. 1–. **American Public Health Association.** New York: American Public Health Association, 1969–. Monthly.

Comprehensive index to current periodical medical literature on the etiology, prevention, and control of diseases. References culled from MEDLARS tapes. Arranged under two sections: selected subject headings and diseases, organisms and vaccines. Geared toward practitioners, investigators, and community health workers.
R: *RSR* 3: 102 (July–Dec. 1975); 4: 110 (Oct.–Dec. 1976); *MRW* S2, pp. 43, 81, 85; Win (EK53; 3EJ9).

Disaster Technology: An Annotated Bibliography. **D. Manning, ed.** Oxford, England: Pergamon, 1976.

Focuses on disasters that have been recorded since 1973 including earthquakes, droughts, cyclones, and famines. A useful subject index lists geographic location, types of disasters, education, ethical considerations, proper organization and planning procedures, etc. Also includes author index. Seven special sections devoted to relief organizations, nutritional, sociological, and physical aspects of disasters. Ninety-six abstracts cover disasters involving clinical nutrition. Geared toward those involved in mass casualty management and catastrophe planning.
R: *American Journal of Clinical Nutrition* 30: 292 (Feb. 1977); Sheehy (EK3).

Environmental Pollution and Mental Health. **John S. Williams, Jr. et al.** Washington, DC: Information Resources Press, 1973.

Long abstracts for highly selective entries culled from such sources as *Psychological Abstracts* and MEDLARS Approximately 100 entries.
R: *ARBA* (1975, p. 692); Chen (p. 45).

Health and Disease of American Indians North of Mexico: A Bibliography, 1800–1969. **Mark V. Barrow, Jerry D. Niswander, and Robert Fortuine, comps.** Gainesville, FL: University of Florida Press, 1972.

Emphasis on clinical medicine and related topics. Arranged into 22 categories. Contains three indexes: author index, a disease subject index, and a tribal index. Omits literature on Indian beliefs about disease and folk medicine and references to Eskimos. Does not claim to be exhaustive. Worthwhile addition to all major reference collections.
R: *ARBA* (1974, p. 623).

Industrial Noise: A Selective Bibliography, 1963–1973. **Mary A. Babyak and Marianne C. Kaschak, comps.** Pittsburgh, PA: Industrial Health Foundation, 1973.

Journal articles comprise most of the 1,163 references to English-language literature. Emphasis on the measurement of industrial noise, effects of laborers, and efforts at control. Entries arranged alphabetically by author. Includes subject index.
R: *MRW* S3, pp. 30, 36.

International Bibliography of Studies on Alcohol. Vols. 1–. **Mark Keller, ed.** New Brunswick, NJ: Publications Division, Rutgers Center of Alcohol Studies, 1966–.

Volume 1: 25,342 references to the literature of 1901–1950. Chronological and alphabetical author arrangements. Volume 2: Index to volume 1 (in preparation). Volume 3: References and Indexes to literature of 1951–1960 (in preparation).
R: *MRW* S1, p. 18.

Low and Very Low Dose Influences of Ionizing Radiation on Cells and Organisms, Including Man: A Bibliography. **US Bureau of Radiological Health.** Washington, DC: US Government Printing Office, 1972.

An extensive compilation of references to the literature devoted to the effects of low levels of ionizing radiation on biological organisms.
R: *ARBA* (1973, p. 607).

Man and the Environment: A Bibliography of Selected Publications of the United Nations System, 1946–1971. **Harry N. M. Winton, comp.** New York: Unipub, 1972.

Publications of various United Nations agencies are responsible for the 1,200 annotated references. Arrangement of entries by topic and format (e.g. audiovisuals, directories). Useful data such as price and out-of-print status included in entry. Contains indexes of authors, titles, subjects, and series and serials.
R: Chen (p. 43); Mal (8-90); *MRW* S2, pp. 37, 42.

Marihuana: An Annotated Bibliography. **Coy W. Waller et al.** New York: Macmillan, 1976.

Descriptively annotated bibliography covers international scientific publications from 1964 through 1975. The 3,045 citations are mainly scholarly and research material. Some 20 pages of introductory material are provided on chemistry of marijuana. Arrangement is alphabetical with complete bibliographic information, and subject and author index is provided.
R: *Journal of Pharmaceutical Sciences* 66: 909 (June 1977); *LJ* 101: 2471 (Dec. 1, 1976); *WLB* 51: 538 (Feb. 1977); *ARBA* (1977, p. 725).

Marijuana: A Selective Bibliography, 1924–1970. **William H. Rickles, Jr., Benjamin Chatoff, and Charlotte Whitaker.** Los Angeles, CA: Brain Information Service, UCLA Center for Health Sciences, 1970. Issued by the UCLA Brain Information Service as NINDS Neurological Information Network, NIH 70-2063.

Close to 200 annotated references on marijuana. Can be used as a guide to the scientific literature. Annotations provide abstract of paper, outline. Contents are classified by subject; bibliographies are alphabetically arranged.
R: *MRW* S2, p. 16.

Rape and Rape-Related Issues: An Annotated Bibliography. **Elizabeth J. Kemmer.** New York: Garland Publishing, 1977.
R: *LJ* 102: 2050 (Oct. 1977).

Selected Bibliography on Lead Poisoning in Children. Reprint ed. **Jane S. Lin-Fu, comp.** Community Health Services, US Department of Health, Education, and Welfare. Washington, DC: US Government Printing Office, 1975.

First edition, 1971.
R: *RSR* 4: 107 (Oct.–Dec. 1976).

Selected References on Environment Quality as It Relates to Health. **US National Library of Medicine, Bethesda, MD.** Washington, DC: US Government Printing Office, 1971–. Monthly.

Each issue contains approximately 1,000 citations of articles in journals covered by *Index Medicus.* Covers a variety of technical literature concerned with health hazards.
R: Chen (p. 44); Katz (p. 26).

Smoking and Health Bulletin. **Donald R. Shopland, ed.** Atlanta, GA: Technical Information Center, US National Clearinghouse for Smoking and Health, 1967–. Approx. 10/yr.

Formerly *Smoking and Health Bibliographic Bulletin.* Includes index guide to current research.
R: *MRW* S1, p. 24.

RADIOLOGY

Radiological Health Training Resources 1975, DHEW Pub. no. (FDA) 75-8027. **Food and Drug Administration, US Department of Health, Education, and Welfare.** Washington, DC: US Government Printing Office, 1975.

A list by subject of booklets and audiovisual materials concerning radiological health. Publications are free; audiovisuals can be borrowed temporarily.
R: *RSR* 4: 108 (Oct.–Dec. 1976).

UROGENITAL SYSTEM

Abortion Bibliography. Vols. 1–. **Mary K. Floyd, comp.** Troy, NY: Whitston Publishing, 1972–. Annual.

An annual series of bibliographies on abortion; lists all important journal articles and books. Attempts to be internationally comprehensive. Includes subject and author indexes. Useful in school and university libraries.
R: *American Journal of Nursing* 74: 349 (Jan. 1974); *RSR* 2: 122 (Apr.–June 1974); *WLB* 47: 200 (Oct. 1972); *ARBA* (1973, p. 607; 1976, p. 725).

Adverse Effects of Oral Contraceptives, Literature Search no. 74-20. **Geraldine D. Nowak.** US Department of Health, Education, and Welfare. National Library of Medicine. Washington, DC: US Government Printing Office, 1974.

NLM computer-generated bibliography. Contains close to 1,000 citations from 1970 to June 1973. Lists descriptors and subject heading for each entry.
R: *RSR* 3: 102 (July–Dec. 1975).

An Annotated Bibliography of Induced Abortion. **Cunnar af Geijerstam, ed.** Ann Arbor, MI: Center for Population Planning, University of Michigan, 1969.

Contains 1,175 selected references on all aspects of induced abortion with special emphasis on foreign-language and hard-to-get English publications published mostly between 1960 and 1967. Entries arranged by geographical region and epidemiology.
R: *MRW* S2, p. 2.

Artificial Kidney Bibliography. **US National Institute of Arthritis and Metabolic Diseases.** Washington, DC: US Government Printing Office, 1967–.

A quarterly bibliography provided by MEDLARS. Corresponds to *Index Medicus.*
R: *MRW* S1, p. 33.

Methadone and Pregnancy: An Annotated Guide to the Literature, Special Bibliography no. 1. **National Institute on Drug Abuse, US Department of Health, Education, and Welfare.** Washington, DC: US Government Printing Office, 1974.

Alphabetically arranged by author. Bibliography covers period from late 1940s to 1973. Entries include brief annotation.
R: *RSR* 3: 101 (July–Dec. 1975).

Sex and Sex Education: A Bibliography. **Flora C. Seruya, Susan Losher, and Albert Ellis, comps.** New York: Bowker, 1972.

Bibliography includes over 2,000 sources which are divided by subject. Covers literature within the last 25 years. Annotations accompany some references.
R: *MRW* S3, pp. 48, 49.

Sex Education Books For Young Adults 1892–1979. **Patty Campbell.** New York: Bowker, 1979.

An historical survey of sex education handbooks in America.

VETERINARY MEDICINE

Bibliography of Animal Venoms, Envenomations, and Treatments Period 1500–1968. **Gastao Rosenfeld and Eva M. A. Kelen.** Sao Paulo, Brazil: Instituto Butantan, 1969.

Contains over 10,000 references to works by close to 8,000 authors on venom. Entries are from major medical and scientific indexes. Alphabetical by author and ascending chronological order.
R: *MRW* S2, pp. 7, 106.

Bibliography of Reproduction: A Classified Monthly Title List Compiled from the World's Research Literature. Vertebrates, Including Man. Vol. 1. Cambridge, England: Reproduction Research Information Service, 1963–. Monthly.

Over 600 literature sources per issue for such subjects as biology, medicine, agriculture, and veterinary science. Includes author and animal indexes.
R: Chen (p. 30); Mal (9-156); Wal (p. 226).

CHAPTER 4 ENCYCLOPEDIAS

GENERAL

The Book of Health: A Medical Encyclopedia for Everyone. 3d ed. **Randolph L. Clark and Russell W. Cumley, eds.** New York: Van Nostrand Reinhold, 1973.
An encyclopedia for the lay person; provides accessible general information in medicine. Includes a guide to emergency situations, glossary of terms, diagrams, and illustrations. Recommended for both home and public libraries.
R: *ARBA* (1974, p. 636); *RSR* 2: 112 (Apr.–June, 1974); Sheehy (EK16).

The Encyclopedia of Biochemistry. **Roger John Williams.** New York: Van Nostrand Reinhold, 1967.
Alphabetically arranged articles on broad topics.
R: *Bioscience* 18: 58 (1968); *Choice* 4: 644 (1967); *LJ* 92: 2553 (July 1967); *NTB* 52: 201 (1967); *RQ* 6:200 (Summer 1967); Chen (p. 50); Jenkins (D104); Mal (9-61); Wal (p. 201); Win (2EC8).

Encyclopedia of Bioethics. 4 vols. **Warren T. Reich, ed.** New York: Macmillan, 1978.
A four-volume reference; covers topics in medical bioethics including abortion, euthanasia, human experimentation, patient rights, environmental health, etc. Articles arranged alphabetically; includes bibliographies, cross-references. Concise, comprehensive reference work; recommended to all health sciences personnel.

Encyclopedia of Enzyme Technology. **Yale Meltzer.** Flushing, NY: Future Stochastic Dynamics, 1973.
R: Chen (p. 51).

Encyclopedia of Medical Sources. **Emerson C. Kelly.** Baltimore, MD: Williams & Wilkins, 1948.
Covers major medical discoveries in an alphabetical arrangement. Also lists the location of the original descriptions of their discoveries.

Encyclopedia of Sociology. Guilford, CT: Dushkin, 1974.
Comprehensive encyclopedia which includes references. Articles alphabetically arranged, cover major areas of sociology.
R: *MRW* S3, p. 51.

The Encyclopedia of the Biological Sciences. 2d ed. **Peter Gray, ed.** New York: Van Nostrand Reinhold, 1970.
First Edition, 1961.
Intended as a brief reference for biologists seeking information outside their field of specialty. Perhaps the only comprehensive one-volume encyclopedia in the field. Contains 800 signed articles.
R: *Nature* 227: 208 (July 1970); *Science* 134: 93–94 (1961); *Choice* 7: 818 (Sept. 1970); *LJ* (Mar. 15, 1970); *Subscription Books Bulletin* 58: 585 (1962); *ARBA* (1971,

p. 493); Chen (p. 51); Jenkins (G41); Mal (9-17); Wal (p. 192); Win (EC18; 3EC3).

Family Health Encyclopedia: An International Reference in the Health Sciences. 2 vols. Philadelphia, PA: J. B. Lippincott, 1970.

Short articles written for the lay person, covering a wide range of subjects. Also includes a brief history of medicine, information on child development, glossary, and directory of community health services. Provides brief definitions of medical terms. Alphabetically arranged, in two volumes.
R: *ARBA* (1972, p. 628).

Kingzett's Chemical Encyclopedia: A Digest of Chemistry and Its Industrial Applications. 9th ed. **D. Hey, ed.** New York: Van Nostrand Reinhold, 1966.

Provides definitions of chemical terms, properties of chemical substances, and their industrial applications.

Kirk-Othmer Encyclopedia of Chemical Technology. 3d ed. **Raymond Eller Kirk and Donald F. Othmer, eds.** New York: Wiley-Interscience, 1978-.
Second revised edition, 1963-1971; 22 vols.
Volume 9, *Enamels to Felts,* 1980.
Third edition published in 1979. A multivolume set written by experts in the field. Authoritative primary reference for producers and users of chemical products.
R: *British Chemical Engineering* 10: 50 (Jan. 1965); *Choice* 4: 966; *ARBA* (1970, p. 160); Chen (p. 58); Jenkins (D65); Mal (11-88); Wal (p. 470); Win (EI56; 1EI9; 2EI11; 3EI8).

McGraw-Hill Encyclopedia of Science and Technology. 4th ed. 15 vols. New York: McGraw-Hill, 1977.
First edition, 1960; third edition, 1971.
A comprehensive (7,600 articles) reference intended primarily for the intelligent layman. Many of the longer articles are signed and contain bibliographies. Kept up to date since 1972 by the *McGraw-Hill Yearbook of Science and Technology.*
R: *American Scientist* 59: 253-254 (Mar./Apr. 1971); *Journal of Chemical Education* 48: 463 (July 1971); *Scientific American* 214: 138-140 (June 1966); *Australian Library Journal* 20: 325 (Mar. 1971); *LJ* 92: 2146 (1967); *RQ* 10: 274 (Spring 1971); *Subscription Books Bulletin* 64: 793-802 (1968); Chen (p. 47); Mal (3-15); Wal (p. 17); Win (EA86, 1EA11).

The Mothers' and Fathers' Medical Encyclopedia. **Virginia E. Pomeranz and Dodi Schultz.** Boston, MA: Little, Brown, 1977.

Revised and expanded version of the *Mother's Medical Encyclopedia.* Over 2,000 entries. Includes many illustrations, useful appendixes, room for charting medical histories. An excellent source for home ready reference. Includes particulary helpful section on poisonous household substances with appropriate antidotes.
R: *ARBA* (1973, p. 617; 1978, p. 726).

The New Illustrated Medical Encyclopedia for Home Use: A Practical Guide to

Good Health. 4 vols. **Robert E. Rothenberg, ed.** New York: Abradale Press, 1974.
In four volumes, geared toward the lay person, aims to answer frequently asked medical questions. Succinct, authoritative information, detailed index. Cross-referenced, up-to-date, and extensive. Recommended for students and consumers.
R: *ARBA* (1976, p. 737).

The Practical Encyclopedia of Natural Healing. **Mark Bricklin.** Emmaus, PA: Rodale Press, 1976.
Cumulated discussions on natural healing; comprises a volume of folk medicine and nondrug therapies. Recommended more for curiosity reading than for ready-reference information. For public libraries.
R: *ARBA* (1978, p. 728).

The Reston Encyclopedia of Biomedical Engineering Terms. **Rudolf F. Graf and George J. Whalen.** Reston, VA: Reston Publishing Co., 1977.
Alphabetically arranged biomedical and engineering terms. Definitions are brief, though cross-references are supplied; many interdisciplinary terms are included. Not overly technical, the work is suitable for medical libraries as a reference in this fast-growing field.
R: *Choice* 14: 832 (Sept. 1977); *LJ* 102: 1170 (May 15, 1977); *RQ* 17:76 (Fall 1977); *ARBA* (1978, p. 710).

Symptoms: The Complete Home Medical Encyclopedia. **Sigmund S. Miller, ed.** New York: Thomas Y. Crowell, 1976.
Helps reader to identify symptoms of disease. In two main parts: symptoms and diseases, arranged systematically. Also includes glossary. Thorough, helpful for home reference.
R: *ARBA* (1977, p. 721).

Van Nostrand's Scientific Encyclopedia. 5th ed. **Douglas M. Considine, ed.** Princeton, NJ: Van Nostrand Reinhold, 1976.
First edition, 1938; second edition, 1947; third edition, 1958; fourth edition, 1968.
A well-received one-volume work. Definitions provide both basic and technical information. Dated, however, as concerns topics of current interest.
R: *New Scientist* 41: 188–189 (Jan. 23, 1969); *SJ* 5: 117 (May 1969); *Choice* 5: 1417 (1969); *CRL* 30: 84 (1969); *RQ* 10: 28 (Fall 1970); Chen (p. 47); Jenkins (A49); Mal (3-17); Wal (p. 18); Win (EA88; 2EA17).

The World Book Illustrated Home Medical Encyclopedia. 4 vols. Chicago, IL: World Book, 1979.
Volume 1, *Medical Reference Guide (A–H) and Index of Symptoms*; volume 2, *Medical Reference Guide (I–Z)*; volume 3, *First Aid, Safety, and Care of the Sick*; volume 4, *Guide to Health and Fitness; Index.*
A family medical reference set prepared under the direction of 25 internationally respected medical specialists. Contains some 2,500 question-and-answer articles and nearly 70 high-interest articles on cancer, arteriosclerosis, heart disease,

etc. Complete with color illustrations and anatomical drawings. Includes index and cross-references.

ANESTHESIOLOGY AND GENERAL SURGERY

Clincal Surgery. Vols. 1–16. **Charles Rob and Rodney Smith, eds.** Philadelphia, PA: J. B. Lippincott, 1964–1970.

Encyclopedic approach. Each volume covers a specialized branch of surgery. Contributors include many of the most eminent surgeons of our time. Medical aspects with main essentials of diagnosis and treatment are stressed. Sample volumes include volume 13, *Orthopaedics,* 1968; volume 14, *Vascular Surgery and Reticulo-Endothelial Systems,* 1967; volume 15, *Gynaecology, Obstetrics,* 1968, and volume 16, *Neurosurgery,* 1970. An index volume is available (1970). Volumes 1–12 are out of print.

Principles of Anesthesiology. 2d ed. **Vincent J. Collins.** Philadelphia, PA: Lea & Febiger, 1976.

First edition, 1950.

Encyclopedic coverage of anesthesiology. Volume consists of four main sections. Section 1 records the history of anesthesia and discusses the theoretical basis of the use of drugs and techniques. Section 2 deals with the anatomical, physiological, and pharmacological aspects of regional analgesia. Section 3 outlines the physiology of the respiratory, circulatory, autonomic nervous systems, and functional kidney. Section 4, entitled "Pharmacological Considerations" discusses the liver. An American version of the application of SI units concludes the volume.
R: *Anaesthesia* 32: 395 (Apr. 1977).

INTERNAL MEDICINE

Biochemical Values in Clinical Medicine: The Results Following Pathological or Psychological Change. 5th ed. **R. D. Eastham.** Bristol, England: John Wright, 1975.

Condensed clinical chemistry encyclopedia. Includes new sections of polypeptide hormones, amniocentesis, autoimmune antibody tests. Handy pocket reference.
R: *ABL* 40: entry 285 (July 1975).

The Encyclopedia of Common Diseases. **Staff of Prevention Magazine.** Emmaus, PA: Rodale Press, 1976.

In 63 sections, covers major diseases of men, women, and children. Nontechnical approach to subject, emphasizes natural healing methods. Extensive discussions, well-referenced and indexed. Helpful for the lay person.
R: *ARBA* (1977, p. 711).

Pears Medical Encyclopedia, Illustrated. **J. A. C. Brown; rev. by A. M. Hastin Bennett.** London: Pelham, 1971.

American edition entitled *Stein and Day International Medical Encyclopedia,* 1972. An encyclopedia for laymen and allied health personnel. Cross-referenced, illustrated. Entries vary from brief to lengthy.
R: *MRW* S2, p. 65.

The Penguin Medical Encyclopedia. 2d ed. **Peter Wingate.** Baltimore, MD: Penguin Books, 1976.
First edition, 1972.
A paperback encyclopedia which consists of brief definitions and biographical sketches. Adequate for the paraprofessional and layman. An expensive reference tool for the home or public library.
R: *ARBA* (1973, p. 610; 1977, p. 713).

The Stein and Day International Medical Encyclopedia. **J. A. C. Brown; rev. by A. M. Hastin Bennett.** New York: Stein & Day, 1972.
Originally published in England under the title *Pears Medical Encyclopedia.* For both laymen and allied health professionals.
R: *ARBA* (1973, p. 608).

Vascular Disorders of the Extremities. 2d ed. **David I. Abramson.** New York: Harper & Row, 1974.
An encyclopedia of peripheral vascular disorders. Cross-referenced; recommended to the family physician, dermatologists, orthopedists. Contains a great deal of useful information.
R: *Archives of Surgery* 110: 353 (Mar. 1975); *JAMA* 231: 420 (Jan. 27, 1975).

NUTRITION

Encyclopedia of Food Science. **Martin S. Peterson and Arnold H. Johnson.** Westport, CT: Avi Publishing, 1978.

McGraw-Hill Encyclopedia of Food, Agriculture and Nutrition. **Daniel N. Lapedes, ed.** New York: McGraw-Hill, 1977.
Presents an overview of the world food problem. Contains 400 signed, alphabetically arranged articles, with cross-references. Includes tables of food composition. A handy, authoritative ready reference for general libraries.
R: *American Scientist* 66: 500 (July–Aug. 1978); *WLB* 52: 647 (Apr. 1978); Sheehy (EK32).

OPHTHALMOLOGY

System of Ophthalmology. Vols. 1–15. **Sir Stewart Duke-Elder and Peter A. MacFaul, eds.** St. Louis, MO: C. V. Mosby, 1958–1975.
Praised to be the definitive work and the most complete treatise on its subject. A unique and monumental encyclopedia for every ophthalmologist.
R: *American Journal of Ophthalmology* 79: 891 (May 1975); *British Journal of Ophthalmology* 60: 392 (May 1976); *Archives of Ophthalmology* 93: 1067 (Oct. 1975); Allyn.

PATHOLOGY

Encyclopedia of Microscopic Stains. **Eduard Gurr.** Baltimore, MD: Williams & Wilkins, 1960.
A guide to the materials used for staining microscopic tissue preparations, in-

cluding properties and applications. Alphabetical by name of dye, with relevant information.
R: *Nature* 188: 817 (Dec. 3, 1960); *Science* 132: 614 (1960): Chen (p. 51); Jenkins (G53); Mal (9-48); Wal (p. 204).

The Encyclopedia of Microscopy and Microtechnique. **Peter Gray, ed.** New York: Van Nostrand Reinhold, 1973.

An extensive reference providing information on the apparatus and technique of microscopic examination. Contains diagrams, photographs, tables. A useful reference source for biologists, mineralogists, chemists. Well-indexed.
R: *American Scientist* 62: 490 (July–Aug. 1974); *Microchemical Journal* 19: 219 (June 1974); *Quarterly Review of Biology* 50: 368 (1975); *Science* 184: 55 (Apr. 5, 1974); *TBRI* 40: 297 (Oct. 1974); *ARBA* (1974, p. 565); Chen (p. 51); Mal (9-47); *MRW* S3, p. 34.

PEDIATRICS

Child Health Encyclopedia: The Complete Guide for Parents. **The Boston Children's Medical Center and Richard I. Feinbloom.** New York: Delacorte Press, 1975.

Primary emphasis on childrens' diseases and conditions from infancy to adolescence.
R: Sheehy (EK15).

The Encyclopedia of Baby and Child Care. **Lendon H. Smith.** Englewood Cliffs, NJ: Prentice-Hall, 1972.

A comprehensive encyclopedia for all parents. Systematic presentation. Detailed index. For the lay person, a thorough, though not overly technical, encyclopedia.
R: *ARBA* (1973, p. 618).

Neonatal Emergencies and Other Problems. **John Black.** New York: Appleton-Century-Crofts, 1972.

A pocket-reference encyclopedia for pediatric emergencies.
R: *Clinical Pediatrics* 12: 17A (Apr. 1973).

The Parents' Encyclopedia of Infancy, Childhood, and Adolescence. **Milton I. Levine and Jean H. Seligmann.** Philadelphia, PA: Harper & Row, 1978.

Contains substantial contributions from prominent pediatricians and pediatric professors. Covers some 1,000 outstanding topics in the field. Appendixes provide useful directory information: poison control centers, community mental health and genetic counseling agencies. Extensive bibliography aimed at the beginner. No index, but adequate cross-references.
R: *LJ* 98: 2264 (Aug. 1973); *ARBA* (1974, p. 639).

PHARMACY AND PHARMACOLOGY

Encyclopedia of Antibiotics. 2d ed. **John S. Glasby, ed.** New York: John Wiley, 1979.

First edition, 1976.

An alphabetical arrangement of well over 1,000 antibiotics. Provides brief information concerning structure, chemical properties, clinical use, toxicity. An extensive reference for pharmacists, physicians, medical investigators.
R: *Archives of Internal Medicine* 137: 1262 (Sept. 1977); *Journal of the American Chemical Society* 99: 5840 (Aug. 17, 1977); *Lancet* 1: 784 (Apr. 9, 1977); *Nature* 265: vi (Feb. 3, 1977); *Unlisted Drugs* 31: 157 (Oct. 1979); *ARBA* (1978, p. 730).

Hypersensitivity to Drugs. 2 vols. **Max Samter and C. W. Parker, eds.** New York: Pergamon, 1972.

Section 75: *The International Encyclopedia of Pharmacology and Therapeutics.*
A two-volume encyclopedia which surveys current knowledge in pharmacology. Comprehensive, valuable to research workers, physicians.
R: *Brain* 97: 221 (Mar. 1974); *BMJ* 1: 55 (Jan. 6, 1973).

The International Encyclopedia of Pharmacology and Therapeutics. New York: Pergamon, 1973–.

A multivolume reference encyclopedia. Contains articles by authorities in their fields. For researchers in medicine and pharmacology.
R: *Annals of Internal Medicine* 78: 807 (1973); *Brain* 96: 210 (Jan. 1973); *JAMA* 229: 1925 (Sept. 30, 1974); *NEJM* 290: 61 (Jan. 3, 1974); *Pharmaceutical Journal* 212: 498 (1974).

Pharmaceutical Manufacturing Encyclopedia. **Marshall Sittig.** Park Ridge, NJ: Noyes Data, 1979.

Describes drug manufacturing processes. Arranged alphabetically by generic name.

Potter's New Cyclopaedia of Medicinal Herbs and Preparations. Reprint ed. **R. C. Wren.** New York: Harper & Row, 1972.

Original edition, *New Cyclopaedia of Botanical Drugs and Preparations,* 1907.
A classic work on medicinal herbs. This is an updated version of a work originally published in 1907. Contains valuable information on herbal compounds, glossary of botanical and medical terms. Indexed. Recommended to public libraries.
R: *ARBA* (1973, p. 618).

Psychedelics Encyclopedia. **Peter Stafford.** Berkeley, CA: And/Or Press, 1977.

Complete account of pyschedelic substances which are divided into eight groups (mushrooms, LSD, etc.). Lists botanical, pharmacological, physiological information. Both scholarly and scientific, well illustrated. Of contemporary and historical value.
R: *ARBA* (1978, p. 733).

Psychopharmacology: A Generation of Progress. **Morris A. Lipton, Alberto Di Mascio, and Keith F. Killam, eds.** New York: Raven Press, 1978.

An extensive one-volume encyclopedia of basic and clinical psychopharmacology. Covers ethics and strategy of administering psychotropic drugs; describes commonly dealt with syndromes. A thorough and comprehensive reference work;

recommended to all those involved with the study and use of psychotropic drugs.
R: *Lancet* 1: 1292 (June 17, 1978); *Nature* 274: 406 (July 27, 1978).

PHYSICAL MEDICINE AND REHABILITATION

Encyclopedia of Sport Sciences and Medicine. **Albert S. Hyman, Leonard A. Larson, and Donald E. Herrmann, eds.** New York: Macmillan, 1971.

Pulls together international literature relating to sports medicine; provides data on the changes that affect sports participants, covering a wide range of subjects such as intellect, disease, environment, rehabilitation. Contributions from over 500 authors. A well-written encyclopedia; indexed. Recommended for general and medical libraries.
R: *ARBA* (1972, p. 614).

The Physical Fitness Encyclopedia. **Charles T. Kuntzleman, Paul F. Eyanson, and Arne L. Olson, eds.** Emmaus, PA: Rodale Books, 1970.

Alphabetically arranged terms. Provides comprehensive coverage, detailed illustrations and tables. Shows how daily routines improve physical fitness.
R: *MRW* S2, pp. 50, 79.

PSYCHIATRY AND PSYCHOLOGY

A Concise Encyclopedia of Psychiatry. **Denis Leigh, C. M. B. Pare, and John Marks, eds.** Baltimore, MD: University Park Press, 1977.

Provides a concise summary of psychiatry. Includes biographical as well as conceptual information. Includes charts and diagrams.

Encyclopaedic Handbook of Medical Psychology. **Stephen Krauss.** London: Butterworths, 1976.

Contains over 200 articles written by psychiatrists, neurologists, and psychologists. Arranged alphabetically, covers a wide range of topics. Most useful to students of psychiatry and psychology, small libraries.
R: *BMJ* 1:1509 (Dec. 18, 1976).

Encyclopedia of Human Behavior: Psychology, Psychiatry, and Mental Health. 2 vols. **Robert M. Goldenson, ed.** Garden City, NY: Doubleday, 1970.

In two volumes, includes terms, theories, biographies, treatment techniques. Alphabetically arranged, cross-referenced.
R: Win (3EH7).

Encyclopedia of Mental Health. 6 vols. **Albert Deutsch, ed.** New York: Watts, 1963.

In six volumes, includes bibliography, index, and list of mental health agencies.

Encyclopedia of Psychoanalysis. **Ludwig Eidelberg, ed.** New York: Macmillan, 1968.

Highly specialized encyclopedia. Includes bibliographies, definitions, interpretations. For medical libraries.

R: *American Scientist* 57: 357A (Winter 1969); Win (2EH3).

Encyclopedia of Psychology. 3 vols. **Hans J. Eysenck and W. A. R. Meili, eds.** London: Search Press, 1972.

A three-volume, alphabetically arranged encyclopedia of terms and concepts in psychology. Articles vary in length, depending on subject, but are well-referenced. Authors from 22 different countries. A fundamental reference for all science and psychology libraries.
R: *Brain* 96: 207 (Jan. 1973); *Contemporary Psychology* 19: 279 (Apr. 1974); *Psychological Medicine* 3: 535 (Nov. 1973); *LJ* 97: 3889 (Nov. 1972); *MRW* S2, p. 83.

International Encyclopedia of Psychiatry, Psychology, Psychoanalysis, and Neurology. 12 vols. **Benjamin B. Wolman, ed.** New York: Van Nostrand Reinhold, 1977.

A twelve-volume encyclopedia with contributions from 1,500 international authorities. Articles are both biographical and conceptual in nature, and contain bibliographies. This is an extensive specialized work with clear and methodological format. It is recommended as a standard reference for its scientific approach and its thorough coverage of the study of the mind.
R: *American Journal of Psychiatry* 135: 1443 (Nov. 1978); *BL* 75: 318 (Oct. 1978); *LJ* 102: 2049 (Oct. 1977).

Reference Encyclopedia of American Psychology and Psychiatry. **Barry T. Klein, ed.** Rye, NY: Todd Publications, 1975.

A thorough compilation of associations, research centers, periodicals, audiovisual aids, hospitals appropriate to psychologists and psychiatrists. Alphabetically arranged sections. A useful directory-encyclopedia recommended for college, medical, and public libraries.
R: *RSR* 4: 45 (Jan.–Mar. 1976).

PUBLIC HEALTH

Encyclopaedia of Occupational Health and Safety. 2d ed. 2 vols. **International Labour Office.** New York: McGraw-Hill, 1972.

First edition, 1934.
Two-volume encyclopedia which is a major reference source on all aspects of occupational safety and health. Material is taken from international standards. New edition emphasizes industrial medicine. Includes helpful appendixes and bibliographies, comprehensive analytic index.
R: *BL* 70: 161 (1974); *IBID* 1: 198 (Sept. 1973); *MRW* S2, p. 57; Allyn.

Occupational Health and Safety. 2 vols. **International Labour Office.** Washington, D.C.: International Labour Office, 1972.

Contains 900 articles which deal with the health and safety of people at work. International contributions cover occupations, industrial processes, chemical hazards, statistics. A worthwhile reference for medical libraries.
R: *Lancet* 1: 752 (Apr. 7, 1973).

RADIOLOGY

Encyclopedia of Medical Radiology. Handbuch der Medizinischen Radiologie. **O. Olsson et al., eds.** New York: Springer-Verlag, 1963–.

Volume 1 (2 parts), *Physical Principles and Techniques*; volume 2 (3 parts), *Radiation Biology*; volume 4 (2 parts), *Anatomy of the Skeletal System*; volume 5, *Diseases of the Skeletal System*, 1973; volume 6 (3 parts), *Roentgen Diagnosis of the Vertebral Column*; volume 7 (2 parts), *Skull*; volume 8, *Roentgen Diagnosis of the Soft Tissue*; volume 9 (multiple parts) on respiratory tract; volume 10 (6 parts), *Roentgen Diagnosis of the Heart and Blood Vessels* (volume 10/2a, 1977); volume 11/1, *Digestive Tract*; volume 11/2, *Digestive Tract and Abdomen*; volume 12/1, *Roentgen Diagnosis of the Liver and Biliary System*; volume 12/2, *Roentgen Diagnosis of the Pancreas & Spleen*; volume 13/1, *Roentgen Diagnosis of the Urogenital System*; volume 14/2, *Roentgen Diagnosis of the Central Nervous System*; volume 15/2, *Nuclear Medicine—Diagnosis, Therapy, Clinical Research*; volume 16 (2 parts), *Methods and Procedures of Radiation Therapy*; volume 17, *Radiation Therapy of Benign Diseases*; volumes 18–19, *Radiation Therapy of Malignant Tumors*.

A multivolume series, each volume devoted to a specific aspect of radiology in medicine. The series contains comprehensive references and high-quality illustrations; in-depth coverage of each specific topic, written in German with English-German vocabulary lists provided. Highly recommended.

R: *American Heart Journal* 91: 407 (1976); *Archives of Surgery* 108: 252 (Feb. 1974); 108: 255 (Feb. 1974); *British Journal of Radiology* 52: 152 (1979); *Quarterly Review of Biology* 49: 281 (1975).

RESPIRATORY SYSTEM

Bronchial Asthma: Mechanisms and Therapeutics. **Earle B. Weiss and Maurice S. Segal, eds.** Boston, MA: Little, Brown, 1976.

Summarizes the history, epidemiology, genetics, pharmacology, and immunology of bronchial asthma. Discusses newer therapies. Extensively referenced and indexed. An asthma encyclopedia of merit. Recommended to practitioners and investigators.

R: *Canadian Medical Association Journal* 117: 1011 (Nov. 5, 1977); *NEJM* 296: 1303 (1977).

UROGENITAL SYSTEM

Encyclopaedia of Urology. 15 vols. New York: Springer-Verlag, 1959–1977.

A multivolume encyclopedia for urologists. Articles written by authorities in their respective field. Well illustrated and well referenced.

R: *Lancet* 1: 339 (Feb. 4, 1970).

VETERINARY MEDICINE

Animal Cytology and Evolution. 3d ed. **M. J. D. White.** New York: Cambridge University Press, 1973.

An up-to-date review of major issues in evolution and cytology. Gives basic chromosomal information for over 1,500 animal species, answers common questions. Useful to human geneticists and evolutionists.

R: *American Journal of Human Genetics* 26: 531 (July 1974).

Dog Owner's Encyclopedia of Veterinary Medicine. **Allan H. Hart.** Hong Kong: T. F. H. Publications; distr. New York: Crown, 1971.

An encyclopedia of canine diseases, grouped topically rather than alphabetically. Covers a wide range of topics, includes photos and line drawings. A helpful book for dog owners.
R: *ARBA* (1972, p. 634).

Encyclopedia of Animal Care. 12th ed. **Geoffry P. West, ed.** Baltimore, MD: Williams and Wilkins, 1977.

Ninth edition, 1971.
Modeled after *Blacks Veterinary Dictionary*, a continually revised encyclopedia of veterinary science. Covers all major topics, cross-referenced. Includes drawings, photographs. For medical and public libraries.
R: *ARBA* (1973, p. 624; 1974, p. 645); *MRW* S3, p. 54; Win (EK232).

Grzimek's Animal Life Encyclopedia. 13 vols. **Bernhard Grzimek.** New York: Van Nostrand Reinhold, 1972–1975.

Earlier edition in German, 1967.
The set is arranged by animal groups, with the material in each volume arranged by animal orders and families. Includes a systematic classification index and multilingual glossary.
R: *American Scientist* 61: 486–487 (July/Aug. 1973); 62: 484 (July/Aug. 1974); *Science* 177: 1184 (Sept. 29, 1972); *ARBA* (1976, p. 675; 1975, p. 689; 1973, p. 569); Chen (p. 54); Mal (9-167).

Livestock Health Encyclopedia. 3d ed. **Rudolph Seidon.** W. James Gough, ed. New York: Springer-Verlag, 1968.

A nonspecialist's compendium of information on disease and parasite control in farm livestock.
R: Chen (p. 54).

CHAPTER 5   DICTIONARIES

ABBREVIATIONS AND ACRONYMS

Abbreviations Dictionary. 4th ed. **Ralph DeSola.** New York: American Elsevier, 1974.

Full identification of acronyms, initials, abbreviations, symbols, etc. Myriad features such as weather symbols, atomic numbers, astronomical constellations, etc.
R: *LJ* 93: 535 (1968); Chen (p. 64); Jenkins (A58); Mal (3-28).

Acronym Handbook. **Donald D. Spencer.** Englewood Cliffs, NJ: Prentice-Hall, 1974.

An alphabetical list of over 4,500 acronyms and abbreviations, with definitions. Poorly received because of inconsistencies in arrangement.
R: *ARBA* (1975, p. 792); Chen (p. 64).

Acronyms, Initialisms, & Abbreviations Dictionary. 6th ed. 3 vols. **Ellen T. Crowley, ed.** Detroit, MI: Gale Research, 1978–.

Volume 1, *Acronyms, Initialisms, and Abbreviations Dictionary,* 1978; volume 2, *New Acronyms, Initialisms, and Abbreviations,* 1979 and 1980 annual supplement to volume 1; volume 3, *Reverse Acronyms, Initialisms, and Abbreviations Dictionary,* 1978. First edition, 1960.
Lists over 178,000 entries altogether (with 48,000 new entries in this edition). Major areas of expansion include periodical titles, chemical and medical terms, etc. An essential reference tool.
R: *Data Processing Digest* (Nov. 1976); *Engineering Societies Library* (Dec. 1976); *Military Review* (Jan. 1977); *Society of Motion Picture and Television Engineers* (May 1977); *BL* (Feb. 15, 1977); *ARBA* (1977); Chen (p. 64).

British Initials and Abbreviations. 3d ed. **I. H. Wilkes.** London: Hill, 1971.

Concise Dictionary of Soviet Terminology, Institutions, and Abbreviations. **Barry Crowe.** New York: Pergamon Press, 1969.
R: *ARBA* (1970, p. 101); Chen (p. 64).

Internationales Woerterbuch der Abkuerzungen von Organisationen Pt. 1: A–H. International Dictionary of Abbreviations of Organizations. **P. Spillner.** Muenchen-Pullach, Germany: Dokumentation, 1970.

Subject

Abbreviations and Acronyms in Medicine and Nursing. **Solomon Garb, Eleanor Krakauer, and Carson Justice.** New York: Springer Publishing, 1976.

An up-to-date compilation of medical abbreviations and acronyms. Includes 400 terms, with brief explanations, Greek and Roman abbreviations. A convenient ready-reference for libraries.
R: *BMLA* 64: 339 (July 1976); *Choice* 13: 646 (July–Aug. 1976); *ARBA* (1977, p. 712).

Abbreviations in Medicine. 2d ed. **Albrecht Schertel.** Basel: S. Karger, 1977.

Abbreviations in Medicine. 4th ed. **Edwin B. Steen.** New York: Macmillan, 1978.
Previous editions have title *Dictionary of Abbreviations in Medicine and the Related Sciences.*
The new edition contains over 13,000 abbreviations in common use in medicine and the related sciences.

Diagnostic and Statistical Manual of Mental Disorders, DSM-III. 3d ed. **American Psychiatric Association.** Washington, DC: American Psychiatric Association, 1978.
Completely revised edition of psychiatric nomenclature.

Dictionary of Abbreviations in Medicine and the Health Sciences. **Harold K. Hughes.** Lexington, MA: Lexington Books, 1977.
Considered a highly useful collection of abbreviations used in every field of the health sciences. There are more than 12,000 entries which include varying definitions as they apply to each field. Contains a handy guide to construction and use. A valuable tool for health and allied professionals.
R: *Modern Healthcare* 7: 67 (June 1977); *Physics in Medicine & Biology* 22: 1215 (Nov. 1977); *ARBA* (1978, p. 711); Sheehy (EK12).

Medical Abbreviations. 3d ed. **Edwin B. Steen.** Philadelphia, PA: F. A. Davis, 1971.
Alphabetical arrangement of nearly 4,600 medical abbreviations. Includes abbreviations for societies, organizations, government agencies, and over 200 journal titles. No critical evaluation of terms.
R: *ARBA* (1972, p. 627); *MRW* S2, p. 64.

Medical Abbreviations: A Cross Reference Dictionary. 2d ed. **Special Studies Committee of the Michigan Occupational Therapy Association.** Ann Arbor, MI: Michigan Occupational Therapy Association, 1967.
First edition, 1961.
Lists abbreviations from all areas of medicine and allied health fields. Part 1 gives abbreviation and full meaning; part 2 indicates the full form followed by the accepted abbreviation.
R: Win (EK88).

Medical Abbreviations and Acronyms. **Peter Roody, Robert E. Forman, and Howard B. Schweitzer.** New York: McGraw-Hill, 1976.
A compilation of abbreviations and acronyms used in medicine and related health fields (e.g. dentistry, audiology, psychology). Indexes 14,000 terms in an alphabetical manner with corresponding definitions. Cross-referenced; heavy emphasis on American terminology. One glaring weakness is the lack of a section listing full terms followed by the corresponding shortened form. A "must" for every core reference collection in hospitals, medical laboratories, pharmaceutical

companies, government health agencies, and nursing, dental, and medical schools.
R: *Annals of Internal Medicine* 88: 139 (Jan. 1978); *Choice* 14: 834 (Sept. 1977); *ARBA* (1978, p. 719); Sheehy (EK13).

Medical Hieroglyphs: Abbreviations and Symbols. **Avice Kerr.** Chicago, IL: Clissold, 1970.

Over 8,400 abbreviations and 300 symbols of official and unofficial designation. Abbreviations and symbols extracted from medical records.
R: *MRW* S2, pp. 1; 64; 101.

THESAURI AND NOMENCLATURES

GENERAL

Biological Nomenclature. 2d ed. **Charles Jeffrey.** New York: Crane Russak, 1977.

International codes of biological, zoological, and bacterial nomenclature. Includes glossary, index, and bibliography. Informative and easy to use.
R: *Annals of Human Genetics* 43: 83 (July 1979).

Biomedical Thesaurus and Guide to Classification. **Michael S. Koch.** New York: CCM Information, 1972.

A compilation of medical terms from the National Library of Medicine, the Library of Congress, and Medical Subject Heading List. Thesaurus includes 5,000 headings and cross-references; emphasizes clinical terms; works as a guide to classification schemes. Recommended to all types of libraries.
R: *Bibliography, Documentation, Terminology* 13: 181 (May 1973); *ARBA* (1974, p. 627); *MRW* S3, pp. 8, 32, 51.

Handbook of Chemical Synonyms and Trade Names. 8th ed. **William Gardner, Edward I. Cooke, and Richard W. I. Cooke.** Cleveland, OH: Chemical Rubber Company Press, 1978.
R: *ABL* 33: entry 334 (July 1968); *Choice* 8: 1317 (Dec. 1971); *ARBA* (1973, p. 543); Chen (p. 83); Jenkins (D73); Mal (11-89); Wal (p. 472); Win (ED33).

Medical and Health Related Sciences Thesaurus, Public Health Service Pub. no. 1031. 2d ed. **Research Documentation Section, US National Institutes of Health.** Washington, DC: US Government Printing Office, 1969.

Entries compiled and maintained as indexing authority list for research grants index. Contains 9,200 terms, alphabetically arranged. Includes cross-references and notations under terms.
R: *MRW* S2, pp. 64, 100.

Roget's International Thesaurus. 4th ed. **Peter M. Roget.** Scranton, PA: Thomas Y. Crowell, 1977.

Third edition, 1962.
Comprehensive source of synonyms and antonyms in American and British usage.

Subject

American Medical Ethnobotany: A Reference Dictionary. **Daniel E. Moerman.** New York: Garland Publishing, 1977.

Over 3,500 entries arranged according to standardized contemporary botanical nomenclature. Lists plants with medical properties; includes full bibliographical citation for each entry.

Anatomical Dictionary With Nomenclatures and Explanatory Notes. **Tibor Donath. English ed. edited by G. N. C. Crawford.** New York: Pergamon, 1970.

English translation of a classic Hungarian dictionary. Presents terms both systematically and alphabetically in two separate sections. Contains complete etymology; current internationally-accepted nomenclature.
R: *Lancet* 1: 756 (Apr. 11, 1970); *MRW* S2, p. 6.

CIS Thesaurus. **Occupational Safety and Health Information Centre.** Washington, DC: International Labour Office, 1976.

French-English dictionary of more than 10,000 terms relating to occupational safety and health. Includes systematic and alphabetical sections. Also published under title *Thesaurus CIS*.
R: *IBID* 5: 355 (Dec. 1977).

Classification and Nomenclature of Viruses: 2nd Report of the International Committee on Taxonomy of Viruses. **F. Fenner, ed.** Basel: S. Karger, 1976.

Updates work of International Committee on Taxonomy of Viruses. Describes in detail the properties of each virus group and their classification into families, genera, and species. Published as issue 1-2 of the journal *Intervirology*.

CTFA Cosmetic Ingredient Dictionary. **Norman F. Estrin, ed.** Washington, DC: The Cosmetic, Toiletry, and Fragrance Association, 1973.

Compiles pertinent data on substances frequently used in the cosmetic industry. Attempts to standardize cosmetic ingredient nomenclature. Monograph format lists adopted names, synonyms, CAS registry numbers, structural formulas, and reference sources. Complete reference source for cosmetic industry and consumer.
R: *Journal of Pharmaceutical Sciences* 63: 477 (Mar. 1974).

Diseases of the Heart and Blood Vessels; Nomenclature and Criteria for Diagnosis. 7th ed. **New York Heart Association.** Boston, MA: Little, Brown, 1973.
Sixth edition, 1964.

Fertility Modification Thesaurus with Focus on Evaluation of Family Planning Programs. **Kathryn H. Speert and Samuel M. Wishik.** New York: International Institute for the Study of Human Reproduction, Columbia University, 1973.

Thesaurus focuses on terms relating to family planning program development and evaluation. Follows the MeSH tree structure. Nearly 2,000 items divided into

four neat sections. Includes three appendixes: descriptors, categories, and hierarchy. Limited application; intended primarily as an indexing tool.
R: *ARBA* (1974, p. 629); *MRW* S3, pp. 24, 51.

Food: Multilingual Thesaurus. 4 vols. New York: K. G. Saur, 1978.

In four volumes, an English, German, French, and Italian index to controlled vocabulary for information on food. Complies to UNISIST/ISO guidelines.

Illustrated Tumor Nomenclature. 2d rev. ed. **H. Hamperl, ed.** International Union Against Cancer. New York: Springer-Verlag, 1969.

Lists 270 accepted terms in English, French, Spanish, German, and Russian, describing common neoplasms. Black and white illustrations complement terminology. Terms and illustrations arranged by histological section.
R: *MRW* S2, p. 70.

International Code of Nomenclature of Bacteria: Bacteriological Code. **S. P. Lapage et al., eds.** Washington, DC: American Society for Microbiology, 1975.

Approved code of the First Congress for Bacteriology, 1973.
Detailed description of "principles," "rules," and "recommendations." All taxa listed in Latin. Intended as a standard for bacteriological nomenclature.
R: *Journal of Clinical Pathology* 30: 393 (1977).

Nomenclature and Criteria for Diagnosis of Diseases of the Heart and Great Vessels. 7th ed. **New York Heart Association Criteria Committee.** Boston, MA: Little, Brown, 1973.

First edition, 1928; sixth edition, 1964.
Emphasis on definitions and descriptions of cardiovascular symptoms. Arranged under five sections: etiology, anatomy, physiology, cardiac status and prognosis, and uncertain diagnosis. Concludes with miscellaneous appendixes and subject index.
R: *MRW* S3, p. 8; Allyn.

Nomenclature Dermatologica. **F. E. Rabello.** Rio de Janeiro: Impressora Brasileira, 1974.

Attempts to establish a uniform, universal nomenclature in dermatology. Geared toward those involved in dermatology.
R: *International Journal of Dermatology* 14: 229 (Apr. 1975).

Veterinary Multilingual Thesaurus. 4 vols. **Commission of the European Communities, Directorate-General for Research, Science and Education.** New York: K. G. Saur, 1979.

In four languages: English, German, Italian, and French. Provides controlled veterinary vocabulary designed for indexing and retrieving bibliographical references in documentation systems. Indexed. Complies to UNISIST/ISO guidelines.

Visual Science Information Center Thesaurus. Berkeley, CA: Visual Science Information Center, University of California, 1971–. Annual.

Essentially the authority list for subject terms appearing in the *Vision Index*. Re-

flects terminology in the current literature on vision. Includes alphabetical permuted section.
R: *MRW* S3, pp. 51, 54.

DRUG NAMES

American Pharmaceutical Association Drug Names. 2d ed. **American Pharmaceutical Association.** Washington, DC: American Pharmaceutical Association, 1979.

Continues *Proprietary Names of Official Drugs,* 3d ed., 1965.
Alphabetical listing of drug names. A cross-reference to proprietary and nonproprietary drugs, best used in conjunction with the *National Formulary* and the *United States Pharmacopoeia.*

Nonproprietary Names for Pharmaceutical Substances, WHO Technical Report Series no. 581. Geneva: World Health Organization, 1975.

Report reviews general principles of name selection for pharmaceutical substances. Discusses some of the relevant literature; provides helpful illustrations.
R: *JAMA* 236: 2449 (Nov. 22, 1976); *RSR* 4: 107 (July–Sept., 1976).

Trademarks Listed with the Pharmaceutical Manufacturers Association. Rev. ed. **Pharmaceutical Manufacturers Association.** Washington, DC: Pharmaceutical Manufacturers Association, 1974.

USAN and the USP Dictionary of Drug Names. 1st ed.–. Rockville, MD: United States Pharmacopoeial Convention, 1963–. Annual.

Eighteenth edition, 1980.
The new edition is a continuation of *United States Adopted Names* and its cumulations, with each edition replacing the previous edition. Lists USAN (US Adopted Names), USP and NF official names, FDA approved names, brand names, abbreviations, and trivial names of drugs, including over 12,000 entries.
R: *Journal of Pharmaceutical Sciences* 62: 177 (Jan. 1973); 63: 311 (Feb. 1974); 64: 180 (Jan. 1975); 65: 1268 (Aug. 1976); 67: 144 (Jan. 1978); *JAMA* 230: 907 (Nov. 11, 1974); 235: 2542 (June 7, 1976); *Pharmaceutical Journal* 219: 181 (1977).

MULTILINGUAL

BIBLIOGRAPHIES

Bibliography of Interlingual Scientific and Technical Dictionaries. 5th ed. Paris: Unesco, 1969.

Fourth edition, 1961.
Approximately 2,500 entiries.
R: *NTB* 56: 4 (1971); Chen (p. 68); Wal (p. 20); Win (EA96; 1EA14; 3EA15).

A Bibliography of Scientific, Technical and Specialized Dictionaries, Polyglot, Bilingual, Unilingual. **C. W. Rechenbach and E. R. Garnett.** Washington, DC: Catholic University Press, 1969.

Includes 1,257 titles classified by subject. Entries do not include annotations.

Should be used in conjunction with *Unesco's Bibliography of Interlingual Scientific and Technical Dictionaries,* 1969.
R: *LJ* 95: 4244 (1970); *ARBA* (1971, p. 471); Chen (p. 68); Mal (3-24); Wal (p. 19); Win (3EA14).

Dictionaries of English and Foreign Languages: A Bibliographical Guide to Both General and Technical Dictionaries with Historical and Explanatory Notes and References. Rev. and enl. **Robert L. Collison.** New York: Hafner, 1971.
R: Chen (p. 69); Mal (3-26).

ENGLISH-FRENCH

Dictionnaire Médical. **André Duranteau.** Paris: Seuil, 1971.
A French medical dictionary which includes over 1,500 terms. Intended for the layman. Includes illustrations. Indexed.
R: *MRW* S3, p. 15.

English-French French-English Dictionary of Medical and Biological Terms. 2d ed. **P. Lepine and P. R. Peacock.** Paris: Flammarion, 1975.
Technically oriented medical terminology. Contains information on eponyms. Helpful when used in conjunction with a standard French or English dictionary.
R: *BMJ* 4: 174 (Oct. 18, 1975).

French-English Dictionary of Physical Medicine and Rehabilitation. **H. & G. Kamenetz.** Paris: Librairie Maloine, 1972.
Concise edition which will be helpful to students and instructors of physical therapy who use English-French language.
R: *Archives of Physical Medicine & Rehabilitation* 58: 187 (Apr. 1977).

Vocabulary of Medicine and Related Sciences Principally Containing Terms Not Found in Bilingual and Multilingual Dictionaries, and Terms that May Present Special Problems of Translation: English-French, French-English. 2d ed. **William J. Gladstone.** New York: New York Press, 1970.
Emphasis on medical jargon and words not covered in standard bilingual or multilingual dictionary. Abbreviations listed.
R: *MRW* S2, p. 30.

ENGLISH-GERMAN

Dental-Wörterbuch. Dictionary of Dental Practice. **Herbert Bucksch.** München, Germany: Verlag Neuer Merker, 1970.
A bilingual dictionary for English- and German-speaking dentists. Includes equivalent terms and definitions but no pronunciation.
R: *MRW* S3, p. 14.

Medical Dictionary of the English and German Languages. 6th rev. ed. **Dieter W. Unseld.** Stuttgart: Wissenschaftliche Verlagsgesellschaft, 1971.
Contains 20,000 entries with no definitions or derivatives. Includes useful appendix of measures, weights, and temperatures. Intended audience: practicing and

research physicians, dentists, psychologists, pharmacists, chemists, physicists, and veterinarians.
R: *MRW* S2, p. 30.

Wörterbuch der Medizin. **Maxim Zetkin.** Berlin: Verlag Volk und Gesundheit, 1973.
East German publication. Reflects the present state of medical terminology. Includes expanding fields of nuclear medicine, biochemistry, and cybernetics. Entries consist of word and origin, gender, number, and part of speech. Lists additional biographical entries and eponyms.
R: *MRW* S3, p. 89.

Wörterbuch der Neurophysiologie. **Dietrich Burkhardt and Ingrid de la Motte.** Jena: G. Fischer, 1969.
German neurophysiology dictionary. Consists of 1,239 words and definitions. Entry includes English and Russian equivalents. Features diagrams, bibliography, and English and Russian indexes.
R: *MRW* S2, pp. 31, 71.

Wörterbuch der Psychiatrie und Medizinischen Psychologie. **Uwe H. Peters.** Munich: Urban & Schwarzenberg, 1971.
German psychiatry and psychology dictionary. Features 6,000 terms along with a definition and French and English equivalents of the term. Incorporates English-German and French-German glossaries in volume.
R: *MRW* S2, pp. 82, 84.

ENGLISH-HEBREW

New Medical Dictionary. **Joseph Even-Odem and Yaacov Rotem.** Jerusalem, Israel: Rubin Mass, 1967.
English-Hebrew medical dictionary.
R: *MRW* S1, p. 4.

ENGLISH-JAPANESE

Ika, Shika, Waei Hatsuon Bunrei Jiten: Japanese-English Medical-Dental Dictionary. **Ryutaro Yamauchi.** Tokyo: Perikan, 1965.
Medical and dental dictionary in Japanese and English. Has phonetic signs and practical usage guide.
R: *MRW* S1, p. 4.

ENGLISH-RUSSIAN

Klinik Terminler Lugeti (Ruscha-Latyncha-Azerbaichancha). **Akademiia nauk Azerbaidzhanskoi SSR. Terminologicheskii komitet.** Baky: Elm, 1970.
Over 9,000 alphabetically arranged Russian terms with Latin equivalents. Also includes Azerbaijani equivalents.
R: *MRW* S2, p. 29.

Russian-English Medical Dictionary. **U. B. Eliseenkov et al.** Moscow: Russian Language Publishers, 1975.

Lists 50,000 terms covering all areas of medical and allied sciences. A one-way dictionary (Russian-English) written primarily for Russian speakers and those who have access to Russian medical literature but do not speak the language.
R: *Lancet* 1: 286 (Feb. 7, 1976).

Russian-English Translators Dictionary: A Guide to Scientific and Technical Usage. **Mikhail G. Zimmerman.** New York: Plenum, 1967.

Alphabetical listing of common word combinations and expressions frequently encountered in scientific and technical sources.
R: *MRW* S1, p. 30.

Russian-English Veterinary Dictionary. **Roy Mack.** Farnham Royal, Slough, England: Commonwealth Agricultural Bureaux, 1972.

Covers 6,000 terms on veterinary and relevant biological sciences. Includes names of diseases, pathogens, drugs, and poisons. Entries consist of Russian entry followed by English equivalent. Includes abbreviations and acronyms. No pronunciation given.
R: *ABL* 38: entry 81 (Feb. 1973); *MRW* S3, p. 54.

Slovar-minimum Po Angliiskomu Iazyku Dlia Studentov Meditsinskikh Vuzov. **Alevtina M. Maslova and Zinaida I. Vainshtein.** Moskva: Vysshaia shkola, 1969.

Contains 1,200 English medical terms alphabetically arranged with their Russian equivalents. Provides a list of suffixes and abbreviations. No definitions.
R: *MRW* S2, p. 31.

English-Spanish

Communicating in Spanish for Medical Personnel. **Julia J. Tabery, Marion R. Webb, and Beatriz V. Mueller.** Boston, MA: Little, Brown, 1975.

R: *Annals of Internal Medicine* 85: 556 (Oct. 1976).

Southwestern Medical Dictionary: Spanish/English, English/Spanish. **Margarita A. Kay et al.** Tucson, AZ: University of Arizona Press, 1977.

Described as a bilingual, technical, regional, and colloquial dictionary. Lists about 1,200 English terms and over 1,300 Spanish terms. Words or phrase incorporated into sentence to indicate usage. Sample sentence translated into English. Includes three appendixes: food items, kinship terms, and other sources of Spanish medical terminology. Highly recommended to those involved with health care of Spanish-speaking patients.
R: *ARBA* (1978, p. 711).

More than Two Languages

Dictionary of Bacteriological Equivalents: French-English, German-English, Italian-English, Spanish-English. **W. Partridge.** London: Bailliere Tindall, 1927.

Elsevier's Dictionary of Pharmaceutical Science and Techniques in Five Languages: English, French, Italian, Spanish, German. 2 vols. **A. Sliosberg, comp.** New York: American Elsevier, 1968.

Volume 1, *Pharmaceutical Technology.*
Lists some 10,000 terms. Applicable to both pharmacy proper and the pharmaceutical industry. Useful reference tool for pharmacists, chemists, and technologists.
R: *American Scientist* 57: 64A (Spring 1969); *MRW* S1, p. 23.

Elsevier's Dictionary of Public Health: In Six Languages, English-French-Spanish-Italian-Dutch and German. **Nic J. I. Deblock.** New York: Elsevier Scientific, 1976.

Provides translations of public health words and phrases in six basic European languages. Initial section lists all terms alphabetically under English format with translations in five languages. Following is an index for each of other five languages. Very useful for all health-related libraries.
R: *Bibliography, Documentation, Terminology* 16: 329 (Nov.–Dec. 1976); *ARBA* (1978, p. 710).

Elsevier's Medical Dictionary in Five Languages. 2d ed. **A. Sliosberg, comp.** Amsterdam, Holland: Elsevier, 1975.

About 20,000 medical, biological, pharmacological, and anatomical terms arranged alphabetically. English word is followed horizontally by French, Italian, Spanish and German equivalents. Second edition includes 2,500 more terms than the first. Text has thumb-indexing.
R: *Lancet* 1: 1226 (May 31, 1975); *Pharmaceutical Journal* 215: 563 (Nov. 19, 1975); *RSR* 4: 48 (Jan.–Mar. 1976); *TBRI* 42: 67 (Feb. 1976).

Glossary of Genetics in English, French, Spanish, Italian, German, Russian. **Francoise Biass-Ducroux, comp.** Amsterdam: Elsevier, 1970.

Features nearly 3,000 genetic terms in English with equivalents in French, Spanish, German, Italian, and Russian. Includes various spellings and synonyms. Concludes with indexes in each language.
R: *Lancet* 2: 1118 (Nov. 28, 1970); Chen (p. 75); Mal (9-20); *MRW* S2, p. 49; Wal (p. 197).

Lexicon Medicum: Anglicum, Russicum, Gallicum, Germanicum, Latinum, Polonum. Warszawa: Panstwowy Zaklad Wydawnictw Lekarskich, 1971.

Approximately 20,000 terms arranged alphabetically in English with Russian, French, German, Latin, and Polish equivalent terms in parallel columns. Includes indexes.
R: Win (EK86).

A Lexicon of English Dental Terms With Their Equivalents in Espanol, Deutsch, Francais, Italiano. **International Dental Federation.** The Hague, Netherlands: Sijthoff, 1966.

Dental terms in English listed alphabetically, followed by their equivalents in Spanish, German, French, and Italian. Includes index.
R: Win (EK148).

Medical Dictionary: Medizinisches Wörterbuch: Dictionnaire Medical. 5th ed. **Emanuel Veillon, ed. Revised and enlarged by Albert Nobel.** New York: Springer-Verlag, 1969.

First edition, 1950; fourth edition, 1964.
Three-language medical dictionary consisting of over 40,000 numbered terms. Main body is English vocabulary with German and French terms running parallel. A German and French index refers back to the English entries. No definitions included. A Spanish supplement accompanies the fifth edition of the Veillon/Nobel dictionary. Recommended to medical libraries.
R: *Choice* 7: 530 (June 1970); *ARBA* (1970, p. 133; 1971, p. 533; 1972, p. 616); *MRW* S2, pp. 30, 31; Win (EK87).

Multilingual Medical Dictionary: Lexicon Medicum Polyglottum. Enlarged and rewritten ed. **Aleksandar D. Kostic.** Belgrade, Yugoslavia: Medicinska knjiga, 1971.

Includes 125,000 entries in seven languages: Latin, English, French, Italian, German, Russian, and Serbo-Croatian. An etymological description and brief definition accompanies each term. Includes an eponymous dictionary.
R: *MRW* S3, pp. 14, 16.

Polyglot Medical Questionnaire in Twenty-Seven Languages with Digital System of Communication. 2d ed. **Shedden C. Parry.** London: Heinemann Medical, 1972.

First edition, 1953.
Lists 193 common questions and answers, each bearing the same numerical identification through all 27 languages. Helpful for physician and patient encountering a language barrier.
R: *MRW* S2, pp. 29, 32.

Steinbichler's Lexikon für die Apothekenpraxis in Sieben Sprachen. **Eveline Steinbichler.** Frankfurt/Main, Germany: Govi-Verlag G.M.B.H.-Pharmazeutischer Verlag, 1963.

Multilingual listing of pharmaceutical terms in French, Spanish, English, German, Italian, Greek, and Russian. No corresponding definitions.
R: Win (EK193).

SPELLING DICTIONARIES

Analyzer of Medical-Biological Words. **Jacob E. Schmidt.** Springfield, IL: Charles C. Thomas, 1973.

Over 1,000 medical and biological words with clarifying dissection. Includes Greek or Latin origin. Helpful to medical students, paramedics.
R: *ARBA* (1974, p. 628); *MRW* S3, pp. 7, 37.

How to Divide Medical Words: Over Twenty-Five Thousand Words in Common Usage Showing Their Spellings and Combinations into Syllables. **Richard V. Lee and Doris J. Hofer.** Carbondale, IL: Southern Illinois University Press, 1972.

Two sections: "Drugs and Medication" and "Medical Terms." Handy reference tool for the medical secretary and technical publisher.
R: *Journal of Pharmaceutical Sciences* 62: 1909 (Nov. 1973); *ARBA* (1974, p. 627).

Instant Spelling Medical Dictionary. **Donald O. Bolander, comp.** Wandelein, IL: Career Institute, 1970.
Spelling aid provides handy list of 20,000 of the most commonly used medical, biological, and pharmaceutical words. Includes spelling, word division, and accent but no definitions.
R: *ARBA* (1971, p. 533).

Medical Secretary Medi-Speller: A Transcription Aid. **Harriette L. Carlin.** Springfield, IL: Charles C. Thomas, 1973.
Designed as a spelling book. Includes few definitions. Arrangement of entries by main areas of transcription. Sections arranged as follows: general terminology, anatomy, surgical pathology, radiology, disease/syndromes, surgical procedures, instruments, clinical pathology, and commonly misspelled English words. Geared toward medical secretaries.
R: *ARBA* (1974, p. 626).

The Medical Word Book: A Spelling and Vocabulary Guide to Medical Transcription. **Sheila B. Sloane.** Philadelphia, PA: W. B. Saunders, 1973.
Alphabetically lists medical terms in nineteen convenient sections. Five sections are general and fourteen are specialty or organ systems. Accurately spells and organizes entries; no definitions given. Provides cross references from phonetic to correct spelling. The initial section, "Anatomy," begins with a series of eighteen color plates of anatomical structures. Most useful section entitled "Abbreviations and Symbols." Compiled especially for those engaged in medical transcription.
R: *ARBA* (1974, p. 628); *MRW* S3, p. 37.

Webster's Medical Speller. **Merriam Webster Editorial Staff, eds.** Springfield, MA: G. & C. Merriam, 1975.
Handy reference tool of 35,000 medical and technical terms alphabetically arranged. Emphasis on broad areas of medicine including pharmacology, biochemistry and microbiology. Indicates syllabication, hyphenation in compound words, and common plurals. Features Latin abbreviations used in prescription writing, along with their full Latin forms and English equivalents; 1,500 medical abbreviations and a list of medical symbols. Geared toward all health care professionals.
R: *Journal of Pharmaceutical Sciences* 65: 1268 (Aug. 1976).

SUBJECT DICTIONARIES

GENERAL

Bioscientific Terminology: Words from Latin and Greek Stems. **Donald M. Ayers.** Tucson, AZ: University of Arizona Press, 1972.
More a treatise than a dictionary on the use of these languages in scientific terminology. Organized in a logical sequence of lessons for students' use.
R: *Choice* 9: 1277 (Dec. 1972); *ARBA* (1973, p. 550); Chen (p. 77); Mal (3-30).

Chambers Dictionary of Science and Technology. **T. C. Collocott, ed.** New York: Barnes & Noble, 1972.

Expanded edition of *Chambers Technical Dictionary.* Best one-stop technical dictionary available. Appendixes include "Table of Chemical Elements," "Periodic Table," etc. Over 40,000 terms.
R: *Nature* 236: 246 (Mar. 31, 1972); *New Scientist* 45: 577–578 (Mar. 19, 1970); *Choice* 9: 623 (July/Aug. 1972); *WLB* 47: 293 (Nov. 1972); *ARBA* (1973, p. 534); Chen (p. 78); Mal (3-18); Wal (p. 22).

Chemical Dictionary (American and British Usage). 4th rev. ed. **Julius Grant, ed.** New York: McGraw-Hill, 1969.

Third edition, 1944.
Close to 55,000 definitions of words used in chemistry and the related fields of physics, agriculture, biology, engineering, etc. Oriented toward British and American usage.
R: *MRW* S2, p. 28.

Chemical Synonyms and Trade Names: A Dictionary and Commercial Handbook. 7th rev. ed. International Scientific Series. **William Gardner.** Cleveland: Chemical Rubber Company, 1971.

This latest edition adds 4,600 entries principally in the fields of minerals, plastics, and pharmaceuticals. Most comprehensive list of 32,500 terms and proprietary trade names for those involved in the marketing and applications of chemicals.
R: *ABL* 33: entry 334 (July 1968); *Choice* 8: 1317 (Dec. 1971); *ARBA* (1973, p. 543); Chen (p. 83); Jenkins (D73); Mal (11-89); Wal (p. 472); Win (ED33).

Dictionary of Biochemistry. **J. Stenesh.** New York: John Wiley, 1975.

Approximately 12,000 entries drawn from reference books, textbooks, and the research literature in biochemistry.
R: Chen (p. 82).

Dictionary of Biological Terms. 8th ed. **Isabella Ferguson Henderson and W. D. Henderson.** Edinburgh: Oliver and Boyd, 1963.

Provides pronunciation, derivation, and brief technical definitions for approximately 18,000 terms in biology and related subjects.
R: Chen (p. 82); Jenkins (G30); Mal (9-18); Wal (p. 193; 207; 224); Win (EC12).

A Dictionary of Biology. 6th ed. **Michael Abercrombie, C. J. Hickman, and M. L. Johnson.** Baltimore, MD: Penguin Books, 1973.

Fifth edition, 1966.
Over 3,000 biological terms. Basic definitions, intended primarily for the lay person. Cross-referenced. Illustrations.
R: *Choice* 10: 1168 (Oct. 1973); *ARBA* (1974, p. 564; 1972, p. 564); *MRW* S3, p. 7; Chen (p. 83); Jenkins (G27); Mal (9-15); Wal (p. 193); Win (EC10; 1EC2).

Dictionary of the Biological Sciences. **Peter Gray.** New York: Reinhold, 1967.

Contains terms excluded from the author's *Encyclopedia of the Biological Sciences.*

Intended for use at the college level. An abridged version, *Student Dictionary of Biology,* 1973, is also available.
R: *American Scientist* 56: 90A–91A (1968); *Choice* 4: 1224 (Jan. 1968); *LJ* 93: 1585 (Apr. 1968); 92: 4491 (1967); Chen (p. 84); Jenkins (G29); Mal (9-16); Wal (p. 193); Win (2EC4).

Gardner's Chemical Synonyms and Trade Names. 8th ed. **E. I. Cooke and R. W. I. Cooke.** Oxford, England: Technical Press, 1978.
Seventh edition, 1971.
Concise listing of materials accompanied by chemical name and definition. Emphasis on products such as alloys, plastics, medicines, and industrial chemicals. Insignificant amount of space paid to revision of older items. Comprehensive list of manufacturers numbers almost 400 names. Duplication, omission, and limitations may lead pharmacists to other reference sources.
R: *Pharmaceutical Journal* 220: 531 (1978).

McGraw-Hill Dictionary of Scientific and Technical Terms. New York: McGraw-Hill, 1974.
An abundantly illustrated dictionary of over 100,000 definitions intended for use by scientists and intelligent laymen. Appendixes include information on SI conversion factors, tables in mathematics, chemistry, electronics, etc. Explanatory notes designate the areas of science to which each term applies.
R: *AIChE J* 21: 206 (Jan. 1975); *Journal of the American Chemical Society* 97: 2308 (April 16, 1975); *TBRI* 41: 331 (Nov. 1975); *ARBA* (1975, p. 640); Chen (p. 78).

McGraw-Hill Dictionary of the Life Sciences. New York: McGraw-Hill, 1976.
Designed as a practical guide to the vocabulary of the biological sciences. Lists 20,000 terms and definitions covering 49 fields of science. Good cross-referencing and over 800 complementary illustrations. Serves both the specialist and general public.

A Source-Book of Biological Names and Terms. 3d ed. 6th printing. **Edmund C. Jaeger.** Springfield, IL: Charles C. Thomas, 1978.
A listing of 12,000 terms of biological and scientific importance. Entries also include names, word elements, combining forms, prefixes, and suffixes. Entries consist of origin of the work (Greek, Latin, etc.), literal meaning, and examples of usage in the biological sciences. Addenda includes a 1,000-word supplement and brief biographies.

Trade Name Dictionary. 2d ed. 2 vols. **Ellen T. Crowley, ed.** Detroit, MI: Gale Research, 1979.
Supplemented by *New Trade Names,* 1980 and 1981. Companion volume, *Trade Name Dictionary: Company Index.*
A comprehensive and convenient guide to consumer-oriented trade names, brand names, product names, coined names, model names, and design names, with addresses of their manufacturers, importers, marketers, or distributors. Well indexed. The new edition includes more than 130,000 entries, with over 8,000 revisions. The new supplements include more than 20,000 new entries each year.

R: *Chemical Marketing Reporter* (Dec. 4, 1978); *Business Journal* (July 27, 1977); *Choice* (July/Aug. 1976); *The Counselor* (Dec. 1974); *LJ* (June 1, 1976); *RQ* (Summer 1975); *Serial News* (May 1975); *WLB* (June 1976); *ARBA* (1977); Chen (p. 79).

Webster's New Collegiate Dictionary. Rev. ed. **Merriam-Webster Editorial Staff.** Springfield, MA: G. & C. Merriam, 1973.

A standard English usage dictionary.
R: Stearns & Ratcliff (*AJN*).

GENERAL—MEDICINE

Black's Medical Dictionary. 31st ed. **William A. R. Thomson.** New York: Barnes & Noble, 1976.

First edition, 1906; twentieth edition, 1951; twenty-eighth edition, 1969; twenty-ninth edition, 1971; thirtieth edition, 1974.
A standard ready-reference for authoritative definitions of medical terms. Editions are frequently revised and updated. Definitions include information on therapy and diagnosis. Provides illustrations and tables. A standard dictionary in the medical field.
R: *Choice* 11: 1602 (Jan. 1975); *RSR* 2: 119 (July–Sept. 1974); *ARBA* (1970, p. 133; 1972, p. 615; 1976, p. 728; 1977, p. 710); *MRW* S2, p. 29; Sheehy (EK7); Win (EK68).

Blakiston's Gould Medical Dictionary: A Modern Comprehensive Dictionary of the Terms Used in All Branches of Medicine and Allied Sciences; With Illustrations and Tables. 3d ed. **Arthur Osol, ed.** New York: McGraw-Hill, 1972.

First edition, 1949; second edition, 1956.
Over 75,000 terms, alphabetically arranged, are listed in this medical dictionary which has been published since 1949. Provides etymology, biographical data, meaning of eponyms. Includes plates and tables.
R: *ARBA* (1973, p. 607); *MRW* S2, p. 28; Win (EK69).

Blakiston's Pocket Medical Dictionary. 4th ed. **Arthur Osol, ed.** New York: McGraw-Hill, 1979.

Third edition, 1973.
A shortened version of *Blakiston's Gould Medical Dictionary*, arranged alphabetically. Includes anatomical tables, acronyms, abbreviations. Important to nurses, paramedics, medical secretaries, dental assistants.
R: *ARBA* (1974, p. 627); *MRW* S3, p. 14.

Butterworths Medical Dictionary. 2d ed. **Macdonald Critchley, ed.** London: Butterworths, 1978.

A comprehensive and standard British medical dictionary. The new edition has 8,000 new entries. Clear format; thorough definitions. It ignores American conventions.
R: *Annals of Internal Medicine* 89: 1020 (Dec. 1978); *British Journal of Surgery* 66: 68 (Jan. 1979); *Journal of Bone and Joint Surgery* 60B: 449 (Aug. 1978); *Lancet* 1: 536 (Mar. 11, 1978); Sheehy (EK8).

Computer Glossary for Medical and Health Sciences. **William T. Blessum and Charles J. Sippl.** New York: Funk & Wagnalls, 1973.

Alphabetically arranged glossary of over 2,900 computer terms. Definitions are brief but concise. Includes two appendixes: acronyms, essays on the impact of the computer on medicine.
R: *ARBA* (1974, p. 626); *MRW* S3, pp. 5, 12, 31.

A Concise Dictionary of Medicine. **M. W. Martin.** Middle Village, NY: Jonathan David, 1975.

A medical dictionary intended for the lay public. Contains concise but accurate definitions. This book will serve public librarians who need to disseminate information quickly.
R: *ARBA* (1976, p. 729).

Current Medical Information and Technology. 4th ed. **American Medical Association.** Chicago, IL: American Medical Association, 1971.

First edition, 1963; third edition, 1966.
Includes over 3,000 medical terms preferred by the AMA. Cross-references French, Spanish, and German names of diseases. Provides a KWIC Index and a classification of diseases.
R: Win (EK67).

Dictionary of Medical Ethics. **A. S. Duncan, R. B. Welbourn, and G. R. Dunstan, eds.** London: Darton, Longman & Todd, 1977.

A necessary and valuable dictionary; editors have compiled alphabetically arranged terms which include detailed, though undogmatic, explanations. Recommended to physicians as a helpful tool.
R: *British Journal of Haematology* 38: 581 (1978); *British Journal of Radiology* 51: 219 (1978); *BMJ* 2: 1208 (Nov. 5, 1977); *Canadian Medical Association Journal* 117: 1377 (Dec. 17, 1977); *Lancet* 2: 1112 (Nov. 26, 1977).

The Dictionary of Medical Folklore. **Carol Ann Rinzler.** New York: Crowell, 1979.

A collection of some 500 medical old wives' tales.
R: *LJ* 105: 572 (Mar. 1, 1980).

Dictionary of Medical Syndromes. **Sergio Magalini.** Philadelphia, PA: J. B. Lippincott, 1971.

An alphabetical listing of over 1,800 entries which define medical syndromes. Includes eponyms. Provides reference to etiology, pathology, symptoms, therapy, and prognosis of each disease. Includes bibliography and index. Comprehensive.
R: *ARBA* (1972, p. 615); *MRW* S2, pp. 28, 32; Win (EK81).

Dorland's Illustrated Medical Dictionary. 25th ed. Philadelphia, PA: W. B. Saunders, 1974.

First edition, 1900; twenty-third edition, 1957, twenty-fourth edition, 1965.
A standard medical dictionary for over 70 years; contains over 120,000 entries with contributions from 80 authorities. Contains illustrations and plates; now available on computer tape. A high-quality dictionary; recommended.

R: *Annals of Internal Medicine* 84: 623 (May 1976); *Archives of Surgery* 110: 226 (Feb. 1975); *Lancet* 2: 700 (Sept. 21, 1974); *Plastic & Reconstructive Surgery* 62: 608 (1978); *Choice* 2: 471 (Oct. 1965); *RSR* 2: 129 (Oct.–Dec. 1974); Sheehy (EK9); Win (EJ47; EK70; 1EJ8); Stearns & Ratcliff *(AJN; NEJM,* 1970).

Dorland's Pocket Medical Dictionary. 22d ed. Abridged from *Dorland's Illustrated Medical Dictionary.* Philadelphia, PA: W. B. Saunders, 1977.

First edition, 1898; twenty-first edition, 1968.
A handy pocket-size edition of the classic *Dorland's.* Contains essential definition, spelling, punctuation. Includes plates, anatomical information, pharmaceutical trade names. A fine ready-reference tool.
R: *ARBA* (1978, p. 710).

The Faber Medical Dictionary. 2d ed. **Cecil Wakeley, ed. John Bate, rev.** Philadelphia, PA: J. B. Lippincott, 1975.

First edition, 1953.
Revised edition contains updated terms and eponyms. Lists drugs by approved names. Contains essential, concise terms including etymological information. A handy reference tool for health science personnel.
R: *British Journal of Surgery* 62: 753 (Sept. 1975); *Lancet* 1: 1226 (May 31, 1975); *RSR* 3: 38 (July–Dec. 1975); *ARBA* (1976, p. 728).

The Faber Pocket Medical Dictionary. 2d ed. **Patrick A. Riley and P. J. Cunningham.** London: Faber & Faber, 1974.

First edition, 1966.
Over 6,500 entries which include pronunciation, concise definitions, and occasional cross references. Excludes drugs except in appendix.
R: *MRW* S1, p. 4; *MRW* S3, p. 14.

Familiar Medical Quotations. **Maurice B. Strauss, ed.** Boston, MA: Little, Brown, 1968.

Contains more than 7,000 quotations.
R: *MRW* S1, p. 5.

Glossary of Molecular Biology. **Anthony Evans, comp.** New York: Halsted Press, 1975.

About 350 entries of terms related to molecular biology. Cross-references and bibliography of 139 citations. Useful for molecular biologists as well as individuals with backgrounds in biology and chemistry.
R: *Lancet* 1: 434 (Feb. 22, 1975).

Harbeck's Glossary of Medical Terms. **Evelyn Harbeck Rimer.** Menlo Park, CA: Pacific Coast Publishers, 1967.

Identifies correct spelling of terms and phrases associated with medical specialties.

An Illustrated Guide to Medical Terminology. **Helen R. Strand.** Baltimore, MD: Williams & Wilkins, 1968.

Emphasis on human anatomy, diseases, radiology, pathology, and anesthesiology. Lists roots, prefixes, suffixes, etc., of various terms.
R: *MRW* S1, p. 3.

Illustrated Medical Dictionary. 25th ed. **William A. N. Dorland.** Philadelphia, PA: W. B. Saunders, 1974.

First edition, 1900.
Standard biomedical dictionary. Lists current terminology as well as eponyms, acronyms, abbreviations. Each entry describes derivation, pronunciation, plural form, definition, and subentries. Numerous illustrations complement text.
R: *MRW* S3, p. 14.

Index of Paramedical Vocabulary: An Index-Indicator Enabling the User Not Versed in Greek and Latin to Locate the Terminology of Any Given Subject in a Paramedical, Medical, or Biological Dictionary. **Jacob E. Schmidt.** Springfield, IL: Charles C. Thomas, 1974.

To be used as a key to alphabetical medical dictionaries. Cross-references English to Latin prefixes. Helpful to paramedics and to those seeking to acquaint themselves with medical vocabulary.
R: *ARBA* (1975, p. 738).

The Inverted Medical Dictionary: A Method of Finding Medical Terms Quickly. **Waldo A. Rigal.** Westport, CT: Technomic Publishing, 1976.

Includes almost 13,000 medical terms. Each definition has been reduced to a brief key phrase. Arranged alphabetically by descriptive subject. Reference tool for medical writers. Does not contain cross-references.
R: *Nation's Health* 6: 5 (Nov. 1976); *Choice* 14: 1194 (Nov. 1977); *ARBA* (1978, p. 712); Sheehy (EK11).

Livingstone's Pocket Medical Dictionary. 12th ed. **Nancy Roper, ed.** London: Churchill Livingstone, 1974.

First edition, 1933; tenth edition, 1966; eleventh edition, 1969.
Pocket medical dictionary intended for nurses, medical assistants, students, pharmacists, and secretaries. Illustrated; appendixes of prefixes and suffixes, poison information, measurements, and abbreviations.
R: *ARBA* (1975, p. 737); *MRW* S2, p. 29; *MRW* S3, p. 80.

The Medical & Health Sciences Word Book. **Ann Ehrlich, comp.** Boston, MA: Houghton Mifflin, 1977.

Alphabetical arrangement of 60,000 medical, nursing, and allied health terms. Provides pronunciation of each term; no definitions included. Useful appendixes list information on surgical equipment and procedures, drug names, medical symbols and signs, and medical abbreviations used by the American Medical Association. Pronunciation information valuable for secretaries and record keepers in medical setting; of little value to the general public or health professionals who primarily require definition assistance.
R: *ARBA* (1978, p. 712).

Medical Legal Dictionary. **Edward J. Bander and Jeffrey J. Wallach.** Dobbs Ferry, NY: Oceana, 1970.

Selective list of 400 terms geared toward the legal and medical professions. Stresses practical definitions. Most useful material found in the appendix (e.g. lists of reference sources, the text of the Uniform Anatomical Gift Act).
R: *LJ* 95: 2651 (Aug. 1970); *ARBA* (1971, p. 531); Win (EK159).

Melloni's Illustrated Medical Dictionary. **Ida D. Melloni, Biagio J. Melloni, and Gilbert M. Eisner.** Baltimore, MD: Williams & Wilkins, 1979.

Consists of 2,500 illustrations prepared by the distinguished medical illustrators Biagio and Ida Melloni. Features color details. Concise definitions. Useful for allied health personnel.
R: Brandon (*NO*).

The Origin of Medical Terms. 2d ed. **Henry A. Skinner.** Baltimore, MD: Williams & Wilkins, 1961.

Paramedical Dictionary: A Practical Dictionary for the Semi-medical and Ancillary Medical Professions. **Jacob E. Schmidt.** Springfield, IL: Charles C. Thomas, 1969.

Includes some 10,000 words and nontechnical definitions. Indicates pronunciation. Useful information found in appendix (e.g. prescription symbols, tables of communicable diseases, medical abbreviations). Geared toward paramedical professionals.
R: *ARBA* (1970, p. 134); *MRW* S2, p. 29.

Stedman's Medical Dictionary: A Vocabulary of Medicine and Its Allied Sciences, With Pronunciations and Derivations. 23d ed. Baltimore, MD: Williams & Wilkins, 1976.

First edition, 1911, seventeenth edition, 1949; twentieth edition, 1962; twenty-first edition, 1966; twenty-second edition, 1972.
A truly classic work since 1911. Enjoys a lofty place among medical dictionaries. Features an exhaustive, comprehensive, and current vocabulary. Includes pharmacological and dental terms as well as purely medical ones. Entries also include pronunciation and derivation. Contains many pertinent illustrations (color plates, sketches, drawings, charts, and graphs). A gold mine of information found in the indexes and appendixes. Definitions are accurate, crisp, and technical. Deserves a special position on every physician's bookshelf.
R: *Anesthesiology* 45: 699 (Dec. 1976); *Archives of Dermatology* 107: 130 (Jan. 1973); *Archives of Internal Medicine* 132: 459 (Sept. 1973); *JAMA* 237: 1623 (Apr. 11, 1977); *RSR* 3: 46 (Jan.–Mar. 1975); *ARBA* (1973, p. 608; 1977, p. 712); *MRW* S2, p. 29; Sheehy (EK10); Win (EJ50; EK74; 1EJ11).

Structural Units of Medical and Biological Terms. **Jacob E. Schmidt.** Springfield, IL: Charles C. Thomas, 1969.

A guide to the dissection of the medical vocabulary. Each of the 1,000 main entries includes definition, origin, combining stem, and examples of compound words. Abundant cross-references. Useful appendix lists 56 suffixes common to medical and biological terminology. Helpful reference tool for physicians, medi-

cal researchers, paramedical personnel, and students in medicine, nursing, and biology.
R: *Choice* 7: 370 (May 1970); *ARBA* (1971, p. 532); *MRW* S2, pp. 13, 65.

Taber's Cyclopedic Medical Dictionary. 13th ed. **Clayton L. Thomas, ed.** Philadelphia, PA: F. A. Davis, 1977.

First edition, 1940; ninth edition, 1962; tenth edition, 1965; eleventh edition, 1969; twelfth edition, 1973.

High-quality dictionary aimed primarily at nurses and allied health professionals. Contains current medical terms and phrases arranged alphabetically. Definitions are concise. Entries also include phonetic spellings, derivations, and abbreviations where necessary. Synonyms generously added. Features a limited number of tables and two-color line drawings. Appendix provides useful information not readily found in a dictionary (e.g. first aid procedures, addresses of poison control centers, and common queries in several foreign languages). The simple, straight-forward presentation should meet the demands of health professionals and laymen.
R: *Archives of Internal Medicine* 133: 323 (Feb. 1974); *MRW* S2, p. 29; *ARBA* (1974, p. 629; 1978, p. 713); Win (EJ51; EJ112; EK75; 1EJ12; 3EJ12a).

20,000 Medical Words. **Robert W. Prichard and Robert E. Robinson.** New York: McGraw-Hill, 1972.

Consists of 20,000 medical words accompanied by their spelling and syllabication. Proper names and drug terms omitted. No definitions.
R: *ARBA* (1973, p. 609); *MRW* S2, pp. 64, 72.

Understanding Medical Terminology. 6th ed. **Agnes C. Frenay.** St. Louis, MO: Catholic Hospital Association, 1977.

First edition, 1958; fourth edition, 1970; fifth edition, 1973.

An easy-language dictionary divided into two sections. Section 1 consists of sixteen chapters devoted to terms covering numerous biological disorders. Section 2 encompasses four chapters, treating terms relating to various fields of medicine. Contains illustrations and charts. Includes bibliography and index. Written primarily for students of pharmacy, nursing, medical technology, physical therapy, and hospital administration and the general public.
R: *ARBA* (1971, p. 531); *MRW* S2, p. 71; *MRW* S3, p. 37.

Visual Aids for Paramedical Vocabulary. **J. E. Schmidt.** Springfield, IL: Charles C. Thomas, 1973.

Aims to provide a simplified means of learning medical vocabulary through visual aids. Provides discussions, illustrations (largely anatomical), which are presented by body system. Especially useful for paramedics and lay people.
R: *ARBA* (1974, p. 632).

A Word-Part Book for Medical Terminology. **Leo G. Gosser.** Auburn, AL: Auburn University, 1973.

Emphasis on definitions of parts of medical words and identification of origins. Alphabetical arrangement under prefixes, suffixes, roots, and derivatives. Designed as a study guide in learning and spelling medical terms.
R: *MRW* S3, p. 37.

Allergy and Immunology

A Dictionary of Immunology. 2d ed. **W. J. Herbert and P. C. Wilkinson, eds.** Oxford, England: Blackwell Scientific Publications, 1977.

First edition, 1971.
A pocket-size dictionary of over 1,500 terms. Definitions are brief but pertinent and helpful to those needing immunological vocabulary. Includes abbreviations and symbols.
R: *British Journal of Haematology* 38: 581 (1978); *Immunology* 35: 857 (Nov. 1978); *Nature* 273: 254 (May 18, 1978); *ARBA* (1973, p. 551); *MRW* S2, p. 56.

Glossary of Immunological Terms. **W. J. Halliday.** London: Butterworths, 1971.

Word, definition, and numerical code referring to separate bibliography comprise each entry. Useful glossary for immunologists, clinicians, and biologists.
R: *MRW* S2, p. 56.

Anatomy

A Systematic Guide to Medical Terminology. 2d ed. **Nathaniel Weiss.** Madison, WI: National Shorthand Reporters Association, 1971.

Provides definitions of medical roots of words according to their use in anatomy and physiology. Entries consist of word, Greek or Latin origin, terse definition, and pronunciation. Includes indexes to Latin and Greek roots and English equivalents.
R: *MRW* S2, p. 72.

Anesthesiology and General Surgery

Guide to Surgical Terminology. **Frances Coleman.** Oradell, NJ: Medical Economics Co., 1971.

Lists common terms associated with physical examination, laboratory results, symptoms, diagnosis, instruments and equipment, and surgical procedures and findings. Alphabetical arrangement. Aids court reporters, transcribers, and medical clerical personnel.
R: *MRW* S2, p. 100.

Brain and Nervous System

Desk Reference for Neuroanatomy: A Guide to Essential Terms. **Isabel Lockard.** New York: Springer-Verlag, 1977.

A reference of essential terms for neuroanatomists.

Dictionary of Epilepsy. **Henri Gastaut.** Geneva: World Health Organization, 1973.

Simultaneously published in French, Spanish, and English. Includes over 750 entries related to clinical aspects of epilepsy. Compiled by international authorities. Entries include definition, synonym, cross-references.
R: *Lancet* 2: 646 (Sept. 22, 1973); *IBID* 1: 275 (Dec. 1973); *MRW* S3, p. 24; Win (EK77).

DENTISTRY

Current Clinical Dental Terminology: A Glossary of Accepted Terms in all Disciplines of Dentistry. 2d ed. **Carl O. Boucher, ed.** St. Louis, MO: C. V. Mosby, 1974.
First edition, 1963.
Includes over 10,000 clinical dental terms; definitions supplied by over 40 contributors are concise and cross-referenced. Includes appendixes of chemical names and miscellaneous information. Recommended for clinicians and students.
R: *RSR* 2: 119 (July–Sept. 1974); *MRW* S3, p. 13; Win (EK147).

Heinemann Modern Dictionary for Dental Students. 3d ed. **Jenifer E. H. Fowler, comp.** Paris: Prélat, 1973.
Second edition, 1957.
Over 2,000 brief definitions, English terms, explanation in French. Contains historical terms, list of periodicals and abbreviations.
R: *MRW* S3, p. 14.

DERMATOLOGY

A Dictionary of Dermatological Words, Terms and Phrases. **Morris Leider and Morris Rosenblum.** New York: McGraw-Hill, 1968.
Close to 3,000 brief explanations of dermatological diseases, theories, and concepts. Includes pronunciation key, vernacular terms.
R: *MRW* S1, p. 12; Win (EK80).

GENETICS

A Dictionary of Genetics. 2d ed. **Robert C. King.** New York: Oxford University Press, 1974.
First edition, 1968.
Includes historical and recent terms. Also lists periodicals, directory of genetic laboratories in North America.
R: *Choice* 9: 792 (Sept. 1972); 12: 818 (Sept. 1975); *TBRI* 39: 163 (Apr. 1973); *ARBA* (1976, p. 655; 1973, p. 551); Chen (p. 84); Jenkins (G165); Mal (9-21); *MRW* S2, p. 49; Wal (p. 197); Win (3EC20).

Glossary of Genetics and Cytogenetics, Classical and Molecular. 4th rev. ed. **R. Rieger, A. Michaelis, and M. M. Green.** New York: Springer-Verlag, 1976.
Third edition, 1968.
Comprehensive glossary which is valuable to workers in the field for quick reference purposes. Includes some outdated terms as well as some with indirect genetic implications. Comprehensive cross-referencing system. Useful appendix is bibliography of papers in which a word was first used.
R: *Annals of Human Genetics* 41: 517 (May 1978); *Heredity* 41: 115 (Aug. 1978).

Mendelian Inheritance in Man. 3d ed. **V. A. McKusick.** Baltimore, MD: Johns Hopkins University Press, 1971.

First edition, 1966; second edition, 1969.
First extensive dictionary of genetic disease. Computer-generated listing accounts for the precision, speed, and economy in publishing. However, also produces an aesthetic problem. Includes various valuable summaries (e.g. classification of disease of hands, bones and hearing; linkages and enzymopathies). Definite omission from the volume is data on incidence. Worthy purchase for hospital and university libraries and for departments of clinical genetics, clinical biochemistry, hematology, and radiology.
R: *Annals of Human Genetics* 36: 364 (Jan. 1973).

HEALTH SERVICES ADMINISTRATION

A Discursive Dictionary of Health Care. **Subcommittee on Health and the Environment of the Committee on Interstate and Foreign Commerce, US House of Representatives.** Washington, DC: US Government Printing Office, 1976.

Close to 1,000 entries of terms relating to health, health administration, welfare programs, legal matters. All are government-related terms and government definitions. Clearly printed and illustrated.
R: *Annals of Internal Medicine* 84: 767 (June 1976); *Medical Care* 15: 446 (May 1977); *NEJM* 294: 853 (Apr. 8, 1976); *ARBA* (1977, p. 713).

Glossary of Health Care Terminology, Public Health in Europe No. 4. **James Hogarth.** Copenhagen: World Health Organization, Regional Office for Europe, 1975.

Glossary of 350 health care terms used in documents inssued by the WHO and other international health organizations. Includes index and references.
R: *Bibliography, Documentation, Terminology* 16: 329 (Nov.–Dec. 1976); *IBID* 4: 354 (Dec. 1976).

Simplified Medical Records System: A Directory of Medical Terminology. **Burgess L. Gordon.** Acton, MA: Publishing Sciences Group, 1975.

Alphabetically lists descriptors and qualifiers covering symptoms, physical and radiologic signs, laboratory determinations, and drugs. Also provides corresponding codes for computerization.
R: *JAMA* 233: 1113 (Sept. 8, 1975).

INFECTIOUS DISEASES

Ainsworth & Bisby's Dictionary of the Fungi. 6th ed. **Geoffrey C. Ainsworth.** Kew, England: Commonwealth Mycological Institute, 1971.

First edition, 1943; fifth edition, 1961.
A dictionary of lichens and fungi. Includes generic, common, taxonomic names, biographical notes.
R: *MRW* S2, p. 48.

A Dictionary of Microbial Taxonomy. **S. T. Cowan. L. R. Hill, ed.** Cambridge, England: Cambridge University Press, 1978.

Started as a revision of *A Dictionary of Taxonomic Usage* but greatly enlarged. Four

introductory chapters include early history, philosophical background material, taxonomic source material, and various codes of microbial nomenclature. Accurate guide to taxonomic microbial terminology for taxonomists and general readers.
R: *Abstracts on Hygiene* 44: 85 (Jan. 1969); *Journal of Clinical Pathology* 32: 309 (Mar. 1979); Chen (p. 84); Mal (9-46); Wal (p. 199); Win (3EC19a).

Dictionary of Microbiology. **P. Singleton and D. Sainsbury.** New York: John Wiley, 1978.
Provides definitions of terms, techniques, and concepts in microbiology. Also includes descriptions of over 1,000 taxa. Concise definitions, extensively cross-referenced.

Glossary of Bacteriological Terms. **P. Sampson.** London: Butterworths, 1975.
A glossary of over 1,000 medical laboratory terms and their definitions. Entries are alphabetically arranged with copious cross-references included. Drawings and an extensive bibliography are provided. Useful tool for those interested in medical bacteriology.

NURSING

Bailliere's Nurses Dictionary. 18th ed. **Barbara F. Cape, ed.** Baltimore, MD: Williams & Wilkins, 1974.
Seventeenth edition, 1968.
R: *British Book Notes* p. 190 (Mar. 1975); *RSR* 3: 49 (Apr./June 1975).

Duncan's Dictionary For Nurses. **Helen A. Duncan.** New York: Springer Publishing, 1971.
Defines 11,000 terms from nursing, medicine, and related disciplines. Definitions are clear and include pronunciation guide. Etymology and chemical formulae are omitted. Contains small line drawings. For use by professional nurses, paramedical personnel, and students.
R: *Choice* 10: 1283 (Oct. 1973); *ARBA* (1972, p. 629; 1973, p. 619).

Encyclopedia and Dictionary of Medicine, Nursing and Allied Health. 2d ed. **Benjamin F. Miller and Claire B. Keane.** Philadelphia, PA: W. B. Saunders, 1978.
First edition, *Encyclopedia and Dictionary of Medicine and Nursing,* 1972.
Geared toward nursing professionals. Alphabetically arranges terms and definitions with brief but appropriate explanation for each. Contains photographs, line drawings, and anatomic plates. A useful book for the nurse, paramedic, or lay person.
R: *Archives of Internal Medicine* 132: 461 (Sept. 1973); *Journal of Nursing Administration* 4: 10 (Jan.–Feb. 1974); *ARBA* (1973, p. 619); *MRW* S2, pp. 29, 72; Sheehy (EK27); Win (EK168); Brandon (*NO*).

Livingstone's Dictionary for Nurses. 14th ed. **Nancy Roper.** Edinburgh: Churchill Livingstone; distr. New York: Longman, 1973.

Thirteenth edition, 1969.
Over 5,000 entries reflect current usage of words which represent new advances in medicine. Pronunciation aid. Etymology for majority of entries. Appendixes of common prefixes and suffixes and their meanings; procedures for urine and blood tests; and common toxic substances. For use by practicing nurses.
R: *MRW* S2, pp. 29, 72; *MRW* S3, p. 37; *ARBA* (1975, p. 737).

The Macmillan Dictionary for Practical and Vocational Nurses. **Grace E. Fitch and Mary J. Dubiny, eds.** New York: Macmillan, 1966.
R: *MRW* S1, p. 20.

McGraw-Hill Nursing Dictionary. New York: McGraw-Hill, 1979.
R: Brandon (*NO*).

NUTRITION

The Barbara Kraus Dictionary of Protein. **Barbara Kraus.** New York: Harper's Magazine Press, 1975.
A quick reference on the protein and caloric content of a broad range of foods.
R: *LJ* 100: 1112 (June 1, 1975); *WLB* 50: 126 (Oct. 1975); *ARBA* (1976, p. 750); Chen (p. 87).

Dictionary of Nutrition and Food Technology. 4th ed. **Arnold E. Bender.** New York: Chemical Publishing, 1976.
First edition, 1960; second edition, 1965; third edition, 1968.
Authoritative definitions that apply to food study. Includes appropriate terms from medicine, chemistry, home economics, etc.
R: *Nutrition* 29: 387 (Nov.–Dec. 1975); *Nutrition Reviews* 35: 29 (Jan. 1977); *Choice* 6: 991 (Oct. 1969); *ARBA* (1970, p. 152); Chen (p. 87); Jenkins (J113); Wal (p. 485); Win (EJ118; EK173; 1EJ23). Additional reviews in *Food Science and Technology Abstracts*.

A Dictionary of Sodium, Fats, and Cholesterol. **Barbara Kraus.** New York: Grosset & Dunlap, 1974.
Comprehensive listing of sodium, fat, and cholesterol content in most foods. Somewhat technical, hence most likely to be used by physicians, dieticians, and nutritionists.
R: *Choice* 12: 370–372 (May 1975); *RSR* 2: 130 (Oct.–Dec. 1974); *ARBA* (1976, p. 750); Chen (p. 87).

Food and Nutrition Terminology: Definitions of Selected Terms and Expressions in Current Use, FAO Terminology Bulletins, no. 28. Rome, Italy: Food and Agriculture Organization, 1974.
Contains definitions, in English only, intended to facilitate the work of organizations and agencies of the UN system and should not be considered as official or definitive. Prepared by FAO and WHO in collaboration with the International Union of Nutritional Sciences.
R: *IBID* 4: 36 (Mar. 1976); Chen (p. 88).

The Health Food Dictionary with Recipes. **Anstice Carroll and Embree De-Persiis Vona.** Englewood Cliffs, NJ: Prentice-Hall, 1973.
Brief and superficial information on identifying and buying "health foods."
R: *LJ* 98: 1572 (May 15, 1973); *ARBA* (1974, p. 654); Chen (p. 88).

Nutrition and Diet Therapy; Reference Dictionary. 2d ed. **Rosalinda T. Lagua, Virginia S. Claudio, and Victoria F. Thiele.** St. Louis, MO: C. V. Mosby, 1974.
Lists some 3,500 terms and their definitions. Concentrates on biochemistry, nutrition, dietetics physiology, and related topics. Contains some terms of historic value. Outlines valuable information in appendixes: classification of carbon hydrates, lipids and proteins and description of minerals, vitamins, and enzymes. Geared toward the American student and public.
R: *Nutrition* 29: 919 (Mar./Apr. 1975); *RSR* 3: 43 (Jan.–Mar. 1975).

OPHTHALMOLOGY

An Annotated Glossary of the Terms Used in Electroretinography. **Lucia Ronchi and Giovanni del Signore.** Firenze, Italy: Baccini & Chiappi, 1969.
A glossary of annotated terms pertaining to the physics of electroretinography. Includes illustrations, references, and subject index.
R: *MRW* S2, p. 41.

Ophthalmic Eponyms: An Encyclopedia of Named Signs, Syndromes, and Diseases in Ophthalmology. **Spencer P. Thornton.** Birmingham, AL: Aesculapius, 1967.
Consists of two sections: diseases, signs, and syndromes in medical, pediatric, and neuro ophthalmology, and eponyms in ophthalmic surgery. Alphabetical arrangement within each section. Includes references with most terms.
R: Win (EK82).

OTORHINOLARYNGOLOGY

A Comprehensive Dictionary of Audiology. **James H. Delk.** Sioux City, IA: Hearing Aid Journal, 1973.
A dictionary of wide scope; includes 5,500 entries which provide definitions, pronunciations, abbreviations. Illustrates hearing equipment. Provides word equivalent list.
R: *MRW* S3, p. 28.

Dictionary of Speech & Hearing, Anatomy & Physiology. **Joseph F. Brown.** Sacramento, CA: Speech and Hearing Service, 1974.
Intended for the specialist. Alphabetically arranged terms covering a broad spectrum of anatomy and physiology related to speech and hearing. Clear format; includes excellent line drawings. A handy ready reference tool; does not include pronunciation.
R: *Choice* 13: 955 (Oct. 1976); *ARBA* (1976, p. 728; 1977, p. 710).

Terminology of Communication Disorders: Speech, Language, and Hearing. **Lu-**

cille Nicolosi, Elizabeth Harryman, and Janet Kreschek. Baltimore, MD: Williams & Wilkins, 1978.

Comprehensive coverage of the terminology of audiology, otolaryngology, neurology, and psychology. Over 10,000 terms, followed by definitions and descriptions, cover language, voice, rhythm, structure, and hearing. Intended for speech, language, and hearing professionals.

Pathology

Glossary of Histopathological Terms. **John W. Law and H. John Oliver.** London: Butterworths, 1973.

Focuses on histopathology terminology frequently encountered in laboratory. Besides 500 terms, includes biographical references. No pronunciation key.
R: *MRW* S3, pp. 28, 39.

Illustrated Dictionary of Eponymic Syndromes and Diseases and Their Synonyms. **Stanley Jablonski.** Philadelphia, PA: W. B. Saunders, 1969.

Lists alphabetically 10,000 eponymic names of pathological conditions. Used in naming clinical entities, animal diseases, experimental diseases, diagnostic signs, and pathological conditions. Entries consist of eponyms, synonyms, definitions, and citations. Cross-referenced, photographs.
R: *Lancet* 1: 596 (Mar. 21, 1970); *ARBA* (1970, p. 133); *MRW* S2, p. 28; Win (EK78, 3EJ12).

Pharmacy and Pharmacology

Drugs from A to Z: A Dictionary. 2d ed. **Richard R. Lingeman.** New York: McGraw-Hill, 1974.

First edition, 1969.
Reference tool which lists drug terms, including slang, defined from both a pharmacological and sociological point of view. Entries include synonyms, cross-references, and quotations from authors. Four appendixes of legal classifications of drugs. For medical, public, and college libraries.
R: *Choice* 6: 486 (June 1969); *LJ* 94: 3041 (Sept. 15, 1969); *RSR* 4: 89 (Apr.–June 1976); *ARBA* (1970, p. 139); *MRW* S2, pp. 33, 50; Win (EK191; 3EJ26).

Modern Drug Encyclopedia, 1975–76. New York: Yorke Medical Books, 1975.

Continued by *Modern Drug Encyclopedia & Therapeutic Index,* 14th ed., Arthur J. Lewis, ed., 1977.

Modern Drug Encyclopedia and Therapeutic Index. 15th ed. New York: Yorke Medical Books, 1979. Annual.

First edition, 1934; tenth edition, 1965; eleventh edition, 1970; twelfth edition, 1973; fourteenth edition, 1977.
Monographs on drugs, listed alphabetically by nonproprietary names or drug groups, giving description, indicators, contraindications, dosage, and administration. Also availability information, which includes trademark, packaging, dose

forms, and manufacturer. Index includes therapeutic manufacturer and nomenclature.
R: *MRW* S3, p. 20; Sheehy (EK39); Win (EJ130; EK198; 3EJ29).

Pharmacological and Chemical Synonyms; A Collection of Names of Drugs and Other Compounds Drawn from the Medical Literature of the World. 6th ed. **E. E. J. Marler, comp.** Amsterdam: Excerpta Medica Foundation, 1976.

Fifth edition, 1973.
Alphabetically lists nonproprietary drugs and related agents. Provides cross-references among trade names, nonproprietary synonyms, and research codes. Emphasis on American spellings, no official status.
R: *Clinical Pharmacology and Therapeutics* 15: 227 (1974); *MRW* S3, pp. 13, 16; Sheehy (EK35); Win (EK192).

PSYCHIATRY AND PSYCHOLOGY

A Critical Dictionary of Psychoanalysis. **Charles Rycroft.** Totowa, NJ: Littlefield, Adams, 1973.

Over 600 terms, cross-referenced. Emphasizes conceptual and theoretical usage. Includes medical, Jungian, anthropological, biological terms.
R: *MRW* S3, p. 43.

Dictionary of Behavioral Science. **Benjamin B. Wolman, ed.** New York: Van Nostrand Reinhold, 1973.

Covers terms used in psychology and related fields such as biochemistry, neurology, endocrinology. Includes over 12,000 entries, compiled by 29 international specialists. Concise definitions, cross-references, disease classification are provided. Highly recommended. Does not include pronunciation.
R: *Contemporary Psychology* 19: 660 (Sept. 1974); *Neuropsychology* 13: 384 (Sept. 1975); *MRW* S3, pp. 5, 44.

Glossary of Mental Disorders and Guide to Their Classification. 8th Revision. **World Health Organization.** Geneva: World Health Organization, 1974.

A WHO publication which attempts to codify the terminology and classification of mental disorders. Intended for use in conjunction with the *International Classification of Diseases.* Alphabetically arranged by category. Lists synonyms as well. Helpful for psychiatrists.
R: *American Journal of Psychiatry* 132: 881 (Aug. 1975); *Social Biology* 22: 294 (Fall 1975); *IBID* 3: 52 (Mar./June 1975).

Handbook of Psychological Terms. **Philip L. Harriman.** Totowa, NJ: Rowman & Littlefield, 1977.

Interdisciplinary Glossary on Child Abuse and Neglect: Legal, Medical, Social Work Terms, DHEW Pub. no. (OHDS) 78–30137. **Office of Human Development Services, Administration for Children, Youth and Families, Children's Bureau, US National Center on Child Abuse and Neglect.** Washington, DC: US Government Printing Office, 1978.

The Mental Retardation Dictionary. **Alexander J. Tymchuk.** Los Angeles, CA: Western Psychological Services, 1973.

Contains 2,000 entries with corresponding, terse definitions selected from various areas within the realm of exceptional children. Terms include persons, organizations, tests, abbreviations, eponyms, and acronyms. No pronunciation. Fourteen references cited.
R: *MRW* S3, p. 34.

1971 Drug Abuse Reference: General Terms, Drug Abuse Terms, User Slang, Drugs, Chemicals, Education Source Guide. **Charles L. Winek.** Bridgeville, PA: Bek Technical Publications, 1971.

Includes over 600 terms relating to drug use and abuse. Brief definitions include interpretations by both users and doctors. Topically arranged. Intended for use by parents, teachers, physicians.
R: *MRW* S3, p. 17.

Psychiatric Dictionary. 4th ed. **Leland E. Hinsie and Robert J. Campbell.** New York: Oxford University Press, 1970.

First edition, 1940; third edition, 1960.
Considered a standard psychiatric dictionary, this revised edition includes over 1,400 new words, provides pronunciations, illustrations, references, and maintains a multidisciplinary approach to psychiatry.
R: *ARBA* (1971, p. 542); *MRW* S2, p. 82.

A Psychiatric Glossary. 5th ed. Washington, DC: American Psychiatric Association, 1980.

Reflects the major and important changes in psychiatric terminology. Includes numerous new entries, especially terms in biologic psychiatry and neurosciences; table of commonly abused drugs; and a list of widely used abbreviations in the mental health field. Indispensable reference tool for physicians, psychologists, lawyers, social workers, students, and editors.

PUBLIC HEALTH

Common Environmental Terms: A Glossary. **Gloria J. Studdard.** Washington, DC: US Environmental Protection Agency, 1973.

A compilation of over 400 words which provides concise definitions of words and terms essential to understanding environmental terms. Intended primarily for students.
R: *MRW* S3, p. 23.

A Dictionary of Midwifery and Public Health. 2d ed. **G. B. Carter et al.** Salem, NH: Faber & Faber, 1963.

Dictionary of the Environmental Sciences. **Robert W. Durrenberger.** Palo Alto, CA: National Press Books, 1973.

Includes approximately 4,000 terms related to the environmental sciences; concise definitions, illustrations. Also includes appendix of geologic time and equiva-

lents and conversion table. Useful. Recommended to professionals as well as students from the junior high school level through college.
R: *ARBA* (1974, p. 600); Chen (p. 99); Mal (8-93); *MRW* S3, pp. 20, 22.

The New York Times Encyclopedia Dictionary of the Environment. **Paul Sarnoff.** New York: Quadrangle Books, 1971.
Comprehensive listing of terms and phrases related to the environment and its preservation. Includes drawings, tables, and photographs.
R: *MRW* S2, pp. 4, 42, 109.

RADIOLOGY

Dictionary of Radiologic Terminology. **Alphons Jacob and Herbert L. Jackson.** St. Louis, MO: Warren H. Green, 1979.
A comprehensive, complete dictionary which defines terms used in all specialized branches of radiology. Among branches covered are pediatric, diagnostic, therapeutic, and anatomic radiology.

Glossary of Words and Phrases Used in Radiology, Nuclear Medicine, and Ultrasound. 2d ed. **Lewis E. Etter.** Springfield, IL: Charles C. Thomas, 1970.
First edition, 1960.
Over 5,500 words and definitions which include abbreviations, cross-references, and footnotes. Prepared for medical secretaries, X-ray technicians, medical students and residents.
R: *MRW* S2, pp. 72, 87, 105; Win (EK76; 3EJ11).

A Radiographic Index. 6th ed. **Myer Goldman and David Cope.** Baltimore, MD. Williams & Wilkins, 1978.
First edition, 1961; third edition, 1968; fourth edition, 1970.
Features an A-Z glossary of terms of radiographic positioning and techniques. Includes appendixes on medical terms, abbreviations, average exposure tables, and named views of the skull. Updated. Appendix on contrast media.
R: *ABL* 43: entry 397 (Sept. 1978); *MRW* S2, p. 102.

RESPIRATORY SYSTEM

Dictionary/Reference Guide for Respiratory Therapy. **J. Owen Krasowski.** Chicago, IL: Year Book Medical Publishers, 1977.
A quick reference guide for respiratory therapists.

UROGENITAL SYSTEM

Obstetric-Gynecologic Terminology with Section on Neonatology and Glossary of Congenital Anomalies. **Edward C. Hughes, ed.** American College of Obstetricians and Gynecologists, Committee on Terminology. Philadelphia, PA: F. A. Davis, 1972.
Represents a serious attempt to standardize terminology in obstetrics and gynecology. Alphabetical arrangement of terms in nine sections. Each entry includes

the following information: preferred term, definition, synonyms, eponyms, and abbreviations. Work produced by the American College of Obstetricians and Gynecologists with the aid of a grant from the Maternal and Child Health Service of the Health Services and Mental Health Administration. Recommended purchase for physicians and medical and health sciences libraries.
R: *ARBA* (1973, p. 609); *MRW* S2, pp. 1, 46, 50, 57, 74.

VETERINARY MEDICINE

Black's Veterinary Dictionary. 10th ed. **William C. Miller and Geoffrey P. West.** London: Black, 1972.
Ninth edition, 1970.
Encyclopedic dictionary of veterinary care; similar to *Black's Medical Dictionary* in format. Includes causes, symptoms, and treatment of disease. Illustrated.
R: *MRW* S2, p. 107; *MRW* S3, p. 54.

CHAPTER 6 HANDBOOKS

INDEX

Composite Index for CRC Handbooks. **Robert C. Weast, ed.** Cleveland: Chemical Rubber, 1977.

Earlier edition, 1971.
R: *Aslib Proceedings* 24: 273 (May 1972): Chen (p. 101); Wal (p. 49).

GENERAL

Agriculture Handbook: Food Yields Summarized by Different Stages of Preparation, Agriculture Handbook no. 102 (Revised). Rev. ed. **Ruth H. Matthews and Young J. Garrison.** Consumer and Food Economics Institute, Survey Statistics Group, Agricultural Research Service, US Department of Agriculture. Washington, DC: US Government Printing Office, 1975.

First edition, 1956.
Updates the information in the 1956 Handbook. Records recent developments affecting food yields. Data used for research purposes and practical purposes such as estimating food costs, developing food plans, assigning food allotments, etc. Will form basis for values to be compiled in next edition of Agriculture Handbook No. 8: *Composition of Foods . . . Raw, Processed, Prepared.* Specialists in dietetics, nutrition, and institutional food management will directly benefit from this work.
R: *American Journal of Clinical Nutrition* 29: 320 (Mar. 1976).

Chemical Abstracts Service Registry Handbook. Number Section. Columbus, OH: American Chemical Society, 1965/1971–. Annual Supplement.
R: *MRW* S3, p. 9.

Chromatography: A Laboratory Handbook of Chromatographic and Electrophoretic Methods. 3d ed. **Erich Heftmann, ed.** New York: Van Nostrand Reinhold, 1975.

R: *Clinical Chemistry* 22: 128 (Jan. 1976); *Journal of the American Chemical Society* 98: 308 (Jan. 7, 1976); *TBRI* 42: 84 (Mar. 1976); Chen (p. 107).

The Complete Handbook for Medical Secretaries and Assistants. 2d ed. **Robert L. Dennis and Jean M. Doyle.** Boston, MA: Little, Brown, 1978.

First edition, 1971.
A succinct revised edition, containing all essential information pertinent to medical secretaries; scope covers all aspects of daily office routine. A standard reference for both the hospital record department and the doctor's office.
R: *Archives of Internal Medicine* 132: 143 (July 1973); *ARBA* (1972, p. 617).

Enzyme Handbook. 2 vols. **Thomas E. Barman.** New York: Springer-Verlag, 1969.

A concise guide to molecular data on enzymes.
R: *Science* 167: 860 (Feb. 6, 1970); Chen (p. 107); Wal (p. 203); Win (3EC4).

Enzyme Handbook Supplement 1. **Thomas E. Barman.** New York: Springer-Verlag, 1974.
R: Chen (p. 107).

Handbook for Foreign Medical Graduates. **Education Council for Foreign Medical Graduates.** Philadelphia, PA: Education Council for Foreign Medical Graduates, 1972.
Helpful to newly educated physicians from foreign countries. Contains practical information, stresses the need to acquire command of the English language, and covers all major problems encountered by foreign-educated physicians.
R: *Journal of Medical Education* 48: 876 (Sept. 1973).

Handbook for the Medical Secretary. 4th ed. **Miriam Bredow.** New York: McGraw-Hill, 1963.
Useful tool for experienced medical and dental secretaries and beginners. Includes Gregg shorthand drills.

Handbook of Biochemistry and Molecular Biology. 3d ed. **Gerald D. Fasman, ed.** Cleveland: Chemical Rubber, 1975–1976.
First edition, 1968; second edition, 1970.
The third edition appears in several sections: *Lipids, Carbohydrates, and Steroids Section,* volume 1, 1975; *Nucleic Acids Section,* 2 volumes, 1975; *Physical and Chemical Data Section,* 2 volumes, 1976; *Proteins Section,* 3 volumes, 1976.
A specialized supplement to the *Handbook of Chemistry and Physics* providing critical physical/chemical data, abbreviations and nomenclature for amino acids, peptides and proteins, purines, steroids, pyrimidines, nucleic acid, etc. Intended for use by researchers and graduate students.
R: *Journal of Chemical Education* 48: 5563 (Sept. 1971); *ARBA* (1971, p. 491); Chen (p. 107); Mal (9-63); Wal (p. 202); Win (2EC7; 3EC6).

Handbook of Engineering in Medicine and Biology. **David G. Fleming and Barry N. Feinberg, eds.** Cleveland: Chemical Rubber, 1976.
R: Chen (p. 109).

Handbook of Medical Library Practice. 3d ed. **Gertrude L. Annan and Jacqueline W. Felter, eds.** Chicago, IL: Medical Library Association, 1970.
First edition, 1943; second edition, 1956; fourth edition, forthcoming.
A basic handbook for medical librarians. Details administration, technical services, automation, archiving, planning, etc. Includes references, glossary of acronyms. Considered an indispensable reference.
R: *MRW* S2, p. 62; Win (EJ1; EK1; EK2; 2EJ2; 3EJ1; 3EJ3); Stearns & Ratcliff (*NEJM,* 1971).

Markets for the Medical Author: A Handbook of Over 500 Journal, Book and Paramedical Publishing Markets for the Medical Writer. **John G. Deaton.** St. Louis, MO: Warren H. Green, 1971.
Over 300 scientific journals alphabetically arranged by titles under 25 medical fields. Entries include address, types of materials suitable, and format for refer-

ences. Provides information on paramedical journals, house organs, medical newspapers, and book publishers. Appendix covers bibliographical preparation and MEDLARS. General index.
R: *MRW* S2, pp. 86, 110.

The Medical Transcriptionist Handbook. **Charles T. McConnico.** Springfield, IL: Charles C. Thomas, 1972.
Aimed at assisting medical transcriptionists with their training. Text is suitable for self-instruction. Familiarizes the transcriptionist with medical terms, the content of medical reports, medical synonyms, various medical procedures and instruments, etc. Material is somewhat oversimplified. Useful reference work also for individuals in the paramedical field.
R: *ARBA* (1973, p. 613).

1975 Handbook on Women Workers, US Department of Labor, Women's Bureau, Bulletin 297. **US Department of Labor, Women's Bureau.** Washington, DC: US Government Printing Office, 1975.
Collection of statistics on women outside the home. Twelve chapters document the progress made by women students and workers in the last decade. Also, clearly indicates inequalities still in existence. Part I deals with the status of women both in the labor force and enrolled in educational institutions. Laws governing women's employment are included in Part II. Final section describes existing institutions currently working on improving the plight of women outside the home. This handbook has much practical use for workers whose aim it is to eliminate employment and educational discrimination on the basis of sex.
R: *JAMWA* 32: 233 (June 1977).

Physicians' Desk Reference. 1st ed–. Oradell, NJ: Medical Economics, 1947–. Annual.
Thirty-fourth edition, 1980.
Outlines essential pharmaceutical information on some 2,500 products. Produced in cooperation with listed manufacturers. Volume concludes with pertinent data on signs, symptoms, and treatments of overdose. Valuable reference for physicians, nurses, pharmacists, and other allied health professionals.

Serving Physically Disabled People. **Ruth A. Velleman.** New York: Bowker, 1979.
Provides guidelines for librarians, helping them to provide information to the physically disabled.

Training of Medical Laboratory Technicians: A Handbook for Tutors, WHO Offset Publications, 21. **Alex McMinn and Graham J. Russell.** Geneva: World Health Organization, 1975.
Specifically designed as an aid for training medical laboratory tutors and as an instructional tool for medical laboratory personnel. Collection of data on theory, objectives, curriculum. Choice of media, assessment, and examinations. Additional discussions of proposed programs for training, examples of programmed learning schemes, and safety in the medical laboratory. References to additional reading listed.

R: *IBID* 3: 267 (Dec. 1975); *RSR* 4: 89 (Apr.–June 1976).

The UFAW Handbook on the Care and Management of Laboratory Animals. 5th ed. **Universities Federation for Animal Welfare.** Edinburgh: Churchill Livingstone, 1976.

First edition, 1949.
Practical guide to the care and management of laboratory animals. General information included in chapters 1–15: genetics, anesthesia, transportation, housing, euthanasia. Chapters 16–51 deal with specific animals. Includes data on husbandry, feeding, diseases, and treatment. Useful list of references complete the text.
R. Sheehy (EK45).

ALLERGY AND IMMUNOLOY

Handbook of Experimental Immunology. 3d ed. **D. M. Weir, ed.** Philadelphia, PA: J. B. Lippincott, 1978.

Second edition, 1973.
Volume 1, *Immunochemistry*; volume 2, *Cellular Immunology*; volume 3, *Application of Immunological Methods*.
New third edition. Emphasizes established and innovated techniques in comprehending and measuring the body's resistance to disease. Background immunological data enhances the "how-to" presentation of laboratory procedures.
Thoroughly revised chapters. Twelve additional contributors. New information on immunological methods in bacteriology, measurement of graft (vs. host) activity, tumor immunology. Added appendixes on mouse breeding techniques and biometrics.
R: *Archives of Pathology & Laboratory Medicine* 103: 368 (July 1979); *Immunology* 27: 341 (1974); 37: 288 (May 1979); *Lancet* 2: 1178 (November 24, 1973); *NEJM* 290: 637 (Mar. 14, 1974).

ANATOMY

Growth, Including Reproduction and Morphological Development. **Philip L. Altman and Dorothy S. Dittmer, comps. and eds.** Bethesda, MD: Federation of American Societies for Experimental Biology, 1962.

Handbook of Microscopic Anatomy for the Health Sciences. **Annabelle Cohen.** St. Louis, MO: C. V. Mosby, 1975.

Designed to acquaint nurses, technicians, and paramedical personnel with the introductory features of microscopic anatomy. Photomicrographs and diagrams of normal organs and tissues form the core. The usefulness of the book is enhanced by a comprehensive index. No references included. Helpful in public and high school libraries.
R: *RSR* 3: 34 (July–Dec. 1975).

Handbuch der Mikroskopischen Anatomie des Menschen. **W. V. Mollendorf and W. Bargmann, eds.** Berlin: Springer-Verlag, 1975.

Indispensable source of information on the structure of the allocortex. Bulk of book devoted to microscopical anatomy. The fields of comparative and quantita-

tive histology receive greater emphasis due to author's expertise. Although published in German, the outstanding micrographs, diagrams, and tables will make it widely accessible. Provides sound basis for further research in neuroscience fields dealing with the allocortex.
R: *Electroencephalography & Clinical Neurophysiology* 41: 448 (Oct. 1976).

Kimber-Gray-Stackpole's Anatomy and Physiology. 17th ed. **Marjorie A. Miller, Anna B. Drakontides, and Lutie C. Leavell.** Riverside, NJ: Macmillan, 1977.

A classic textbook for nurses and paramedics. Numerous excellent illustrations, emphasizes clinical subjects.

ANESTHESIOLOGY AND GENERAL SURGERY

The Anesthesiologist's Handbook. 2d ed. **Donald G. Catron.** Baltimore, MD: University Park Press, 1977.

Small paperback written for practicing anaesthetists. Does not bog reader down with unnecessary basic maneuvers or apparatus. Incorporates pharmacological, physiological, and pathological background material. Particularly useful to the specialist faced with an abnormal situation. Basic American publication; knowledge of transatlantic synonyms (especially for drugs) is desirable. Forty-three basic references adequately cover the subject matter.
R: *Anaesthesia* 32 (7): 682 (July 1977).

Handbook of Surgery. 5th ed. **John L. Wilson, ed.** Los Altos, CA: Lange Medical Publications, 1973.

Fourth edition, 1969.
Pocket-size handbook for students and physicians. Intended as a concise summary and quick reference to basic information in several specific areas of surgery, excluding technique. Includes many valuable tables and charts.
R: *American Family Physician* 10: 263 (Oct. 1974); *British Journal of Surgery* 61: 927 (Nov. 1974).

Principles and Practice of Obstetric Anaesthesia. 4th ed. **J. Selwyn Crawford.** Oxford, England: Blackwell Scientific Publications, 1978.

Authoritative and comprehensive compendium of all information on obstetric anesthesia. An exhausting list of references follow each of the eight chapters. Numerous diagrams, tables, and figures compliment the text. Handbook ends with details on personnel and equipment. Truly encyclopedic in scope; should be read by all practicing obstetric anesthesiologists and junior anesthetists.
R: *Anaesthesia* 34: 91 (Jan. 1979).

Standard Nomenclature of Diseases and Operations. 5th ed. **Edward T. Thompson and Adaline C. Hayden, eds.** National Conference on Medical Nomenclature. New York: Blakiston, 1961.

Preliminary printing, 1932; first edition, 1933; fourth edition, 1952.
Topographic and etiologic arrangement. Includes a disease and operations index.
R: Win (EK97).

Trauma Surgery. **Kimball I. Maull and Ward O. Griffen, Jr.** Garden City, NY: Medical Examination Publishing, 1977.

Brief explanations and ample references accompany the 1,000 multiple-choice questions in this handbook. Covers all areas of trauma surgery including general management, predictable complications, and obvious syndromes. Both text and journal article input guarantee its reasonable currency. Serves as an excellent review for surgical board examinations as well as an update for all levels of surgeons. Good self-assessment tool.
R: *Archives of Surgery* 112: 904 (July 1977).

BRAIN AND NERVOUS SYSTEM

Anatomy of the Central Nervous System in Review. **Donald H. Ford.** New York: American Elsevier, 1975.

A concise handy reference which presents information pertinent to the central nervous system. Contains numerous black and white illustrations helpful in emphasizing anatomical relationships. Clearly presented information, most helpful to neuroanatomists.
R: *Journal of Neurosurgery* 45: 239 (Aug. 1976).

Diagnostic Neuroradiology. 2d ed. 2 vols. **Juan M. Taveras and Ernest H. Wood.** Baltimore, MD: Williams & Wilkins, 1976.

Golden's Diagnostic Radiology Series, section 1.
Additional and elaborated information on neuroradiologic diagnosis, including procedures required in daily practice in this second edition. Covers pathology of cerebral angiograms, angiography of spinal cord, computerized axial tomography. Presents a state of the art of invasive neuroradiologic techniques.
R: *JAMA* 236: 2906 (Dec. 20, 1976).

Electrodiagnosis: A Handbook for Neurologists. **Mario P. Smorto and John V. Basmajian.** Hagerstown, MD: Harper & Row, 1977.

This is a handbook of electrodiagnosis. Subjects included are electromyography (EMG), equipment needs, comparison of EMGs, neuropathies, polymyositis, nerve conduction time, motor disturbance tests, among others. This handbook is considered one of the best available, and is recommended to all neurologists, psychiatrists, and medicial librarians for its clear style and excellent illustrations.
R: *Archives of Neurology* 36: 390 (June 1979); *Archives of Physical Medicine and Rehabilitation* 59: 102 (Feb. 1978); *Canadian Medical Association Journal* 116: 1125 (May 21, 1977); *Journal of Neurosurgery* 47: 303 (Aug. 1977).

Electronics for Neurobiologists. **Paul B. Brown, Bruce W. Maxfield, and Howard Moraff.** Cambridge, MA: MIT Press, 1973.

This handbook for neurobiologists explains basic electronics and electronic circuit theory. Emphasizes integrated circuits and modules as well as construction and maintenance of neurobiological testing equipment. Enables the researcher to adapt and construct equipment according to his/her needs.

Epilepsy Handbook. 2d ed. **Louis D. Boshes and Frederic A. Gibbs.** Springfield, IL: Charles C. Thomas, 1972.

This concise handbook of 33 chapters contains valuable information concerning various conditions of epilepsy. The chapters are short and serve to outline diagnosis and treatment of epilepsy. There are seventeen graphs which review facts of epilepsy through 1972. This compact handbook is recommended for specialists, general practitioners, and lay people who desire a source of useful knowledge concerning epilepsy.
R: *Archives of Internal Medicine* 131: 614 (Apr. 1973); 131: 758 (May 1973); *Journal of Neurosurgery* 38: 396 (Mar. 1973).

Handbook for Differential Diagnosis of Neurologic Signs and Symptoms. **Kenneth M. Heilman, Robert T. Watson, and Melvin Greer.** New York: Appleton-Century-Crofts, 1977.
Covers common neurological symptoms along with their respective pathological, anatomical, and physiological characteristics. Numerous tables accurately point to appropriate diagnostic possibilities. Three sections dominate: weakness; abnormalities of tone, coordination, posture, and movement; and cranial nerve dysfunction. Tabular information will serve as ready-reference for clinicians and residents faced with neurological deficits.
R: *Journal of Neurosurgery* 48: 660 (Apr. 1978).

Handbook of Clinical Neurology. Vols. 1–. **P. J. Vinken and G. W. Bruyn, eds.** Amsterdam: North Holland, New York: American Elsevier, 1969–.
Volume 36, 1979.
Comprehensive multivolume set (originally intended to be 36 volumes) on the subject. Covers such topics as sensation, pain, motor function, reflexes, eye movements, electromyography, autonomic nervous system, etc. Extensive bibliography follows each chapter. To facilitate usage, titles of selected volumes are Volume 1, *Disturbances of Nervous Functions*, 1969; volume 2, *Localization in Clinical Neurology*; volume 3, *Disorders of Higher Nervous Activity*, volume 4, *Disorders of Speech, Perception, and Symbolic Behaviour*; volume 24, *Metabolic and Deficiency Diseases of the Nervous System*, 1977; volume 25, *Injuries of the Spine and Spinal Cord*; volume 31, *Congenital Malformations of the Brain and Skull*, 1977.
R: *American Scientist* 62: 232 (Mar.–Apr. 1974); *Archives of Internal Medicine* 132: 459 (Sept. 1973); *Brain* 96: 44 (June 1973); 97: 811 (Dec. 1974); 98: 183 (Mar. 1975); 99: 160 (Mar. 1976); 99: 604 (Sept. 1976); 99: 795 (Dec. 1976); 101: 376 (June 1978); *Journal of Clinical Pathology* 32: 94 (Jan. 1979); 32: 312 (Mar. 1979); *Journal of Neurosurgery* 46: 694 (May 1977); *Neurology* 24: 99 (Jan. 1974); 27: 1184 (Dec. 1977); *Choice* 6: 996 (Oct. 1969); *ARBA* (1970, p. 135); Win (3EJ15).

Handbook of Drug and Chemical Stimulation of the Brain: Behavioural, Pharmacological and Physiological Aspects. **R. D. Myers.** New York: Van Nostrand Reinhold, 1974.
This excellent handbook provides a gold mine of information on the current knowledge of local application of drugs and chemicals to specific areas of the brain. Various aspects are reviewed including the theoretical, methodological, hormonal, reproductive. The roughly 1,400 references cover 61 pages. Contains many carefully selected figures, tables, and a subject and author index. The master summary tables are particularly useful; they provide critical data on volume, dose, species, site of application, the state of animals, and response. Provides a

comprehensive survey of clinical brain "stimulation" and is recommended to neuroscientists and all serious students in this field.
R: *American Scientist* 63: 105 (Jan/Feb 1975); *Electroencephalography & Clinical Neurophysiology* 40: 437 (Apr. 1976); 40: 555 (May 1976); *Journal of Nervous and Mental Disease* 162: 222 (1976); *Nature* 256: 242 (July 1975); *Quarterly Review of Biology* 51: 182 (1976); *Science* 190: 1196 (Dec. 19, 1975); *RSR* 3: 44 (Jan–March 1975).

Handbook of Neurochemistry. 7 vols. **Abel Lajtha, ed.** New York: Plenum, 1969–1972.

Volume 1, *Chemical Architecture of the Nervous System*, 1969; volume 2, *Structural Neurochemistry*, 1969; volume 3, *Metabolic Reactions in the Nervous System*, 1970; volume 4, *Control Mechanisms in the Nervous System*, 1970; volume 5A, 1971; volume 5B, *Metabolic Turnover in the Nervous System*, 1971; volume 6, *Alterations of Chemical Equilibrium in the Nervous System*, 1971; volume 7, *Pathological Chemistry of the Nervous System*, 1972.
An outstanding series for serious students of neurochemistry.
R: *Lancet* 1: 702 (Apr. 4, 1970); *New Scientist & Science Journal* (Dec. 9, 1971); *Choice* 6: 994 (Sept. 1969); *ARBA* (1973, p. 612); Win (EK93, 3EJ16).

Handbook of Neurologic Emergencies. **Desmond S. O'Doherty & Joseph L. Fermaglich.** Garden City, NY: Medical Examination Publishing, 1977.
Concise handbook which covers a wide variety of neurological problems. Emphasizes promptness of action in emergency situations, focusing on problem and disease orientation. Well illustrated, easy to use. Of value to family physicians.
R: *American Family Physician* 18: 255 (Nov. 1978).

Handbook of Sensory Physiology. Vols. 1–9. New York: Springer-Verlag, 1971–1978.
Volume 1, *Principles of Receptor Physiology*. W. R. Loewenstein, ed., 1971; volume 2, *Somatosensory System*. A. Iggo, ed., 1973; volume 3/1, *Enteroceptors*. E. Neil, ed., 1971; volume 3/2, *Muscle Receptors*. C. C. Hunt et al., eds., 1971; volume 3/3 *Electroreceptors and Other Specialized Receptors in Lower Vertebrates*. A. Fessard, ed., 1975; volume 4, *Chemical Sense*. L. M. Beidler, ed., 1971; volume 4/1, *Olfaction*, 1971; volume 4/2, *Taste*, 1971; volume 5/1, *Auditory Systems*. W. D. Keidel and W. D. Neff, eds., 1974; volume 5/2, 1975; volume 5/3, *Auditory System: Clinical and Special Topics*. W. D. Keidel and W. D. Neff, eds., 1976; volume 6/1, *Vestibular System*. H. H. Kornhuber, ed., 1974; volume 6/2, *Vestibular System: Psychophysics, Applied Aspects and General Interpretations*. H. H. Kornhuber, ed., 1975; volume 7/1, *Photochemistry of Vision*. H. J. Dartnell, ed., 1972; volume 7/2, *Physiology of Photoreceptor Organs*. M. G. Fuortes, ed., 1972; volume 7/3, *Central Processing of Visual Information*. R. Jung, ed., 1973; volume 7/4, *Visual Psychophysics*. D. Jameson and L. M. Hurvich, eds., 1972; volume 7/5, *The Visual System in Vertebrates*. F. Crescitelli, ed., 1978; volume 8, *Perception*. H. L. Teuber, ed., 1978; volume 9, *Development of Sensory Systems*. H. L. Teuber et al., 1978.
A multivolume, comprehensive, authoritative, and complete reference source book in the field of neurophysiology for researchers and graduate students in the field. Designed as an advanced text on the vestibular system and its disorders. Thorough coverage of various aspects of psychophysics, physiological responses to motion and vestibular system disorders. Extensive bibliography

follows each chapter. Useful textbook for advanced students, the specialist, and the researcher.
R: *American Journal of Ophthalmology* 77: 124 (Jan. 1974); *American Scientist* 61: 225 (Mar./Apr. 1973); 63: 108 (Jan.–Feb. 1975); 63: 582 (Sept.–Oct. 1975); 63: 712 (Nov.–Dec. 1975); *Annals of Otology, Rhinology and Laryngology* 84: 563 (1975); 84: 720 (1975); 85: 422 (1976); 87: 114 (1978); 87: 447 (1978); *Archives of Neurology* 28: 142 (Feb. 1973); 30: 424 (May 1974); *Brain* 96: 892 (Dec. 1973); 97: 420 (June 1974); 97: 612 (Sept. 1974); 98: 334 (June 1975); *British Journal of Ophthalmology* 58: 562 (May 1974); *Journal of Neurosurgery* 42: 736 (June 1975); *JAMA* 223: 1217 (Sept. 15, 1975); 234: 541 (Nov. 3, 1975); 238: 1413 (Sept. 6, 1977); *Nature* 254: 230 (Mar. 20, 1975); 275: 257 (Sept. 21, 1978); *NEJM* 291: 857 (Oct. 17, 1974); 293: 1375 (Dec. 25, 1975); *Physical Therapy* 55: 810 (1975); 56: 879 (1976); *Psychological Medicine* 14: 122 (Feb. 1974); *RSR* 3: 36 (July–Dec. 1975); Chen (p. 110).

Medical Neurology. 2d ed. **John Gilroy and John S. Meyer.** New York: Macmillan, 1975.

First edition, 1969.
Covers diseases and disorders of the nervous system and muscles. Great emphasis placed on pathogenesis, treatment, and diagnosis. Of particular value is the section on the neurologic examination. This second edition completely revises the chapters on pediatric neurology demyllinating diseases, muscle diseases, and degenerative diseases. Numerous charts, tables, and illustrations add value to this handbook. Recommended readings and extensive references are useful. Ready source of information for medical students and practicing physicians.
R: *Physical Therapy* 56: 760 (1976); *Choice* 7: 50 (Mar. 1970); *RSR* 4: 88 (Apr.–June 1976); *ARBA* (1971, p. 532); Allyn.

CARDIOVASCULAR SYSTEM

Basic Electrocardiography Handbook. **Leonard J. Lyon.** New York: Van Nostrand Reinhold, 1977.

A useful handbook for emergency electrocardiographic diagnosis, both acute and potentially fatal. Contains an appendix of well-explained terms, tips for recognizing common heart attack symptoms, how to detect a malfunctioning pacemaker. Recommended for physicians and paramedics in emergency room situations.
R: *ARBA* (1978, p. 718).

Cardiovascular Dynamics. 4th ed. **R. F. Rushmer.** Philadelphia, PA: W. B. Saunders, 1977.

Third edition, 1970.
A classic handbook of cardiologic physiology, with helpful illustrations. Covers normal functional aspects of the cardiovascular system.
R: *American Heart Journal* 92: 677 (1976); Allyn.

The EKG: Basic Techniques for Interpretation. **Jerome Passman and Constance Drummond.** New York: McGraw-Hill, 1976.

This book is useful for medical, nursing, and allied health personnel who desire a practical, self-instructional book which systematically outlines the procedure for analyzing the electrocardiogram. Two indexes, listing cardiac disorders and EKG abnormalities. One format facilitates quick, ready reference.

The Heart Attack Handbook: A Commonsense Guide to Treatment, Recovery, and Prevention. **Joseph S. Albert.** Boston, MA: Little, Brown, 1978.

DENTISTRY

Complete Dental Assistant's, Secretary's, and Hygienist's Handbook. **Charles A. Reap, Jr.** West Nyack, NY: Parker, 1973.

Essential information for the dental assistant, covering a wide spectrum of dental office practices. Includes worksheets, photographs.
R: *ARBA* (1974, p. 631).

Dental Practitioner Handbooks. No. 1–. Chicago, IL: Year Book Medical Publishers, 1965–.

Second edition, 1976–.
Number 1, *Silver Amalgam in Clinical Practice,* 1976; number 2, *Gingivitis,* 1977; number 4, *Orthodontic Diagnosis,* 1975; number 8, *Orthodontic Treatment for the Adult,* 1969; number 13, *Full Dentures,* 1977; number 18, *The Maxillary Sinus and Its Dental Implications,* 1977; number 22, *Preventive Dentistry,* 1976; number 24, *Endodontics in Clinical Practice,* 1976; and, number 25, *Orthodontic Treatment With Removable Appliances,* 1977.

Handbook for Dental Identification: Techniques in Forensic Dentistry. **Lester L. Luntz and Phyllys Luntz.** Philadelphia, PA: J. B. Lippincott, 1973.

A concise, well-illustrated guide to forensic dental techniques.

Handbook For Dental Surgery Assistants and Other Ancillary Workers. 2d ed. **S. Gelbier and M. A. H. Copley.** Chicago, IL: Year Book Medical Publishers, 1978.

Handbook of Dental Photography. **Troy E. Daniels and Claude A. Sherrill.** San Francisco, CA: University of California, 1974.

Intended for beginners interested in clinical photography. Sections deal with selection of equipment, principles of photography, and clinical use of camera. Valuable references to literature on more complex techniques are included. Also contains a glossary of technical terms.
R: *Journal of Oral Surgery* 33(4): 311 (Apr. 1975).

Handbook of Medical Emergencies in the Dental Office. **Stanley F. Malamed.** St. Louis, MO: C. V. Mosby, 1978.

Summarizes pertinent medical information on emergencies occurring in the dental office. Six specific situations are scrutinized: unconsciousness, respiratory difficulty, convulsive seizures, local anesthetic reactions, drug reactions, and chest pains. Each emergency is organized by patient's symptoms.

Handbook of Orthodontics. 3d ed. **Robert E. Moyers.** Chicago, IL: Year Book Medical Publishers, 1973.

Oral Diagnosis: A Handbook of Modern Diagnostic Techniques Used to Investigate Clinical Problems in Dentistry. 2d ed. **W. R. Tyldesley.** Oxford, England: Pergamon, 1978.

Covers techniques of examination and laboratory tests in dentistry.
R: *Nature* 274: 294 (July 20, 1978).

Swenson's Complete Dentures. 6th ed. **Carol O. Boucher, ed.** St. Louis, MO: C. V. Mosby, 1970.

Describes the process of making a complete set of dentures from patient counseling to relining old dentures. Integrates theory and technique in step-by-step illustrated instructions. Extensive subject bibliographies, glossary, index.

DERMATOLOGY

Funktionelle Dermatologie. **G. Stuttgen and H. Schaefer.** Berlin: Springer-Verlag, 1974.

Summarizes enormous amounts of information pertaining to skin. Tables are extremely helpful in providing normal values for almost every chemical constituent. Embraces the development, morphology, pharmacology, pathology, and therapy of skin. Diagnostic index included. Reviews information gathered over the past twenty years. Sections on endocrinology, enzymology, and nucleic acid metabolism are well written. Useful work for the beginner and expert reader.
R: *Journal of Anatomy* 122: 479 (Nov. 1976).

ENDOCRINOLOGY

Diagnostic Endocrinology. **Philip E. Cryer.** New York: Oxford University Press, 1976.

Timely handbook of current diagnostic procedures in endocrinology; emphasizes radioimmunoassay techniques and systematic accounts of the endocrine glands. Summarizes gland disorders, although thorough discussion of treatment is absent from this book. Recommended as an accurate, up-to-date reference for the field of diagnostic endocrinology.
R: *American Family Physician* 15: 291 (Mar. 1977).

Endocrinology. Vol. 6. **American Physiological Society.** Baltimore, MD: Williams & Wilkins, 1975.

Handbook of Endocrine Tests in Adults and Children. **Robert N. Alsever and Ronald W. Gotlin.** Chicago, IL: Year Book Medical Publishers, 1975.

Handbook of Endocrinology: Diagnosis and Management of Endocrine and Metabolic Disorders. 2d ed. **Richard S. Dillon.** Philadelphia, PA: Lea & Febiger, 1973.

Originally prepared for the University of Pennsylvania house staff. Encyclopedic coverage of the diagnosis and treatment of endocrine and metabolic disorders. Includes excellent chapter on diabetes. Presents multiple viewpoints and a strong bibliography. Contains exhaustive tables. Quick reference source for student, general internist and specialist in diabetes or thyroidology.
R: *Annals of Internal Medicine* 80: 436 (Mar. 1974); *BMJ* 2: 736 (June 29, 1974).

Handbuch des Diabetes Mellitus. **Ernst F. Pfeiffer, ed.** Munich, Germany: J. F. Lehmanns Verlag, 1971.

A two-volume publication written in German and English. Volume I, published in 1968, deals with theoretical foundations for the study of diabetes. Volume II approaches the scientific and clinical aspects of diabetes mellitus. Volume II consists of 56 chapters. A note-worthy detail deals with the epidemiology of diabetes. This encyclopedic coverage of diabetes mellitus covers 1,400 pages of which 100 pages serve as an index. Contains up-to-date references, well-reproduced illustrations and tables. Valuable tool for departments of pathology, obstetrics, pediatrics, internal medicine, and public health.
R: *Archives of Internal Medicine* 131: 311 (Feb. 1973).

Metabolism. **Philip L. Altman and Dorothy S. Dittmer, comps. and eds.** Bethesda, MD: Federation of American Societies for Experimental Biology, 1968.

GASTROINTESTINAL SYSTEM

The Esophagus Handbook and Atlas of Endoscopy. **M. Savary and G. Miller.** Solothurn, Switzerland: Verlag Gassmann AG, 1978.

This handbook, intended for use by gastroenterologists, contains information of diagnosis and treatment of esophageal disorders. There are 310 endoscopic photographs, which are of high quality, as well as 71 instructive anatomical drawings. These illustrations are frequently accompanied by pertinent radiographic and pathological materials. The book has copious references, many from foreign texts and journals. It is recommended to gastroenterologists of all levels for its instructiveness and easily deciphered text.
R: *Gastroenterology* 75: 926 (Nov. 1978).

GENETICS

Biochemical Methods in Medical Genetics. **S. Kelly.** Springfield, IL: Charles C. Thomas, 1977.

An excellent laboratory handbook of biochemical procedures for diagnosing genetic disorders of metabolism. Includes chromatographic techniques, reviews basic terminology, and gives detailed descriptions of test procedures. There are tables useful for summary. Recommended for laboratory technicians.
R: *American Journal of Human Genetics* 30: 451 (July 1978).

Catalog of Teratogenic Agents. **T. H. Shepard.** Baltimore, MD: Johns Hopkins University Press, 1973.

Emphasis on special toxic mechanisms. Represents the printout type of publication.
R: *Clinical Pharmacology and Therapeutics* 15: 227 (1974).

Handbook of Enzymes Electrophoresis in Human Genetics. **Harry Harris and D. A. Hopkinson.** Amsterdam: North-Holland, 1976.

Practical laboratory guide for all concerned with enzyme electrophoresis. Concise discussions of more than 70 enzymes, with additional chapters on staining tech-

niques, principles of electrophoresis, and interpretation of enzyme patterns. Photographs of stained gels provided. Loose-leaf format.
R: *American Journal of Human Genetics* 29: 115 (Jan. 1977); *BMJ* 1: 515 (Feb. 1977); *Nature* 263: 534 (Oct. 7, 1976); Chen (p. 109).

Handbook of Genetics. 5 vols. **R. C. King, ed.** New York: Plenum, 1974–1976.

Volume 1, *Bacteria, Bacteriology, and Fungi*; volume 2, *Plants, Plant Viruses and Protists*; volume 3, *Invertebrates of Genetic Interest*; volume 4, *Vertebrates of Genetic Interest*; volume 5, *Molecular Genetics.*
Considered a valuable reference on topics in genetics. Volumes are uniformly high in quality and serve as useful information sources for a wide range of medical and biological researchers.
R: *American Journal of Human Genetics* 28: 429 (July 1976); *Heredity* 41: 246 (Oct. 1978); *Nature* 256: 153 (July 10, 1975); 266: 570 (Apr. 7, 1977); *Science* 188: 283 (July 25, 1975); 189: 283 (July 1975); Chen (p. 109).

Handbook of Mutagenicity Test Procedures. **B. Kilbey et al., eds.** New York: Elsevier, 1977.

Handbook of Teratology. 4 vols. **James G. Wilson and F. Clarke Fraser, eds.** New York: Plenum, 1977–1979.

Volume 1, *General Principles and Etiology*, 1977; volume 2, *Mechanisms and Early Pathogenesis*, 1977; volume 3, *Maternal, Comparative and Epidemiologic Aspects*, 1978; volume 4, *Research Procedures and Data Analysis*, 1979.
This four-volume treatise offers an integrated source of facts, concepts, methods, and references in the broad field of teratology. Provides the graduate student and investigator with a background of the major areas of current research interest.
R: *American Journal of Human Genetics* 30: 93 (Jan. 1978); 30: 669 (1978); *American Scientist* 66: 374 (May–June 1978); *Heredity* 41: 409 (Dec. 1978); *Lancet* 2: 336 (Aug. 13, 1977); *Nature* 273: 325 (May 25, 1978).

GERONTOLOGY

Geriatric Psychiatry: A Handbook for Psychiatrists and Primary Care Physicians. **Leopold Bellak and Toksoz B. Karasu.** New York: Grune & Stratton, 1976.

Handbook of Aging and the Social Sciences. Robert H. Binstock & Ethel Shanas, eds., 1976; *Handbook of the Psychology of Aging.* James E. Birren & K. Warner Schaie, eds., 1977; *Handbook of the Biology of Aging.* Caleb E. Finch & Leonard Hayflick, eds., 1977.
R: *Journal of Gerontology* 33: 769 (Sept. 1978); 33: 770 (Sept. 1978); *Quarterly Review of Biology* 53: 20 (1978).

Handbook of Aging Series. 3 vols. **James E. Birren, ed.** New York: Van Nostrand Reinhold, 1976–1977.

The Management of Geriatric Cardiovascular Disease. **Raymond Harris.** Philadelphia, PA: J. B. Lippincott, 1970.

Focuses on cardiology problems connected with age, particularly of the elderly. Highlights the differences between the young and the old cardiac patient. Well-chosen illustrations and tables compliment the text. Fills a void in the literature for many allied health personnel and all professionals who handle aging patients.
R: *Journal of the American Geriatrics Society* 19: 652 (1971); *JAMA* 216: 523 (Apr.–June 1971); Brandon.

HEALTH SERVICES ADMINISTRATION

Consent Handbook. **H. Rutherford Turnbull, ed.** Washington, DC: American Association on Mental Deficiency, 1977.

Delivers information on consent issues, particularly those which deal with mentally retarded citizens. The book has a conceptual approach, presenting an outline of the purposes of informed consent doctrines and reviews the framework applicable to consent decisions. Recommended to both consumers and professionals.
R: *American Journal of Psychiatry* 135: 148 (Jan. 1978); *Physical Therapy* 58: 1409 (1978).

Control of Hospital Infection: A Practical Handbook. **E. J. L. Lowbury et al., eds.** London: Chapman & Hall, 1975.

Emphasizes practical aspects on the control of hospital infection such as sterilization, disinfection, and cleaning procedures. This excellent book is recommended for doctors, nurses, physiotherapists for its convenient layout and good coverage of subject matter.
R: *British Journal of Surgery* 63: 838 (Oct. 1976); *Lancet* 1: 727 (April 3, 1976); *ABL* (May 1976).

Crisis Center/Hotline: A Guidebook to Beginning and Operating. **Ursula Delworth, Edward H. Rudow, and Janet Taub.** Springfield, IL: Charles C. Thomas, 1972.

The Design of a Health Maintenance Organization: A Handbook for Practitioners. **Allan Easton, ed.** New York: Praeger Publishers, 1975.

An economic and sociological survey of health maintenance organizations, geared to future planning of additional HMOs. Certain limitations are present in the marketing approach to the subject presented here. Intended for students, though price is high considering the quality.
R: *Medical Care* 15: 265 (Mar. 1977).

Discharge Planning Handbook. **Bernita M. Steffl and Imogene Eide.** Thorofare, NJ: Charles B. Slack, 1978.

Attempts to provide guidelines for implementing patient discharge. Includes sample protocols, managerial strategies. Educationally oriented; for nurses, social workers, and administrators.
R: *Supervisor Nurse* 10: 73 (May 1979).

Handbook of Biomedical Instruments and Measurement. **Harry E. Thomas.** New York: Appleton-Century-Crofts, 1974.

Updates Thomas's 1967 *Handbook*. Technical information on hospital electronic instrumentation. Amply illustrated with diagrams, charts, and tables. Geared toward operating personnel as well as biomedical engineers and attending physicians.

A Handbook of Human Service Organizations. **Harold W. Demone, Jr., and Dwight Harshbarger.** New York: Behavioral Publications, 1974.

Details organizational and administrative theories as they relate to human service organizations. Discusses planning of medical facilities, bringing together a broad scope of information. A notable source, useful to administrators of health organizations.
R: *Journal of Allied Health* 4: 35 (Winter 1975); *NEJM* 291: 1198 (Nov. 28, 1971).

Handbook on Hospital-Associated Infections. Vol. 1–. **Willson J. Fahlberg & Dieter Groschel, eds.** New York: Marcel Dekker, 1978–.

Volume 1, *Occurrence, Diagnosis, and Sources of Hospital-Associated Infections*, 1978; volume 3, *Hospital-Associated Infections in the General Hospital Population and Specific Measures of Control*, 1979.
A treatise which surveys aspects of hospital related infections, contributions coming from international sources. Provides historical background of subject, methods of quality control. Includes references. Useful for students involved in all levels of health care. Intended to be a ten-volume series.
R: *Journal of Clinical Pathology* 32: 637 (June 1979).

HMO Handbook: A Guide for Development of Prepaid Group Practice HMOs. **John R. Kress and James Singer.** Germantown, MD: Aspen Systems Corp., 1975.

Outlines the planning of health maintenance organizations. Written by experienced planners. Helpful in establishing guidelines in setting up health maintenance and prepaid medical care organizations.
R: *Nation's Health* 6: 6 (1976); 7: 5 (1977).

Hospital Engineering Handbook. Chicago, IL: American Hospital Association, 1974.

Contains information on staff organization, management, and health care facility maintenance.

Infection Control in the Hospital. 4th ed. Chicago, IL: American Hospital Association, 1979.

A handbook of hospital infection control.

Insurance Handbook for the Medical Office. **Marilyn T. Fordney.** Philadelphia, PA: W. B. Saunders, 1977.

Designed as a learning tool and reference source for those involved in medical or dental insurance billing. Introductory material is followed by various forms of insurance: Blue Cross and Blue Shield, Medicaid, Medicare, etc. A listing of review questions and principal consultants with their affiliations concludes each chapter. More than 150 illustrations in the form of tables, line drawings, and

sample letters enhance its usefulness. A handy tool for all medical office personnel.
R: *ARBA* (1978, p. 717).

HEMATOLOGY

Blood and Other Body Fluids. **Dorothy S. Dittmer, ed.** Bethesda, MD: Federation of American Societies for Experimental Biology, 1961.

Blood Disorders Due to Drugs and Other Agents. **R. H. Girdwood, ed.** Amsterdam, Holland: Excerpta Medica Foundation, 1973.

A useful handbook of drug interactions. Helpful for legal and humanistic matters.
R: *Clinical Pharmacology and Therapeutics* 15: 227 (1974).

Clinical Hematology. 7th ed. **Maxwell M. Wintrobe, et al.** Philadelphia, PA: Lea & Febiger, 1974.

First edition, 1942; sixth edition, 1967.
Seventh revised edition of this classic hematology text, reorganized into six major sections which accommodate new material. The coverage is encyclopedic: classification of anemias, pathology, disorders and normalities of the hematopoietic system, morphological classification, among other subjects. Recommended to both student and teacher.
R: *American Journal of Diseases of Children* 129: 1364 (Nov. 1975); *JAMA* 232: 759 (May 19, 1975); Allyn; Stearns & Ratcliff (*NEJM*, 1969); Stearns & Ratcliff (*NEJM*, 1970).

Current Haematology. 5th ed. **R. D. Eastham.** Chicago, IL: Year Book Medical Publishers, 1977.

A pocket-size handbook containing brief information on the main aspects of hematology: definitions, classifications, pathology. Does not discuss laboratory techniques or clinical symptoms. Intended for rapid reference, listing specific abnormalities of hematology.
R: *Canadian Medical Association Journal* 119: 698 (Oct. 7, 1978).

Handbook of Hemophilia. 2 vols. **K. M. Brinkhous and H. C. Hemker, eds.** Amsterdam: Excerpta Medica, 1975. Distributed by New York: American Elsevier.

In two volumes, topics are divided into well-organized chapters. The handbook covers a wide range of topics within hematology, employs useful graphs and tables. A multi-authored reference book, recommended especially for teaching hospitals.
R: *American Journal of Human Genetics* 28: 430 (July 1976); *Annals of Internal Medicine* 84: 512 (Apr. 1976); *Journal of Clinical Pathology* 29: 468 (1976); *NEJM* 294: 1244 (May 27, 1976).

INFECTIOUS DISEASES

Catalogue of Arthropod-Borne Viruses of the World: A Collection of Data on Registered Arthropod-Borne Animal Viruses, Public Health Service Pub. no.

1760. **Richard M. Taylor, comp.** US Public Health Service. Washington, DC: US Public Health Service, 1967.
A handbook which contains standardized information of 204 arthropod-borne viruses. Includes physical, chemical, antigenic, and pathogenetic factors as well as geographic distribution and symptoms of human infection. Helpful to allergists, specialists in infectious disease.
R: *MRW* S1, p. 15.

Communicable and Infectious Diseases: Diagnosis, Prevention, Treatment. 8th ed. **Franklin H. Top and Paul F. Wehrle, eds.** St. Louis, MO: C. V. Mosby, 1976.
Seventh edition, 1972.
Complete, ready reference handbook dealing with communicable disease vectors, diagnosis, treatment, and prevention. Includes helpful tables and illustrations.
R: *American Family Physician* 16: 161 (Aug. 1977); *TBRI* 43: 308 (Oct. 1977); Allyn; Stearns & Ratcliff (*AJN*).

Craig and Faust's Clinical Parasitology. 8th ed. **Ernest C. Faust et al.** Philadelphia, PA: Lea & Febiger, 1970.
R: Allyn.

Handbook for the Differential Diagnosis of Infectious Disease. **Jonas A. Shulman.** New York: Appleton-Century-Crofts, 1979.
Consists of extensive charts listing causes, clinical course, and suggested treatment for common infectious diseases. Symptom-oriented for quick reference.

Handbook of Microbiology. **Morris B. Jacobs and Maurice J. Gerstein.** Princeton, NJ: Van Nostrand Reinhold, 1960.

Handbook of Microbiology. 4 vols. **Allen I. Laskin and Hubert A. Lechevalier, eds.** Cleveland, OH: Chemical Rubber Company, 1973–1974.
Volume 1, *Organismic Microbiology*, 1973; volume 2, *Microbial Composition*, 1973; volume 3, *Microbial Products*, 1974; volume 4, *Microbial Metabolism, Genetics and Immunology*, 1974.
A handbook of four volumes providing current data on microbiology; covers a wide range of subjects in varying depth. Topics included are taxonomy, metabolism, genetics, and immunology of microbiological organisms.
R: *American Scientist* 62: 490 (July/Aug. 1974); *Journal of the Medical Society of New Jersey* 71: 241 (Mar. 1974); *New Scientist* 41: 88 (Jan. 10, 1974); *TBRI* 40: 155 (Apr. 1974); 40: 199 (May 1974); Chen (p. 109); Mal (9-53).

Toxic and Hallucinogenic Mushroom Poisoning: A Handbook for Physicians and Mushroom Hunters. **Gary Lincoff, D. H. Mitchel, and Wilbur K. Williams, eds.** New York: Van Nostrand Reinhold, 1977.

Tropical Diseases: A Handbook for Practitioners. **Kevin M. Cahill.** Westport, CT: Technomic Publishing, 1976.
Contains core knowledge on tropical infections. Covers selected bacterial, viral treponemal, and richettsial infections, with pertinent information on life cycles.

Pathology, epidemiology, clinical symptoms, and therapy. Aimed at primary physicians and residents unfamiliar with common parasitic diseases.
R: *American Family Physician* 16: 307 (Nov. 1977); *Nation's Health* 6: 4 (Aug. 1976); *Nation's Health* 6: 5 (Nov. 1976).

Zinsser Microbiology. 16th ed. **Wolfgang K. Joklik and Hilda P. Willett, eds.** New York: Appleton-Century-Crofts, 1976.

First edition, 1910; 15th edition, 1972.
Sixteenth edition of Zinsser's original 1910 work. Introductory material arranged in seven basic sections: immunology, medical bacteriology, basic virology, clinical virology, bacterial physiology, medical mycology, and parasitology. Selected reading list follows each chapter. Lucid charts, graphs, and illustrations enhance the volume. Extensive index. Aimed at medical students, instructors, and practicing physicians.
R: *ARBA* (1977, p. 719); Allyn.

INTERNAL MEDICINE

Accidents and Emergencies: A Practical Handbook for Personal Use. 2d ed. **R. H. Hardy.** London: Oxford University Press, 1978.

First edition, 1976.
Covers common conditions encountered in accident departments. Excellent handbook, arranged in alphabetical order. Useful for medical students, nurses, general practitioners, and emergency room staff.

Acupuncture and Moxibustion: A Handbook for the Barefoot Doctors of China. **Wei Sheng T'ing. Martin E. Silverstein et al., trans.** New York: Schocken Books, 1975.

Discusses common techniques and usages of acupuncture and moxibustion. An authoritative translation of one of the instruction manuals used by Chinese medical practitioners. Recommended for medical libraries with interest on this topic.
R: *Choice* 12: 1332 (Dec. 1975).

American Red Cross Advanced First Aid and Emergency Care. **American National Red Cross.** Garden City, NY: Doubleday, 1973.

Standard textbook of advanced emergency care and first aid measures. Comprehensive coverage of simple first aid for shock, wounds, poisoning, burns, emergency rescue, etc., as well as additional specialized topics like childbirth. Eighteen chapters; complete index.
R: *ARBA* (1974, p. 1629).

American Red Cross Standard First Aid and Personal Safety. **American National Red Cross.** Garden City, NY: Doubleday, 1973.

Standard reference for emergency care and first aid measures. Contains basic instruction for the general care of emergency cases: burns, wounds, shock, poisoning, etc. Information gleaned from the division of Medical Sciences, National Academy of Sciences–National Research Council and numerous medical authorities. More than 200 simple color drawings. Despite some discrepancies in proce-

dure, the handbook contains reliable information. Ready reference for general public.
R: *ARBA* (1974, p. 630).

CRC Handbook Series in Clinical Laboratory Science. Cleveland, OH: Chemical Rubber Company, 1977–.
Section F: *Immunology*, Vol. 1. 1978.
Section I: *Hematology*, Vol. 1. 1979.

Clinical and Biochemical Analysis Series. 8 vols. New York: Marcel Dekker, 1974-1978.
Volume 1, *Colorimetric and Fluorimetric Analysis of Organic Compounds and Drugs.* M. Pesez and J. Bartos, 1974; volume 2, *Normal Values in Clinical Chemistry: Determination, Definition and Use.* H. F. Martin et al., 1975; volume 3, *Continuous Flow Analysis: Theory and Practice.* William B. Furman, 1976; volume 4, *Handbook of Enzymatic Methods of Analysis.* George Guibault, 1976; volume 5, *Handbook of Radioimmunoassay.* Guy E. Abraham, ed., 1977; volume 6, *Hemoglobinopathies: Techniques of Identification.* Titus H. J. Huisman and J. H. P. Jonxis, 1977; volume 7, *Automated Immunoanalysis.* Robert F. Ritchie, ed., 1978; volume 8, *Computers in the Clinical Laboratory: An Introduction.* E. Clifford Toren, Jr., and Arthur A. Eggert, 1978.
R: *Journal of Clinical Pathology* 31: 503 (May 1978) (pertains only to volume 5).

Critical Care Medicine Handbook. **M. H. Weil and H. Shubin, eds.** Baltimore, MD: Williams & Wilkins, 1974.
A compendium of information on crises in critical care medicine, more a reference work than a handbook. This volume is divided into eight sections, each of which deal with a specific crisis. Sections vary in quality, but the book will be useful to those who familiarize themselves with the information that is well organized and detailed.
R: *Anaesthesiology* 45: 373 (Sept. 1976).

Drug Dosage in Laboratory Animals: A Handbook. **C. D. Barnes and L. G. Eltherington.** Berkeley, CA: University of California Press, 1973.
Furnishes toxicologic dosage information for over 200 drugs used in biomedical research. Drugs listed have major pharmacological classification and are listed largely in alphabetical order. Trade and common names are supplied and cross-referenced in the index. The handbook contains a good sampling of available data and is recommended to the investigator and graduate student as a source of reference.
R: *Archives of Pathology & Laboratory Medicine* 97: 404 (June 1974).

Emergency Care Handbook: How to Deal With People in Emergencies. **Arthur R. Ciancutti.** Westport, CT: Technomic Publishing, 1978.
Contains much vital information for those who deal with emergency care. Written succinctly, the author describes many situations, symptoms, and treatments for emergency situations. Recommended to nurses, physicians, firefighters, and police officers.

R: *Canadian Medical Association Journal* 119: 1284 (Dec. 9, 1978); *Occupational Health Nursing* 27: 62 (Jan. 1979).

Emergency-Room Care. 3d ed. **Charles Eckert, ed.** Boston, MA: Little, Brown, 1976.

A ready reference handbook of emergency room care. Well illustrated, covers a wide range of emergency situations. Considered one of the best such handbooks available in both hardcover and paperback.
R: *JAMA* 236: 1296 (Sept. 13, 1976).

Handbook of Automated Electronic Clinical Analysis. **Harry E. Thomas.** Reston, VA: Reston Publishing, 1979.

State of the art handbook on medical instrumentation. Covers a wide range of methods, including hemodialysis, electrolyte measurements, continuous flow analysis, and chromatography.
R: *Choice* 16: 1057 (Oct. 1979).

Handbook of Laboratory Safety. 2d ed. **Norman V. Steere.** Cleveland, OH: Chemical Rubber Company, 1971.

First edition, 1967.
Comprehensive reference on the methods of recognizing and preventing laboratory hazards.
R: *Journal of Chemical Education* 48: A676 (Oct. 1971); *TBRI* 38: 20 (Jan. 1972); Chen (p. 101); Win (2ED11).

Handbook of Medical Treatment. 16th ed. **Milton J. Chatton, ed.** Los Altos, CA: Lange Medical Publications, 1979.

Thirteenth edition, 1972; fourteenth edition, 1974.
A handy general reference tool for those involved in patient care. Updated from earlier editions. Includes concise and recent information on a wide range of diseases. Well recommended as a ready source of information.
R: *Annals of Internal Medicine* 79: 477 (Sept. 1973); *ARBA* (1974, p. 630; 1975, p. 739); Allyn.

Handbook of Microbiological Investigations for Laboratory Animal Health. **J. R. Needham.** New York: Academic Press, 1979.

Contains a complete laboratory and animal health care program.

Handbook of Micromethods for the Biological Sciences. **Georg Keleti and William H. Lederer.** New York: Van Nostrand Reinhold, 1974.

A handbook of laboratory methods which deal specifically with biochemical or microbiological techniques. Comprises a handy compilation of data. Highly recommended for researchers in biochemistry, pharmacology, and microbiology.
R: *Clinical Chemistry* 20: 634 (1974); *Growth* 38: 395 (Sept. 1974).

Handbuch der Inneren Medizin. Vols. 1–. New York: Springer-Verlag, 1968–.

Volume 3, 1974.
R: *Gastroenterology* 70: 143 (Jan. 1976).

Human Health and Disease. **Philip L. Altman and Dorothy D. Katz, eds.** Bethesda, MD: Federation of American Societies for Experimental Biology, 1977–.

Volume 2, *Biological Handbooks,* 1977.

A general reference for clinical medicine, intended to be published one volume per year. Numerous tables, graphs, and diagrams. Multiple contributors.

R: *Gastroenterology* 74: 637 (Mar. 1978); *Nature* 272: 472vi (Mar. 30, 1978); Sheehy (EK14).

The International Handbook of Medical Science. 2d ed. **David Horrobin and Alexander Gunn, eds.** Baltimore, MD: University Park Press, 1972.

First edition, 1970.

Billed as a fine introduction to general medicine. Contains reviews of advances in clinical medicine and some basic sciences; succinct essays on many common drugs; an extensive guide to modern treatment and a section on general information (many tables). Each topic is handled by a respected international authority in that field. Recommended for a medical library collection and junior and senior clinicians.

R: *Annals of Internal Medicine* 78: 161 (Jan. 1973); *Archives of Internal Medicine* 132: 772 (Nov. 1973); *JAMA* 215: 646 (1971); *Lancet* 2: 346 (Aug. 15, 1970); *Choice* 8: 202 (Apr. 1971); *ARBA* (1972, p. 618).

Interpretation of Diagnostic Tests: A Handbook Synopsis of Laboratory Medicine. 3d ed. **Jacques B. Wallach.** Boston, MA: Little, Brown, 1978.

Second edition, 1974.

Designed as a practical aid to the physician in the proper selection and correct interpretation of clinical laboratory tests. This unique volume covers all areas of clinical pathology. Second edition contains extensive pediatric material. The mass of information is organized into 68 tables. The 59-page subject index efficiently helps retrieve this vital data.

R: *Gastroenterology* 68: 420 (Feb. 1975).

Physician's Handbook. 18th ed. **Marcus A. Krupp et al.** Los Altos, CA: Lange Medical Publications, 1976.

Seventeenth edition, 1973.

Mini-encyclopedia on diagnostic and therapeutic information and procedures. Work is arranged in 33 chapters, covering many disease conditions. Minimum amount of theory; instead stresses diagnosis. Appropriate data on examinations, laboratory tests, and procedures included. Appendix outlines information on staining methods, desirable weight tables, conversion charts, and normal laboratory values. Superior pocket reference for practicing physicians and medical students.

R: *Annals of Internal Medicine* 81: 280 (Aug. 1974); *Clinical Pediatrics* 15: 909 (Oct. 1976); *ARBA* (1977, p. 718); Allyn.

Travel Medicine: A Handbook for Practitioners. **Anthony C. Turner.** Edinburgh: Churchill Livingstone, 1975.

Provides the physician with practical advice for his traveling patients.

R: *Lancet* 2: 486 (Sept. 13, 1975); *Journal of the Royal Society of Health* 96: 137 (June 1976); *TBRI* 42: 350 (Nov. 1976).

NURSING

Army Medical Department Handbook of Basic Nursing. **US Department of the Army.** Washington, DC: US Government Printing Office, 1972.

Intended for Army medical personnel, but also helpful for civilians, this book serves as a ready reference to such basic medical topics as anatomy, disease, physiology, pharmacology.
R: *ARBA* (1973, p. 619).

Comprehensive Cardiac Care: A Text For Nurses and Other Health Professionals. 4th ed. **Kathleen Andreoli et al.** St. Louis, MO: C. V. Mosby, 1979.
R: Stearns & Ratcliff (*AJN, NEJM,* 1970).

The Drug, the Nurse, the Patient. 6th ed. **Mary W. Falconer et al.** Philadelphia, PA: W. B. Saunders, 1978.

The sixth edition of this handbook keeps pace with the current changes in the nursing field, taking a patient-centered approach. The 1978–1980 drug handbook, which provides ready reference to 1,500 drugs, is included at the end of the text.
R: *Nursing Care* 9: 30 (Aug. 1976); *ARBA* (1978, p. 729).

Fundamentals of Public Health Nursing. **Kathleen M. Leahy and Marguerite Cobb.** New York: McGraw-Hill, 1966.
R: Stearns & Ratcliff (*AJN*).

Handbook for Radiologic Technologists and Special Procedures Nurses in Radiology. **Nieta W. Powell.** Springfield, IL: Charles C. Thomas, 1974.

Ready reference to patient care, instrumentation, and sterile techniques. Outlines basic radiologic procedures for technologists and special procedures nurses in radiology.

Handbook of Cardiology For Nurses: Heart Disease and Its Treatment, the Patient and His Nursing Care. 5th ed. **Walter Modell et al.** New York: Springer Publishing, 1966.
R: Stearns & Ratcliff (*AJN*).

Intravenous Medications: A Handbook For Nurses and Other Allied Health Personnel. 2d ed. **Betty L. Gahart.** St. Louis, MO: C. V. Mosby, 1977.
R: *American Journal of Nursing* 74: 85 (Jan. 1974).

McGraw-Hill Handbook of Clinical Nursing. **Margaret E. Armstrong et al.** New York: McGraw-Hill, 1979.
R: Brandon (*NO*).

Modern Intravenous Therapy Procedures: A Handbook for Nurses and Other

Allied Health Personnel. **William J. Kurdi.** Century City, CA: Medical Education Consultants, 1976.

The Nurse's Drug Handbook. 2d ed. **Suzanne Loebl et al.** New York: John Wiley, 1980.

Handbook deals comprehensively with pharmacological concepts in nursing. Describes drugs, includes all details on contraindications, dosage, etc. Well written and organized. Useful for both the student and the practicing nurse.
R: *Modern Health Care* 7: 67 (June 1977); *Nurse Educator* 3: 28 (July–Aug. 1978).

Nurses' Handbook of Fluid Balance. 3d ed. **Norma Metheny and William D. Snively.** Philadelphia, PA: J. B. Lippincott, 1979.

First edition, 1967; second edition, 1974.
Updated edition presents basic knowledge of fluid balance problems in patients. Emphasizes practical applications. Reviews physiology, systematic discussions of fluid disturbances. A good reference source for recent developments in the field.
R: Brandon (*NO*).

The Nurse's Materia Medica. 3d ed. **John Gibson.** Oxford, England: Blackwell Scientific Publications, 1973.

Lists over 400 drugs including name, dosage, action, and side effects. Also provides abbreviations, metric system equivalents, and children's dosage chart. Index is included.
R: *MRW* S3, p. 20.

Pharmacological Basis of Patient Care. 3d ed. **Mary K. Asperheim and Laurel A. Eisenhauer.** Philadelphia, PA: Saunders, 1977.

Pharmacology in Nursing. 14th ed. **Betty S. Bergerson.** St. Louis, MO: C. V. Mosby, 1979.

Thirteenth edition, 1976.

NUTRITION

CRC Handbook of Food Additives. 2d ed. **Thomas E. Furia, ed.** Cleveland, OH: Chemical Rubber Company, 1972.

First edition, 1968.
Covers various data on additives based on FDA standards. Each chapter, written by chemists, includes definitions, chemical properties and reactions, representative uses, and safety inhibitors. Also includes a guide to current regulations for frequently used additives.
R: *Food Technology* p. 108 (Apr. 1973); *Journal of Food Technology* 9: 125 (Mar. 1974); *TBRI* 40: 269 (Sept. 1974); *ARBA* (1974, p. 655); Chen (p. 117); Wal (p. 485).

Handbook of Diet Therapy. 5th ed. **Dorothea Turner.** Chicago, IL: University of Chicago Press, 1970.

Contains data on food composition and nutritional requirements. Clearly presented, concise information emphasizes optimal nutrition regiments in normal

and therapeutic situations. Includes references, suggestions for food preparation. Recommended to dietitians, science and public libraries.
R: *ARBA* (1972, p. 634); Stearns & Ratcliff (*AJN*).

Handbook of Food Preparation. 7th ed. Washington, DC: American Home Economics Association, 1975.
First edition, 1946; fifth edition, 1964; sixth edition, 1971.
Practical guide to food preparation. Buying guides, baking temperatures, cooking instructions, government meat standards, etc.
R: *ARBA* (1976, p. 748); Chen (p. 111); Win (3EK11).

Handbook of Human Nutritional Requirements. New York: Unipub, 1974.
R: Chen (p. 111).

Handbook of Lipid Research. **H. F. DeLuca, ed.** New York: Plenum, 1978.
Volume 2, *The Fat-Soluble Vitamins.*
Review of current research concerning fat-soluble vitamins, including mechanisms of absorption, distribution in nature, metabolism, mechanisms of action, and relationships to disease states.
R: *American Journal of Clinical Nutrition* 32: 1555 (July 1979); *Nutrition Reviews* 36: 316 (Oct. 1978).

Handbook of Nutrition and Food: Diets, Culture Media and Food Supplements Section. **Miloslav Rechcigl, Jr., ed.** Cleveland: Chemical Rubber, 1976.

Handbook of the Nutritional Content of Foods. **US Department of Agriculture.** New York: Dover, 1963. Reprint. 1975.
Original title, *Composition of Foods.*
R: *ARBA* (1976, p. 750); Chen (p. 111).

Handbook of Vitamins and Hormones. **R. Kutsky.** New York: Van Nostrand Reinhold, 1973.
A summary of information about vitamins and hormones, and their place in the drug industry.
R: Chen (p. 111).

Handbook on Human Nutritional Requirements, FAO Nutritional Studies No. 28; WHO Monograph Series No. 61. **R. Passmore et al.** New York: United Nations Bookshop, 1974.
Monograph sponsored jointly by Food and Agriculture Organization of the United Nations and World Health Organization reviews human nutritional requirements for individuals at various stages of the life cycle. Summarizes recommendations regarding intake of energy, protein, vitamins, and minerals in layman's terms. Useful for instructors and students of nutrition, nursing, sociology. Data are accurate and put together in a handy volume.
R: *American Journal of Clinical Nutrition* 32: 501 (Feb. 1979); *JAMA* 233: 825 (Aug. 18, 1975); *Nutrition* 29: 120 (Mar.–Apr. 1975); *Choice* 12: 1598 (Feb. 1976); *IBID* 3: 35 (Mar./June 1975); Chen (p. 111).

The Heinz Handbook of Nutrition. 2d ed. **Benjamin T. Burton.** New York: McGraw-Hill, 1965.
Comprehensive treatise on nutrition in health and disease. Introductory material on principles of nutrition.

Laboratory Handbook of Methods of Food Analysis. 2d ed. **R. Lees.** Cleveland, OH: Chemical Rubber Company, 1971.
A practical guide for the food industry worker or anyone learning the rudiments of food analysis. Gives methods of sampling, lab techniques, and testing procedures.
R: *Chemistry and Industry* (Oct. 2, 1971); *Food Engineering* (Oct. 1973); Chen (p. 118).

Modern Food Analysis. **Frank Leslie Hart and Harry J. Fisher.** New York: Springer-Verlag, 1971.
A laboratory handbook for the testing of food composition, including food analysis, standards, adulteration tests, etc. Aimed at the food chemist and analyst.
R: *Food Technology* 25: 86 (Oct. 1971); Chen (p. 118).

A Physician's Handbook on Orthomolecular Medicine. 2d printing. **Roger J. Williams and Dwight K. Kalita, eds.** New York: Pergamon, 1977.
Discusses optimum concentration of minerals, trace elements, hormones, amino acids, and other nutritional substances in the body. This handbook presents the latest review in the field; maintains a multidisciplinary approach. Useful to physicians in all branches of medicine.

Recommended Dietary Allowances. 8th ed. **Dietary Allowances Committee & Food & Nutrition Board, US National Academy of Sciences.** Washington, DC: National Academy of Sciences, 1974.
First edition, 1943; seventh edition, 1968.
Includes a table of recommended daily dietary allowances, listing calories and nutrients according to sex and age. Relates the physiological and biochemical bases for dietary allowances of each specific nutrient. References included.
R: Sheehy (EK33); Win (EK177).

ONCOLOGY AND NUCLEAR MEDICINE

Cancer Chemotherapeutic Agents: Handbook of Clinical Data. **Mike R. Sather et al., eds.** Boston, MA: G. K. Hall, 1979.
Details the significant effects, toxicities, solubilities, stabilities, and pharmacokinetics of 37 cancer chemotherapeutic agents. Outlines various drug acronyms and protocols used in cancer chemotherapy. Quick reference format aimed at physicians, pharmacists, and nursing personnel.

Cancer Handbook of Epidemiology and Prognosis. **J. A. H. Waterhouse.** Edinburgh: Churchill Livingstone, 1974.
A worthy book which provides facts concerning the incidence of cancer in the United Kingdom. Material is succinctly presented, with helpful graphs and classifications of disease. Data is from the Birmingham Regional Cancer Registry. A

handy reference, which will provide answers to the questions of both the researcher and the clinician.
R: *British Journal of Radiology* 47: 629 (1974); *British Journal of Surgery* 62: 168 (Feb. 1975); *BMJ* 3: 182 (July 20, 1974); *Journal of Obstetrics and Gynaecology of the British Commonwealth* 81: 655 (Aug. 1974); *Proceedings of the Royal Society of Medicine* 67: 1196 (Nov. 1974); *TBRI* 41: 57 (Feb. 1975); 41: 111 (Mar. 1975).

Handbook of Cancer Immunology. 5 vols. **Harold Waters, ed.** New York: Garland Publishing, 1978.

Volume 1, *Basis Cancer-Related Immunology*; volume 2, *Cellular Escape From Immune Destruction*; volume 3, *Immune Status in Cancer Treatment and Prognosis, Part A*; volume 4, *Immune Status in Cancer Treatment and Prognosis, Part B*; volume 5, *Immunotherapy.*
A five-volume treatise written by established authorities. Presents an overview of cancer immunology in animal and human systems. Thorough, comprehensive, detailed.
R: *Immunology* 37: 914 (Aug. 1979); *Nature* 279: 742 (June 21, 1979).

WHO Handbook for Standardized Cancer Registries, WHO Offset Publications, 25. **World Health Organization.** Geneva: World Health Organization, 1976.

Handbook based on recommendations of three WHO expert consultations which are concerned with recording cancer data. Core data is that concerned with identification of the patient and description of the cancer, while optional data is important for hospital needs such as planning.
R: *IBID* 4: 349 (Dec. 1976).

OPHTHALMOLOGY

Handbook of Lasers with Selected Data on Optical Technology. **Robert J. Pressley, ed.** Cleveland, OH: Chemical Rubber Company, 1971.

Published and unpublished works concerned with laser research and development. Data presented as of summer 1970. Charts, tables, and graphs illustrate the handbook. Index of wavelengths is a special feature.
R: *MRW* S2, p. 61.

Handbook of Pediatric Ophthalmology. **Stephen S. Feman.** New York: Grune & Stratton, 1978.

Management of Ocular Injuries. **David Paton and Morton F. Goldberg.** Philadelphia, PA: W. B. Saunders, 1976.

Superb working handbook to the most current and best management procedures for diagnosis and treatment of ocular trauma. Eleven sections containing 22 handy tables and a bibliography of 255 references make up this timely book. Many step-by-step diagrams and well-chosen headings point to a practical and efficient handbook. Provides a practical resource for nonophthalmologists in industrial health or emergency situations and for practicing ophthalmologists.
R: *American Journal of Ophthalmology* 82: 805 (Nov. 1976).

Ocular Differential Diagnosis. 2d ed. **Frederick H. Roy.** Philadelphia, PA: Lea & Febiger, 1975.

Ready reference to almost 600 signs and symptoms of ocular diagnosis.

ORTHOPEDICS

Orthopaedic Surgery. **Edward L. Compere.** Chicago, IL: Year Book Medical Publishers, 1974.

Essentially a handbook of basic orthopedic surgical procedures. Reflects the author's personal preference of surgical techniques. Although some reviewers question the narrowness of this publication, the high-quality illustrations reinforce its usefulness. Good orthopedic surgical material for physical medicine and rehabilitation personnel.

R: *Archives of Physical Medicine and Rehabilitation* 56: 462 (Oct. 1975); *British Journal of Surgery* 62: 415 (May 1975).

Shands' Handbook of Orthopaedic Surgery. 9th ed. **H. Robert Brashear.** St. Louis, MO: C. V. Mosby, 1978.

Collection of fundamental principles and facts of orthopedic surgery. Reflects recent advances in chronic arthritis, tumors, congenital deformities, cerebral palsy, etc. The bibliography lists the most recent references available. Includes new illustrations.

R: *Physical Therapy* 59: 925 (July 1979).

OTORHINOLARYNGOLOGY

The Artificial Larynx Handbook. **Shirley Salmon and Lewis P. Goldstein.** New York: Grune & Stratton, 1978.

An informative book which present facts concerning the use of artificial communication devices. Provides much information not found elsewhere. For otolaryngologists and speech therapists.

R: *Lancet* 1: 1062 (May 19, 1979).

Audiological Handbook of Hearing Disorders. **Stephen V. Prescod.** New York: Van Nostrand Reinhold, 1978.

PATHOLOGY

A Beginner's Handbook in Biological Electron Microscopy. **Brenda S. Weakley.** Baltimore, MD: Williams & Wilkins, 1972.

A concise handbook for the electron microscope technician, this book emphasizes practice rather than theory: it covers embedding and thin sectioning techniques, routine maintenance, darkroom techniques. Includes references. Intended primarily for the beginner.

R: *NEJM* 288: 110 (Jan. 11, 1973).

Cell Biology. **Philip L. Altman and Dorothy D. Katz, comps. and eds.** Bethesda, MD: Federation of American Societies for Experimental Biology, 1976.

Handbook of Histology. 5th ed. **Karl A. Stiles.** New York: McGraw-Hill, 1968.

Handbook of Molecular Cytology. **A. Lima-de-Faria, ed.** New York: Wiley-Interscience, 1969.
Frontiers of Biology, volume 15.
R: *American Scientist* 59: 765 (Nov./Dec. 1971); Chen (p. 110).

Handbuch der Allgeminen Pathologie. Vols. 1–. Berlin: Springer-Verlag, 1955–.

A comprehensive, multivolume compendium with massive information. Chapters are mostly in German. An excellent reference tool for those who can read German with ease. A monumental work.
R: *Growth* 39: 553 (Dec. 1975); 40: 203 (June 1976); *Journal of Gerontology* 28: 516 (Oct. 1973).

PEDIATRICS

Accident and Emergency Paediatrics. **H. B. Valman.** Philadelphia, PA: J. B. Lippincott, 1976.

Emphasis on readily available information on the management of emergency and accident cases for medical and nursing staffs working in these departments. Convenient, pocket-size book.
R: *Clinical Pediatrics* 17: 717 (Sept. 1978).

Current Pediatric Therapy. 8 vols. **Sydney S. Gellis and Benjamin M. Kagan, eds.** Philadelphia, PA: W. B. Saunders, 1976.

Ready access to such topics as pediatric pharmacology, bronchial asthma, and contact dermatitis are included in this pediatric handbook. Issued biennially, this edition will be helpful to the practicing pediatrician.
R: *American Family Physician* 9: 197 (June 1974); *Canadian Medical Association Journal* 102: 1114 (May 23, 1970); Allyn; Stearns & Ratcliff (*NEJM,* 1969; *NEJM,* 1970).

Handbook of Common Poisonings in Children, DHEW Pub. no. (FDA) 76-7004. **US Food and Drug Administration.** Washington, DC: US Government Printing Office, 1977.

Incorporates materials provided by the American Academy of Pediatrics. Lists only 73 toxic substances; however, these account for seventy to eighty percent of all pediatric poisonings. Handbook contains an excellent section on general management of acute poisonings and a detailed index (lists both generic and trade names of substances). Useful information for pediatricians, emergency room personnel, pharmacists, and parents.
R: *ARBA* (1978, p. 726).

Handbook of Neonatal Respiratory Care. **Thomas J. Williams, ed.** Riverside, CA: Bourns, 1975.

Handbook of Pediatrics. 13th ed. **Henry K. Silver, C. Henry Kempe, and Henry B. Bruyn.** Los Altos, CA: Lange Medical Publications, 1979.
Ninth edition, 1971; tenth edition, 1973; eleventh edition, 1975.
A pocket-size handbook with concise and ready information on subjects related to pediatrics. Intended for the practicing physician and medical student. A good supplement to pediatric texts.
R: *American Journal of Diseases of Children* 126: 862 (Dec. 1973); *Archives of Internal Medicine* 134: 791 (Oct. 1974); *British Journal of Surgery* 63: 167 (Feb. 1976); *Clinical Pediatrics* 15: 352 (Apr. 1976); *Physical Therapy* 54: 552 (1974); *ARBA* (1972, p. 620; 1977, p. 717).

The Harriet Lane Handbook: A Manual for Pediatric House Officers. 8th ed. **Jerry A. Finkelstein, ed.** Chicago, IL: Year Book Medical Publishers, 1978.
Revised edition contains standard laboratory values, drug dosages, growth tables. Also includes many charts, outlines of procedures. Pocket-size edition; considered an indispensable ready reference.
R: *American Journal of Diseases of Children* 128: 267 (Aug. 1974).

Pediatric and Adolescent Echocardiography: A Handbook. **Stanley J. Goldberg, Hugh D. Allen, and David J. Sahn.** Chicago, IL: Year Book Medical Publishers, 1975.
Emphasizes pediatric echocardiography, but much of the material is equally applicable to adult echocardiography. The volume critically analyzes the echocardiogram, differentiates between normal and abnormal results, and stresses pitfalls in technique and interpretation. All illustrations are authentic strip-recorder echocardiograms of the highest quality. Tables of measurable criteria appear in appropriate sections. Provides a self-assessment section to test reader's knowledge of diagnosis. Light, breezy style makes for very easy reading. Long list of references encourages supplemental reading. Recommended as a practical manual for beginning echocardiographers and a reference source for experienced echocardiographers.
R: *American Journal of Diseases of Children* 130: 1283 (Nov. 1976); *Annals of Internal Medicine* 83: 918 (Dec. 1975); *Archives of Internal Medicine* 137: 539 (Apr. 1977); *NEJM* 295: 845 (Oct. 7, 1976).

Pediatric Dosage Handbook. 2d ed. **Harry C. Shirkey.** Washington, DC: American Pharmaceutical Association, 1979.
First edition, 1973.
Concentrates on the dosage requirements for infants and children. "Table of Pediatric Drugs, Their Dosage, Cautions and Contradictions for Use, and Their Available Dosage Forms" comprises the bulk of the volume. Indexed by subject. Aimed at physicians, nurses, dentists, and pharmacists.
R: *ARBA* (1972, p. 632).

Pediatric Neurology Handbook. 2d ed. **J. T. Jabour et al., eds.** Flushing, NY: Medical Examination Publishing, 1976.
First edition, 1973.
Contains much basic information presented in a simplified manner. Discusses all

major topics, provides photographs. Most useful to residents seeking quick, unreferenced information.
R: *American Journal of Diseases of Children* 126: 718 (Nov. 1973); *Archives of Neurology* 29: 286 (Oct. 1973); *Neurology* 27: 597 (June 1977).

Quick Reference to Pediatric Emergencies. 2d ed. **Delmer J. Pascoe and Moses Grossman, eds.** Philadelphia, PA: J. B. Lippincott, 1978.

First edition, 1973.
A ready reference handbook for pediatricians confronted with emergency situations. Arranged topically, covers commonly confronted situations such as coma, smoke inhalation, battered child syndrome. Provides, for each listed condition, definition, clinical diagnosis, names of drugs used in treatment. Includes complete index, appendixes of essential equipment, emergency resources, etc.
R: *American Journal of Diseases of Children* 128: 428 (Sept. 1974); *ARBA* (1975, p. 741).

PHARMACY AND PHARMACOLOGY

American Drug Index. Philadelphia, PA: J. B. Lippincott, 1956–. Annual.

An annual listing of American pharmaceuticals. Alphabetically arranged by generic name. Correlates proprietary information, dosage, forms, manufacturers information. A handy ready reference for those who work with pharmaceuticals. A basic tool.
R: *Annals of Internal Medicine* 91: 344 (Aug. 1979); *RSR* 3: 38 (July–Dec. 1975); 4: 108 (July–Sept. 1976); *ARBA* (1971, p. 541; 1972, p. 632; 1973, p. 623; 1974, p. 644; 1978, p. 728); Win (EK201).

Clinical Handbook of Psychopharmacology. **Albert DiMascio and R. I. Shader, eds.** New York: Science House, 1970.

Readable text offering a collection of articles by authoritative clinicians in psychopharmacology. Based on accepted practices in the Massachusetts mental health system, this work compares and examines theoretical and clinical aspects of the field. Suitable for student and professional.

The Compleat Herbal: Being a Description of the Origins, the Lore, the Characteristics, the Types, and the Prescribed Uses of Medicinal Herbs, Including an Alphabetical Guide to All Common Medicinal Plants. **Ben C. Harris.** Barre, MA: Barre Publishers, 1972.

A reliable guide to herbal medicine, outlines history of use and lore of medicinal plants. Includes directions for preparing herbs.
R: *ARBA* (1973, p. 617).

Cutting's Handbook of Pharmacology: The Actions and Uses of Drugs. 6th ed. **T. Z. Csaky.** New York: Appleton-Century-Crofts, 1979.

A ready reference guide to important drugs, listing drugs according to therapeutic group. The handbook supplies information on chemistry, history, toxicity, structural formula, and mechanisms of drugs arranged so that compounds can be easily compared.

Drug Interactions. 4th ed. **Philip D. Hansten.** Philadelphia, PA: Lea & Febiger, 1979.

First edition, 1971; second edition, 1973.
Outstanding source of information on drug-drug interactions. Arranged in two sections: drug-drug interactions, and effects of drugs on clinical laboratory results. New fourth edition features important drug-food interactions.
R: *Pharmaceutical Journal* 212: 473 (1974); Win (EK182).

Drug Interactions: A Handbook of Clinical Use. **Stanley N. Cohen and Marsha F. Armstrong.** Baltimore, MD: Williams & Wilkins, 1974.

Contains detailed information on drug interactions and mechanisms, which is outlined in table form. Information is pertinent to clinicians, pharmacists, physicians and is easily retrieved.

Drug Interactions Index 1978/79. **Eric W. Martin.** Philadelphia, PA: J. B. Lippincott, 1979. Annual.

An up-to-date manual which, in outline form, presents interactions of 900 widely prescribed drugs. Cross references drugs with reactable substances, provides brief descriptions. Flexible binding for convenient handling. The first edition, 1978/79, is a reprint from Martin's book, *Hazards of Medication.*
R: *Annals of Internal Medicine* 91: 342 (Aug. 1979).

The Drugs Handbook. **Paul Turner and Glyn Volans.** New York: Macmillan, 1977.

Alphabetical listing of therapeutic drugs gives both generic and approved names. Describes briefly drug uses and effects. A cross-referenced index. Intended primarily for nurses, medical secretaries, and other auxiliary staff.
R: *Nature* 274: 624iv (Aug. 10, 1978); *ABL* 13: entry 395 (Sept. 1978).

Drugs in Current Use and New Drugs. 25th ed. **Walter Modell, ed.** New York: Springer Publishing, 1979. Annual.

First edition, 1955.
Annual alphabetical listing of drugs in compact handbook form. Classic compendium contains information on description, preparation, uses of drugs. The handbook is concise and comprehensive but has limitations; one might find it necessary to use other drug indexes along with the latest edition.
R: *ARBA* (1971, p. 540; 1972, p. 631; 1973, p. 621; 1976, p. 739).

Facts and Comparisons. St. Louis, MO: Facts and Comparisons, 1979.

In three formats: loose-leaf format, updated monthly; microfiche, updated monthly; and hardbound, updated annually.
Supplies comprehensive information on all drugs. Organized by therapeutic use, contains much current information including cost index, dosage information, contraindications, patient information.
R: *American Journal of Nursing* 79: 1321 (July 1979); *Journal of School Health* 49: 232 (Apr. 1979).

Handbook of Clinical Drug Data. 4th ed. **James E. Knoben, Philip O. An-**

derson, and **Arthur S. Watanabe.** Hamilton, IL: Drug Intelligence Publications, 1978.

Third edition, 1973.

Excellent tabular presentation of drugs and their indications, contraindications, and reactions. Convenient size makes it clearly a handbook. Data compilations and drug reviews comprise the two parts. References to more in-depth topics are of special value. Superb index.

R: *American Journal of Nursing* 74: 758 (Apr. 1974); *Annals of Internal Medicine* 81: 135 (July 1974); 89: 582 (Oct. 1978).

Handbook of Drug Interactions. 3d ed. **Edward A. Hartshorn.** Hamilton, IL: Drug Intelligence Publications, 1976.

Handbook of Drug Interactions. **Gerald Swidler.** New York: John Wiley, 1971.

This handbook is a compilation of useful information about drug-drug interactions. Although not comprehensive, it includes 1,300 drugs, arranged alphabetically usually by trade name of the drug. Some drawbacks: unpopular in foreign countries due to American proprietary names; information supplied by pharmaceutical manufacturers; and usefulness is questionable unless there are frequent revisions. Despite these inherent shortcomings, it will serve as a quick reference source for a busy pharmacist or physician.

R: *Archives of Internal Medicine* 132: 302 (Aug. 1973); *ARBA* (1972, p. 632).

Handbook of Nonprescription Drugs. 6th ed. Washington, DC: American Pharmaceutical Association, 1979.

Fourth edition, 1973; fifth edition, 1977.

Comprehensive reference source for data, guidance, and product composition on over-the-counter drugs. Covers some 1,500 drugs and related products. Thirty-two chapters feature illustrations, tables, and anatomical drawings. Of special interest are the 50 product tables supplying data on some 2,000 frequently used products. Includes literature references. Intended primarily for pharmacists and allied health professionals.

R: *Modern Health Care* 7: 83 (March 1977); *ARBA* (1978, p. 731); Sheehy (EK37).

Handbook of Practical Pharmacology. **Sheila A. Ryan and Bruce D. Clayton.** St. Louis, MO: C. V. Mosby, 1977.

Handbook of Psychopharmacology. Vol. 1–. **Leslie L. Iverson, Susan D. Iverson, and Solomon H. Snyder, eds.** New York: Plenum, 1975–.

Section 1, *Basic Neuropharmacology*: volume 1, *Biochemical Principles and Techniques in Neuropharmacology*, 1975; volume 2, *Principles of Receptor Research*, 1975; volume 3, *Biochemistry of Biogenic Amines*, 1975; volume 4, *Amino Acid Neurotransmitters*, 1975; volume 5, *Synaptic Modulators*, 1975; volume 6, *Biogenic Amine Receptors*, 1975. Section 2, *Behavioral Pharmacology in Animals*: volume 7, *Principles of Behavioral Pharmacology*, 1977; volume 8, *Drugs, Neurotransmitters, and Behavior*, 1977; volume 9, *Chemical Pathways in the Brain*, 1978. Section 3, *Human Psychopharmacology*: volume 10, *Neuroleptics and Schizophrenia*, 1978; volume 11, *Stimulants*, 1978; volume 12, *Drugs of Abuse*, 1978; volume 13, *Biology of Mood and*

Antianxiety Drugs, 1978; volume 14, *Affective Disorders: Drug Actions in Animals and Man,* 1978.
R: *American Journal of Psychiatry* 136: 470 (Apr. 1979); 136: 1003 (July 1979); 136: 1005 (July 1979); *Brain* 100: 204 (Mar. 1977); *Lancet* 2: 352 (Aug. 12, 1978); 2: 972 (Nov. 4, 1978); *Nature* 264: 299 (Nov. 18, 1976); 267: 292 (May 19, 1977); 277: 674 (Feb. 22, 1979); *Pharmaceutical Journal* 222: 90 (1979); 222: 117 (1979); *Quarterly Review of Biology* 54: 216 (June 1979).

Handbook on Injectable Drugs. **Lawrence A. Trissel.** Washington, DC: American Society of Hospital Pharmacists, 1977.
Handbook of over 150 injectable drugs available in the United States. Arranged alphabetically by generic name.
R: *Pharmaceutical Journal* 220: 184 (Feb. 25, 1978).

Handbuch der Experimentellen Pharmakologie/Handbook of Experimental Pharmacology. Vols. 1–. New York: Springer-Verlag, 1950–.
Volume 51, 1978.
R: *American Heart Journal* 98: 139 (July 1979); *American Scientist* 64: 222 (Mar.–Apr. 1976); *BMJ* 1: 1008 (Apr. 14, 1979); 2: 487 (Aug. 25, 1979); *Journal of Pharmaceutical Sciences* 67: 744 (May 1978); *Pharmaceutical Journal* 223: 45 (July 14, 1979); *Quarterly Review of Biology* 54: 76 (Mar. 1979).

Index-Handbook of Ototoxic Agents 1966–1971. **E. Louisa Worthington et al.** Baltimore, MD: Johns Hopkins University Press, 1973.
A compilation of all information concerning ototoxic agents that was published between 1966 and 1971. It is truly an index, containing well-organized summaries of 732 papers on ototoxic agents. Part I is a categorical arrangement of ototoxic agents. Part II deals with the effects of ototoxic agents, and part III outlines the species affected by ototoxic agents. Additional bibliographic information to entire papers can be found in the extensive citation section (732 references). Especially written to alert physicians to potential dangers of ototoxic drugs.
R: *Archives of Otolaryngology* 99: 156 (Feb. 1974); *Clinical Pharmacology and Therapeutics* 15: 227 (1974); *Pediatrics* 53: 774 (May 1974).

Index Nominum 1978/79. 1st ed.–. **Swiss Pharmaceutical Society, ed.** Berne, Switzerland: Swiss Pharmaceutical Society, 1956–. Irregular.
Ninth edition, 1978.
R: *Journal of Pharmaceutical Sciences* 63: 1176 (July 1974); 65: 162 (Jan. 1976); *Pharmaceutical Journal* 222: 16 (1979).

Martindale: The Extra Pharmacopoeia. 27th ed. **Ainley Wade and James E. F. Reynolds, eds.** London: Pharmaceutical Press, 1977.
Comprehensive reference source of information on drugs used throughout the world. Sections cover drugs in current use, over-the-counter medicine, directory of manufacturers, index to clinical use, and general index. Valuable for pharmacists as well as professionals and students in health-related and scientific fields. Recommended for all library collections.
R: *Journal of Pharmaceutical Sciences* 66: 1664 (Nov. 1977).

The Merck Index: An Encyclopedia of Chemicals and Drugs. 9th ed. **M. Windholz et al., eds.** Rahway, NJ: Merck and Co., 1976.

First edition, 1889.
Alphabetical listing of some 10,000 chemicals, drugs, and related biological products. Index characterized by descriptive monographs outlining structural forms, chemical properties, toxicity, medical and veterinary uses, and dosages. Includes literature references. Geared toward chemists, biochemists, pharmacists, botanists, and other health science professionals.
R: *Pharmaceutical Journal* 219: 357 (1977).

Pharmaceutical Handbook. 19th ed. London: Pharmaceutical Press, 1979.

Eighteenth edition, 1970.
Incorporates the *Pharmaceutical Pocket Book.*

Physicians Desk Reference to Pharmaceutical Specialties and Biologicals. Oradell, NJ: Medical Economics, 1946–. Annual.

Provides prescription information on major pharmaceutical products. Lists over 2,500 products. Includes manufacturers index.
R: Win (EK199).

Prescriber's Guide to Drug Interaction. **Jack M. Rosenberg.** Oradell, NJ: Medical Economics, 1978.

Up-to-date, handy guide to various categories of drug interactions. Drugs are divided into 23 categories, including alcohol, vitamins, and barbiturates. Categories are prefaced with general introductory material. Intended for physicians, nurses, and pharmacists.
R: *Modern Healthcare* 9: 74 (Jan 1979).

Toxicology of Drugs and Chemicals. 4th ed. **William B. Deichmann and Horace W. Gerarde.** New York: Academic Press, 1969.

Third edition, 1964.
Concentrates on the toxicity of industrial chemicals and drugs. Ready reference source of information on adverse effects, treatments, and overdoses. Complete with index outlining organs particularly affected.
R: Win (EK222; 3EJ34).

The United States Dispensatory. 27th ed. **A. Osol et al.** Philadelphia, PA: J. B. Lippincott, 1978.

First edition, 1833.
A classic reference for physicians, pharmacists. Alphabetically arranged, supplies technical information on drugs and drug compounds.
R: *Pharmaceutical Journal* 212: 221 (1974); *ARBA* (1974, p. 643); Win (EK208).

PHYSICAL MEDICINE AND REHABILITATION

Disability and Rehabilitation Handbook. **Robert M. Goldenson, Jerome R. Dunham, and Charles S. Dunham, eds.** New York: McGraw-Hill, 1978.

Handbook of Adult Rehabilitative Audiology. **Jerome G. Alpiner, ed.** Baltimore, MD: Williams & Wilkins, 1978.

Brings together material relating to adult hearing loss and the rehabilitative process. Includes Dr. Alpiner's famous "Denver Scale of Communication Function" and the "Denver Scale of Communication Function for Senior Citizens Living in Retirement Centers." Students will find the sample tests and measurement scales particularly helpful for a complete examination of the hearing handicapped.

Handbook of Physical Medicine and Rehabilitation. 2d ed. **Frank H. Krusen et al., eds.** Philadelphia, PA: W. B. Saunders, 1971.

First edition, 1965.
A basic reference source in physical medicine. Considered essential in core reference collections.
R: Allyn; Brandon; Stearns & Ratcliff (*AJN*; *NEJM*, 1969; *NEJM*, 1970).

Handbook of Speech Pathology and Audiology. Rev. ed. **Lee E. Travis, ed.** New York: Appleton-Century-Crofts, 1971.

First edition, 1957.
Revised and updated handbook of speech pathology in five parts: concepts of communication, multifaceted discussion of hearing loss, processes of voice communication, extensive explanation of speech disorders, language and related disorders. Well recommended for beginners in the field.
R: *Choice* 8: 1649 (Feb. 1972); *ARBA* (1972, p. 622); Stearns & Ratcliff (*NEJM*, 1970).

Sexual Options for Paraplegics and Quadriplegics. **Thomas O. Mooney, Theodore M. Cole, and Richard A. Chilgren.** Boston, MA: Little, Brown, 1975.

Presents information on sexuality and sexual techniques for disabled persons. Five chapters written in easily understood terms. Tasteful illustrations and a glossary of terms increase the handbook's usefulness. Much useful information for disabled persons as well as health team members faced with this sensitive area of rehabilitation.
R: *Canadian Nurse* 72: 63 (Aug. 1976).

PSYCHIATRY AND PSYCHOLOGY

Adult Assessment: A Source Book of Tests and Measures of Human Behavior. **Richard S. Andrulis.** Springfield, IL: Charles C. Thomas, 1977.

A complete source book of adult behavior, emphasizes important issues in testing and assessment. Includes legal guidelines, reference materials, tools, and strategies. Recommended primarily for practitioners and counselors.

American Handbook of Psychiatry. 2d ed. 6 vols. **Silvano Arieti, ed.** New York: Basic Books, 1974.

Volume 1, *The Foundations of Psychiatry*; volume 2, *Child and Adolescent Psychiatry, Sociocultural and Community Psychiatry*; volume 3, *Adult Clinical Psychiatry*; volume 4, *Organic Disorders and Psychosomatic Medicine*; volume 5, *Treatment*; volume 6, *New Psychiatric Frontiers*.
Editors of great distinction have contributed toward this massive review of the

state of modern psychiatry. Psychological, biological, and sociological factors related to mental health are highlighted. Since many articles are reprinted from the first edition, a comparison of the state of psychiatry in the late 1950s and in the mid-1970s is possible. These six volumes are vital references for any psychiatrist or student of human behavior.
R: *American Journal of Psychiatry* 133: 1211 (Oct. 1976); *JAMA* 235: 2244 (May 17, 1976); Stearns & Ratcliff (*AJN*).

The Annual Handbook for Group Facilitators. **J. William Pfeiffer and John E. Jones, eds.** La Jolla, CA: University Associates, 1971–. Annual.
In *Series in Human Relations Training.*
In five sections, aims to inform the user of new methods of group interaction. Maintains a practical approach, can be used as a handbook which describes, evaluates, and classifies human behavior.
R: *American Journal of Nursing* 77: 72 (Jan. 1977).

Basic Handbook of Child Psychiatry. 2 vols. **Joseph Noshpitz et al., eds.** New York: Basic Books, 1979.
Volume 1, *Development*; volume 2, *Disturbances in Development.*
An extensive handbook with over 250 contributors. Systematically arranged; includes up-to-date references. Articles are in depth. Considered a major and essential reference work for medical and university libraries.
R: *LJ* 104: 1465 (July 1979).

Behavioral Pediatrics and Child Development: A Clinical Handbook. **Thomas J. Kenny and Raymond L. Clemmens.** Baltimore, MD: Williams & Wilkins, 1975.
A complete survey of child care and development which takes an interdisciplinary approach. Topic range is from communication problems to physical growth. Written for those who take a holistic approach to child care.

Bibliotherapy: Methods and Materials. **Mildred T. Moody and Hilda K. Limper.** Chicago, IL: American Library Association, 1971.
A survey of the progress in bibliotherapy. This handbook is in two parts: therapeutic program suggestions and a bibliography appropriate to the subject. The bibliography is annotated and separated into subjects such as sibling rivalry, alcoholism, sexual maladjustments. Recommended to clinical psychologists, social workers, teachers as well as most library collections.
R: *ARBA* (1973, p. 603).

The Biofeedback Syllabus: A Handbook for the Psychophysiologic Study of Biofeedback. **Barbara B. Brown.** Springfield, IL: Charles C. Thomas, 1975.
Abstracts of journal articles in the field of biofeedback research from 1965 to 1973. Arranged in six sections for comprehensive understanding of biofeedback framework. Summary studies and additional (pre-1965) references are listed.
R: *Physical Therapy* 57: 222 (1977).

Child Health in the Community: A Handbook of Social and Community Paediatrics. **Ross G. Mitchell, ed.** Edinburgh: Churchill Livingstone, 1977.

Contains information on many facets of child health: physical, epidemiological, social, and biological. Recommended to all those who work with health and children and their well-being.
R: *Lancet* 2: 17 (July 2, 1977).

The Child Protection Team Handbook; A Multidisciplinary Approach to Managing Child Abuse and Neglect. **Barton D. Schmitt.** New York: Garland Publishing, 1978.
An inclusive handbook with a multidisciplinary approach to child protection. Evaluates each role the various professions can play in treatment of child neglect. Well organized, an indispensable aid to those concerned.
R: *American Journal of Nursing* 78: 1106 (June 1978).

Clinical Diagnosis of Mental Disorders: A Handbook. **Benjamin B. Wolman, ed.** New York: Plenum, 1978.
A readable source for details on psychological testing. Both theoretical and practical procedures in assessments and diagnosis are included. A helpful tool for psychiatrist's library.
R: *American Journal of Psychiatry* 136: 1240 (Sept. 1979).

Drugs and Therapy: A Psychotherapist's Handbook of Psychotropic Drugs. **Alvin K. Swonger and Larry L. Constantine.** Boston, MA: Little, Brown, 1976.
Spiral-bound handbook, 300 pages, useful as a desk reference for mental heath workers. Explains mechanisms of all major psychotropic drugs with an integrated medical, psychological, and physiological approach.
R: *American Journal of Occupational Therapy* 31: 270 (Apr. 1977).

Effective Psychotherapy: A Handbook of Research. **Alan S. Gurman and Andrew M. Razin, eds.** New York: Pergamon, 1977.

A Handbook For Specific Learning Disabilities. **William C. Adamson and Katherine K. Adamson, eds.** New York: John Wiley, 1979.
Maintains a multidisciplinary approach to various aspects of learning disabilities. Describes different therapies clearly. For use by therapists and teachers as well as interested parents.
R: *American Journal of Psychiatry* 136: 1238 (Sept. 1979).

A Handbook for the Study of Suicide. **Seymour Perlin, ed.** New York: Oxford University Press, 1975.
Result of a postgraduate fellowship program in suicidology at Johns Hopkins in 1967. Provides historical and philosophical perspectives on suicidal behavior. Adequate index. Aimed at medical students, doctoral students in social science and psychiatric residents.
R: *American Journal of Psychiatry* 132: 1094 (Oct. 1975); *RSR* 3: 37 (July–Dec. 1975). Also reviewed in *Contemporary Psychology.*

Handbook of Behavior Modification and Behavior Therapy. **Harold Leitenberg, ed.** Englewood Cliffs, NJ: Prentice-Hall, 1976.
Considered a much needed handbook, well written with contributions from au-

thorities in their field. A valuable reference and research tool for both professionals and graduate students.
R: *Journal of Nervous and Mental Disease* 167: 317 (May 1979); *Choice* 13: 1213 (Nov. 1976).

Handbook of Biological Psychiatry. **Herman M. van Praag et al., eds.** New York: Marcel Dekker, 1979–.

Volume 1 of *Experimental and Clinical Psychiatry* series.
Six-part summary and evaluation of the entire range of biological determinants of abnormal human behavior. Presents both laboratory and clinical results. A textbook of research strategies and technologies and a useful bibliography of key papers, reviews, and books for the specialized laboratory worker, general psychiatrist, and mental health worker.

Handbook of Perception. Vols. 1–10. **Edward C. Carterette and Morton P. Friedman, eds.** New York: Academic Press, 1973–1978.

Volume 1 *Historical and Philosophical Roots of Perception,* 1974; volume 2, *Psychophysical Judgement and Measurement,* 1974; volume 3, *Biology of Perception Systems,* 1973; volume 4, *Hearing,* 1978; volume 5, *Seeing,* 1975; volume 6A, *Tasting and Smelling,* 1978; volume 6B, *Feeling and Hurting,* 1978; volume 7, *Language and Speech,* 1976; volume 8, *Perceptual Coding,* 1978; volume 9, *Perceptual Processing,* 1978; volume 10, *Perceptual Ecology,* 1978.
R: *Choice* 12: 1502 (Jan. 1976).

Handbook of Psychobiology. **Michael Gazzaniga.** New York: Academic Press, 1975.
R: Chen (p. 110).

Massachusetts General Hospital Handbook of General Hospital Psychiatry. **Thomas P. Hackett & Ned H. Cassem, eds.** St. Louis, MO: C. V. Mosby, 1978.

A multi-authored compendium which covers a diverse range of topics in hospital psychiatry, emphasizing liaison consultation psychiatry. Represents a basic reference source, more a monograph than a typical handbook.
R: *American Journal of Psychiatry* 136: 1237 (Sept. 1979); *Annals of Internal Medicine* 91: 340 (Aug. 1979).

A Multidisciplinary Approach to Learning Disability, Handbook for the Classroom Teacher. **P. Ackerman et al.** Kent, OH: American School Health Association, 1978.

Eleven professionals have contributed to this volume dealing with learning disabled children. Essentially describes the function of different professionals in the detection, assessment, and treatment of learning disabilities. Emphasizes practical advice for classroom teachers, psychologists, ophthalmologists, and school nurses. Outlines specific behaviors and differences peculiar to children with learning disabilities. Comprehensive source of information for all those with an interest in understanding and helping these children.
R: *Journal of School Health* 48: 373 (June 1978).

Private Practice: A Handbook for the Independent Mental Health Practitioner. **R. M. Pressman.** New York: Halsted Press, 1979.

Focuses on building and maintaining a successful private practice. Ten topics on record keeping, fees, association and state laws, licensing, personal relations with community, and expanding the practice; provides valuable suggestions and strategies. Worthwhile addition to collections in chemical and social psychology.

Psychological Disorders of Children: A Handbook for Primary Care Physicians. **Mark A. Stewart and Ann Gath.** Baltimore, MD: Williams & Wilkins, 1978.

Serves as an introduction to psychiatric disorders in children. Most data derived from recent British research. Bulk of handbook consists of accounts of the main syndromes found in disturbed children. Special highlights include factual descriptions of psychological disorders, diagnostic criteria, treatment, concise definitions, and a review of research on natural history. Handy summary of facts for all clinicians working with disturbed children.
R: *Lancet* 2: 242 (July 29, 1978).

Serial Handbook of Modern Psychiatry. Vols. 1–. New York: Intercontinental Medical Books, 1974–.

Volume 1, *The Psychiatric Examination,* Jules Masserman and John J. Schwab, 1974; volume 2, *Psychiatric Syndromes and Modes of Therapy,* Jules Masserman, 1974.
R: *American Journal of Psychiatry* 132: 304 (1975); *JAMA* 230: 285 (Oct. 14, 1974).

PUBLIC HEALTH

Alcoholism: A Handbook. **L. R. H. Drew, J. R. Moon, and F. H. Buchanan.** London: Heinemann, 1974.

Introductory text geared toward the layman. Information based on authors' vast wealth of clinical experience.
R: *Lancet* 1: 1364 (June 21, 1975).

Dangerous Properties of Industrial Materials. 4th ed. **N. Irving Sax.** New York: Van Nostrand Reinhold, 1975.

Third edition, 1968.
The fourth and largely revised edition of this handbook details the labeling, toxicity levels, chemical formulas, and other pertinent information concerning the properties of industrial chemicals. The book also describes the handling of hazardous wastes and government standards for labeling them, carcinogenesis, and industrial hygiene. The handbook is recommended to all public, research, and university libraries.
R: *Occupational Health Nursing* 23: 57 (June 1975); *RSR* 4: 91 (Apr.–June 1976).

Disaster Handbook. 2d ed. **Solomon Garb and Evelyn Eng.** New York: Springer Publishing, 1969.

First edition, 1964.
Second edition of this paperback handbook contains new information on rescue, first aid, and emergency care. Intended to assist doctors, nurses, and others in-

volved with disaster prevention and management, the handbook details emergency care in major types of disasters (including thermonuclear). Index and bibliography are included.
R: *ARBA* (1970, p. 138).

The Diseases of Occupations. 4th ed. **Donald Hunter.** Boston, MA: Little, Brown, 1969.

Environmental Biology. **Philip L. Altman and Dorothy S. Dittmer, comps. and eds.** Bethesda, MD: Federation of American Societies for Experimental Biology, 1971.
A handbook of biological effects on the environment, intended for the specialist. Compendium of tables, graphs, and diagrams arranged according to major environmental factors.
R: Chen (p. 142); Win (1EC3).

Environmental Radiation Measurements, NCRP Report No. 50. **National Council on Radiation Protection.** Washington, DC: National Council on Radiation Protection, 1976.
A comprehensive documentation of radiation in the environment; assesses radiation measurements and identification. Material is directed towards health physicists, discussing practical methods of understanding and improving measures of radiation. Considered a standard reference.
R: *Health Physics* 34: 281 (Mar. 1978).

Environment Regulation Handbook: Air Pollution, Land Use, Mobile Sources, NEPA, Noise, Pesticides, Radioactive Materials, Solid Wastes, Water Pollution. New York: Environmental Information Center, 1973.
Eclectic information on environmental topics in loose-leaf format. Includes comprehensive regulatory sections and directory information. Duplicates some material in *Environment Reporter* and the *Environmental Law Reporter.*
R: *ARBA* (1975, p. 697); Chen (p. 143).

Good Health Abroad—A Traveller's Handbook. **W. H. Jopling.** Chicago, IL: Year Book Medical Publishers, 1975.

Handbook of Community Health. 2d ed. **Murray Grant.** Philadelphia, PA: Lea & Febiger, 1975.
First edition, *Handbook of Preventive Medicine and Public Health,* 1967.
Covers environmental health, occupational diseases and accidents, maternal and child health, food and nutrition, and disaster planning. Second edition features updated material on mental health, alcoholism, and drug addiction. Expanded section on dental health. Comprehensive index refers to illustrations as well as text. Useful addition to medical, college, many public, and pertinent specialized libraries.
R: *RSR* 3: 35 (July–Dec. 1975).

A Handbook of Community Medicine. **A. M. Nelson et al.** Chicago, IL: Year Book Medical Publishers, 1975.

Handbook of Emergency Toxicology. 3d ed. **Sidney Kaye.** Springfield, IL: Charles C. Thomas, 1970.

Second edition, 1961.
Alphabetical listing of almost 170 poisons. Pertinent information includes minimum lethal dosage, symptoms, treatment, synonyms, derivatives. Also a list of common, botanical, and trade names with ingredients.
R: Win (EK225; 3EJ37).

Handbook of Epidemiology and Prognosis. **J. A. H. Waterhouse.** Edinburgh: Churchill Livingstone, 1974.

Provides information on cancer incidence and on survival rates for patients. It is an essential reference book for all those working in epidemiological and clinical tumor studies.
R: *Lancet* 2: 28 (July 6, 1974).

Handbook of Industrial Toxicology. 2d ed. **Edmond R. Plunkett.** New York: Chemical Publishing, 1976.

A ready source for information on industrial toxicology. Subjects listed alphabetically. Includes synonyms, descriptions, toxicity levels, suggested therapies in case of exposure. A practical and useful book.
R: *Pharmaceutical Journal* 220: 206 (1978); Sheehy (EK42); Win (EK99; 1EJ14).

Handbook of Medical Sociology. 2d ed. **Howard Freeman, Sol Levine, and Leo G. Reeder.** Englewood Cliffs, NJ: Prentice-Hall, 1972.

Presents twenty articles with emphasis on types of illnesses, medical education, methods of research, etc.
R: *ARBA* (1973, p. 611).

Handbook of Poisoning: Diagnosis and Treatment. 9th ed. **Robert H. Dreisbach.** Los Altos, CA: Lange Medical Publications, 1977.

Seventh edition, 1971; eighth edition, 1974.
Pocket-size handbook intended as a vital resource for clinical use. Lists over 6,000 poisonous compounds and summarizes diagnosis and treatment. Includes detailed indexes, appendixes, and tables. Emphasizes preventive measures.
R: *American Family Physician* 17: 260 (May 1978); *Archives of Internal Medicine* 131: 758 (May 1973); *NEJM* 291: 1313 (Dec. 12, 1974); *TBRI* 41: 62 (Feb. 1975); *ARBA* (1972, p. 617; 1973, p. 611; 1975, p. 739); Sheehy (EK40).

Handbook on Alcoholism and Its Treatment. **W. Poley, G. Lea, and G. Vibe.** New York: Halsted Press, 1979.

Deals with the practical aspects of alcoholism. Focuses on various treatments, methods, programs and, current research.

A Handbook on Drug and Alcohol Abuse: The Biomedical Aspects. **Frederick G. Hofmann.** New York: Oxford Press, 1975.

Detailed source of pharmacological and medical data on drug and alcohol abuse. Copiously illustrates all drugs subjected to abuse. Includes findings from various experimental studies and clinical research reports. Authoritative and well-organized source book for practitioners and students.

Handbook on Environmental Monitoring. **Frank L. Cross, Jr.** Westport, CT: Technomic, 1974.

Information on the monitoring of air and water pollution, meterological and noise monitoring, solid waste management, and the measurement of radioactivity. Has been poorly received because of high cost and uneven quality.
R: *ARBA* (1975, p. 696); Chen (p. 143).

Nuclear Air Cleaning Handbook, ERDA 76-21. **C. A. Burchsted, A. B. Fuller, and J. E. Kahn.** Oak Ridge, TN: US Energy Research and Development Administration, Oak Ridge National Laboratory, 1976.

Authoritative coverage of high-efficiency (HEPA) filters. Updates and expands the highly acclaimed publication *ORNL-NSIC-65, Design, Construction and Testing of High Efficiency Air Filtration Systems for Nuclear Applications.* Contains valuable information on pre-filters, deep bed glass fiber filters, sand filters, and activated carbon absorbers. Consideration is given to the whole system, not only the filter alone. Handbook has strong applications for situations beyond the nuclear industry. Indispensable reference source for the tester or designer of air cleaning systems in nuclear facilities.
R: *Health Physics* 34: 117 (Jan. 1978).

Nuclear Power Reactor Instrumentation Systems Handbook, TID-25952-P1. Vol. 1. **Joseph M. Harrer and James Buckerley, eds.** Springfield, VA: National Technical Information Service, 1973.

Volume 1 presents a lucid understanding of the technical and practical aspects of reactor instrumentation systems. Twenty-five prominent authors from the U.S. Atomic Energy Commission, its national laboratories, and private industry, have prepared its contents. A collection of data on in-core and out-of-core nuclear radiation sensors, process instrumentation, control rod systems, power supplies, and quality assurance. In spite of some deficiencies in style, the listing of references, and the index, the handbook contains a wealth of information for the health physicist at a power reactor site.
R: *Health Physics* 26: 587 (June 1974).

Public Health Law Manual: A Handbook on the Legal Aspects of Public Health Administration and Enforcement. 2d ed. **Frank P. Grad.** New York: American Public Health Association, 1970.

Published by the United States Public Health Service and the American Public Health Association, designed as a planning guide for public health administrators and officers. Supplies legal reference to public health administration.
R: Win (EK217; 1EJ25).

Toxicologic Emergencies: A Handbook in Problem Solving. **Lewis R. Goldfrank and Robert Kirstein.** New York: Appleton-Century-Crofts, 1978.

Succinct presentation of principles for the emergency management of pharmaceutical, chemical, or food overdose. Uses twenty problem-oriented case histories to illustrate the complexity and perplexity of the emergency situation. Common poisonings include cyanide, carbon monoxide, barbiturates, etc. Tables, charts, and lists are easy to read and understand. Excellent references follow each chapter. Includes index. Main feature of this handbook is its readability. Invaluable

reference for practicing physician, medical student, and emergency room personnel.
R: *American Family Physician* 17: 225 (June 1978); *Annals of Internal Medicine* 89: 734 (Nov. 1978); *JAMWA* 34: 51 (Jan. 1979); *Lancet* 1: 858 (Apr. 22, 1978).

RADIOLOGY

CRC Handbook of Radioactive Nuclides. **Yen Wang, ed.** Cleveland, OH: Chemical Rubber Company, 1969.

A handy reference source of essential information on radioactive nuclides, including instrumentation and measurements. Much of the handbook consists of tables and graphs, with textual explanation, and is arranged conveniently for information retrieval.
R: Chen (p. 140); Wal (p. 310).

Golden's Diagnostic Radiology. 22 sections. Baltimore, MD: Williams & Wilkins, 1976–.

Section 1, *Diagnostic Neuroradiology,* J. Taveras, ed., 1976; section 4, *Radiology of the Heart and Great Vessels,* R. N. Cooley, ed., 1978; section 8, *Urologic Radiology,* Mary Sussman, ed., 1976.
R: *American Journal of Roentgenology* 133: 170 (July 1979).

Handbook of Clinical Ultrasound. **M. de Vlieger.** New York: John Wiley, 1978.

Emphasizes applications of ultrasound. Features over 1,000 excellent illustrations.
R: *NEJM* 301: 448 (Aug. 23, 1979).

Internal Radiation Dose in Diagnostic Nuclear Medicine. **Hans D. Roedler, Alexander Kaul, and Gerald J. Hine.** Berlin: Verlag H. Hoffmann, 1978.

Based on the recommendations of the International Commission on Radiological Protection. Essentially a compilation of data concerning biokinetics of pharmaceuticals and physical characteristics of radionuclides. Information supplied for critical and investigated organs, testes, ovaries, and red bone marrow. Arranged topically by eight specialties in nuclear medicine (endocrinology, neurology, etc.). Intended for physicians inexperienced in the nuclear medicine field, technical assistants, and hospital physicists.

Medical Radiation Exposure of Pregnant and Potentially Pregnant Women, NCRP Report no. 54. **National Council on Radiation Protection.** Washington, DC: National Council on Radiation Protection, 1977.

A handbook which quantitatively surveys the effect of radiation on pregnant and fertile women. Emphasizes the hazard of radiation exposure in early pregnancy. Contains an appendix of data of estimated embryo-fetus radiographic examination exposure.
R: *British Journal of Radiology* 51: 380 (1978).

Physicians' Desk Reference for Radiology and Nuclear Medicine. 1st ed.–. Oradell, NJ: Medical Economics, 1971–. Annual.

Discusses current practices in nuclear medicine. Provides product information and information on specialized instruments. Indexed.
R: *MRW* S2, pp. 72, 87.

Positioning and Technique Handbook for Radiologic Technologists. **Sylvester B. Conte and Douglas H. Kemme.** St. Louis, MO: C. V. Mosby, 1978.
Pocket-size reference for the radiologic technologist. Describes approximately 100 positioning procedures frequently incorporated in a clinical setting. Illustrations of every procedure. Additional space provided for notes for future reference.

Safe Handling of Radiation Sources. **Martin Oberhofer. Translated by James E. Turner and Renate G. Turner.** Munich, Germany: Verlag Karl Thiemig, 1974.
Intended as a practical guide to radiological protection. Consists of five basic sections: elementary principles, working in areas of radiation devices, handling sealed radioactive substances, handling unsealed radioactive substances, and accidents. Includes tables of basic health physics data. Nearly 120 diagrams and photographs complement the text. Numerous references, complete index, and high quality translation add up to an excellent reference source. Geared toward health physicist, radiologist, nurse, and student.
R: *Health Physics* 30: 151 (Jan. 1976); *Physics in Medicine & Biology* 20: 670 (July 1975).

Uranium, Plutonium, Transplutonic Elements: Handbook of Experimental Pharmacology. **H. D. Hodge, J. N. Stannard, and J. B. Hursh, eds.** New York: Springer-Verlag, 1973.
An acclaimed handbook covering present knowledge of the biology and toxicology of uranium, plutonium, and the transplutonic elements. Published as vol. XXXVI of the *Handbook of Experimental Pharmacology* series. Summarizes pertinent historical data, physical and chemical properties, concentrations in water and air, uses and hazards of these elements, and maximum permissible body burdens. Valuable source to original works and to persons actively involved in this field. This massive handbook consists of contributions from 23 notable authors with a *Who's Who* reputation in this field. The definitive work for health physicists, toxicologists, and everyone concerned with the protection aspects of these elements.
R: *British Journal of Radiology* 47: 569 (1974); *Health Physics* 29: 887 (Dec. 1975).

RESPIRATORY SYSTEM

A Concise Handbook of Respiratory Diseases. **Sattar Farzan, Doris L. Hunsinger, and Mary L. Phillips.** Englewood Cliffs, NJ: Prentice-Hall, 1978.
A handbook for respiratory therapists; discusses different pathologic states, physical and radiographic examination. Focuses also on respiratory failure because of the subject's importance. Concise, well presented information.

Respiration and Circulation. **Philip L. Altman and Dorothy S. Dittmer, comps. and eds.** Bethesda, MD: Federation of American Societies for Experimental Biology, 1971.

UROGENITAL SYSTEM

Female Reproductive System. 2 vols. **R. O. Greep, ed.** Washington, DC: American Physiological Society, 1973.
Volume 1, 1959.
Overflows with significant information on the female reproductive system. Fifty chapters deal with ovary, pregnancy, effects of hormones on sexual behavior, fertility control, etc. Illustrations are all excellent reproductions. Since references only include works published to early 1971, current areas of interest (prostaglandins) are likely to be outdated or modestly covered. Students of reproductive physiology will find this volume a worthwhile investment.
R: *Nature* 250: 170 (July 12, 1974).

Female Sterilization: A Handbook for Women. **M. H. Saidie and Carla M. Zainie.** New York: Garland, 1979.
Comprehensive, medically accurate survey of methods of female sterilization. Begins with an historical account. Incorporates operative procedures, complication rates, and psychological reactions. Outlines newer, experimental methods. Well illustrated.
R: *LJ* 105: 626 (Mar. 1, 1980).

Handbook of Obstetrical and Gynecological Data. **Robert C. Goodlin.** Los Altos, CA: Geron-X, 1972.
Comprehensive pocketbook of obstetric and gynecologic data. Features current information with well-annotated references. Handy reference and statistical databook for hospitals, doctor's offices, and training programs.
R: *Archives of Internal Medicine* 132: 143 (July 1973).

Munro Kerr's Operative Obstetrics. 9th ed. **P. R. Myerscough.** London: Bailliere Tindall, 1977.
Standard British text for the obstetrician. The handbook's approach is basically conservative; serves as an excellent contrast to some of the controversial obstetric handbooks in the library's collection.
R: *British Journal of Obstetrics & Gynaecology* 84: 559 (July 1977).

Pathology of Toxaemia of Pregnancy. **Harold L. Sheehan and J. B. Lynch.** Baltimore, MD: Williams & Wilkins, 1973.
Scholarly work devoted to the examination and synthesis of the pathology of toxemia of pregnancy. Definitive source of information on eclampsia. Valuable addition to every hospital library.
R: *British Journal of Surgery* 60: 986 (Dec. 1973); *JAMA* 226: 1574 (Dec. 24, 1973); *Obstetrics and Gynecology* 45: 119 (Jan. 1975); *South African Medical Journal* 47: 2092 (Nov. 3, 1973); *TBRI* 40: 80 (Feb. 1974); 40: 119 (Mar. 1974); 40: 160 (Apr. 1974).

VETERINARY MEDICINE

Complete Desk Reference of Veterinary Pharmaceuticals and Biologicals 78/79. **Carl E. Aronson, ed.** Harwal, PA: Media, 1978.

Lists some 2,000 biologicals, pharmaceuticals, diets and nutritional supplements, parasiticides, and diagnostic aids designed for veterinary use.
R: *Cornell Veterinarians* 69: 213 (April 1979).

Handbook of Laboratory Animal Science. 3 vols. **Edward C. Melby, Jr., and N. H. Altman, eds.** Cleveland, OH: Chemical Rubber Company, 1974–1975.

R: *Journal of the American Veterinary Medical Association* 166: 924 (May 1, 1975); *Journal of Veterinary Research* 36: 715 (May 1975); *TBRI* 41: 260 (Sept. 1975); Chen (p. 112).

A Handbook of Veterinary Parasitology: Domestic Animals of North America. **Henry J. Griffiths.** Minneapolis, MN: University of Minneapolis Press, 1978.

Concise, well organized handbook which serves as an easily used reference book. Supplies taxonomic details of common parasites. For each parasite discussed, information included is common name, disease, host, habitat, identification, life cycle, and transmission. Appendixes of laboratory techniques, host, chemotherapeutic agents and glossary. Highly recommended for veterinary students.
R: *Journal of the American Veterinary Association* 173: 112 (July 1, 1978); *Quarterly Review of Biology* 54: 102 (Mar. 1979).

Handbook of Veterinary Surgical Instruments and Glossary of Surgical Terms. **Leonard Hurov, ed.** Philadelphia, PA: W. B. Saunders, 1978.

A basic ready reference of surgical terms and procedures in veterinary medicine.
R: *Journal of the American Veterinary Medical Association* 173: 1521 (Dec. 1, 1978).

CHAPTER 7　　　TABLES, ALMANACS, DATABOOKS, STATISTICAL SOURCES

TABLES

SI Units

Conversion Tables for SI Metrication. **William J. Semioli and Paul B. Schubert.** New York: Industrial Press, 1974.

Compendium of logically grouped tables, intended for engineers and related technicians. Tables included pertain to length, mass, volume, flow-rate, mass, etc. All tables are preceded by conversion instructions and examples.
R: *ARBA* (1975, p. 774); Chen (p. 145).

International and Metric Units of Measurement. **Marvin H. Green.** New York: Chemical Publishing, 1973.
R: Chen (p. 145).

Metric Conversion Tables and Factors. New York: Industrial Press, 1973.

Data needed for any English/metric conversions. Emphasis on the international system of units.
R: Chen (p. 145).

SI Units. **B. Chiswell.** New York: John Wiley, 1971.
R: Chen (p. 145).

SI Units and Nomenclature in Soil Science. **P. R. Hesse.** Rome, Italy: Food and Agriculture Organization of the United Nations, 1975.

Provides soil scientists working in many different countries with a commonly understood system of physical units and nomenclature.
R: *IBID* 4: 124 (June 1976); Chen (p. 145).

Units of Weight and Measure, International (Metric), and US Customary. Washington, DC: US National Bureau of Standards, 1967.

Conversion tables are simplified for laymen, with some tables providing instant conversion answers.
R: Chen (p. 145).

Other Tables

Activation and Decay Tables of Radioisotopes. **E. Bujdoso, I. Feher, and G. Kardos.** Amsterdam: Elsevier, 1973.

A collection of radioisotopic data tables which has been arranged by atomic numbers, gamma ray energies, or half-life values. Authors have added data on irradiation and saturation activities. These tables will assist those involved with

neutron calculation work and will be particularly valuable to laboratories without computers.
R: *Health Physics* 27: 233 (Aug. 1974).

Composition of Foods, US Department of Agriculture, Agriculture Handbook No. 8-1-. **US Consumer and Food Economics Institute, Agricultural Research Service.** Washington, DC: US Department of Agriculture, 1976–1977.
First edition, 1950.
Consists mainly of data tables on the nutritive value of food. A major revision of the 1963 edition of USDA Agriculture Handbook No. 8: *Composition of Foods: Raw, Processed, and Prepared.*
R: Sheehy (EK30); Win (EK179).

Human Haemoglobin Variants and Their Characteristics. **H. Lehmann and P. A. M. Kynoch.** New York: North-Holland Publishing, 1976.
Essentially a book of tables. Focuses on structural and functional features of the several hundred normal and abnormal human hemoglobins. Covers the literature prior to and during 1976. Features 327 pertinent references. Arrangement of entries according to positions of structural abnormalities in the polypeptide chains. Includes separate chapters for variants characterized by deletions, amino acid substitutions, and elongated chains. Useful only to investigators engaged in the study of variants of human hemoglobins.
R: *Quarterly Review of Biology* 53: 500 (1978).

Life Table and Mortality Analysis. **Chin L. Chiang.** Geneva: World Health Organization, 1978.
Focuses on the following topics: elements of probability, standard error of mortality rates, the life table and its construction, and death rates and adjustment of rates.
R: *IBID* 6: 433 (Dec. 1978).

ALMANACS, DATABOOKS

GENERAL

Biological Laboratory Data. 2d ed. **Leslie J. Hale.** New York: John Wiley, 1965.
Covers only the most basic data and supplements this with references to sources containing more specialized information. Includes data from math, physics, and chemistry.
R: Chen (p. 158).

Biology Data Book. 2d ed. 3 vols. **Philip L. Altman and Dorothy S. Dittmer, comps. and eds.** Bethesda, MD: Federation of American Societies for Experimental Biology, 1972–1974.
Presents basic, established data in the biological and medical sciences. Each volume covers different aspects and subject areas of biology and is independently indexed. Tables include contributor's name and a list of references. Intended as a comprehensive laboratory reference.

R: *Nature* 206: 971 (1965); *ARBA* (1974, p. 566); Chen (p. 158); Jenkins (G49); Mal (9-23); Wal (p. 194); Win (EC19).

Data for Biochemical Research. 2d ed. **R. M. C. Dawson et al., eds.** Oxford, England: Clarendon Press, 1969.

First edition, 1959.
Basic reference for biochemists, containing information on compounds and reagents.
R: Chen (p. 157); Win (3EC5).

A Growth Chart for International Use in Maternal and Child Health Care: Guidelines for Primary Health Care Personnel. **World Health Organization.** Geneva: World Health Organization, 1978.

Describes the initial development of a standardized system for listing and interpreting growth data. Includes a model chart (adaptable to local needs) with simplified instructions. Geared toward service and research use.
R: *IBID* 6: 434 (Dec. 1978).

International Critical Tables of Numerical Data, Physics, Chemistry and Technology. 7 vols. **US National Research Council.** New York: McGraw-Hill, 1926–1930.

"Critical" in the sense that each contributing specialist was requested to give in each case the "best" value that could be derived from information available. Vast compilation of quantitative information.
R: Chen (p. 145); Jenkins (A83); Mal (3-35); Win (EA139).

Journal of Physical and Chemical Reference Data. Vols. 1–. Washington, DC: American Chemical Society and the American Institute of Physics for the US National Bureau of Standards, 1972–. Quarterly.

Provides quantitative numerical data. Includes bibliographies, abstracts. Updates the *International Critical Tables.*
R: *MRW* S2, pp. 17, 79.

Medical Care Chart Book. 6th rev. ed. **S. J. Axelrod, A. Donabedian, and D. W. Gentry.** Ann Arbor, MI: Department of Medical Care Organization, School of Public Health, University of Michigan, 1976.

NIH Almanac 1969. **US National Institutes of Health.** Bethesda, MD: US National Institutes of Health, US Public Health Service, US Department of Health, Education, and Welfare, 1969. Annual updates.

Updates all historical information and reference material annually. Divided into eight sections: historical data, appropriations, organization, support of medical research, staff, facilities, field units, and lecture series. Also includes current NIH events and legislation, biographical essays of directors, and statistics relevant to all activities in one volume.
R: *ARBA* (1970, p. 131).

NSF Factbook. **US National Science Foundation.** Orange, NJ: Academic Media, 1976. Annual.
R: Chen (p. 153).

Reference Data on Socioeconomic Issues of Health. Vol. 1–. Chicago, IL: Center For Health Services Research and Development, American Medical Association, 1971–.
Compiles statistics and analyses from AMA's research center and U.S. Bureau of the Census. Provides data in charts; contains tables and graphs on characteristics of US population, mortality, health services, supply and distribution of physicians, expenditures on medical care and similar topics.
R: *ARBA* (1973, p. 613).

Reference Data on the Profile of Medical Practice. Vol. 1–. Chicago, IL: Center for Health Services Research and Development, American Medical Association, 1971–.

Standard Medical Almanac. 2d ed. Chicago, IL: Marquis Who's Who, 1979.
First edition, 1977.
Comprehensive overview of the health care industry in the United States. Divided into six sections: manpower, income, education, facilities, diseases, and federal government role. Reproduces exactly many government and private publications and reports. Graphic and tabular format for most data. Broad spectrum of data includes association/organization rosters, statistics, research findings, and legislative surveys. Choice of subject, organization, and geographic indexes. Indispensable tool for health sciences collection.
R: *WLB* 52: 503 (Feb. 1978); *ARBA* (1978, p. 720).

Nursing

The Impact of Health System Changes on the Nation's Requirements for Registered Nurses in 1985, DHEW Pub. no. (HRA) 78-9. **Timothy C. Doyle, George E. Cooper, and Ronald G. Anderson.** Division of Nursing, Bureau of Health Manpower, Health Resources Administration, Public Health Service, US Department of Health, Education, and Welfare. Washington, DC: US Government Printing Office, 1978.

NLN Nursing Data Book. New York: Division of Research, National League for Nursing, 1978–.
Source book on nursing education and work situations of recently licensed nurses. Some 90 statistical tables outline information on positions, kind of employer, status of job, demographic data, etc. Sponsored by the National League for Nursing.
R: *Modern Healthcare* 9: 73 (Feb. 1979).

The Nurse's Almanac. **Howard S. Rowland and Beatrice L. Rowland, eds.** Germantown, MD: Aspen Systems Corp., 1978.
A reference for nurses of all levels. Divided into 38 sections which cover inten-

sive topics in nursing. Examples are nursing and the law, cost of health care, hospitals, unions, etc. Also includes useful appendixes which include glossary of terms, medical abbreviations. A useful reference tool.
R: *Supervisor Nurse* 10: 56 (Feb. 1979); Brandon (*NO*).

Nurse's Drug Reference. **Stewart M. Brooks, Anna T. Manseau, and William Principe, eds.** Boston, MA: Little, Brown, 1978.
Emphasizes nursing implications of drug therapy. Provides explanations of drug classifications, combinations, dosage, and administration. Includes ten appendixes: legalities, poisons, pediatric dosages, latin phrases, medical terms, etc.

Nursing Homes: A County and Metropolitan Area Data Book. **US National Center for Health Statistics.** Washington, DC: US Government Printing Office, 1970.
Presents statistics related to nursing homes. Covers data on number of beds, personnel and ownership. Tables arranged by state, metropolitan area, and county.
R: *ARBA* (1972, p. 630).

NUTRITION

Eater's Digest: The Consumer's Factbook of Food Additives. **Michael F. Jacobson.** New York: Doubleday, 1972.
A popular treatment of the chemicals that are added to foods.
R: Chen (p. 158).

Laboratory Indices of Nutritional Status in Pregnancy. **Committee on Nutrition of the Mother and Preschool Child, Food and Nutrition Board, National Research Council.** Washington, DC: US National Academy of Sciences, 1978.
Scientific review of current state of knowledge regarding laboratory indices reflecting nutritional and metabolic status during normal pregnancy. Seven chapters written by experts cover such topics as physiological adjustments, hematologic indices, and electrolytes. Timely publication for research scientist.
R: *American Journal of Public Health* 68: 911 (Sept. 1978); 68: 913 (Sept. 1978); *Lancet* 2: 242 (July 29, 1978); *Nutrition Reviews* 36: 160 (May 1978).

McCance and Widdowson's The Composition of Foods. 4th ed. **A. A. Paul and D. A. T. Southgate.** London: Her Majesty's Stationery Office, 1978.
Tables include composition, proximate analysis, inorganic constituents, major vitamins and minor B-vitamins/100 g of food commodities. This edition features cooked dishes and foods common to immigrants and dietary fibre content of cereals and cereal products. Separate section on amino acid composition. Appendixes appropriately cross-referenced.
R: *Journal of Food Technology* 13: 487 (Oct. 1978); *Journal of Human Nutrition* 33: 238 (June 1979); *Quarterly Review of Biology* 54: 125 (Mar. 1979).

Nutrition Almanac. **J. D. Kirschman.** New York: McGraw-Hill, 1975.

Nutritive Value of American Foods: In Common Units, **Agriculture Handbook**

No. 456. **Catherine F. Adams.** US Agricultural Research Service. Washington, DC: US Government Printing Office, 1975.
Based on Agriculture Handbook No. 8: *Composition of Foods: Raw, Processed, Prepared.*
R: Sheehy (EK29).

Ten-State Nutrition Survey, 1968–1970, DHEW Pub. no. (HSM) 72-8130–72-8133. 4 vols. **Center for Disease Control.** Atlanta, GA: Center for Disease Control, 1972.
Selective survey of malnutrition in the states. Concentrates on low income groups. Intended to identify the prevalence, magnitude, and distribution of malnutrition.
R: Win (EK175).

Pharmacy and Pharmacology

Catalog of Teratogenic Agents. **Thomas H. Shepard.** Baltimore, MD: Johns Hopkins University Press, 1973.
Concise and informative introduction to the literature on drugs and chemicals which may or may not cause abnormalities in experimental animals. Four main sections: introduction (explains the needs and defines the context); endpapers table (comparative time table of 38 embryonic and fetal developmental stages in man and experimental animals); catalog proper and two indexes (author and subject). Catalog proper alphabetically lists nearly 650 chemical and pharmacological agents which have been tested for teratogenic effects. Entries include synonyms, relevant studies, data on species, dose, sensitive gestational age, kind of defect, and carefully chosen references. Generally poor illustrations. Computer printout format accounts for ease in production, low cost, and updating. Invaluable desk reference for practicing genetic counselor, clinician, and experimental teratologist.
R: *American Journal of Diseases of Children* 128: 121 (July 1974); *Growth* 39: 178 (Mar. 1975); *Journal of Pharmaceutical Sciences* 63: 1344 (Aug. 1974); *Teratology* 13: 106 (Feb. 1976).

Pocketbook of Pediatric Antimicrobial Therapy. **John D. Nelson.** Philadelphia, PA: J. B. Lippincott, 1975.
Ready reference for antibiotic usage in pediatrics. Booklet is divided into nine sections, including sections on recommendations for antimicrobial, antifungal and antiparasitic therapy. Information on clinical syndromes, indications, doses and trade and generic names is listed in tabular form. A welcome addition to the pediatric therapeutic literature. Medical students, house officers, and pediatricians will benefit most from this handbook.
R: *American Journal of Diseases of Children* 130: 105 (Jan. 1976); *Annals of Internation Medicine* 84: 376 (Mar. 1976); *Clinical Pediatrics* 16: 451 (May 1977); 16: 708 (Aug. 1977).

Poisoning by Drugs and Chemicals, Plants and Animals: An Index of Toxic Effects and Their Treatment. 3d ed. **Peter Cooper.** Chicago, IL: Year Book Medical Publishers, 1974.

First edition, 1958; second edition, 1962.
Bulk of text devoted to poisonous substances. Alphabetically arranged entries yield pertinent information on action, toxic effects, results of overdose, aids to identification, and possible treatment. Main index lists nonproprietary drug names, generic names, and common and popular terms.
R: *RSR* 3: 35 (July–Dec. 1975).

Prescription Drug Industry Fact Book. Washington, DC: Pharmaceutical Manufacturers Association, 1976.

Psychiatric Drugs: A Desk Reference. 2d ed. **Gilbert Honigfeld and Alfreda Howard.** New York: Academic Press, 1978.

Discusses all aspects of psychotropic drugs. Includes appendixes and subject index.
R: *American Scientist* 62: 362 (May–June, 1974).

Undesirable Drug Interactions, 1974–1975. Rev. ed. **Solomon Garb.** New York: Springer Publishing, 1974.

First edition, 1971.
Valuable guide to undesirable interactions between drugs, foods, and/or diagnostic tests. Presented in tabular form, listing code letters for particular interaction and numbers to specific literature references. Most of 1,500 reference sources are journal articles. A second table outlines drugs under certain pharmacologic groups. Ready reference for doctors and pharmacists.
R: *Pharmaceutical Journal* 214: 182 (1975); *ARBA* (1975, p. 750); *MRW* S3, pp. 19, 20.

RADIOLOGY

Data for Protection Against Ionizing Radiation From External Sources: Supplement to ICRP Publication 15, ICRP Publication 21. **The International Commission on Radiological Protection.** New York: Pergamon, 1973.

Represents current recommendations of The International Commission on Radiological Protection against ionizing radiation from external sources. Should be available to every radiological and health physicist involved in protection problems.
R: *International Journal of Applied Radiation Isotopes* 19: 74 (Jan. 1968); *Radiology* 111: 716 (1974).

Gamuts in Radiology: Comprehensive Lists of Roentgen Differential Diagnosis. **Maurice M. Reeder and Benjamin Nelson.** Cincinnati, OH: Audiovisual Radiology of Cincinnati, 1975.

A comprehensive listing of possible diseases, arranged according to a particular roentgenographic abnormality. Volume consists of eight sections, each boasting its own table of contents. Should be available to all clinicians and medical students.
R: *American Journal of Roentgenology* 124: 677 (Aug. 1975); *JAMA* 235: 950 (Mar. 1, 1976).

Protection Against Ionizing Radiation From External Sources, ICRP Publication 15, **The International Commission on Radiological Protection.** New York: Pergamon, 1970.

Radiation Dosimetry Data: Catalogue 1976: A Catalogue of Data Sheets Available From the International Atomic Energy Agency, MDS/CAT/1976. 3d ed. **International Atomic Energy Agency.** Vienna: International Atomic Energy Agency, 1976.

Second edition, 1970.
An excellently revised catalog of radiological data, covering current standards and techniques. Highly recommended to all departments of medical physics; especially useful as a planning guide.
R: *Physics in Medicine & Biology* 21: 1001 (Nov. 1976).

OTHER SUBJECTS

Algal Physiology and Biochemistry. **William D. P. Stewart, ed.** Oxford, England: Blackwell Scientific Publications, 1974.

An essential reference for plant physiologists. Contains data summaries, formulae, and tables.
R: *Nature* 254: 232 (Mar. 20, 1975); *TBRI* 41: 220 (June 1975).

Catalogue of Strains. 11th ed. **American Type Culture Collection.** Rockville, MD: American Type Culture Collection, 1974.

First edition to seventh edition, *Catalogue of Cultures*; ninth edition, 1970.
A listing of 15,000 strains of algae, bacteria, bacteriophages, fungi, and protozoa. Alphabetical arrangement under broad categories by species name. Introductory material outlines the collection, storage, and ordering of strains. Each entry lists ATCC accession number, description, and data on the strain and references to the literature. Includes miscellaneous appendixes.
R: *MRW* S3, p. 5.

Index of Suspicion in Treatable Diseases. **Orville Horwitz & Joseph H. Magee, eds.** Philadelphia, PA: Lea & Febiger, 1975.

Lists diseases which require a specialized early treatment. Provides physiological background, pertinent references. A concise reference source.

Registry of Toxic Effects of Chemical Substances. **National Institute for Occupational Safety and Health. US Department of Health, Education, and Welfare.** Washington, DC: US Government Printing Office, 1977–. Annual.

Continues *Toxic Substances List.*
R: Sheehy (EK43).

World Health Environmental Surveys. London, IMSworld Publications, 1978.

Compiles pertinent information on the health situations and pharmaceutical policies in 60 countries. Provides data in three sections: health statistics, medical services, and health economics. Ideal for health administrators, corporate planning personnel, academic research groups, health consultants, and information specialists.

STATISTICAL SOURCES

Guide to Sources of Statistical Information

American Statistics Index; A Comprehensive Guide and Index to the Statistical Publications of the United States Government. Washington, DC: Congressional Information Service, 1974–. Monthly.

The 1974 edition contains retrospective information. Identifies statistical data published by the federal government. Index and abstract sections.
R: Chen (p. 164).

Bibliography of Statistical Bibliographies. **Henry Oliver Lancaster.** Edinburgh: Oliver & Boyd, 1968.
R: Chen (p. 164).

Bibliography of Statistical Literature. 3 vols. **Maurice G. Kendall and Alison G. Doig.** Edinburgh: Oliver & Boyd, 1962–1968.
Retrospective guide to sources dating back to the sixteenth century.
R: Chen (p. 164).

Federal Statistical Directory. 22d ed. **Executive Office of the President, Office of Management and Budget.** Washington, DC: US Government Printing Office, 1970.
R: Chen (p. 164).

Guide to US Government Statistics. 4th ed. **John Andriot.** McLean, VA: Documents Index, 1973.
Third edition, 1961.
An annotated guide to recurring statistical publication of US agencies. Arranged by Sudocs classification scheme. While many publications of interest to scientists are included, primary emphasis is on economic and social statistics.
R: Chen (p. 164).

Statistics Sources. 5th ed. **Paul Wasserman and Jacqueline Bernero.** Detroit, MI: Gale Research, 1977.
First edition, 1971; fourth edition, 1974.
Identifies primary sources of statistical data, especially in American publications, of national rather than regional scope. Includes over 20,000 citations to sources of statistical data on nearly 12,000 subjects.
R: Chen (p. 165).

Governmental Statistical Sources

Government publications from both international and national organizations are an ever-increasing source of statistical information. At present nearly all government agencies generate some sort of numerical audit.

In most cases, these organizations are the most important and up-to-date sources of statistical information. It is impossible to list all pertinent statistical sources available. The following are a few sample tools from international and non-US governmental agencies.

Cancer Mortality, England and Wales 1911–1970, Studies on Medical and Population Subjects No. 29. **Great Britain. General Registry Office.** London: Her Majesty's Stationery Office, 1975.

Volume extends most of the tables in original 1957 publication of General Registry Office which summarized statistics relating to cancer mortality and survival. Should prove useful to oncologists as source of information of changes that have occurred in cancer mortality at different ages in this century.
R: *British Journal of Radiology* 49: 449 (1976).

Demographic Yearbook. **United Nations. Statistical Office.** Lake Success, NY: Demographic Yearbook, 1948–.

Prepared in cooperation with the Department of Social Affairs, 1948–1954. Since 1955, with the Department of Economic and Social Affairs.

Health. United States 1978, DHEW Pub. no. (HRA) 76-1232. Rockville, MD: US Department of Health, Education, and Welfare, US Public Health Service, US Health Resources Administration, US National Center for Health Statistics, 1978.

This publication consists of reports to Congress required by the Public Health Service Act. The publications consist of four parts: Part A: *Financial Aspects of the Nation's Health Care*; Part B: *Health Resources*; and Parts C and D: *Health Status and Use of Health Services.*

Statistical Indices of Family Health, WHO Technical Report Series, 587. **World Health Organization Study Group** (Geneva, February 17–21, 1975). Geneva: World Health Organization, 1976.

Statistical demographic, epidemiologic, and social/economic approaches to family health. Includes selective bibliography, references, and development of statistical indicators of family health.
R: *IBID* 4: 355 (Dec. 1976).

Statistics on Narcotic Drugs for 1976 Furnished by Governments in Accordance With the International Treaties and Maximum Levels of Opium Stocks, E/INCB/39. Annual update. **International Narcotics Control Board.** New York: United Nations, 1977.

Reports on trends in the licit movement of narcotic drugs during 1971 to 1975, with ten tables, covering production and manufacture, international trade, licit consumption, and seizures in illicit traffic.
R: *IBID* 1: 201 (Sept. 1973); 6: 276 (Sept. 1978).

World Health Statistics Annual. 3 vols. **World Health Organization.** Geneva: World Health Organization, 1962–.

Latest edition, 1977. Volume 1, *Vital Statistics and Causes of Death*; volume 2, *In-*

fectious Diseases: Cases and Deaths; volume 3, *Health Personnel and Hospital Establishments.*
The three-volume yearbook summarizes vital statistics and causes of death in both English and French. Contains statistical data on causes of and deaths from infectious diseases as well as number of immunizations performed. Also reports material on the number of persons working in various health occupations as well as ratio of medical personnel to population of various countries.
R: *IBID* 1: 52 (Mar. 1973); 1: 117 (June 1973); 1: 199 (Sept. 1973); 3: 57 (Mar/June 1975); 4: 145 (June 1976); 4: 355 (Dec. 1976); 5: 50 (Mar. 1977); 6: 74 (Mar. 1978).

In the United States, The Office of Management and Budget's Statistical Policy Division exists solely for the purpose of coordinating the statistical collection and dissemination functions of the federal government. Other government agencies involved primarily in statistical activities are the DHEW's National Center for Health Statistics and National Center for Educational Statistics, the Department of Commerce's Bureau of the Census, and many others. The following is a sample list of essential American governmental statistical publications of interest to health scientists and professionals.

Annual Report of the Council on Environmental Quality, EX 14.1: date. Washington, DC: US Government Printing Office. Annual.
R: Chen (p. 165).

Food Consumption Statistics, 1970–1975. **Organization for Economic Cooperation and Development.** Washington, DC: Organization for Economic Cooperation and Development, 1978.
Bilingual edition: English/French. Provides annual food consumption data in OECD member countries. Covers the 1970–1975 period. Separate chapters devoted to food balance sheets of individual countries. Chapters also include commodity tables, total daily calories, and protein and fat intake per capita in a particular country.
R: *IBID* 6: 288 (Sept. 1978).

Health Manpower Source Book. Sections 1–. **Manpower Resources Staff, US Public Health Service.** Washington, DC: US Government Printing Office, 1952–. Irregular.
Compilation of statistics on manpower in the health sciences professions. Arranged by occupation (medical, dental, nursing, veterinary). Aimed to evaluate trends in training, employment, utilization, and demand for these professionals. Includes numerous tables and figures. Gives present trends and traces historical data from the nineteenth century. Future projections for demand, educational requirements, and employment levels outlined.
R: *ARBA* (1970, p. 115).

Health Resources Statistics: Health Manpower and Health Facilities, 1975. **US National Center for Health Statistics.** Washington, DC: US Government Printing Office, 1976.

Provides necessary statistics for the planning, administration, and evaluation of health programs. Part 1 deals with the statistical data and analysis on the status of manpower in the health fields (physicians, dentists, nurses, etc.); part 2 focuses on the status and operations of inpatient health facilities (hospitals, nursing care); and part 3 concentrates on outpatient and nonpatient health services (family planning services, clinical laboratories, etc.). Statistical data gleaned from various sources: National Center for Health Statistics, professional associations, voluntary health organizations, experts in the field, and government agencies. Incorporates footnote references for further study. Annual compilation.
R: *ARBA* (1978, p. 721).

NONGOVERNMENTAL STATISTICAL SOURCES

Besides government publications, statistical information is also available from many international, national, and local professional and trade organizations; commercial publishers; private interest groups; and so on. Much of the information on these types of sources can be found also in the chapters on yearbooks, directories, guides, data books, and so forth, in this work. The following is only a sample list of statistical sources produced by nongovernmental agencies. The importance of professional organizations as sources of statistical information is apparent.

Annual Statistics of Medical School Libraries in the United States and Canada, 1978–1979. Houston, TX: Houston Academy of Medicine, Texas Medical Center Library, 1980.

Applied Statistics for Food and Agricultural Scientists. **Subhash C. Puri and Kenneth Mullen.** Boston, MA: G. K. Hall, 1979.
Invaluable guide to the analysis and organization of statistical data. Presents basic statistical techniques in food and related sciences. Geared toward students, researchers, and professionals in the field of food and agricultural science and technology.

Biometrika Tables for Statisticians. Vol. 2. **E. S. Pearson and H. O. Hartley, eds.** New York: Cambridge University Press, 1972.
Volume 1, 1966.
Designed to supplement volume 1 (1966); however, tables of volume 2 are quite comprehensive alone. Lengthy introduction and much theoretical data precede tables. Aimed at statisticians who are unable to work with computers.
R: *JAMA* 69: 577 (June 1974); *Journal of the Royal Statistical Society* 136: 267 (1973).

Countdown. Canadian Nursing Statistics. Ottawa, Canada: Canadian Nurses' Association, 1967–. Annual.

Facts About Nursing. New York: American Nurses' Association, 1935–. Annual.
Latest edition, 1976/1977.
Annual statistical summary of nursing distribution, education, economic status,

professional organization, and allied health professionals.
R: Win (EK166).

Hospital Statistics. 1979 ed. **American Hospital Association.** Chicago, IL: American Hospital Association, 1979. Annual.

A reference manual provides a statistical profile of hospitals in the United States and Puerto Rico. Data are compiled from the annual survey of more than 7,000 hospitals. Highlights in graphs and tables data on utilization, personnel, finances, facilities and services, approvals, affiliations, and revenue for over 7,000 hospitals in the United States. A must for every hospital and medical library.

Key Facts on the U.S. Prescription Drug Industry. Washington, DC: Pharmaceutical Manufacturers Association.

Pamphlet, frequently revised.

Medical Risks: Patterns of Mortality and Survival. **Richard B. Singer and Louis Levinson, eds.** Lexington, MA: D. C. Heath, Lexington Books, 1976.

Consists of a compilation of mortality and survival statistics. Compiled under the direction of the Association of Life Insurance Medical Directors of America and the Society of Actuaries. Includes author and subject indexes.
R: Sheehy (EK17).

Pocket Book of Statistical Tables. **Robert E. Odeh et al., comps.** New York: Marcel Dekker, 1977.

Highlights relevant tests and related topics such as power functions and sample size. Useful to determine quality control, tolerance limits, and critical values. Numerous tables concentrate on most reasonable application.
R: *Annals of Human Genetics* 41: 517 (May 1978).

Socioeconomic Issues of Health. **Robert J. Walsh, comp.** American Medical Association. Center for Health Services Research and Development. Chicago, IL: American Medical Association, 1971–.

Relates statistical data on many aspects of the U.S. population. Gathers information from U.S. Bureau of Census, AMA's research division, and various private sources. Includes data on mortality figures, supply and distribution of physicians, financial aspects of health care and services. Format concentrates on tables, charts, and graphs.
R: *ARBA* (1973, p. 613).

Statistical Tables for Biological, Agricultural and Medical Research. 6th rev. ed. **Ronald Aylmer Fisher and Frank Yates.** New York: Hafner, 1974.

Sixth edition, 1963.
Comprehensive collection of tables and bibliography of sources on statistical method.
R: *Choice* 6: 994 (Oct. 1969); Chen (p. 148); Jenkins (C62); Mal (9-24); Wal (pp. 76, 195); Win (EC20).

Vital and Health Statistics Monographs. 16 vols. **American Public Health**

Association. Cambridge, MA: Harvard University Press, 1968–1974. (Sponsored by the American Public Health Association.)

Examines status of American public health based on recent findings, clinical evidence, and awareness of the major trends occurring in the twentieth century. Important monographs for those instrumental in planning the future of American health care system.
R: *RSR* 3: 42 (Jan.–Mar. 1975).

COMMERCIAL MEDICAL MARKET RESEARCH SERVICES

While not directly a statistical source, it should be noted here that medical marketing surveys can be useful services for physicians and allied health professionals. There are numerous market research corporations which provide these services. For example, the Theta Technology Corporation publishes *Complete Market Research Service,* and Frost and Sullivan publishes *Wall Street and F&S Reports.* These publications provide marketing data on numerous products such as skin care aids, laboratory equipment, diagnostic imaging products, energy conservation systems, and ophthalmological products.

Commercial medical marketing services are highly sophisticated and expensive. Thus, smaller health science libraries and institutions will most likely not be able to afford their services. For example, studies published by Theta on medical laboratory disposable and cardiovascular diagnostic instruments cost $600 and $495, respectively, in 1979, while Frost and Sullivan has published such surveys as institutional energy conservation and ophthalmological products marketing which each cost $800. These research services, therefore, will be most helpful to allied health professionals involved in large-scale commercial production and marketing or medical and medical-related products. Most institutions probably will purchase a specific report to meet their needs rather than subscribe to the complete service program.

CHAPTER 8 MANUALS, LABORATORY MANUALS AND WORKBOOKS, AND SOURCE BOOKS

MANUALS

STYLE MANUALS

Bibliographic Guide for Editors & Authors. **American Chemical Society.** Washington, DC: American Chemical Society, 1974.

A bibliographic compilation of serials by BioSciences Information Service, Chemical Abstracts, and Engineering Index. Citations are from over 27,700 scientific and technical journals and contain complete information. Valuable for all library collections.
R: *RSR* 3: 42 (Jan.–Mar. 1975).

The Careful Writer: A Modern Guide to English Usage. 2d ed. **Theodore M. Bernstein.** New York: Atheneum, 1977.

First edition, 1965.
Emphasizes the improvement of medical writing. Deals with the language of physiology, anatomy, and pathology. Provides hints in assembling logical and practical guidelines for manuscript writing. Specifically helpful to those needing answers to grammatical and stylistic problems.
R: *JAMA* 239: 767 (Feb. 20, 1978).

CBE Style Manual. 4th ed. **Council of Biology Editors, Committee on Form and Style.** Arlington, VA: American Institute of Biological Sciences, 1978.

Original title: *Style Manual for Biological Journals.*
A commonly used guide to acceptable forms of abbreviations and citation formats in the biological sciences. For students and researchers.
R: Chen (p. 171)

Guide to Medical Writing: A Practical Manual for Physicians, Dentists, Nurses, Pharmacists. **Henry A. Davidson.** New York: Ronald Press, 1957.

Introductory material on medical writing. Practical approach to basic skills: outlining, revision, summaries, the choice of a dynamic vocabulary, research procedures, and arrangement of illustrations.
R: Win (EK101).

How to Write Scientific and Technical Papers. **Sam F. Trelease.** Cambridge, MA: MIT Press, 1969.

Medical Secretary's Manual. 2d ed. **Myreta Eshom.** New York: Appleton-Century-Crofts, 1977.

Revised edition of a manual for medical secretaries and secretarial students. Teaches terminology and transcription. Shorthand outlines are Diamond-Jubilee Shorthand. A useful self-teaching guide, helpful for training secretaries.

Medical Writing: The Technic and the Art. 4th ed. **Morris Fishbein.** Springfield, IL: Charles C. Thomas, 1972.

First edition, 1938.
A practical guide to medical writing. Comprehensive information on manuscript writing, grammatical usage, Latin words in medicine. Can be used like a dictionary for ready reference. A comprehensive and helpful guide.
R: *Clinical Pediatrics* 12: 624 (Oct. 1973); Win (EK102).

The Scientific Journal: Editorial Policies and Practices; Guidelines for Editors, Reviewers, and Authors. **Lois DeBakey.** St. Louis, MO: C. V. Mosby, 1976.

Synthesizes medical editorial policies of prominent editors. Details format, organization, responsibilities of editors, guidelines in handling manuscripts. Considered an indispensable source for editors.
R: *JAMA* 237: 809 (Feb. 21, 1977).

Stylebook/Editorial Manual. 6th ed. **Scientific Publications Division, American Medical Association.** Littleton, MA: Publishing Sciences Group, 1976.

A style manual for medical authors. Manual published in conjunction with the American Medical Association. Covers such topics as footnotes, abbreviations, copy editing, and proofreading marks. Includes index. Helpful in the writing of medical papers or journal articles.
R: *Journal of Nursing Administration* 7: 48 (Sept. 1977); *Nurse Educator* 2: 24 (Nov.–Dec. 1977); *ARBA* (1978, p. 705).

Technical Literature Search and the Written Report. **D. J. Maltha.** London: Pitman Medical, 1976.

Nine chapters devoted to all phases of literature searching and report writing. Researchers, librarians, and information and documentation workers are its intended audience.
R: *Quarterly Bulletin of the International Association of Agricultural Librarians and Documentalists* 21: 138 (1976).

Why Not Say It Clearly? A Guide to Scientific Writing. **Lester S. King.** Boston, MA: Little, Brown, 1978.

Written by a respected authority in the field of medical editing, this book provides guidelines for clear scientific writing. Considered an excellent reference, providing appropriate examples for many situations.
R: *Archives of Surgery* 114: 756 (June 1979); *Lancet* 1: 1170 (June 2, 1979); *Plastic and Reconstructive Surgery* 64: 92 (July 1979).

Writer's Guide to Medical Journals. **Nancy D. Lane and Kathryn L. Kammerer.** Cambridge, MA: Ballinger, 1975.

Useful reference tool for medical writers contemplating publication of their work. Lists over 300 general and research-oriented journals in the medical field

and a brief summary of their fields of interest. Accurate, full information provided for each journal. Contains a convenient bibliography of reference publications.
R: *Journal of Gerontology* 31: 487 (July 1976); *ARBA* (1976, p. 733).

Writing For Nursing Publications. **Andrea O'Connor.** Thorofare, NJ: Charles B. Slack, 1976.
A complete "how-to" book for nurses interested in writing for nursing publications.
R: Brandon (*NO*).

Writing Scientific Papers in English: An ELSE-Ciba Foundation Guide for Authors. **Maeve O'Connor and F. Peter Woodford.** New York: Associated Scientific Publishers, 1975.
Considered the "Bible" of scientific (primarily medical) writing. Prepared by skillful writers and editors at a meeting of the European Association of Editors of Biological Periodicals (ELSE). Engages the reader in the complete process of writing a paper in English. Contains countless practical hints to guide the writer through all situations. Useful information on units of measure, English usage, abbreviations, and "expressions to avoid" included in five appendixes. General readers, authors, and editors will find the material impressive. Valuable addition to scientific, medical, college, and special libraries.
R: *British Medical Bulletin* 32: 98 (1976); *International Journal of Radiation Biology* 24: 409 (1975); *Physics in Medicine & Biology* 21: 156 (Jan. 1976); *RSR* 4: 89 (Apr.–June 1976).

General

Manual of History Taking, Physical Examination and Record Keeping. 2d ed. **Elmer E. Raus and Madonna M. Raus.** Philadelphia, PA: J. B. Lippincott, 1974.
A pocket-size manual. The loose-leaf format provides necessary information for doctors needing to communicate with patients speaking another language. Phrases used are approved by the American Hospital Association. Includes drawings of body parts with corresponding terms and conversion tables.

A Manual on Medical Literature for Law Librarians: A Handbook and Annotated Bibliography. **Roy M. Mersky, David A. Kronick, and Leslie W. Sheridan.** Dobbs Ferry, NY: Oceana, 1973.
A manual for librarians in the medicolegal field; includes terminology, medical bibliography, indexing tools, citation style. Essential for all library collections.
R: *LJ* 99: 1525 (June 1, 1974); *RQ* 14: 76 (Fall 1974); *SL* 65: 160 (1974); *ARBA* (1975, p. 732).

Scope and Coverage Manual of the National Library of Medicine, PB-271 252. **US National Library of Medicine. Technical Services Division.** Bethesda, MD: US National Library of Medicine, 1977.
Official policy statement of the US National Library of Medicine on the range of

subjects pertinent to medicine and the extent to which certain material should be collected.
R: *RSR* 6: 55 (Apr./June 1978).

ALLERGY AND IMMUNOLOGY

Allergy Management in Clinical Practice. **Louis Tuft.** St. Louis, MO: C. V. Mosby, 1973.

A manual useful for treating allergic patients. Handy size, provides practical assistance.
R: *The Eye, Ear, Nose and Throat Monthly* 53: 90 (Apr. 1974); *Lancet* 1: 1200 (June 15, 1974); *TBRI* 40: 286 (Sept. 1974).

A Manual of Clinical Allergy. 3d ed. **John M. Sheldon et al.** Philadelphia, PA: W. B. Saunders, 1974.

Second edition, 1967.
Contains detailed information not readily available to physicians in the standard medical literature. Includes useful appendix on "Preparation of Allergenic Extracts for Testing and Treatment."
R: Allyn; Stearns & Ratcliff (*NEJM,* 1969; *NEJM,* 1970).

Manual of Clinical Immunology. **Noel R. Rose and Herman Friedman, eds.** Washington, DC: American Society for Microbiology, 1976.

Derived from a combined effort by the American Society for Microbiology and the American Association of Immunologists. Serves as a companion volume to the *Manual of Clinical Microbiology.* Manual covers nearly 1,000 pages. Intended as a comprehensive guide to immunology as it relates to clinical procedures. Essentially an up-to-date source of step-by-step laboratory procedures. Additional space given to inherent complications and pitfalls in procedures and advice and alternate methods. Photographs, tables, and charts help visualize test results. Suggestions and useful information on reagent and equipment suppliers. Manual deals with basic immunology, transplant immunology, autoimmunity, and allergy. Each section has a separate editor who is a recognized expert in his field. The quality of writing is good. Ample references to extensive reviews provided. Manual will define standard procedures for many of these techniques. Aimed mainly at laboratory directors and technologists but will serve as a useful reference source for graduate and medical students, residents, and clinicians.
R: *American Journal of Tropical Medicine and Hygiene* 26: 335 (1977); *Annals of Internal Medicine* 84: 359 (Mar. 1976); 86: 370 (Mar. 1977); *BMJ* 1: 717 (Mar. 12, 1977); *Clinical Chemistry* 23: 619 (1977); *Clinical Immunology and Immunopathology* 7: 442 (1977); *Clinical Pediatrics* 17: 375 (Apr. 1978); *Journal of Pharmaceutical Sciences* 66: 910 (June 1977); *Lancet* 1: 784 (Apr. 9, 1977); *Nature* 265: 282 (Jan. 20, 1977); *NEJM* 296: 458 (Feb. 24, 1977); *Yale Journal of Biology and Medicine* 50: 691 (1977); Brandon.

ANATOMY

Cunningham's Manual of Practical Anatomy. 14th ed. **G. J. Romanes, ed.** New York: Oxford University Press, 1976–1978.

Volume 1, *Upper and Lower Limbs,* 1976; volume 2, *Thorax and Abdomen,* 1977; volume 3, *Head, Neck and Brain,* 1978.
This revised edition of Cunningham's manual presents a regional approach to the study of human anatomy. There are new illustrations, many colored, and explanatory diagrams. Includes dissection instructions. In three volumes. Well written manual for medical and other students.
R: *Physical Therapy* 57: 754 (1977); 58: 237 (1978).

Experiments in Physiology. 3d ed. **Gerald D. Tharp.** Minneapolis: Burgess, 1976.

Anesthesiology and General Surgery

Anesthesiology: A Manual of Concept and Management. 2d ed. New York: Appleton-Century-Crofts, 1979.
Expanded second edition of anesthesia manual, contains most recent developments in diverse areas of one field. Includes up-to-date bibliographies referencing each chapter.

Clinical Anesthesia Procedures of the Massachusetts General Hospital. **Philip W. Lebowitz.** Boston, MA: Little, Brown, 1978.
Outlines basic information about anesthetic drugs and techniques. Particularly strong in problems relating to general and local anesthesia. Section on anesthesia for burn patient helpful to plastic surgeon. Written by the house staff of the Anesthesia Department of the Massachusetts General Hospital. List format recommended for inexperienced anesthesiologist.
R: *Plastic and Reconstructive Surgery* 63: 419 (1979).

Manual of Anesthesia. **John C. Snow.** Boston, MA: Little, Brown, 1977.
In practical format, this pocket-size manual offers the essentials of modern-day anesthesiology practice. Useful reference for those involved with the administration of anesthetic agents. Useful for clinical anesthesiologists, residents, nurses, and students.
R: *Anaesthesia* 34: 93 (Jan. 1979); *Anesthesiology* 49: 381 (Nov. 1978); *Plastic and Reconstructive Surgery* 63: 260 (1979).

Manual of Operating Room Technology. 4th printing. **Frances Ginsberg, Lillian S. Brunner, and Vernita Cantlin.** Philadelphia, PA: J. B. Lippincott, 1966.
R: Stearns & Ratcliff (*AJN*).

Manual of Surgical Intensive Care. **John M. Kinney, ed.** American College of Surgeons. Committee of Pre- and Post-Operative Care. Baltimore, MD: Williams & Wilkins, 1977.
Comprehensive guide to the development and management of surgical intensive care unit. Topics range from architectural to ethical problems.

Manual of Surgical Therapeutics. 4th ed. **Robert E. Condon and Lloyd M. Nyhus.** Boston, MA: Little, Brown, 1978.

First edition, 1969; second edition, 1972; third edition, 1975.
Companion to the *Manual of Medical Therapeutics*. Practical guide to the management and treatment of surgical patients. Twenty-five concise chapters touch on topics like trauma, surgical infections, burns, cardiac arrest, and renal failure. Designed to be available in the intern's and surgical house officer's pocket.
R: *Archives of Internal Medicine* 131: 943 (June 1973); *Archives of Surgery* 106: 118 (Jan. 1973); *British Journal of Surgery* 60: 670 (Aug. 1973); *Canadian Medical Association Journal* 103: 309 (Aug. 1, 1970); *Gastroenterology* 64: 145 (Jan. 1973): 71: 175 (July 1976).

Manual on Control of Infection in Surgical Patients. **American College of Surgeons. Commitee on Control of Surgical Infections and the Committee on Pre- and Post-Operative Care.** Philadelphia, PA: J. B. Lippincott, 1976.
Comprehensive treatment covering the prevention and control of infections. Organized and compiled by the Board of Regents of the American College of Surgeons. Considerable detail allotted to techniques of cleaning. Useful for all levels of patient care in a modern hospital. Should be compulsory reading for new personnel, medical students, interns, and infection control committees.
R: *Journal of Neurosurgery* 46: 840 (June 1977).

A Practice of Anaesthesia. 4th ed. **H. C. Churchill-Davidson, ed.** Philadelphia, PA: W. B. Saunders, 1978.
Considered a classic manual of anesthesiology, extensively revised and updated; cross-referenced.
R: *NEJM* 300: 933 (Apr. 19, 1979).

Quick Reference to Surgical Emergencies. **Gerald W. Shaftan, ed.** Philadelphia, PA: J. B. Lippincott, 1974.
A ready reference manual in outline form, supplies information on all aspects of surgical emergencies. Comprehensive coverage, strongly recommended for physicians in the emergency room as well as paramedical staff. Contains illustrations, easy to use, flexibly bound.
R: *British Journal of Surgery* 62(7): 587 (July 1975); *Journal of Neurosurgery* 43(2): 248 (Aug. 1975).

Synopsis of Surgery. 2d ed. **Richard D. Liechty and Robert T. Soper.** St. Louis, MO: C. V. Mosby, 1972.
A reference manual which offers definitive information concerning the wide range of topics in the field of surgery. Chapters are divided into subject by organ system. Also includes chapters on fluids, electrolytes, shock, infections. Well-illustrated, reliable guide. Useful for medical students and physicians.
R: *American Family Physician* 7: 205 (Mar. 1973).

Washington University Department of Surgery Manual on Techniques of Emergency and Outpatient Surgery. **Allen P. Klippel and Charles B. Anderson.** Boston, MA: Little, Brown, 1978.
Provides essential information on emergency care measures. Illustrates emergency room methods of patient handling in routine and uncommon situations.

Detailed illustrations of all anatomic regions accompany the text. Useful mini-atlas for physicians, surgeons, and students.

BRAIN AND NERVOUS SYSTEM

Aphasia Therapy Manual. **Joseph C. Aurelia.** Danville, IL: Interstate, 1974.
A manual for the treatment of speech dysfunction. Well organized, describes clinical treatment techniques, provides both comprehensive and specific information. Helpful for professionals who deal with speech therapy treatment of neurologically handicapped adults.
R: *Archives of Physical Medicine and Rehabilitation* 56: 184 (Apr. 1975).

Comprehensive Management of Epilepsy in Infancy, Childhood, and Adolescence. **Samuel Livingston.** Springfield, IL: Charles C. Thomas, 1972.
A reference manual which emphasizes attention to drug therapies and side effects, differential diagnosis, epilepsy in children. Handy tables, up-to-date bibliographies are included. Well organized, comprehensive manual.
R: *Clinical Pediatrics* 12: 508 (Aug. 1973).

The Diagnosis and Treatment of Diseases of the Nervous System. 2 vols. **Frederick Lees.** New York: American Elsevier, 1970.
A two-volume manual which covers diseases of the nervous system. A basic reference source which includes description, treatment, investigations, and illustrations of diseases. Recommended for medical libraries.

Electrical Activity of the Nervous System. 4th ed. **Mary A. B. Brazier.** Baltimore, MD: Williams & Wilkins, 1977.
First edition, 1951; third edition, 1967.
Well organized, concise presentation of select neuroelectric fundamentals. Introductory book which is recommended for students in neuroscience and practicing clinicians in neurological areas.
R: *Journal of Neurosurgery* 48: 842 (May 1978).

Manual of Basic Neuropathology. 2d ed. **Raymond Escourolle and Jacques Poirier. Lucien J. Rubinstein, trans.** Philadelphia, PA: W. B. Saunders, 1978.
First edition, 1973.
Up-to-date introductory manual of neuropathology. Includes recent advances in the field, a survey of neuropathological techniques. High-quality black and white photographs and drawings; numerous tables and diagrams which convey fundamental anatomic and pathological concepts. Organization by specific disease categories. Extensive revisions and accurate English translation add to its worth. Invaluable as a teaching tool; also recommended for residents in neurology, neurosurgery, pathology, and neuropathology.
R: *Archives of Neurology* 31: 216 (Sept. 1974); 36: 183 (Mar. 1979); *Journal of Clinical Pathology* 32: 95 (1979); *Journal of Neurosurgery* 41: 780 (Dec. 1974); *Lancet* 1: 16 (Jan. 5, 1974); *NEJM* 289: 1316 (Dec. 13, 1973).

A Manual of Head Injuries in General Surgery. **Graham Martin.** London: Heinemann, 1974.

Straightforward guide to the understanding and treatment of head injuries. Emphasis on the prevention of complications after the damage is done. Well illustrated. Compact, sturdy manual fits nicely in a coat pocket. Intended for general and orthopedic surgeons, junior staff, nurses, and medical students.
R: *BMJ* 2: 345 (May 10, 1975); *Lancet* 1: 78 (Jan. 11, 1975).

A Manual of Neurosurgery. **Marshall B. Allen et al.** Baltimore, MD: University Park Press, 1977.

Highlights nervous system pathological conditions: CNS lesions, intervertebral disks, neoplasms, etc. Some discussion of CNS infection and surgical relief of pain. Follows a clinical orientation. Some 300 illustrations complement text. Chapters conclude with self-evaluation questions. Good introduction to neurosurgery for the medical student.
R: *Archives of Neurology* 36: 325 (May 1979).

Reflex Testing Methods for Evaluating C. N. S. Development. 2d ed. **Mary R. Fiorentino.** Springfield, IL: Charles C. Thomas, 1973.

A photographic manual which presents CNS reflexes, both normal and abnormal. Discusses motor problems in handicapped children, among other topics. Useful, practical manual for occupational and physical therapists.
R: *American Journal of Diseases of Children* 127: 601 (Apr. 1974).

Cardiovascular System

Atherosclerosis—Is It Reversible? **G. Schettler, E. Stange, and R. W. Wissler, eds.** New York: Springer-Verlag, 1978.

A manual of atherosclerosis, includes tables and illustrations. Recommended for clinicians, specialists, and researchers.

Bedside Cardiology. 2d ed. **Jules Constant, ed.** Boston, MA: Little, Brown, 1976.

A manual of cardiovascular diagnosis, useful for both the student and the practitioner.
R: *Annals of Internal Medicine* 87: 136 (July 1977); *Chest* 72: A-20 (July 1977).

Cardiac Catheterization and Angiocardiography: An Introductory Manual. 3d ed. **David Verel and Ronald G. Grainger.** London: Churchill Livingstone, 1978.

This manual includes photographs of heart disease with accompanying legends. Considered a superior work for cardiologists.
R: *American Heart Journal* 89: 101 (1975).

Hypertension Manual. **John H. Laragh, ed.** New York: Dun-Donnelley, 1974.

Definitive review of hypertension. Nine hundred pages devoted to current research in this field. Contributions include six parts, dealing with epidemiology, methods, mechanisms, management diet, the renin system, and antihypertension

agents. Short, practical drug and diet tables enhance the manual's usefulness. Few illustrations. Manual designed for cardiovascular specialists, researchers in hypertension, libraries. Too complex for average family physician.
R: *American Family Physician* 11: 195 (Jan. 1975); *American Heart Journal* 88: 392 (1974); *Lancet* 2: 441 (Aug. 24, 1974).

Intensive Coronary Care. **Michael F. Oliver, Desmond G. Julian, and Myra G. Brown.** Geneva: World Health Organization, 1974.
Key information on the setup, organization, and operation of coronary care units. Useful for physicians and nurses in training. Based on author's experience at the Royal Infirmary in Edinburgh. Emphasis on disorders of rhythm and conduction. No index or references.
R: *RSR* 3: 36 (July–Dec. 1975).

Intensive Coronary Care: A Manual for Nurses. 3d ed. **Lawrence E. Meltzer, Rose Pinneo, and J. R. Kitchell.** Bowie, MD: Charles Press, 1977.
R: Stearns & Ratcliff (*AJN*; *NEJM*, 1970).

Manual of Coronary Care. **Joseph S. Alpert and Gary S. Francis.** Boston, MA: Little, Brown, 1977.
Authoritative coverage of the management of patients with acute myocardial infarction. Attempts to fill the gap made by the change in character of coronary care units and confusing literature. Avoids ambiguous statements; simple language and few grammatical errors add to the manual's usefulness. A necessity for every coronary care unit (CCU) and its nursing personnel and house officers.
R: *Annals of Internal Medicine* 87: 385 (Sept. 1977).

Peripheral Vascular Surgery. **Martin Birnstingl, ed.** Philadelphia, PA: J. B. Lippincott, 1974.
An authoritative manual for vascular, thoracic, and orthopedic surgeons. Detailed discussions. A good reference source.
R: *Annals of Surgery* 183: 448 (Apr. 1976); *Annals of Thoracic Surgery* 19: 611 (May 1975); *Archives of Surgery* 110: 355 (Mar. 1975); *JAMA* 231: 1397 (Mar. 31, 1975).

Practical Echocardiography: A Basic Manual. 2d ed. **C. David Joffe.** Bowie, MD: Charles Press, 1978.
Written for the beginning student, technician, or physician, this is a basic manual of echocardiography. Discussions are brief; the text outlines such things as recording technique, equipment, diagnosis. Useful in ultrasound departments.
R: *Annals of Internal Medicine* 89: 731 (Nov. 1978); Allyn.

Practical Electrocardiography. 5th ed. **H. J. L. Marriott.** Baltimore, MD: Williams & Wilkins, 1972.

Treatment of Cardiac Emergencies. **Emanuel Goldberger and Myron W. Wheat, Jr.** St. Louis, MO: C. V. Mosby, 1974.
Concise discussion of cardiac emergencies, diagnosis, and management. Outlines the use of pacemakers, other devices, and drugs used in the treatment of cardiac

problems. Practical reference for thoracic and cardiac surgeons, resident, medical student, and general physician.
R: *American Heart Journal* 88: 815 (1974); *Annals of Internal Medicine* 82: 294 (Feb. 1975); *Annals of Thoracic Surgery* 21: 268 (Apr. 1976); *Journal of the Kansas Medical Society* 76: 14A (Jan. 1975); *TBRI* 41: 104 (Mar. 1975); 41: 143 (Apr. 1975).

DENTISTRY

Clinical Dental Anesthesia: A Manual of Principles and Practice. **J. M. Bell.** Philadelphia, PA: J. B. Lippincott, 1975.

A manual which approaches the care of the dental in-patient. Offers guidelines for the dentist and physician-anesthesiologist. Contains information on sedation methods, patient risk, in relation to operating room procedures. Excellent manual for dentists, residents.
R: *Anesthesiology* 45: 109 (July 1976).

Construction and Utilization of Visual Aids in Dental Health Education. **Florean Dearth.** Thorofare, NJ: Charles B. Slack, 1974.
R: *RSR* 3: 35 (July–Dec. 1975).

Dentist's Manual of Emergency Medical Treatment. **Robert J. Braun.** New York: Prentice-Hall, 1979.

A handbook for use in the diagnosis and management of acute medical emergency situations in the dentist's office. A practical tool for both dental professional and paraprofessional.

A Manual of Dissection for Students of Dentistry. **N. J. B. Plomley.** New York: Churchill Livingstone, 1975.

A manual which attempts to codify dissection procedures for dental students. Concise, clear descriptions and line drawings of head and neck dissection, emphasizing orofacial region. Helpful to students and instructors.
R: *Journal of Anatomy* 121: 214 (Feb. 1976); *Journal of Oral Surgery* 34: 1044 (Nov. 1976).

A Manual of Practical Orthodontics. 3d ed. **W. J. Tulley and A. C. Campbell.** Chicago, IL: Year Book Medical Publishers, 1970.

Oral Health Survey, Basic Methods. 2d ed. Geneva: World Health Organization, 1977.

Outlines the design of oral health surveys; new edition includes modifications and presents guidelines of survey methods which can be used more frequently.
R: *Journal of Oral Surgery* 36: 323 (Apr. 1978).

DERMATOLOGY

Current Dermatologic Management. 2d ed. **Stuart Maddin, ed.** St. Louis, MO: C. V. Mosby, 1975.

Alphabetically arranges skin diseases and briefly discusses appropriate therapeutic techniques, diagnostic criteria. Contributions from over 200 dermatologists;

copious references. Recommended to all medical libraries.
R: *JAMA* 235: 2542 (June 7, 1976).

Manual of Contact Dermatitis. **Sigfrid Fregert.** Chicago, IL: Year Book Medical Publishers, 1975.

Precise, reliable coverage of contact dermatitis. Especially useful are tables of patch test concentrations, a compilation of irritants and sensitizers in common occupations, and a survey of areas of greatest concentrations of common allergens. Good index. Highly recommended for clinical dermatologists, industrial medical officers, and employment advisors. Useful for consultation in hospitals, the law, and industry.
R: *Archives of Dermatology* 112: 1346 (Sept. 1976); *Lancet* 1: 78 (Jan. 11, 1975).

Manual of Dermatologic Syndromes. 2d ed. **Thomas Butterworth.** Philadelphia, PA: J. B. Lippincott, 1972.

A pocket-size manual of over 335 syndromes of dermatologic significance. Alphabetical listing with basic descriptions of particular syndrome; enlarged from first edition, a practical source of information recommended for inclusion in all medical libraries.
R: *American Family Physician* 7: 199 (Feb. 1973); *Annals of Internal Medicine* 78: 472 (Mar. 1973); *Archives of Dermatology* 107: 130 (Jan. 1973); *MRW* S2, p. 27.

Manual of Skin Diseases. 3d ed. **Gordon C. Sauer.** Philadelphia, PA: J. B. Lippincott, 1973.

Detailed information on common and not-so-common skin diseases. Good descriptions of the structure of the skin. Laboratory procedures, dermatological diagnosis, and a basic formulary. Treatment of dermatological disorders receives greatest emphasis. Over 400 color and black and white photographs of good quality enhance the manual's usefulness. Innovative and valuable dictionary-index to all known skin diseases is a valuable source of information. Highly recommended for medical students, nurses, paramedicals, and nondermatologist physicians.
R: *American Family Physician* 9: 257 (Jan. 1974); *American Journal of Nursing* 74: 1171 (June 1974); *Annals of Internal Medicine* 81: 142 (July 1974); *Archives of Internal Medicine* 134: 1141 (Dec. 1974).

ENDOCRINOLOGY

Joslin Diabetes Manual. 11th ed. **Leo P. Krall, ed.** Philadelphia, PA: Lea & Febiger, 1978.

First edition, 1918; tenth edition, 1959.
Strongly recommended as a "classic" in the area of diabetic education and self-management. Presents basic facts on the nature and physiology of diabetes as well as specific guidelines for exercise, diet, and insulin intake. Several sections deal with marriage, pregnancy, employment, and complications in simple terms. Makes liberal use of illustrations, photographs, and tabular data. Highly recommended for the diabetic patient and family.
R: *American Family Physician* 19: 257 (May 1979); *Journal of Community Health* 4: 333 (Summer 1979); *Journal of the American Dietetic Association* 74: 715 (June 1979); *Nursing* 9: 108 (Apr. 1979).

MANUALS, WORKBOOKS, AND SOURCE BOOKS

Manual of Endocrine Surgery. **Anthony J. Edis, Luis A. Ayala, and Richard H. Egdahl.** New York: Springer-Verlag, 1975.
A comprehensive manual of endocrine diagnosis and treatment of diseases. Divided into four sections which deal systematically with diseases of thyroid, parathyroid, adrenals, and pancreas. Contains numerous illustrations, references, and a wealth of up-to-date information. Recommended to endocrinological surgeons of all levels.
R: *Annals of Internal Medicine* 85: 705 (Nov. 1976); *Archives of Surgery* 111: 726 (June 1976); *British Journal of Surgery* 64: 381 (Apr. 1977); *JAMA* 235: 2020 (May 3, 1976) *NEJM* 294: 1242 (May 27, 1976).

GASTROINTESTINAL SYSTEM

Manual of Surgery of the Gallbladder, Bile Ducts and Exocrine Pancreas. **R. E. Hermann.** New York: Springer-Verlag, 1978.

GENETICS

Dealing with Dilemma: A Manual for Genetic Counselors. **Patricia T. Kelly.** New York: Springer-Verlag, 1977.
Orients the genetic counselor to the necessary skills of the field, presenting information in outline form. Deals also with social and psychological impact of genetic diagnosis. A commendable manual, linking general counseling skills with clinical genetics.
R: *American Journal of Human Genetics* 30: 233 (Mar. 1978); *Social Biology* 25: 85 (1978).

GERONTOLOGY

Working with the Elderly: A Training Manual. **C. S. Deichman and C. P. O'Kane.** Buffalo, NY: D. O. K. Publishers, 1975.
Instructive manual for persons in charge of developing activity leader training programs. Publication stems from the experiences of the Department of Occupational Therapy, SUNY Buffalo. Contains a substantial index of miscellaneous useful information.
R: *Journal of Gerontology* 31: 617 (Sept. 1976).

HEALTH SERVICES ADMINISTRATION

A Coursebook in Health Care Delivery. **Sidney Shindell, Jeffrey C. Salloway, and Colette M. Oberembt.** New York: Appleton-Century-Crofts, 1976.
A manual which addresses problems in health care delivery in this country, covering a wide range of topics from rehabilitation to malpractice. Timely, instructive book for physicians, residents.
R: *JAMA* 236: 2110 (Nov. 1, 1976).

Health Planning & Manpower Register. Washington, DC: Capitol Publications, 1979.
Lists all federal requirements in the health planning and manpower fields. Pro-

vides full texts of documents affecting state and local health planning grants, grants and loans for medical facility modernization, HSA governing board regulations, and new laws and regulations. Updated monthly.

Health Project Management: A Manual of Procedures for Formulating and Implementing Health Projects, WHO Offset Pub. no. 12. **J. Bainbridge and S. Sapirie.** Geneva: World Health Organization, 1974.

Outlines plans which implement the management of health. Topics include a malaria control plan, water supply systems, recruitment of health care workers. Includes charts, diagrams.
R: *RSR* 4: 42 (Jan.–Mar. 1976).

Hospital Law Manuals. 6 vols. **Paul C. Lasky, ed.** Germantown, MD: Aspen Systems.

Administrators' Set, vols. 1, 1A, 1B; Attorneys' Set, vols. 2, 2A, 2B. Subscription service in binder format. Each set contains identical laws but differing descriptive material.

Manuals For Health Care Institutions. **Frank D. Murphy.** Boston, MA: G. K. Hall, 1979–.

Cost Management Techniques for Hospitals, 1978 rev. ed.; *Model Policy Statements for Hospitals with Job Descriptions,* 1978; *Model Safety, Environmental, and Infection Control Policies,* 1977; *Manual For Review and Update of Hospital Department Safety, Environmental, and Infection Control Policies,* 1979.

A series of manuals to serve as models for hospital policy development. Looseleaf format provides for easy integration with the institutions' own administrative manuals.

Medical Equipment Service Manual: Theory and Maintenance Procedures. **Frank Biloon.** Englewood Cliffs, NJ: Prentice-Hall, 1978.

Staff Development in Geriatric Institutions: A Manual for the Trainer. **M. B. Kinney.** Ann Arbor, MI: University of Michigan-Wayne State University, Institute of Gerontology, 1976.

A manual which serves those who provide care for the elderly. Discusses training of personnel, organizing activities and workshops, and resources. Includes a bibliography.
R: *Journal of Gerontology* 31: 618 (Sept. 1976).

The Volunteer Services Department in a Health Care Institution. **American Hospital Association.** Chicago, IL: American Hospital Association, 1973.

A volunteer's manual. Designed to meet the needs of a developing volunteer services department. Provides guidelines for director. Information on legal aspects and AHA support programs.

Hematology

Lymphocytes, Isolation, Fractionation and Characterisation. **J. B. Natvig, P. Perlmann, and H. Wigzell, eds.** Oslo, Norway: Universitetsforlaget, 1976.

Emphasis on descriptions of procedures for isolation of lymphocytes and granulocytes, fractionation techniques, and affinity fractionation on columns. Clear account of complement receptors. Useful, practical manual in a specific field.
R: *Immunology* 34: 955 (May 1978).

INFECTIOUS DISEASES

Control of Communicable Diseases in Man. 12th ed. New York: American Public Health Association, 1975.

Eleventh edition, 1970.
Standard reference manual listing etiology and epidemiology of over 100 communicable diseases, published by the American Public Health Association. Standard information for laboratory identification, diagnosis, treatment, and prevention is provided. A basic tool.
R: *Occupational Health Nursing* 24: 55 (June 1976); Brandon; Stearns & Ratcliff (*AJN*; *NEJM*, 1970).

Manual of Acute Bacterial Infections: Early Diagnosis and Treatment. **Pierce Gardner and Harriet T. Provine.** Boston, MA: Litte, Brown, 1976.

Quick reference source for physicians in emergency room situations. Encompasses investigation and diagnosis of acute bacterial infections. Noteworthy suggestions on the interpretation of results and rational use of antibiotics. Relevant illustrations; numerous tables which capture diagnostic features, therapeutic application, and the organism. Useful addition to the primary physician's library and emergency room.
R: *Gastroenterology* 72: 187 (Jan. 1977); *Lancet* 1: 840 (Apr. 17, 1976).

A Manual of Antimicrobial Therapy. **Geroge A. Pankey.** Springfield, IL: Charles C. Thomas, 1969.

Primarily concerned with antimicrobial agents, their pharmacokinetic properties, and their role in the treatment of infectious disease. Essentially an objective guide for the practitioner faced with the decision of the best agent for a particular patient. Required reading for medical personnel: students and physicians.
R: *Canadian Medical Association Journal* 102: 878 (Apr. 25, 1970).

Manual of Clinical Microbiology. 2d ed. **Edwin H. Lennette et al., eds.** Washington, DC: American Society for Microbiology, 1974.

Standard handbook covering a wide range of topics in this discipline, including mycology, bacteriology, virology, etc. Similar in scope to Bailey's *Diagnostic Microbiology*, 1974.
R: *Choice* 12: 1798 (Feb. 1975); *ARBA* (1976, p. 658).; Chen (p. 171).

Manual of Practical Entomology in Malaria, WHO Offset Pub. no. 13. **World Health Organization Division of Malaria and Other Parasitic Diseases.** Geneva: World Health Organization, 1975.

Part I, *Vector Bionomics and Organization of Anti-Malaria Activities*; Part II, *Methods and Techniques*.
A valuable publication of entomological vectors of malaria. Discusses methods

and techniques of control. Includes references and illustrations. Recommended for special libraries.
R: *RSR* 4: 46 (Jan.–Mar. 1976).

Manual of Tropical Medicine. 5th ed. **George W. Hunter et al.** Philadelphia, PA: W. B. Saunders, 1976.

Fourth edition, 1966.
Emphasizes the clinical and epidemiological aspects of tropical medicine. Divides chapters according to diseases. Contains over 1,000 photographs, an appendix of the distribution of communicable diseases. Helpful to all those who deal with tropical medicine.
R: Allyn; Stearns & Ratcliff (*NEJM,* 1969; *NEJM,* 1970).

Manual on Control of Infection in Surgical Patients. **Committee on Control of Surgical Infections and the Committee on Pre- and Post-Operative Care, American College of Surgeons.** Philadelphia, PA: J. B. Lippincott, 1976.

Comprehensive treatment covering the prevention and control of infections. Organized and compiled by the Board of Regents of the American College of Surgeons. Considerable detail allotted to techniques of cleaning, preparing, and sterilizing rooms and instruments. A specific weakness is the abundant number of references dating to 1970 and earlier. Due to multi-authored nature, some repetition and personal bias are inevitable but kept to a minimum. Extremely useful for all levels of patient care in a modern hospital. Should be compulsory reading for new personnel, medical students, interns, and infection control committees.
R: *Anesthesiology* 46: 380 (May 1977); *British Journal of Surgery* 64: 379 (May 1977); *Journal of Bone and Joint Surgery* 59B: 522 (Oct. 1977); *Journal of Neurosurgery* 46: 840 (June 1970); *Journal of Oral Surgery* 35: 1005 (Dec. 1977); *JAMA* 237: 808 (Feb. 21, 1977); *Plastic and Reconstructive Surgery* 59: 741 (1977).

Manual on Larval Control Operations in Malaria Programmes. **World Health Organization Division of Malaria and Other Parasitic Diseases.** Geneva: World Health Organization, 1973.

A standard source of information on control of malarial agents. Describes technicalities of antilarval programs, lists insecticides. Also discusses vectors and epidemiology. Highly recommended for the wealth of information it contains. Helpful to those who deal with medical problems in entomology.
R: *BMJ* 2: 566 (June 8, 1974).

Internal Medicine

Acute Drug Abuse Emergencies: A Treatment Manual. **Peter G. Bourne, ed.** New York: Academic Press, 1976.

A manual which updates *A Treatment Manual for Acute Drug Abuse Emergencies,* contains information on drug abuse emergencies of all kinds. Provides an excellent clinical reference; written by a cross-section of 41 specialists. The book has a helpful index and will be useful to all those who deal with drug abuse.
R: *American Journal of Psychiatry* 134: 1061 (Sept. 1977); *Lancet* 1: 402 (Feb. 19, 1977).

A Barefoot Doctor's Manual. **Revolutionary Health Committee of Hunan Province.** London: Routledge & Kegan Paul, 1978.

Focuses on the skill of Chinese "barefoot doctors" and their role in improving public health in China. Introduction outlines human anatomy, hygiene, diagnostic and therapeutic techniques, and birth control. Heart of the manual deals with diseases, their treatment and prevention. Conclusion describes some 500 medicinal herbs with many illustrations and drawings. Includes good indexes. Despite some translation errors, the manual provides welcome information to the Western world. Essentially written for medical auxiliaries of Hunan Province.
R: *Brain* 102: 230 (Mar. 1979).

Bedside Diagnosis. 11th ed. **Charles Seward.** London: Churchill Livingstone, 1979.

Tenth edition, 1974.
A manual which describes symptoms used to detect common diseases; data is collected from various sources: clinical histories, physical examinations, etc. Brief discussions. Useful for students and physicians.
R: *Annals of Internal Medicine* 81: 573 (Oct. 1977).

Bedside Diagnostic Examination. 3d ed. **Elmer L. DeGowin.** New York: Macmillan, 1976.

A pocket-size manual with an integrated approach to bedside diagnosis; includes facts from major fields of medicine. Functional format, numerous illustrations.
R: Allyn.

Current Therapy. **Howard F. Conn, ed.** Philadelphia, PA: W. B. Saunders, 1949–. Annual.

Provides access to up-to-date treatment measures for practicing physicians. Arranged by type of disease, discusses disorder and lists treatment drugs, reactions, dosages, etc. A useful tool in therapeutics, particularly for the primary physician.
R: *American Family Physician* 19: 239 (Nov. 1978); *Annals of Internal Medicine* 79: 323 (Aug. 1973); 91: 148 (July 1979); *Canadian Medical Association Journal* 103: 210 (July 25, 1970); Allyn.

Diagnosis and Early Management of Trauma Emergencies: A Manual for the Emergency Service. **Robert J. Touloukian and Thomas J. Krizek.** Springfield, IL: Charles C. Thomas, 1974.

A ready-reference manual for treatment of emergency trauma; divided into three sections for quick information retrieval. Complete index; concisely written; recommended for residents, medical students, and emergency room personnel.
R: *Plastic and Reconstructive Surgery* 56: 206 (1975).

First Aid Principles and Procedures. **Pamela B. doCarmo and Angelo T. Patterson.** Englewood Cliffs, NJ: Prentice-Hall, 1976.

Comprehensive guide to the correct handling of the injured person in an emergency. Highlights general and specialized techniques. Some 100 illustrations complement text; appendixes chock-full of pertinent diagrams. Geared as a first aid text for students. Transparencies available.

A Manual of Adverse Drug Interactions. 2d ed. **J. P. Griffin and P. F. D'Arcy.** Bristol, England: John Wright, 1979.
First edition, 1975.
R: *Lancet* 1: 344 (Feb. 14, 1976).

Manual of Ambulatory Medicine. **Alan S. Robbins and James A. Tamkin, eds.** Philadelphia, PA: W. B. Saunders, 1979.
Offers guidelines to cover common outpatient problems. Provides primary care physicians with sound and cost-effective diagnosis and therapy.

A Manual of Basic Virological Techniques. **G. C. Rovozzo and C. N. Burke.** Englewood Cliffs, NJ: Prentice-Hall, 1973.
R: *American Scientist* 63: 353 (May/June 1975); Chen (p. 171).

Manual of Clinical Biology. Bethesda, MD: American Society for Microbiology, 1970.
R: Chen (p. 171).

Manual of Clinical Laboratory Methods. 4th ed. **Opal Hepler.** Springfield, IL: Charles C. Thomas, 1973.
R: Chen (p. 171).

Manual of Critical Care Medicine. **M. H. Weil and P. L. da Luz, eds.** New York: Springer-Verlag, 1977.

Manual of Emergency Medical Therapeutics. **Mickey S. Eisenberg and Michael K. Copass.** Philadelphia, PA: W. B. Saunders, 1978.
Handy reference source of emergency therapeutic information. Lists over 70 common emergency situations, each categorized by major body sections. General considerations, diagnosis, therapy, and numerous references follow selected conditions or diseases. Important topics include drug overdose, management of cardiac arrhythmia, and critical drug dosage.

Manual of Medical Therapeutics. 22d ed. **Nicholas V. Costrini and William M. Thomsom, eds.** Boston, MA: Little, Brown, 1977.
First edition, 1943; twentieth edition, 1971; twenty-first edition, 1974.
Twenty-two editions in less than 35 years attest to this manual's popularity. One of the most used references on the management of common problems in general medicine. Prepared by Washington University in St. Louis. Comprehensive coverage in 22 chapters. Includes information on appropriate laboratory tests, non-drug methods of treatment, and logical, organized guidance. Features concise, handy tables. Highly recommended to residents, interns, and senior medical students.
R: *Annals of Internal Medicine* 82: 597 (Apr. 1975); *Archives of Internal Medicine* 131: 306 (Feb. 1973); *Archives of Surgery* 110: 1053 (Aug. 1975); *Canadian Medical Association Journal* 118: 240 (Feb. 4, 1978); *Gastroenterology* 75: 546 (Sept. 1978).

Manual of the International Statistical Classification of Diseases, Injuries, and

Causes of Death. 2 vols. **World Health Organization.** Geneva: World Health Organization, 1977–1978.

Alphabetical index to *Ninth Revision of the International Classification of Diseases* printed in form of tabular list. Essential adjunct to tabular list which has three sections of alphabetical indexes covering diseases and nature of injury, external causes of injury, and drugs and other chemical substances. A corrigenda to vol. 1 is also included.
R: *American Journal of Public Health* 68: 76 (Jan. 1978); 68: 78 (Jan. 1978); *IBID* 5: 351 (Dec. 1977); 6: 427 (Dec. 1978).

Medical Assistant's Manual. **G. B. Wyatt and J. L. Wyatt.** New York: Mc-Graw-Hill, 1973.

Oriented to developing countries. A guide to diagnosis and treatment. Excellent textbook for assistant in training and standard reference for rural area practice.
R: *Lancet* 1: 844 (May 4, 1974).

The Merck Manual of Diagnosis and Therapy. 13th ed. **Robert Berkow, ed.** Rahway, NJ: Merck and Co., 1977.

First edition, 1899; twelfth edition, 1972.
Comprehensive, encyclopedic manual which emphasizes the diagnosis and treatment of disease. Contributions are from more than 250 North American and British doctors from all branches of medicine. Provides a good index and convenient format for quick information retrieval. Concise, accurate, classic guide for doctors in all fields and levels of practice.
R: *American Journal of Digestive Diseases* 23: 575 (June 1978); *American Journal of Ophthalmology* 84: 880 (Dec. 1977); *Archives of Ophthalmology* 90: 423 (Nov. 1973); *JAMA* 239: 1217 (Mar. 20, 1978); *Pediatrics* 51: 325 (Feb. 1973); Sheehy (EK18); Win (EK95, 1EJ13).

Multilingual Manual for Medical History-Taking. **Louis R. M. Del Guercio.** Boston, MA: Little, Brown, 1972.

Compact, spiral-bound manual which contains 100 questions to aid the physician in obtaining a history from non-English speaking patients. Languages included are French, Spanish, German, Russian, Polish, Italian. Most questions can be answered in simple "yes" or "no" fashion. Contains helpful, rudimentary terms in each language.
R: *Annals of Internal Medicine* 78: 993 (June 1973); *Archives of Surgery* 107: 351 (Aug. 1973).

NIOSH Manual of Analytical Methods. **US National Institute for Occupational Safety and Health.** Washington, DC: US Government Printing Office, 1979.

Shock Trauma Manual. **William Gill and William B. Long.** Baltimore, MD: Williams & Wilkins, 1979.

Provides guidelines for care of emergency patients suffering trauma or needing resuscitation. Succinct, up-to-date. Includes effective and detailed procedures of emergency therapy.

Student Manual of Physical Examination. **Marie S. Brown et al.** Philadelphia, PA: J. B. Lippincott, 1977.
A manual of physical examination of children and adults. Designed to work as a companion to selected films and texts. Easy to follow format. Intended for medical students.

NURSING

Ambulatory Care Manual for Nurse Practitioners. **Peter T. Capell and David B. Case.** Philadelphia, PA: J. B. Lippincott, 1976.
A well-organized reference for nurse practitioners; covers diagnosis and treatment of health problems frequent in the adult and adolescent. Includes helpful drawings, tables, and case studies.
R: *American Journal of Nursing* 77: 81 (Jan. 1977); *Nurse Practitioner* 2: 38 (Sept.–Oct. 1976).

Basic Arithmetic Review and Drug Therapy. 4th ed. **Grace E. Fitch, Margaret A. Larson, and Marion P. Mooney.** Riverside, NJ: Macmillan, 1977.
Updated edition of a manual that provides information for nurses who administer drugs. Contains practical administration such as measuring, calculating doses, drugs used in allergies.

Clinical Nursing and Techniques. 4th ed. **Norma Deson.** St. Louis, MO: C. V. Mosby, 1979.
R: Brandon (*NO*).

Illustrated Manual of Nursing Techniques. **Eunice M. King, Lynn Wieck, and Marilyn Dyer.** Philadelphia, PA: J. B. Lippincott, 1977.
Guide to basic nursing procedures. Covers all aspects of nursing from psychosocial aspects to patient education. Each section includes terminology, definitions, equipment, evaluation, and charting. Alphabetical listing of items within the outline format enhances the manual's usefulness. Numerous illustrations. Good discussion of chest drainage, neurological signs, traction, and intra-catheter insertion.
R: *American Journal of Nursing* 78: 150 (Jan. 1978); *Nursing* 7: 12 (June 1977); Brandon (*NO*).

Inservice Education Manual for the Nursing Department. 2d ed. **Monica Mary Wagner.** St. Louis, MO: Catholic Hospital Association, 1978.
Prepared for the inservice education staff of Misericordia Medical Center, New York. Valuable introductory manual for all inservice coordinators contemplating the design or revision of personal inservice manuals. Includes accurate job descriptions, format for annual reports, and sample evaluation forms.
R: *Journal of Nursing Administration* 9: 4 (July 1979).

The Lippincott Manual of Nursing Practice. 2d ed. **Lillian S. Brunner and Doris S. Suddarth.** Philadelphia, PA: J. B. Lippincott, 1978.
First edition, 1974.

Extensive coverage of three major sections of nursing: medical/surgical, maternity, and pediatrics. Presents clinical problems, causes, manifestations, treatments, etc. Includes an index to emergency situations, nursing alerts for critical procedural points, and capsule guidelines to basic nursing action. Includes 300 superb illustrations highlighting treatment and nursing management. Considerable information for instructors, students, practitioners, and returning nurses.
R: Brandon (*NO*).

Manual for Nurses in Family and Community Health. 2d ed. **Helen Cohn and Joyce E. Tingle.** Boston, MA: Little, Brown, 1974.

Written in an outline form. Includes helpful exercises; also guidelines to the instructor for these exercises. Intended to orient instructors, nurses, nursing supervisors, and public health nurses in the field of community health nursing.

Massachusetts General Hospital Manual of Nursing Procedures. **Massachusetts General Hospital Department of Nursing.** Boston, MA: Little, Brown, 1975.

Spiral-bound outline of patient care techniques for nurses. Emphasizes frequently encountered problems. Clearly written in step-by-step manner.

Mosby's Manual of Critical Care. **Linda F. Abells, ed.** St. Louis, MO: C. V. Mosby, 1979.
R: Brandon (*NO*).

Nursing Care of the Cancer Patient. 3d ed. **Rosemary E. Bouchard and Norma F. Owens.** St. Louis, MO: C. V. Mosby, 1976.

Second edition, 1972.
The third edition of this manual specifically outlines problems and principles in caring for cancer patients.
R: Brandon (*NO*); Stearns & Ratcliff (*AJN*; *NEJM,* 1970).

Nursing Diagnosis and Intervention in Nursing Practice. **Claire Campbell.** New York: John Wiley, 1978.

A complete manual which helps nurses to identify patient problems. Lists over 200 diagnoses and evaluations. Written in nursing terms. A good ready reference manual.
R: *Occupational Health Nursing* (Apr. 1978); *Saskatchewan Registered Nurses' Association* (Apr. 7, 1978); Brandon (*NO*).

A Nursing Manual for Care of the Patient with Stroke. **Mary O'Brien and Phyllis Pallett.** Boston, MA: Little, Brown, 1978.

The Pediatric Nursing Skills Manual. **B. J. Whitson and J. McFarlane.** New York: Wiley Medical, 1980.

A Practical Manual for Patient Teaching. **Karen Zander et al.** St. Louis, MO: C. V. Mosby, 1978.

A manual for nurses geared toward patient education. Deals with disorders of all major systems.
R: Brandon (*NO*).

Practical Nurse Nutrition Education. 4th ed. **Alberta D. Shackleton and Charlotte L. Poleman.** Philadelphia, PA: W. B. Saunders, 1978.
Emphasizes maintenance and improvement of nutrition as an integral part of the total patient care. Numerous charts, graphs, and illustrations complement the text. Reliable reference source for practical nurses and students.

Primary Care Nursing: A Manual of Clinical Skills. **Clarke B. Hazlett, ed.** Philadelphia, PA: F. A. Davis, 1977.
Systematic, cross-referenced manual approaching primary health care procedures for nurses. Well organized, spiral bound; objectives of book are easily outlined.
R: Brandon (*NO*).

Psychiatric Nursing: A Basic Manual. 4th ed. **Annie L. Crawford and Barbara B. Buchanan.** Philadelphia, PA: F. A. Davis, 1974.
Handbook of developments in field of mental health and changes which must occur in education of mental health and psychiatric nursing personnel. Important for instructors of nursing students, psychiatric attendants, etc.

Techniques of Patient Care: A Manual of Bedside Procedures. 2d ed. **Clarence E. Zimmerman.** Boston, MA: Little, Brown, 1976.
Concise, practical manual which includes numerous bedside procedure techniques. Chapters include information on respiration therapy, catheterization. Includes clear illustrations, index. Handy ready reference manual which brings together a large amount of useful information.
R: *Archives of Physical Medicine and Rehabilitation* 59: 296 (June 1978).

NUTRITION

Diet Manual. 2d ed. **Dietary Staff of Vanderbilt University Hospital, comp.** Nashville, TN: Vanderbilt University Press, 1969.
First edition, 1961.
A guide for dietitians, dietetics interns, physicians, and professional nursing staff.
R: *Choice* 7: 1018 (Oct. 1970); Win (EK178; 3EJ21).

Diet Manual. **Massachusetts General Hospital. Dietary Department.** Boston, MA: Little, Brown, 1976.
An excellent manual intended for those who plan nutritional needs of hospitalized patients; provides food values, principles of nutrition, and relates these to special groups such as pregnant women, diabetics, etc. Spiral bound. There is an appendix which includes food labeling information, measure conversion charts, dietary preparation for diagnostic procedures.
R: *Gastroenterology* 73: 859 (Oct. 1977).

Manual of Applied Nutrition. 6th ed. **Nutrition Department, Johns Hopkins Hospital et al.** Baltimore, MD: Johns Hopkins University Press, 1973.

Manual of Clinical Dietetics and Physician's Guide. 2d ed. **Chicago Dietetic Association and South Suburban Dietetic Association of Chicago.** Downers Grove, IL: Johnson Printers, 1975.

Aims to assemble information needed to plan an effective diet. Publication is the work of dietitians from eight hospitals in the Chicago area. Various diets are specifically arranged: standard hospital diets; pediatric diets; protein-, fat-, and sodium-controlled diets; and gastrointestinal diets. Loose-leaf binder format allows for a quick, easy reference answer. Practical guide for physicians on ordering special diets for specific diseases included. Valuable library addition for physicians, health professionals involved in nutritional counseling, and nutritionists.

R: *American Journal of Clinical Nutrition* 30: 1197 (July 1977); *Journal of the American Dietetic Association* 68: 190 (Feb. 1976).

Mayo Clinic Diet Manual. 4th ed. **Mayo Clinic.** Philadelphia, PA: W. B. Saunders, 1971.

A manual for dietitians. Contains standard and specialized diets for pregnant women, heart patients, overweight patients, and allergics. Appendix contains data on chemical composition of foods. Recommended for trained dietitians.

Methods of Sampling and Analysis of Contaminants in Food: Report of a Joint FAO/WHO Expert Consultation, 1978. **Food and Agriculture Organization of the United Nations.** New York: Unipub, 1978.

Discusses sampling and analytic methods in food contaminant testing. Standard for WHO committees; includes method for analyzing tin and arsenic. List of documents.

R: *IBID* 4: 332 (Dec. 1976); 6: 289 (Sept. 1978).

Nutritional Support of Medical Practice. **Howard A. Schneider, Carl E. Anderson, and David B. Coursin, eds.** Hagerstown, MD: Harper & Row, 1977.

An excellent manual that emphasizes nutrition as a method of treatment and therapy. Presents, in three sections, basic science of nutrition, metabolic responses in illness, and specific formulas and their clinical applications. A basic reference for the clinical dietitian.

R: *American Family Physician* 17: 299 (Jan. 1978); *Journal of the American Dietetic Association* 72: 344 (Mar. 1978).

Surgical Nutrition. **Committee on Pre- and Post-Operative Care, American College of Surgeons.** Philadelphia, PA: W. B. Saunders, 1975.

An excellent manual which presents nutritional information from history to metabolism of fats, proteins, carbohydrates. Includes instructive diagrams, numerous references. This manual is geared specifically toward the surgeon and is highly recommended.

R: *Archives of Surgery* 111: 833 (July 1976).

ONCOLOGY AND NUCLEAR MEDICINE

Cancer: A Manual for Practitioners. 5th ed. **Blake Cady, ed.** Boston, MA: American Cancer Society, Massachusetts Division, 1978.

A multidisciplinary overview of cancer management. Includes information on melanoma, immunology, pediatric oncology, lung cancer. Emphasizes clinical aspects of treatment, details classification and stages of tumor growth. Provides an authoritative review. Highly recommended to clinicians who care for cancer patients.
R: *NEJM* 301: 280 (Aug. 2, 1979).

Clinical Oncology: A Manual for Students and Doctors. **Committee on Professional Education. International Union Against Cancer.** New York: Springer-Verlag, 1973.

Succinct, covering a wide range of topics in oncology: etiology, epidemiology, pathology, treatment, etc. Includes color illustrations and photomicrographs of specific types of tumors, and classification. Edited by International Union Against Cancer. Excellent index; provides much basic information.
R: *NEJM* 289: 758 (Oct. 4, 1973).

Manual of Tumor Nomenclature and Coding. Washington, DC: American Cancer Society, 1968.

OPHTHALMOLOGY

Anatomy of the Orbit. 2d ed. **Crowell Beard and Marvin H. Quickert.** Birmingham, AL: Aesculapius, 1977.

First edition, 1969.
Superior second edition; a dissection manual of ophthalmologic anatomy containing excellent photographic illustrations. An excellent reference for surgeons who perform ophthalmologic procedures.
R: *American Journal of Ophthalmology* 84: 277 (Aug. 1977); *Archives of Ophthalmology* 95: 1472 (Aug. 1977).

Practical Management of Eye Problems: Glaucoma, Strabismus, Visual Fields. **Frederick H. Roy.** Philadelphia, PA: Lea & Febiger, 1975.

Presents practical advice on the prevention, recognition, and treatment of ocular problems. Comprehensive coverage in outline form. Reviews basic examination procedures, symptoms, and signs. Strongest component of this manual is the differential diagnosis of the three main eye disorders: glaucoma, strabismus, and visual field defects. Useful companion to ophthalmologists, trainees, internists, and general practitioners.
R: *American Journal of Ophthalmology* 80: 307 (1975); *Archives of Ophthalmology* 93: 1379 (Dec. 1975); *NEJM* 294: 175 (Jan. 15, 1976); *TBRI* 42: 66 (Feb. 1976); Brandon.

ORTHOPEDICS

Manual of Acute Orthopaedic Therapeutics. **Larry D. Iverson and D. Kay Clawson.** Boston, MA: Little, Brown, 1977.

Succinct, updated version of the *Orthopaedic Department Manual* used at the University of Washington. Outlines basic management procedures of fractures and joint injuries and their complications. Clear, concise advice on topics such as traction, plaster and bandaging techniques, and emergency splints. Contains es-

sential references, useful appendix, and good quality drawings and diagrams. Strongly recommended for the orthopedic resident.
R: *British Journal of Surgery* 65: 523 (July 1978); *Journal of Bone and Joint Surgery* 59A: 701 (July 1977); *Lancet* 1: 588 (Mar. 18, 1978).

Manual of Mechanical Orthopaedics. **Z. Alfonso Tohen.** Springfield, IL: Charles C. Thomas, 1973.

Profusely illustrated manual which contains information on orthotic and prosthetic devices. Helpful to surgeons and physical therapists. Provides a ready reference to questions concerning prosthetic and orthotic systems.
R: *Journal of Bone and Joint Surgery* 56A: 219 (Jan. 1974); *Physical Therapy* 54: 910 (1974).

Muscle Testing: Techniques of Manual Examination. 3d ed. **Lucille Daniels and Catherine Worthingham.** Philadelphia, PA: W. B. Saunders, 1972.

First edition, 1946.

Classic manual on muscle testing for physical therapists and others. Updated edition includes an illustrated guide to gait analysis. Maintains easy-to-follow format, brief discussions. Spiral bound, useful for elementary techniques of testing muscle strength.
R: *Archives of Physical Medicine and Rehabilitation* 55: 46 (Jan. 1974); *Plastic and Reconstructive Surgery* 53: 342 (1974).

Traction and Orthopaedic Appliances. **John D. M. Stewart.** New York: Churchill Livingstone, 1975.

Comprehensive instruction manual. Covers many important and long neglected aspects of orthopedic appliances and traction. Excellent chapters on foot wear and walking aids. Good quality line drawings. Contains wealth of information not readily available in standard textbooks. Fills a gap in orthopedic literature for trainees, house surgeons, nurses, and physical therapy staff.
R: *Archives of Physical Medicine and Rehabilitation* 59: 201 (Apr. 1978); *Journal of Bone and Joint Surgery* 57B: 408 (Aug. 1975).

Pathology

Autopsy Pathology, Procedure and Protocol. **D. L. Weber, E. P. Fazzini, and T. J. Reagan.** Springfield, IL: Charles C. Thomas, 1973.

A basic manual of postmortem techniques. Explains autopsy procedures, reasons for rules of permission, protocol construction. Some photographs are not easily interpreted, and text varies; however, useful for pathology departments.
R: *Journal of Anatomy* 117: 443 (Apr. 1974).

Histological Typing of Skin Tumours. **R. E. J. ten Seldam and E. B. Helwig.** Geneva: World Health Organization, 1974.

Focuses on the classification of skin tumors according to histological type. One hundred seventy-six color photomicrographs enhance the text. Invaluable reference source for pathologists and dermatologists.
R: *JAMA* 234: 1186 (Dec. 15, 1975).

Manual of Cyto-Technology. **American Society of Clinical Pathology. National Committee for Careers in the Medical Laboratory.** Chicago, IL: American Society of Clinical Pathology, 1975.

A text used for teaching cytotechnology in the Boston Hospital for Women program.

PEDIATRICS

A Manual of Newborn Medicine. **Gerard Van Leeuwen, ed.** Chicago, IL: Year Book Medical Publishers, 1973.

A concise informative manual of neonatology. Includes useful tables and diagrams; fills a necessary gap in the literature of neonatology. Recommended particularly to residents in pediatrics.
R: *BMJ* 1: 462 (Mar. 9, 1974); *Pediatrics* 53: 591 (Apr. 1974).

Manual of Pediatric Therapeutics. 2d ed. **John W. Graef and Thomas E. Cone, Jr., eds.** Boston, MA: Little, Brown, 1978.

First edition, 1974.
Written by the house staff at the Boston Children's Hospital. Basically a prescriptive source of information for the practitioner who encounters single clinical problems infrequently. A compendium of data on drug dosages and common pediatric treatments. All information based on current practice at the Children's Hospital. Usefulness inhibited by several shortcomings: references rarely cited, reference tables lack completeness, and lack of precision in dangerous therapeutics is evident. Welcome reference source for private physicians and house staff.
R: *American Journal of Diseases of Children* 130: 454 (Apr. 1976); *NEJM* 293: 365 (Aug. 14, 1975).

Paediatric Allergy and Clinical Immunology (as applied to Atopic Disease): A Manual for Students and Practitioners of Medicine. 4th ed. **Cecil C. Williams.** New York: Longman, 1973.

A brief manual that discusses allergy problems in children; a useful reference.
R: *Clinical Pediatrics* 14: 803 (Sept. 1975).

The Parents' Medical Manual. **Glenn Austin, ed.** Englewood Cliffs, NJ: Prentice-Hall, 1978.

Introduces parents to basic childhood health problems. Encourages them to take an active role in managing medical situations at home. Contains information on first aid, accident prevention, and nutrition. Illustrated section deals with normal growth and development from infancy to adolescence. Thoroughly explains injury and illness in simple language. Special problems, such as retardation, speech defects, and handicaps, encompass a separate section.

Practical Manual of Pediatrics: A Pocket Reference for Those Who Treat Children. **William W. Waring and Louis O. Jeansonne.** St. Louis, MO: C. V. Mosby, 1975.

Handy collection of facts for the pediatrician. Divided into eleven sections for easy reference; contains methods of treatment, diagnosis, and care in emergency

situations, as well as graphs and charts. Loose-leaf format; contains much useful information.
R: *NEJM* 293: 515 (Sept. 4, 1975).

Practical Paediatric Endocrinology. **C. G. D. Brook.** New York: Grune & Stratton, 1978.
Geared toward the practicing physician who plans and executes the investigation of children with endocrine problems. Recommended to pediatricians and endocrinologists.

Primary Child Care: A Manual for Health Workers. **Maurice King and Felicity King.** New York: Oxford University Press, 1978.
Emphasizes a simple introduction to practical pediatric care in developing countries. Geared toward paramedical workers in third world areas.

Reece-Chamberlain's Manual of Emergency Pediatrics. 2d ed. **Robert M. Reece, ed.** Philadelphia, PA: W. B. Saunders, 1978.
Features alphabetical listings of problems in five major sections: neonatal emergencies, complaints in emergency room pediatrics, specific diagnostic entities, true emergencies, and procedures and therapeutics. Revision concentrates on actual emergencies.

The Whole Pediatrician Catalog. **Julia A. McMillan, Phillip I. Nieburg, and Frank A. Oski.** Philadelphia, PA: W. B. Saunders, 1977.
Assists the pediatrician in diagnosing and treating disease. Organized systematically, a frequently used source of ready reference.
R: *American Family Physician* 17: 323 (Mar. 1978).

PHARMACY AND PHARMACOLOGY

American Hospital Formulary Service. 2 vols. **Mary J. Reilly and Judith A. Kepler, eds.** Washington, DC: American Society of Hospital Pharmacists, 1977.
First edition, 1959–.
Two volumes in loose-leaf format; describes and evaluates drugs including their chemical uses, side effects, dosage, and preparations. Information is arranged by therapeutic category.

AMA Drug Evaluations. 4th ed. **American Medical Association.** Littleton, MA: Publishing Sciences Group, 1980.
First edition, 1971; third edition, 1977.
Provides critical evaluations of various categories of drugs used in medicine. Lists basic information on dosage, adverse reactions, structural formulas, and generic and proprietary names of some 1,300 drugs. Highly recommended to those who prescribe, dispense, or administer drugs.
R: *Canadian Medical Association Journal* 117: 1376 (Dec. 17, 1977); *Clinical Pharmacology and Therapeutics* 15: 227 (1974); *Journal of Oral Surgery* 36: 568 (July 1978); *Journal of Pharmaceutical Sciences* 66: 1512 (Oct. 1977); *Pharmaceutical Journal* 220: 323 (1978); Sheehy (EK36); Win (EK194); Allyn.

Chinese Herbs: Their Botany, Chemistry, and Pharmacodynamics. **John D. Keys.** Rutland, VT: Charles E. Tuttle, 1976.

A compendium of herbal properties. Entries arranged by division, class, order, family, and genera. Provides name(s), habitat, chemical analysis, description. Numerous appendixes and tables are included. Also a glossary and bibliography. A source of scholarly insight into herbal lore.
R: *ARBA* (1977, p. 724).

Clinical Toxicology of Commercial Products: Acute Poisoning. 4th ed. **Robert E. Gosselin et al.** Baltimore, MD: Williams & Wilkins, 1976.

First edition, 1957; second edition, 1963; third edition, 1969.
Provides assistance for physicians dealing with chemical poisoning. Lists all pertinent toxicological information, trade name and chemical formula of drugs, recommendations for treatment. Up-to-date, reliable, authoritative manual.
R: *ARBA* (1977, p. 717); Sheehy (EK41); Win (EK 223; 3EJ35); Allyn; Stearns & Ratcliff (*AJN*; *NEJM,* 1969; *NEJM,* 1970).

Hazards of Medication: A Manual on Drug Interactions, Incompatibilities, Contraindications, and Adverse Effects. 2d ed. **Eric W. Martin, ed.** Philadelphia, PA: J. B. Lippincott, 1978.

Second edition guides the doctor to choice of prescription. Includes tables of drug interactions, laboratory tests. Comprehensively cross-referenced and referenced.

Pharmacy Technicians' Manual. 2d ed. **Jane M. Durgin, Zachary I. Hanan, and Charles O. Ward.** St. Louis, MO: C. V. Mosby, 1978.

A comprehensive manual written for pharmacy support staff training. Examines aspects of pharmacy from history to administration; also discusses such topics as education, job opportunities.

Principles of Drug Information Services. **Arthur S. Watanabe and Christopher S. Conner.** Hamilton, IL: Drug Intelligence Publications, 1978.

Covers all aspects of drug information, emphasizes patient-oriented information. Contains self-assessment information, clinical problems, extensive bibliography. Also contains helpful information on how to do systematic literature search. A valuable manual for pharmacy students.
R: *Lancet* 1: 808 (Apr. 14, 1979).

Techniques of Medication: A Manual on the Administration of Drug Products. **Eric W. Martin et al.** Philadelphia, PA: J. B. Lippincott, 1969.

A comprehensive manual for those who administer or prescribe drugs. Details prescription writing, avoiding legal pitfalls. Under three main sections: dermatology, gastroenterology, and parenterally.

PHYSICAL MEDICINE AND REHABILITATION

Lifting, Moving, and Transferring Patients: A Manual. **Marilyn J. Rantz and Donald Courtial.** St. Louis, MO: C. V. Mosby, 1977.

Photographic description of the activities involved in numerous patient transfers

and lifting and moving techniques. Each pictorial sequence is accompanied by simple instructions and precautions on positioning of therapy assistants and patient. Excellent outline for physical and occupational therapists, nurses, and other health professionals. A learning tool for students, aides, and even patients' families.
R: *Physical Therapy* 57: 1439 (Dec. 1977).

Manual for Physical Therapy Technicians. **Willibald Nagler.** Chicago, IL: Year Book Medical Publishers, 1974.
A basic manual outlining various therapeutic procedures and the types of patients involved. Contains valuable information on transfers and gaits. Excellent step-by-step illustrations. References at end of chapters refer readers to further readings. No detailed coverage of the arthritic patient, the patient with neurological problems, or the physically disabled child. Geared as a study guide for the physical therapy aide or technician. Insufficient reference source for registered physical therapists and physical therapy students.
R: *Archives of Physical Medicine and Rehabilitation* 56: 506 (Nov. 1975).

Rehabilitation: A Manual for the Care of the Disabled and Elderly. 2d ed. **Gerald G. Hirschberg, Leon Lewis, and Patricia Vaughan.** Philadelphia, PA: J. B. Lippincott, 1976.
Revised manual which emphasizes the combination of all health personnel skills in treatment of the elderly. Explains common methods of rehabilitation, discusses the structure and physical plant of rehabilitation units. Helpful to medical personnel and instructors, both academic and clinical.
R: *Physical Therapy* 57: 1090 (1977).

PSYCHIATRY AND PSYCHOLOGY

Manual of Psychiatric Therapeutics: Practical Psychopharmacology and Psychiatry. **Richard I. Shader, ed.** Boston, MA: Little, Brown, 1975.
Written in outline format, this pocket-size manual serves as a quick reference for emergency room psychiatric problems. Topics range from "hypnosis" to "management of violent patients." Special emphasis on the rise of psychotherapeutic drugs. Most of the seventeen authors are recognized authorities in their fields. References are scarce, and controversial subjects are avoided. Designed for the house officer who manages psychiatric patients with drugs.
R: *American Journal of Psychiatry* 135: 139 (Jan. 1978); *NEJM* 294: 1351 (June 10, 1976).

Psychotropic Drugs: A Manual for Emergency Management of Overdosage. **Nathan S. Kline, Stewart F. Alexander, and Amparo Chamberlain.** Oradell, NJ: Medical Economics Co., 1974.
Lists over 120 compounds in alphabetical order, contains color pictures for identification, toxicity information, cross-references, as well as a directory of Poison Control Centers in the United States. Discusses clinical signs and treatment of overdose. Concise, cogent manual for emergency departments.
R: *Annals of Internal Medicine* 82: 130 (Jan. 1975); *JAMA* 229: 1509 (Sept. 9, 1974); *ARBA* (1975, p. 751); *MRW* S3, pp. 4, 22, 41, 42, 53.

Psychotropic Drugs and Related Compounds, DHEW Pub. no. (HSM) 72-9074. 2d ed. **Earl Usdin and Daniel H. Efron.** Washington, DC: US Government Printing Office, 1972.

Exhaustive listing of compounds with psychoactive properties. Discusses their chemical structure, pharmacologic activity, and therapeutic classification. Also a guide to names and addresses of manufacturers and distributors. Contains an index of compounds and combinations. Over 1,750 references included. Useful volume for research worker, clinician, and medical student.
R: Win (EK200).

PUBLIC HEALTH

Accident Prevention Manual for Industrial Operations. 7th ed. **US National Safety Council.** Chicago, IL: US National Safety Council, 1974.

Clinical Toxicology of Commercial Products. 4th ed. **R. Gosselin, ed.** Baltimore, MD: Williams and Wilkins, 1976.

Health Information for International Travel. Atlanta, GA: US Center for Disease Control, US Public Health Service, US Department of Health, Education, and Welfare. Annual.

Annual Supplement to *MMWR, Morbidity and Mortality Weekly Reports.*

Manual of Mortality Analysis: A Manual on Methods of Analysis of National Mortality Statistics for Public Health Purposes. Geneva: World Health Organization, 1977.

A manual which includes graphs, tables, formulae, analysis of population data, which relate to measures of mortality. Data also includes a basic explanatory text
R: *IBID* 6: 434 (Dec. 1978).

A Manual on Drug Dependence. **J. F. Kramer and D. C. Cameron, eds.** Geneva: World Health Organization, 1975.

A summary of scientific patterns of drug dependence. It describes drugs, clinical syndromes, social problems resulting from abuse. Types of drugs included are alcohol, amphetamines, canabis, barbiturates, opiates, hallucinogens. Lists references.
R: *IBID* 3: 151 (Sept. 1975); *RSR* 4: 45 (Jan.–Mar. 1976).

Microorganisms in Foods. 2d ed. **International Commission on Microbiological Specifications for Foods (ICMSF) of the International Association of Microbiological Societies.** Toronto, Ontario: University of Toronto Press, 1978.

Volume 1, *Their Significance and Methods of Enumeration.*
First edition, 1968, F. S. Thatcher and D. S. Clarke, eds.
Updated edition covers entirely new topics (yeasts and molds, foodborne parasitic and viral agents, and bacteria associated with food poisoning). Updating well-balanced by some deletions. Tables list pertinent microbiological values. Sec-

tion on apparatus and materials oversimplified. A comprehensive, international manual on food microorganisms.
R: *Journal of Food Technology* 14: 101 (Feb. 1979).

Plague Manual. **M. Bahmanyar and D. C. Cavanaugh.** Geneva: World Health Organization, 1976.

Comprehensive guidelines for those who work with plague control. Includes epidemiology and characteristics of plague-causing insects and rodents. Referenced, detailed, useful for the epidemiologist, microbiologist, and other lab workers in disease control.
R: *Lancet* 1: 126 (Jan. 15, 1977); *IBID* 5: 46 (Mar. 1977).

RADIOLOGY

An Introduction to Radiation Protection. **Alan Martin and Samuel A. Harbison.** New York: John Wiley, 1973.

Training manual for health physicists and reference source for those without professional guidance. A wealth of technical information on tolerances, shielding, monitors, and related problems.
R: *Physics in Medicine & Biology* 18: 892 (Nov. 1973); *TBRI* 40: 16 (Jan. 1974).

A Manual of Radiographic Positioning. **George B. Greenfield and Steven J. Cooper.** Philadelphia, PA: J. B. Lippincott, 1973.

Designed to provide material on basic positions of radiography. Makes excellent use of photographs, drawings, and radiographs of anatomy and positioning. This core text is organized regionally. Specifically oriented to new students. Due to the elementary nature of its contents, a supplementary textbook is recommended.
R: *Journal of Allied Health* 3: 124 (Spr. 1974); *Radiology* 110: 96 (1974).

Manual on Radiation Protection in Hospitals and General Practice. 4 vols. **International Labour Organization, International Atomic Energy Agency and World Health Organization.** Geneva: World Health Organization, 1974–1977.

Volume 1, *Basic Protection Requirements,* 1974; volume 2, *Unsealed Sources,* 1975; volume 3, *X-ray Diagnosis,* 1975; volume 4, *Radiation Protection in Dentistry,* 1977. Four volumes, each covering essentials of radiation protection. The volumes were written under the authority of the International Labour Organization, the International Atomic Energy Agency, and the World Health Organization. The series is concise, comprehensive, and uniformly authoritative. Highly recommended to those involved in radiation work, hospital administrators, and dentists.
R: *Annals of Internal Medicine* 83: 441 (Sept. 1975); *Archives of Internal Medicine* 136: 628 (May 1976); *British Journal of Radiology* 48: 456 (1975); 51: 57 (1978); *Health Physics* 31: 472 (Nov. 1976); *International Journal of Radiation Biology* 27: 312 (1975); *IBID* 3: 52 (Mar.–June 1975); 3: 267 (Dec. 1975); 5: 249 (Sept. 1977); *RSR* 4: 44 (Jan.–Mar. 1976); 4: 45 (Jan.–Mar. 1976).

Manual on Radiation Sterilization of Medical and Biological Materials, Technical Report Series, no. 149. Vienna: International Atomic Energy Agency. Distr. New York: Unipub, 1973.

Provides information to scientific and technical personnel engaged in radiation sterilization. Individual chapters represent different aspects of the topic.
R: *ARBA* (1975, p. 658); Chen (p. 171); Mal (9–26).

Technical Aspects of Tomography. **M. L. Durizch.** Baltimore, MD: Williams & Wilkins, 1978.

Formerly part of Golden's Diagnostic Radiology, *Tomography: Physical Principles and Clinical Applications.* Working reference to tomographic details such as patient-positioning, film size, and tube movement. Technique charts appear at the end of major sections.

Respiratory System

Cystic Fibrosis: Manual of Diagnosis and Management. **Charlotte M. Anderson and Mary C. Goodchild.** Oxford, England: Blackwell Scientific Publications, 1976.

A complete manual covering the pathogenesis, diagnosis, treatment, and history of cystic fibrosis. Chapters are well referenced and include histologic sections and radiographic reproductions of high quality. For both clinicians and researchers. This book is highly recommended.
R: *Clinical Pediatrics* 17: 656 (Aug. 1978); *Lancet* 2: 1119 (Nov. 20, 1976); *NEJM* 296: 457 (Feb. 24, 1977).

Manual of Respiratory Therapy. 2d ed. **Joan P. Taylor.** St. Louis, MO: C. V. Mosby, 1978.

First edition, 1973.
Reference manual to care for the patient with respiratory problems. Three sections describe the etiology, clinical features, and treatment of respiratory conditions. Recommended as an introductory text for respiratory therapists. Experienced workers will enjoy its handy reference data.
R: *Physical Therapy* 54: 549 (May 1974).

Respiratory Technology: A Procedure Manual. 2d ed. **D. L. Hunsinger et al.** Reston, VA: Reston Publishing Co., 1976.

First edition, 1973.
A study manual for respiration therapists. Presents step-to-step basic procedures and simplified view of anatomy, physiology, chemistry, and gas laws. Over 130 tables and illustrations.
R: *American Journal of Nursing* 74: 8963 (May 1974); *Physical Therapy* 55: 450 (1975).

Respiratory Therapist Manual. **Stanley Pincus.** Indianapolis, IN: Bobbs-Merrill, 1975.

An introductory manual of respiration therapy. Presents technical information at the community college level.
R: *Choice* 12: 1200 (Nov. 1975).

Urogenital System

Clinical Sexuality: A Manual for the Physician and the Professions. 3d ed. **John F. Oliven.** Philadelphia, PA: J. B. Lippincott, 1974.
First edition, 1955.
A manual of sexual behavior covering physiological and psychological aspects. Maintains a clinical approach to the problems of human sexuality.
R: *Annals of Internal Medicine* 81: 720 (Nov. 1974); *JAMA* 230: 616 (Oct. 28, 1974); *NEJM* 291: 1367 (Dec. 19, 1974).

Contraceptive Technology: 1978–1979. 9th ed. **R. A. Hatcher, et al.** New York: Irvington, 1978.
Practical and technological developments in birth control. Discusses contraception, fertility control, abortion, biochemical changes, and drug interactions of contraceptives. Paperback, up-to-date.

Detection, Prevention and Management of Urinary Tract Infections: A Manual for the Physician, Nurse and Allied Health Worker. 2d ed. **Calvin M. Kunin.** Philadelphia, PA: Lea & Febiger, 1974.
A "gem" for allied health professionals involved with the collection of urine specimens.

Manual of Gynecologic and Obstetric Emergencies. **Ben-Zion Taber.** Philadelphia, PA: W. B. Saunders, 1979.
Comprehensive coverage of the management of gynecologic and obstetric emergencies. Alphabetical arrangement of conditions under the following major topics: "General Principles," "Specific Problems," "Procedures and Therapy," and "Emergency Medications." Invaluable reference tool for ob/gyns and emergency personnel.
R: *NEJM* 300: 932 (Apr. 19, 1979).

Manual of Renal Transplantation. **S. N. Chatterjee et al.** New York: Springer-Verlag, 1979.

Manual of Selected Procedures and Treatments. **Vaclav Insler and Roy Homburg.** New York: Kraeger, 1979.
Sets forth guidelines for the diagnosis and management of emergency gynecological and obstetric situations. Nine chapters deal with pregnancy and fetal monitoring. Remaining 23 chapters devoted to various gynecological complications. Valuable reference tool for obstetricians and gynecologists as well as emergency room departments.

Manual on Artifical Organs. 2 vols. **Yukihiko Nose.** St. Louis, MO: C. V. Mosby, 1969–1973.
Volume 1, *The Artificial Kidney: A Guide to Understanding for the Physician and for the Patient,* 1969; volume 2, *The Oxygenator,* 1973.

Practical Obstetrics and Gynecology: Manual of Selected Procedures and Treatment. **Vaclav Insler and Roy Homburg.** Basel: S. Karger, 1979.

Reviews procedures in obstetrics and gynecology. Helpful for residents or interns; well illustrated.
R: *BMJ* 1: 1207 (May 5, 1979).

Problem Pregnancy and Abortion Counseling. **Robert R. Wilson, ed.** Saluda, NC: Family Life Publications, 1973.

A necessary tool, informative for those who counsel women with unwanted or problem pregnancies. Also contains information on birth control, directory of counseling agencies, and bibliography. Recommends counseling methods, deals with abortion and alternatives. A well-balanced book.
R: *American Journal of Diseases of Children* 127: 764 (May 1974); *Annals of Internal Medicine* 79: 615 (Oct. 1973); *Archives of Physical Medicine and Rehabilitation* 55: 99 (Feb. 1974).

Surgical Gynecological Techniques. **F. Novak.** New York: John Wiley, 1978.

A step-by-step manual of techniques in surgical gynecology. Includes all fundamental procedures and new advances. Illustrations are clear, precise, and helpful in understanding each stage of the operation. Recommended for all medical libraries.

VETERINARY MEDICINE

The Merck Veterinary Manual: A Handbook of Diagnosis and Therapy for the Veterinarian. 5th ed. **O. H. Siegmund et al., eds.** Rahway, NJ: Merck and Co., 1979.

First edition, 1955; third edition, 1967; fourth edition, 1973.
Completely revised, this fourth edition covers a wide variety of veterinary subjects. Emphasizes veterinary care in North America; includes diseases, poisons and toxicology, nutrition, care of 200 animals, diagnostic procedures, laboratory diagnosis, and prescriptions. Indexed. Indispensable guide for veterinarians.
R: *ARBA* (1975, p. 753); Sheehy (EK44); Win (EJ146; EK231).

Veterinary Clinical Parasitology. 5th ed. **Margaret W. Sloss and R. L. Kemp.** Ames, IA: Iowa State University, 1978.

A diagnostic manual, considered both a useful teaching tool and practical tool.
R: *Journal of the American Veterinary Medical Association* 173: 1521 (Dec. 1, 1978).

LABORATORY MANUALS AND WORKBOOKS

GENERAL

Medical Terminology and the Body System. **M. A. Collin.** New York: Harper & Row, 1974.

Medical terminology for the layman; provides definitions of relevant terminology in a "teach yourself" format. Does not have an index.
R: *ABL* 41: entry 18 (Jan. 1976).

Terminology and Communication Skills in the Health Sciences. **James Lea.** Englewood Cliffs, NJ: Prentice-Hall, 1975.

Practice exercises in communication skills and techniques for all health professionals. Selected by faculty from medical, dental, nursing, medical technology, pharmacy, and public health schools. Exercises taken from authentic study activities.

ALLERGY AND IMMUNOLOGY

Exercise Manual in Immunology. **Lazar M. and Paula Schwartz.** New York: Medcom, 1975.
R: Chen (p. 181).

Techniques in Clinical Immunology. **R. A. Thompson, ed.** Philadelphia, PA: J. B. Lippincott, 1977.
Covers the most practical laboratory tests in clinical immunology. Methods and problems discussed in detail. Appropriate applications, interpretations, and limitations of methods also listed. Additional references to more detailed techniques.

ANATOMY

Anatomy and Physiology: Workbook and Laboratory Manual. 2d ed. **Anna B. Drakontides, Marjorie A. Miller, and Lutie C. Leavell.** Riverside, NJ: Macmillan, 1977.
Companion volume to the anatomy text by Kimber-Gray-Stackpole, an anatomical and physiological workbook of 18 exercises. Contains outstanding photomicrographs, diagrams. Answer key is provided for instructors.

Grant's Dissector. 8th ed. **E. K. Sauerland.** Baltimore, MD: Williams & Wilkins, 1977.
Seventh edition, 1974.
A well-known guide for physical therapists, covers cadaver dissection and gross anatomy. Visual presentation is clear and concise, and colored slides are available as a supplement. Suggests new dissection procedures. A helpful guide for students of gross anatomy.
R: *British Journal of Surgery* 66: 144 (Feb. 1979); *Physical Therapy* 55: 1171 (1975).

A Laboratory Manual and Study Guide for Anatomy and Physiology. 3d ed. **Kenneth G. Neal and Barbara Kalbus.** Minneapolis: Burgess, 1976.
R: Chen (p. 181).

Laboratory Manual and Study Guide for Clinical Anatomy and Physiology for Allied Health Sciences. **Paul D. Anderson.** Philadelphia, PA: W. B. Saunders, 1976.

Laboratory Manual for Structure and Function in Man. 4th ed. **Stanley W. Jacob, Clarice A. Francone, and Walter J. Lassow.** Philadelphia, PA: W. B. Saunders, 1978.
A basic introductory laboratory text. Provides good orientation to fundamental lab skills and supplements lecture course material.

Laboratory Manual of Human Anatomy and Physiology. 3d ed. **Russell M.**

DeCoursey and Frank Dolyak. New York: McGraw-Hill, 1974.
R: Chen (p. 181).

BRAIN AND NERVOUS SYSTEM

Experimental Models of Epilepsy: A Manual for the Laboratory Worker. **Dominick P. Purpura et al., eds.** New York: Raven Press, 1972.

Sponsored by the National Institute of Neurological Diseases and Stroke and the American Epilepsy Society, this manual describes a wide variety of experimental models used in the detection of epilepsies. Procedures are largely electrophysiological; the manual is recommended for those who do epilepsy and brain research.
R: *American Scientist* 61: 596 (Sept.–Oct. 1973); *Archives of Neurology* 28: 284 (Apr. 1973); *Journal of Neurosurgery* 39: 271 (Aug. 1973); *NEJM* 288: 860 (Apr. 19, 1973); *Yale Journal of Biology and Medicine* 47: 303 (1974).

Histological Processing for the Neural Sciences. **Eileen LaBossiere and Mitchell Gliskstein.** Springfield, IL: Charles C. Thomas, 1976.

Compilation of laboratory procedures for neuroanatomical purposes. Succinct descriptions of fixation, embedding, and histological staining methods. Outline format with some helpful illustration. Short bibliography provided. Valuable addition in laboratories unfamiliar with pathology or anatomy and investigators without prior neuroanatomical experience.
R: *Journal of Neurosurgery* 46: 839 (June 1977).

CARDIOVASCULAR SYSTEM

Principles of Clinical Electrocardiography. 9th ed. **Mervin J. Goldman.** Los Altos, CA: Lange Medical Publications, 1976.

Seventh edition, 1970; eighth edition, 1974.
Outlines basic concepts of electrocardiology. Numerous charts, graphs, and drawings complement the text. A good "how-to-do-it" for students and reference source for the internist.
R: *Postgraduate Medicine* 62: 56 (1977); Allyn; Stearns & Ratcliff (*AJN*; *NEJM*, 1969; *NEJM,* 1970).

DENTISTRY

Manual of Clinical Periodontics. 2d ed. **Howard L. Ward and Marvin R. Simring.** St. Louis, MO: C. V. Mosby, 1978.

Practical, "how-to-do-it" manual of clinical periodontic skills. Over 700 detailed drawings add to the effectiveness of the text. Explores basic procedures ranging from examination to surgical techniques.

GENETICS

Laboratory Technique for the Detection of Hereditary Metabolic Disorders. **Vivian E. Shih.** Cleveland, OH: Chemical Rubber Company, 1974.

Describes routine procedures for the screening of patients with suspected metabolic disorders. Disease-oriented approach to screening. Focuses on detection of

disease rather than an in-depth study of metabolic diseases. Initially presents a series of tables which summarize clinical findings in inborn errors of metabolism. Chapters are arranged categorically according to major groups of disorders and discuss various screening methods, their advantages and limitations, and interpretation of results. Should be of value to physicians faced with abnormal laboratory results on a suspected metabolic disorder case.
R: *Annals of Internal Medicine* 84: 236 (Feb. 1976).

Methods for the Analysis of Human Chromosome Aberrations. **K. E. Buckton and H. J. Evans, eds.** Geneva: World Health Organization, 1973.
A guide to standard methods of chromosome preparation and analysis for screening aberrations. Discusses mutagens, emphasizing ionizing radiation, with succinct descriptions of aberrations. Includes illustrations, outline for recording data. Suitable for all laboratories involved in chromosomal research.
R: *American Journal of Human Genetics* 26: 665 (Sept. 1974).

Methods in Human Cytogenetics. 2d ed. **H. G. Schwarzacher and U. Wolf, eds.** New York: Springer-Verlag, 1974.
First edition, 1970.
A useful and practical manual for conducting human chromosome studies. Discusses cell preparation, culturing blood samples, banding methods. Updated, translated from the German. This book will be useful to geneticists of all levels.
R: *American Journal of Human Genetics* 27: 439 (May 1975); *Journal of Histochemistry and Cytochemistry* 23: 392 (May 1975); *Laboratory Practice* 24: 42 (Jan. 1975).

HEMATOLOGY

Laboratory Evaluation of Hemostasis. 2d ed. **Marjorie S. Sirridge.** Philadelphia, PA: Lea & Febiger, 1974.
General guide to laboratory investigation of hemostasis. Provides insight into coagulation assays. The bulk of the text is devoted to coagulation problems with lucid descriptions of appropriate procedures and interpretations of results.
R: *Annals of Internal Medicine* 81: 284 (Aug. 1974).

A Laboratory Manual of Blood Coagulation. **D. E. G. Austen and I. L. Rhymes.** Oxford, England: Blackwell Scientific Publications, 1975.
Collection of tests used at the Oxford Haemophilia Centre. Essentially a bench manual of tests to determine factors in human blood coagulation. Not intended as a comprehensive survey; minimum amount of theory included. A chapter on graphical calculation of results and the principles involved is very desirable. Necessary apparatus and reagents are given appropriate attention. Valuable working guide for anyone working in coagulation laboratories.
R: *BMJ* 1: 392 (Feb. 5, 1977); *Immunology* 32: 602 (Apr. 1977); *Laboratory Practice* 25: 403 (June 1976).

Manual of Hematology. **Robert E. Mangrum.** New York: Appleton-Century-Crofts, 1975.
Features the origin and development of blood and its components. Lists standard test procedures and related theoretical data. Recent advancements in sickle-

cell anemia, leukemia, and hemophilia are summarized. Step-by-step coverage of hematology adds to its thorough presentation.

Red Cell Manual. 4th ed. **Robert S. Hillman and Clement A. Finch.** Philadelphia, PA: F. A. Davis, 1974.

A manual of experimental and clinical hematology serves as an introduction to the standard hematology tests, which is the emphasis of this revised edition. Text deals with red cell production, oxygen transport, pathology of red blood cell disorders. Includes index and references. Highly recommended.
R: *Annals of Internal Medicine* 80: 682 (May 1974).

White Cell Manual. 3d ed. **Dane R. Boggs and Alan Winkelstein.** Philadelphia, PA: F. A. Davis, 1975.

Compact outline description of the normal function of the human leukocyte systems and the abnormalities associated with disease. Features figures, tables, and normal laboratory values. Good presentation on lymphocytes and immunocyte system. Well-chosen references. Good introductory material for medical and allied health sciences students.
R: *Annals of Internal Medicine* 83: 919 (Dec. 1975).

INFECTIOUS DISEASES

Bergey's Manual of Determinative Bacteriology. 8th ed. **R. E. Buchanan and Norman E. Gibbons.** Baltimore, MD: Williams & Wilkins, 1974.

The classic manual of bacteriology, updated eighth edition has convenient format dividing taxa into nineteen sections. Includes comprehensive key to taxonomy, references, index of scientific names, glossary, 30 micrographs. Companion volume *Index Bergeyana*.
R: *American Journal of Tropical Medicine and Hygiene* 24: 550 (May 1975); *American Scientist* 63: 472 (July–Aug. 1975); *BMJ* 1: 520 (Mar. 1975), Chen (p. 171); Mal (9–110); Win (EC120).

Cowan and Steel's Manual for the Identification of Medical Bacteria. 2d ed. **S. T. Cowan.** New York: Cambridge University Press, 1974.

First edition, 1965.
Updated manual for the identification and classification of bacteria, both gram negative and positive. Includes taxonomy, glossary of terms, extensive bibliography and index. Compact, well-written manual for microbiology laboratories.
R: *ABL* 41: entry 19 (Jan. 1976); *Archives of Pathology & Laboratory Medicine* 100: 288 (May 1976); *Pharmaceutical Journal* 214: 379 (1975); *ARBA* (1976, p. 657).

Diagnostic Parasitology: Clinical Laboratory Manual. **Lynne S. Garcia and Lawrence R. Ash.** St. Louis, MO: C. V. Mosby, 1975.

Emphasizes preparation and recognition of parasites in laboratory samples, intended for the American lab technician. Outlines procedures, includes line drawings, glossary, and index. Useful for common lab diagnosis.
R: *Journal of Parasitology* 62: 572 (Aug. 1976); *Laboratory Practice* 25: 167 (Mar. 1976).

Identification of Medical Bacteria. 2d ed. London: Cambridge University Press, 1974.

First edition, 1965.
Based on reprints from a 1960 paper in the *Journal of Hygiene* by K. J. Steel and S. T. Cowan. Maintains high standards of first edition.
R: *Lancet* 1: 204 (Jan. 25, 1975).

Laboratory Manual and Workbook for General Microbiology. **Frank E. Swatek.** St. Louis: Mosby, 1969.

R: Chen (p. 181).

Laboratory Techniques in Brucellosis. WHO Monograph Series, 55. 2d ed. **G. G. Alton, Lois M. Jones, and D. E. Pietz.** Geneva: World Health Organization, 1975.

First edition, 1967.
Updates 1967 edition. Expanded section on bacteriological methods and necessary precautions to be taken in handling infectious agents. Chapter on seriological methods includes US Department of Agriculture methods for preparation and standardization of antigens. References included.
R: *IBID* 4: 46 (Mar. 1976).

A Manual of Basic Virological Techniques. **Grace C. Rovozzo and Carroll N. Burke.** Englewood Cliffs, NJ: Prentice-Hall, 1973.

Virological methods approached in a step-by-step manner. Numerous straightforward tables and diagrams. Designed as a student manual for virological laboratory techniques.
R: *American Scientist* 63: 353 (May–June 1975).

Manual of Clinical Microbiology. 2d ed. **Edwin H. Lennette, Earle H. Spaulding, and Joseph P. Truant, eds.** Washington, DC: American Society for Microbiology, 1974.

Second edition of the American Society for Microbiology manual. Comprehensive tome covering bacteriology, parasitology, mycology, virology, and immunoserology. Includes practical techniques for the identification and isolation of microorganisms. Volume covers 96 chapters and 970 pages. Very well written sections include anaerobic bacteria and laboratory tests in chemotherapy. Extensive bibliography on each topic. Prepared by 125 authorities in their respective fields. Standard laboratory manual for the Clinical Microbiology Laboratory and undergraduate and graduate students in clinical microbiology.
R: *American Journal of Diseases of Children* 129: 754 (June 1975); *Annals of Internal Medicine* 82: 730 (May 1975); *Archives of Surgery* 110: 763 (June 1975); *Gastroenterology* 68: 834 (Apr. 1975); *Journal of Chronic Diseases* 28: 435 (Aug. 1975); *Choice* 11: 1798 (Feb. 1975).

Manual of Clinical Mycology. **Gary S. Moore and Douglas Jaciow.** New York: Appleton-Century-Crofts, 1979.

Emphasizes clinical methods for the identification of pathogenic and opportunistic fungi. Describes standard tests and measurements. Clear line drawings accompanied by matching photographs support the text. Specific clinical procedures on lab safety, quality control, and mailing and handling of specimens and special features.

Microbes and Man: A Laboratory Manual for Students in the Health Sciences. **I. J. Barnes, H. W. Seeley, Jr., and P. J. VanDemark.** San Francisco, CA: W. H. Freeman, 1974.

Microbiology Laboratory Manual and Workbook. 4th ed. **Alice L. Smith.** St. Louis, MO: C. V. Mosby, 1977.

Revised edition, includes new illustrations, test plates, terminology conforming with *Bergey's Manual of Determinative Bacteriology,* 1974. Up-to-date, helpful in linking microbiology theory and lab applications.

Microbiology Laboratory Manual: A Sequence of Experiments. 2d ed. **Louis P. Gebhardt and Paul S. Nicholes.** St. Louis, MO: C. V. Mosby, 1975.

A companion volume to Gebhardt-Nicholes, *Microbiology*; a basic manual of microbiology, laboratory techniques for students.

Obtencion Y Manejo De Muestras Para Examenes Microbiologicos De Las Enfermedades Transmisibles, Publicaciones Cientificas, 326. **Miguel Kourany.** Washington, DC: Pan American Health Organization, 1976.

A Spanish manual of laboratory techniques in microbiology. Covers preparation of specimens, discusses virology, bacteriology, parasitology.
R: *IBID* 5: 350 (Dec. 1977).

Opportunistic Pathogens. **J. E. Prier and H. Friedman, eds.** Baltimore, MD: University Park Press, 1974.

Both a laboratory and reference manual that discusses disease causing drugs Includes up-to-date reviews and numerous citations of practical value to hospital personnel.
R: *Immunological Communications* 3: 609 (1974).

Practical Clinical Microbiology and Mycology: Techniques and Interpretation. **P. L. Wolf, B. Russell, and A. Shimoda.** New York: John Wiley, 1975.

Lists numerous techniques, media, and flow charts concerned with diagnostic bacteriology and mycology. Outlines established laboratory methods. Intended as a working manual.
R: *Annals of Internal Medicine* 84: 375 (1976).

Principles of Biochemical Tests in Diagnostic Microbiology. **Donna J. Blazevic and Grace M. Ederer.** New York: John Wiley, 1975.

Detailed, comprehensive manual of test procedures used to isolate infectious microorganisms. Contains bibliographies and illustrations which identify bacteria.

INTERNAL MEDICINE

Clinical Chemistry: Conversion Scales for SI Units With Adult Normal Reference Values. **A. M. Bolding and P. Wilding.** Philadelphia, PA: J. B. Lippincott, 1975.

Volume consists of conversion scales, allowing for easy translation of laboratory data from conventional to SI units. Separate section lists reference (normal) values and terse comments on potential areas of error in specimen collection and data interpretation. Although a change to the international system is not imminent, especially in the midst of computerized technology, the volume does provide a complete description of SI units. A pocket-size manual geared toward physicians, nurses, and laboratory workers.
R: *Archives of Pathology & Laboratory Medicine* 100: 509 (Sept. 1976).

Clinical Radioassay Procedures: A Compendium. **P. K. Besch.** Washington, DC: American Association for Clinical Chemistry, 1975.
A compendium of radioassay procedures geared specifically to various fields, including pharmacology, microbiology, enzymology, pathology. Helpful to laboratory researchers.

A Companion to Medical Studies. 3 vols. **Reginald Passmore and J. S. Robson, eds.** Philadelphia, PA: J. B. Lippincott, 1968–1976.
Volume 1, *Anatomy, Biochemistry, Physiology and Related Subjects,* 1968, second edition, 1976; volume 2, *Pharmacology, Microbiology, General Pathology and Related Subjects,* 1970; volume 3, *Medicine, Surgery, Systemic Pathology, Obstetrics, Psychiatry, Paediatrics and Community Medicine,* 1974.
Source of information about modern medicine and the medical sciences. First volume provides foundation for clinical studies covered in second and third volume. Volume 2 discusses principles of medicine, and volume 3 covers practice of medicine.
R: *Lancet* 1: 1374 (June 27, 1970).

The Human Body in Health and Disease. 4th ed. **Ruth L. Memmler and Dena L. Wood.** Philadelphia, PA: J. B. Lippincott, 1977.

Illustrated Manual of Laboratory Diagnosis. 2d ed. **R. Douglas Collins.** Philadelphia, PA: J. B. Lippincott, 1975.
First edition, 1968.
Succinct reference manual containing information on the physical examination, laboratory diagnostic tests, alternative procedures, and final diagnosis. Bulk of text devoted to interpretation of abnormal diagnostic tests in chemistry, hematology, bacteriology, and X-ray. More than 200 full-color illustrations portray the appropriate laboratory test. Four major appendixes and an index of lab tests included. Some brief criticisms: too few references, various outdated procedures, and unusually brief discussions. Written mainly for physicians who deal with data from screening tests.
R: *American Family Physician* 12: 231 (Oct. 1975); *Annals of Internal Medicine* 83: 754 (Nov. 1975); *RSR* 3: 34 (July–Dec. 1975).

Laboratory Manual of Cell Biology. **David C. Hall and S. E. Hawkins.** New York: Crane, Russak, 1975.
R: Chen (p. 181).

Manual of Clinical Laboratory Methods. 4th ed., 20th printing. **Opal E. Hepler.** Springfield, IL: Charles C. Thomas, 1977.

Designed as a step-by-step procedural manual for various laboratory tests. Covers the interpretation and significance of each test. Three previous editions attest to its popularity in hospitals and schools. Consistent revision and technical improvements during the manual's actual use accounts for its currency.

Microanalysis in Medical Biochemistry. 5th ed. **I. D. P. Wootton.** Edinburgh: Churchill Livingstone, 1974.
A laboratory manual of the Royal Postgraduate Medical School detailing biochemical microanalysis. Includes a wide range of procedures, manufacturers' directory; a standard work for the field.
R: *Laboratory Practice* 24: 41 (Jan. 1975).

A Study Guide and Workbook for First Aid and Safety. **Curtis C. Schockmel and M. Miller.** New York: Macmillan, 1978.
A workbook and study guide which serves to review principals and applications of first aid technique. Each chapter outlines pertinent objectives of emergency care. An appendix includes such topics as school emergencies and statutes for "Good Samaritans." This workbook can be a companion volume to standard first aid texts and is helpful in achieving a better understanding of first aid and safety.
R: *Journal of School Health* 49: 50 (Jan. 1979).

Workbook for the Human Body in Health and Disease. 2d ed. **Ruth L. Memmler and Dena L. Wood.** Philadelphia, PA: J. B. Lippincott, 1977.

Workbook to Accompany Medicine for the Paramedical Professions. **Douglas W. Piper.** New York: McGraw-Hill, 1972.
Companion workbook. Enables reader to test his knowledge on symptoms, syndromes, signs, physiological measurements and descriptions. Includes correct answers to all matching and multiple choice questions. Testing material should be advantageous to those without regular instruction.
R: *Archives of Internal Medicine* 134: 185 (July 1974).

Nursing

Basic Medical-Surgical Nursing. 4th ed. **Mildred A. Mason.** New York: Macmillan, 1978.
Accompanying *Workbook* by Bonnie K. Smola and Mildred A. Mason. 2d ed. Excellent introductory text with accompanying workbook. Theoretical and clinical aspects of nursing are developed through use of case studies, review questions, role playing, and study suggestions. Includes brief bibliographies.
R: *American Journal of Nursing* 79: 991 (May 1979).

Clinical Laboratory Tests: A Manual for Nurses. **Marcella M. Strand.** St. Louis, MO: C. V. Mosby, 1976.

A Guide to Nursing Management of Psychiatric Patients. **Sharon O. Dreyer, David Bailey, and Wills Doucet.** St. Louis, MO: C. V. Mosby, 1975.
Bridges gap between learning clinical skills and their practical applications in psychiatric nursing. Workbook covers a wide range of psychiatric disorders. Pro-

vides questions at the end of each chapter that correspond with those found on state board exams. Special sections on death, dying, and special children's problems.

Introductory Medical-Surgical Nursing and Student Work Manual. 2d ed. **Jeanne C. Scherer.** Philadelphia, PA: J. B. Lippincott, 1977.

Lippincott's State Board Examination Review for Nurses. **LuVerne W. Lewis.** Philadelphia, PA: J. B. Lippincott, 1978.

Based on the structure of actual state board examinations. Comprised of 2,568 questions accompanied by answer-recording sheets. Questions follow logical sequence. Covers the five major areas of nursing found on the state board examinations: medical, surgical, obstetric, pediatric, and psychiatric. Integrates nutrition, pharmacology, communicable diseases, and legal and ethical concepts. Answers and rationale for each answer provided after each main section.

Maternity Nursing: Self Study Guide. 4th ed. **Constance Lerch and Virginia J. Bliss.** St. Louis, MO: C. V. Mosby, 1978.

The Nurse Assistant. 2d ed. **Joan E. Donovan, Edith H. Belsjoe, and Daniel C. Dillon.** New York: McGraw-Hill, 1978.

Emphasizes the functions of the nurse assistant. This teaching-textbook discusses such topics as vital signs, the dying patient, emergency room care, etc. Useful in community health and hospital institutions. Loose-leaf format handy for classroom use.

Nursing and Medical Terminology: Workbook. **Ruth K. Radcliff and Sheila Ogden.** St. Louis, MO: C. V. Mosby, 1977.

The Problem-Oriented System in Nursing: A Workbook. **Beth C. Vaughan-Wrobel and Betty Henderson.** St. Louis, MO: C. V. Mosby, 1976.

A problem-oriented workbook for nursing education. Enables student, upon completion of exercises, to list patient care objectives for problems identified and listed.

Student Work Manual for Introductory Medical-Surgical Nursing. **Jeanne C. Scherer.** Philadelphia, PA: J. B. Lippincott, 1977.

This is a workbook of clinical nursing which includes brief textual material accompanied with multiple choice, true/false, discussion, and fill-in questions.

Workbook for Introductory Medical-Surgical Nursing. **Jeanne C. Scherer.** Philadelphia, PA: J. B. Lippincott, 1977.

Brief summary of text opens each chapter. Multiple choice, true/false, and discussion questions follow. Emphasis on clinical nursing.

Workbook for Pediatric Nurses. 2d ed. **Norma J. Anderson.** St. Louis, MO: C. V. Mosby, 1974.

Workbook For the Nurses' Aide. **Charlotte Isler.** New York: Springer Publishing, 1973.

R: *American Journal of Nursing* 74: 350 (Feb. 1974).

Workbook in Basic Medical-Surgical Nursing. **Bonnie K. Smola and Mildred A. Mason.** New York: Macmillan, 1974.

Workbook in Bedside Maternity Nursing and *Answer Key.* 2d ed. **Inge J. Bleier.** Philadelphia, PA: W. B. Saunders, 1974.

Workbook of Solutions and Dosage of Drugs: Including Arithmetic. 10th ed. **Ellen M. Anderson and Thora M. Vervoren.** St. Louis, MO: C. V. Mosby, 1976.

Work Manual For Critical Care Nursing. 2d ed. **Carolyn M. Hudak, Barbara M. Gallo, and Thelma Lohr.** Philadelphia, PA: J. B. Lippincott, 1977.

A self evaluation tool to be used in conjunction with the authors' work, *Critical Care Nursing,* 2d ed., 1977.

NUTRITION

Case Studies in Clinical Nutrition: A Workbook and Study Guide for Students of Nursing and Dietetics. New York: Macmillan, 1977.

A workbook of five case studies which attempts to meet the needs of clinical dietitians and students of dietetics. Includes an answer booklet for instructors. Useful, flexibly written so that workbook will appeal to wide range of dietitians.
R: *Journal of the American Dietetic Association* 71: 355 (Sept. 1977).

ONCOLOGY AND NUCLEAR MEDICINE

Manual for Staging of Cancer, 1977. **American Joint Committee for Cancer Staging and End-Results Reporting.** Chicago, IL: American Joint Commitee, 1977.

Focuses on classification proposals for some 30 cancer areas. Data based on the tumor-nodes-metastases (TNM) system. The TNM system supplies oncologists with a standard method for describing the anatomic extent of cancer. Valuable reference manual for American clinicians.
R: *Canadian Medical Association Journal* 119: 1179 (Nov. 18, 1978).

ORTHOPEDICS

Musculoskeletal Function: An Anatomy and Kinesiology Laboratory Manual. **Dortha Esch and Marvin Lepley.** Minneapolis, MN: University of Minnesota Press, 1974.

A well-organized laboratory manual which emphasizes muscle function and kinesiology. Discusses osteology, anatomy, and kinesiology. Provides question and answer section, references; an excellent manual.
R: *Archives of Physical Medicine and Rehabilitation* 56: 417 (Sept. 1975).

The Radiology of Skeletal Disorders: Exercise in Diagnosis. 2d ed. 4 vols. **Ron-**

ald O. Murray and Harold G. Jacobson. New York: Churchill Livingstone, 1977.

Four-volume set of programmed instruction workbooks in radiological diagnosis. Contains over 4,000 illustrations and photographs, includes thorough discussions of diagnoses. A high-quality encyclopedic work recommended to radiologists, orthopedists, and others who are involved with diseases of the skeletal system.
R: *JAMA* 238: 2544 (Dec. 5, 1977).

PATHOLOGY

A Manual for Histologic Technicians. 3d ed. **Ann Preece.** Boston, MA: Little, Brown, 1972.

Manual of Histopathological Staining Methods. **F. A. Putt.** New York: John Wiley, 1973.

Based on the author's own modification of classic laboratory methods. Lists stains and staining techniques alphabetically according to the most prominent tissue component. Instructions to individual techniques are provided in outline form with no theoretical introduction. Valuable benchside manual.
R: *Laboratory Practice* 23: 27 (Jan. 1974).

Staining Procedures Used by the Biological Stain Commission. **George Clark, ed.** Baltimore, MD: Williams & Wilkins, 1973.

A manual of histological staining procedures in four sections: animal, plant, protozoan, and microbiological. Update of the classic manual by the Biological Stain Commission.
R: *Journal of Histochemistry and Cytochemistry* 22: 1069 (Nov. 1974).

Theory and Practice of Histological Techniques. **John D. Bancroft and Alan Stevens, eds.** Edinburgh: Churchill Livingstone, 1977.

A manual which serves as a reference source for laboratory techniques in histology and histopathology.

PHARMACY AND PHARMACOLOGY

Experimental Pharmaceutics. 4th ed. **Eugene L. Parrott and Witold Saski.** Minneapolis, MN: Burgess, 1977.

A laboratory manual which, in outline form, relates experimental methods in pharmaceutic preparations. There are five sections: solids, metrology, plastic systems, polyphasic systems, and solutions. There is a list of references and an appendix with data appropriate to the book. Recommended for use in beginning pharmaceutical courses.
R: *Journal of Pharmaceutical Sciences* 66: 1514 (Oct. 1977).

PHYSICAL MEDICINE AND REHABILITATION

A Workbook in Auditory Training for Adults. **Clarissa R. Smith and Adrienne Karp.** Springfield, IL: Charles C. Thomas, 1978.

A workbook which emphasizes aiding the hearing-impaired adult. Attempts to help obtain the most efficient use of hearing aids in a normal environment.

PSYCHIATRY AND PSYCHOLOGY

Mental Health Concepts in Medical-Surgical Nursing: A Workbook. 2d ed. **Carol R. Kneisl and Sue A. Ames.** St. Louis, MO: C. V. Mosby, 1979.

PUBLIC HEALTH

Analytical Toxicology Methods Manual. **H. M. Stahr, ed.** Ames, IO: Iowa State University Press, 1977.

Contains specific techniques for the analysis of toxic chemicals: metals, drugs, feed additives, pesticides. Keeps pace with the rapidly changing field of toxicology. Good working manual for diagnostic and research laboratories.
R: *American Journal of Veterinary Research* 38: 1453 (Sept. 1977).

Laboratory Techniques in Rabies, WHO Monograph, Series no. 23. 3d ed. **Martin M. Kaplan and Hilary Koprowski, eds.** Geneva: World Health Organization, 1973.

Guide to diagnosis of rabies and preparation of rabies vaccines from infected avian embryos or brains. Contains details of the preparation of three vaccines from the brains of newborn mammals—mice, rats, and rabbits. Useful compendium of new diagnostic and research methods used in rabies research. The chapter on safety precautions is particularly noteworthy. Recommended as a guide to all workers in the rabies field and virologists.
R: *BMJ* 1: 81 (Jan. 12, 1974).

RADIOLOGY

Laboratory Training Manual on the Use of Radionuclides and Radiation in Animal Research. 3d ed. Vienna: International Atomic Energy Agency. Distr. New York: Unipub, 1972.
R: Chen (p. 181).

Radiologic Science: Workbook and Laboratory Manual. **S. C. Bushong.** St. Louis, MO: C. V. Mosby, 1977.

Loose-leaf format workbook and soft-cover manual useful in training X-ray technologists. Covers basic physics, mathematics, and ten pertinent experiments. Can be used in conjunction with standard textbooks of radiologic physics. Helpful to both the instructor and student.
R: *American Journal of Roentgenology* 129: 960 (Nov. 1977).

RHEUMATOLOGY

Laboratory Diagnostic Procedures in the Rheumatic Diseases. 2d ed. **Alan S. Cohen, ed.** Boston, MA: Little, Brown, 1975.

Outlines methodology, clinical discussions, and interpretation of test results. Required reading for rheumatologists and technicians in clinical pathology laboratories.

R: *JAMA* 232: 1379 (June 30, 1975); *TBRI* 41: 266 (Sept. 1975); Allyn.

UROGENITAL SYSTEM

Specialty Board Review: Obstetrics and Gynecology. **Preston P. Williams.** New York: Arco Publishing, 1975.

Follows a question and answer format. Designed as a study guide for the user anticipating the American Board of Obstetrics and Gynecology examination. Useful guide for medical schools, societies, and hospital libraries.
R: *RSR* 4: 92 (Apr.–June 1976).

VETERINARY MEDICINE

Manual of Standardized Methods for Veterinary Microbiology. **George E. Cottral, ed.** Ithaca, NY: Cornell University Press, 1978.

Fills a gap in veterinary literature. Compiled through the efforts of the Biologics Committee of the Council on Biological and Therapeutic Agents of the American Veterinary Medical Association.
R: *Journal of Parasitology* 65: 245 (Apr. 1979).

SOURCE BOOKS

GENERAL

Family Factbook. Chicago, IL: Marquis Who's Who, 1978.

A broad collection of statistics and articles focus on the family in the United States, with insight to family life in foreign countries. The book consists of six parts: family, adults, children, health, work and income, and housing. Subject index is available.

Health/Medicine Legislation in Congress—How It Works. **Richard E. Vodra.** Bethesda, MD: National Health Directory, 1980.

Comprehensive description of the legislative process in Congress, from the time a bill dealing with medical or health policy is introduced until the time it is signed into law. Appendix lists sample documents from each stage of the legislative process. Includes full explanation of the elements of the *Congressional Record,* details on ordering publications, and description of the Government Printing Office.

The N.I.H.—How It Works. **Guy W. Moore.** Bethesda, MD: National Health Directory, 1980.

Comprehensive description of the National Institutes of Health: operation, organization, grant and contract processes, peer review system, policy development, and advisory committees.

ANESTHESIOLOGY AND GENERAL SURGERY

The Source Book of Plastic Surgery. **Frank McDowell.** Baltimore, MD: Williams & Wilkins, 1977.

Conceived as a history of plastic surgery. Basically a collection of articles gleaned

from *Plastic and Reconstructive Surgery* and previously labeled "Classic Reprints." Topics include cleft palate repairs, facial fractures, and otoplasty. Valuable reference tool for all budding and professional plastic surgeons.
R: *Plastic and Reconstructive Surgery* 63: 117 (1979).

CARDIOVASCULAR SYSTEM

Cardiac Arrest and Resuscitation. 4th ed. **Hugh E. Stephenson.** St. Louis, MO: C. V. Mosby, 1974.

Third edition, 1969.
An informative source book which covers pertinent factors relating to cardiac trauma. Emphasizes risk prevention, mechanism of arrest, resuscitation technique, etc. Close to 400 illustrations; bibliography is included, as is an appendix with standards for emergency care.
R: *American Heart Journal* 89: 408 (1975); *BMJ* 4: 291 (Oct. 31, 1970); *Journal of the American Osteopathic Association* 74: 463 (1975); *Journal of the Kansas Medical Society* 76: 16 (1975); *Plastic and Reconstructive Surgery* 58: 496 (1976); *RSR* 2: 130 (Oct.–Dec. 1974); Allyn; Brandon.

GENETICS

Clinical Genetics: A Source Book for Physicians. **L. G. Jackson and R. N. Schimke, eds.** New York: John Wiley, 1979.

A comprehensive reference on genetic diseases and conditions. Useful as a guide to physicians, genetic counselors. Contains information on prenatal diagnosis, staining and banding techniques, tabular summaries of forms of disease, flow diagrams. Provides references; a practical, clinically relevant book.
R: *John Wiley & Sons Librarians' Newsletter* 18: 16 (July–Aug. 1979).

GERONTOLOGY

Sourcebook on Aging. 2d ed. Chicago, IL: Marquis Who's Who, 1979.

Provides a broad collection of demographic, social, and economic data on problems and programs related to aging. Presents statistical and narrative data gathered from a variety of government and private sources. Extensive bibliography spans 1940 through 1977. Subject, organization, and geographic indexes are available.

HEALTH SERVICES ADMINISTRATION

The HMO Sourcebook. **Health Law Center.** Washington, DC: Science and Health Publications, 1973–. Annual.

An annually published guide to health maintenance organizations. Covers all major fields and plans, insurance regulations. Helpful to administrators and lawyers.

Hospital Organization Research: Review and Sourcebook. **Basil S. Georgopoulos.** Philadelphia, PA: W. B. Saunders, 1975.

Source book and review for those interested in health services management or health administrators' education. From a management point of view, chapter 13 is an excellent overview of trends of hospital organization research. Valuable reference tool for health services administrators.

NURSING

Drugs and Nursing Implications. 3d ed. **Laura E. Govoni and Janice E. Hayes.** New York: Appleton-Century-Crofts, 1978.
Valuable and practical source book detailing pertinent data for proper administration of a particular drug.
R: Brandon (*NO*).

The New Health Professionals: Nurse Practitioners and Physician's Assistants. **Ann A. Bliss and Eva D. Cohen, eds.** Germantown, MD: Aspen Systems Corp., 1977.
A source book which details the new and expanding roles of health professionals. Examines the changing structure of medicine. Useful for nurse practitioners, physician's assistants, health care administrators.
R: *Medical Care* 16: 698 (Aug. 1978); *Nation's Health* 9: 13 (Feb. 1979).

Pain: A Sourcebook for Nurses and Other Professionals. **Ada K. Jacox, ed.** Boston, MA: Little, Brown, 1977.
A comprehensive study providing timely information. Discusses all aspects of pain assessment and alleviation. Annotated bibliography and cross-references are included.
R: *American Journal of Nursing* 78: 62 (Jan. 1978).

Source Book, Nursing Personnel: Health Manpower References, DHEW Pub. no. (HRA) 75-43. **Helen H. Hudson and Margaret D. McCarthy.** Bureau of Health Resources Development. Division of Nursing Manpower Analysis and Resources Branch. Washington, DC: US Government Printing Office, 1975.

A Source Book of Nursing Research. 2d ed. **Florence S. Downs and Margaret A. Newman.** Philadelphia, PA: F. A. Davis, 1977.
First edition, 1973.
An excellent source book of nursing research projects containing a wide variety of investigations. Includes a report article which emphasizes the need for nursing research. An excellent book for both instructors and students.
R: *American Journal of Nursing* 74: 758 (Apr. 1974); *Journal of Nursing Administration* 8: 40 (Mar. 1978); *Nurse Educator* 3: 4 (Sept.–Oct. 1978).

NUTRITION

Source Book For Food Scientists. **H. W. Ockerman.** Westport, CT: Avi Publishing, 1978.

Sourcebook on Food and Nutrition. 2d ed. Chicago, IL: Marquis Who's Who, 1980.
First edition, 1978.

A compendium of statistical and textual nutrition information combined with representative viewpoints on current controversies. The book consists of nine parts: introducton, nutrients, dietary allowances and labeling, nutrition and the life cycle, dieting and weight control, special diets, nutrition and health problems, food additives, etc., and perspectives on world food production. Subject index is available.

ONCOLOGY AND NUCLEAR MEDICINE

Nuclear Medicine Science Syllabus. **Nuclear Medicine Science Syllabus Subcommittee of the Education and Training Committee, Society of Nuclear Medicine.** New York: Society of Nuclear Medicine, 1978.

A bibliographic reference source covering mathematics, physics, radiochemistry, radiation protection, and diagnostic imaging. An excellent source for radiology students.
R: *American Journal of Roentgenology* 133: 527 (Sept. 1979).

OTORHINOLARYNGOLOGY

Sourcebook of Audiology: Speech and Language Terminology. **Lucille Nicolosi, Elizabeth Harryman, and Janet Kreschek.** Baltimore, MD: Williams & Wilkins, 1978.

PHARMACY AND PHARMACOLOGY

Drugs of Choice, 1958/1959–. **Walter Modell, ed.** St. Louis, MO: C. V. Mosby, 1958–. Biennial.

Latest edition, 1978/1979.
Biennial evaluation of pharmaceuticals with authoritative recommendations as to their use and therapeutic value. Discussion of legal and general considerations is followed by chapters dealing with specific drugs including trade names, synonyms, administration, and dosage forms. Includes "Drug Index," which supplies trade and general name, as well as conventional index. A standard reference tool of great value to physicians, pharmacists, medical educators, and librarians.
R: *American Journal of Proctology* 27: 22 (Aug. 1976); *Anesthesiology* 41: 530 (Nov. 1974); *Archives of Internal Medicine* 135: 1411 (Oct. 1975); *Canadian Medical Association Journal* 103: 190 (July 18, 1970); *Pharmaceutical Journal* 214: 337 (1976); *ARBA* (1973, p. 622); Win (EK197).

Evaluations of Drug Interactions. 2d ed. **American Pharmaceutical Association.** Washington, DC: American Pharmaceutical Association, 1976.

First edition, 1973.
A reference source on drug interactions, composed by approximately 200 experts. Consists of 24 chapters covering numerous classes of drugs. Also includes a table of normal values. An excellent and thorough source of information, recommended to all health care personnel involved in drug therapy.
R: *American Journal of Psychiatry* 134: 465 (Apr. 1977); *Anesthesiology* 42: 646 (May 1975); 46: 380 (May 1977); *Clinical Pediatrics* 17: 658 (Aug. 1978); *Journal of Pharmaceutical Sciences* 62: 1744 (Oct. 1973); *Lancet* 2: 646 (Sept. 22, 1973); *ARBA* (1974, p. 642).

Psychiatry and Psychology

The Development of Traditional Psychopathology: A Sourcebook. **Mark D. Altschule.** New York: Halsted Press, 1976.

Consists of articles on the history of psychopathology, including the writings of original thinkers. Illustrates the evolution of psychiatry's concepts. Recommended for students in the field.
R: *Journal of Nervous and Mental Diseases* 164: 142 (1977); *Choice* 13: 589 (June 1976).

The Evolution of Psychoanalytic Technique. **Martin S. Bergmann and Frank R. Hartman, eds.** New York: Basic Books, 1976.

A useful source book which provides historical information on the evolution of psychoanalytic technique. Deals with major psychoanalysts, such as Freud and Reich; covers case studies until the time of Freud's death. An instructive reference for understanding controversies and the history of ideas in psychoanalytic technique.
R: *American Journal of Psychiatry* 134: 592 (May 1977).

Public Health

Toxic Substances Control Sourcebook. **Alexander McRae et al., eds.** Germantown, MD: Aspen Systems Co. (Center for Compliance Information), 1978.

An up-to-date and useful tool for the decision makers in industry, business, government, and others in gaining access to the complex information on toxic substances control. The book includes full texts of the Toxic Substances Control Act of 1976 and other federal laws and regulations, information on toxic and hazardous substances, economic impact on industry, etc.
R: *ARBA* (1980).

Toxic Substances Sourcebook: The Professional's Guide to the Information Sources, Key Literature and Laws of a Critical New Field. **Steven Ross and Monica Pronin.** New York: Environment Information Center, 1978.

A comprehensive source book which identifies and summarizes knowledge of toxic substances. Book includes directory of toxic information centers, tables and charts, OSHA regulations, bibliographic information, abstracts of journal articles, technical papers, and research studies. Includes also EPA registered chemicals and microfiche appendix of all federally labeled toxic chemicals and pesticides.
R: *Choice* (April 1979).

Rheumatology

Gout and Hyperuricemia. **James B. Wyngaarden and William N. Kelley.** New York: Grune & Stratton, 1976.

Classic work in the field of gout and hyperuricemia. Thorough investigation into the physiological, biochemical, pathological, genetic, and clinical aspects. Seven chapters devoted to treatment alone. Each chapter ends with a comprehensive list of references. Well illustrated. A must for every medical library. Bal-

anced presentation for the clinician, biochemist, geneticist, practicing physician, and medical student.
R: *American Journal of Human Genetics* 29: 545 (Sept. 1977); *BMJ* 1: 1654 (June 25, 1977).

CHAPTER 9   GUIDES

For guides to medical and scientific writing, see style manuals section in chapter 8.

GENERAL

Barron's Guide to Medical, Dental, and Allied Health Science Careers. 3d ed. **Saul Wischnitzer.** Woodbury, NY: Barron's Educational Series, 1977.

Second edition, 1974.
Guide for students planning a career in the health field. Provides facts on preparing for medical school, financial aid, applications, etc. Presents information on US and Canadian medical schools in chart form as well as descriptive entries. Covers admission, curriculum, grading, facilities, and special features. Selected medical school application forms all reproduced in the appendix.
R: *BL* 402 (Oct. 15, 1977); *ARBA* (1975, p. 742; 1978, p. 717).

The Doctor's Law Guide: Essentials of Practice Management. **Marc J. Lane.** Philadelphia, PA: W. B. Saunders, 1979.

Aids the doctor in matters of finance and law. Discusses malpractice, partnerships, retirement, tax shelters. Practical and clear presentation.

Dx and Rx: A Physician's Guide to Medical Writing. **John H. Dirckx.** Boston, MA: G. K. Hall, 1977.

Aimed as a guide for the physician who needs practical advice on medical writing and publication.

English-Spanish Guide for Medical Personnel. **Joseph Armengol et al.** Flushing, NY: Medical Examination Publishing, 1966.

A list of Spanish expressions used in physical examination interviewing. Includes pronunciation; helpful in the delivery room, laboratory, etc.
R: *MRW* S1, p. 4.

A Guide to Medical Mathematics. **D. A. Franklin and G. B. Newman.** Oxford, England: Blackwell Scientific Publications, 1973.

Helps to reorient physicians to basic mathematical concepts and also introduces new methods. This guide covers a broad scope of mathematics and also lists references to subjects not covered (one of which is statistics). A high-quality guide which ties together medicine and mathematical models. Well indexed.
R: *BMJ* 4: 620 (Dec. 8, 1973); *ARBA* (1975, p. 740).

A Guidebook to Microscopial Methods. **A. V. Grimstone and R. J. Skaer.** New York: Cambridge University Press, 1972.

Provides insight into the various methods and techniques ordinarily used by researchers and students. References cite sources on less frequently used techniques.
R: *ARBA* (1973, p. 552); Chen (p. 190); Mal (9-51).

How to Pay for Your Health Career Education: A Guide for Minority Students,

DHEW Pub. no. (HRA) 74-8. **US Department of Health, Education, and Welfare.** Washington, DC: US Government Printing Office, 1974.

How to Use A Medical Library. 6th ed. **Leslie T. Morton.** London: Heinemann Medical, 1979.
First edition, 1934; fourth edition, 1964; fifth edition, 1971.
A British guide to medical libraries; succinct and useful.
R: Win (EK4).

Index Bergeyana. **Robert E. Buchanan et al., eds.** Baltimore: Williams & Wilkins, 1966.
An annotated alphabetical listing of names of the taxa of the bacteria. The *Index* evaluates more than 20,000 names of bacteria taxa.
R: Chen (p. 190); Mal (9-88); Wal (p. 200); Win (1EC11).

Laboratory Guide for Biology. 2d ed. **Alfred M. Elliott.** New York: Appleton-Century-Crofts, 1970.
R: Chen (p. 191).

Measuring Medical Education: The Tests and the Experience of the National Board of Medical Examiners. 2d ed. **John P. Hubbard.** Philadelphia, PA: Lea & Febiger, 1978.
Revised edition includes recent changes in the National Board of Medical Examiners. Especially recommended for medical students.

The Microtomist's Formulary and Guide. **Peter Gray.** London: Constable, 1954. Reprint. Huntington, NY: Krieger, 1975.
Guide to methods, techniques, and stains bearing on the use of microscopic slides in biological research.
R: Mal (9-50); Wal (p. 204).

Roe's Laboratory Guide to Chemistry. 7th ed. **Alice Laughlin.** St. Louis, MO: C. V. Mosby, 1976.
A variety of experiments for undergraduate chemistry.

Science: Guide to Scientific Instruments. New York: American Asosciation for the Advancement of Science. Annual.
Provides up-to-date information on scientific instruments; available through subscription to *Science* magazine or separate purchase.

Speaking at Medical Meetings. **James Calnan and Andras Barabas.** London: Heinemann Medical, 1973.
A practical guide to speaking at medical meetings. Discusses many types of presentations: the case demonstration, the fifteen-minute communication, and the longer lecture. Comprehensive coverage of standard techniques. Sections on symposia and chairmanship are extremely relevant. Contains about 40 helpful illustrations and an accurate index. Should be obligatory reading for all doctors who frequently speak at meetings.
R: *Lancet* 1: 920 (Apr. 28, 1973).

Travelers' Guide to U.S.–Certified Doctors Abroad. Chicago, IL: Marquis Who's Who Books, 1976.

An offshoot of the *Directory of Medical Specialists.* Lists over 3,500 English-speaking physicians living in 120 foreign countries and the U.S. overseas territories possessing the credentials required by one of the boards of the American Board of Medical Specialists. Physicians listed by respective specialties and countries of residence. Includes complete biographical data. Excellent guide for American travelers overseas.
R: *WLB* 51: 539 (Feb. 1977); *ARBA* (1977, p. 715).

ALLERGY AND IMMUNOLOGY

Allergy in Children: A Guide to Practical Management. **Jan A. Kuzemko.** Tunbridge Wells, Kent, England: Pitman Medical, 1978.

Reviews etiology and genetic causes of childhood allergies. Comprehensively presents the information with emphasis on care and assessment of the child. Includes helpful charts and illustrations. Highly recommended to pediatricians.
R: *Lancet* 1: 22 (Jan. 6, 1979).

Immunology in Medicine: A Practical Guide to Clinical Immunology. **E. J. Holborow and W. G. Reeves, eds.** New York: Academic Press, 1977.

A comprehensive review of clinical immunology. Discusses mechanisms of immunology, individual system disorders, therapies. An invaluable guide and reference source for physicians, regardless of specialty.

Patch Testing. **S. Fregert and H. J. Bandmann.** New York: Springer-Verlag, 1975.

Devoted to basic procedures of testing and patch test interpretation. Features a unique section on acquisition and availability of diluted patch test substances. Information-packed manual for practicing dermatologists.
R: *Archives of Dermatology* 112: 1806 (Dec. 1976).

Patch Testing Guidelines. **K. E. Malten, W. G. van Ketel, and J. P. Nater.** Netherlands: Royal Vangorcum, 1976.

A more specific approach to patch testing. Reflects the personal viewpoint of the three authors. Essential section on the safe procedure of patch testing with substances of known composition. Well documented with over 200 references. The rambling style and awkward English expressions are two minor criticisms. Recommended for experienced patch testers.
R: *Archives of Dermatology* 112: 1086 (Dec. 1976).

ANATOMY

Gray's Anatomy. 1st ed.–. Henry Gray. 1858–.

Gray's Anatomy. 35th ed. **R. Warwick and P. L. Williams, eds.** Philadelphia, PA: W. B. Saunders, 1973. British ed., London: Longman, 1973.

Gray's Anatomy. 29th ed. **Charles M. Goss, ed.** Philadelphia, PA: Lea & Febiger, 1973.

Numerous editions of the reknowned atlas first published in 1858. Contains over 1,300 illustrations of each region of the body and close to 3,000 references. The one edited by Charles M. Goss is more traditional. Classics of the field, which provides a treasury of information for the surgeon. Recommended to all neophytic anatomists.
R: *BMJ* 3: 505 (Jan. 10, 1973); *Plastic & Reconstructive Surgery* 59: 743 (1977); Stearns & Ratcliff (*NEJM,* 1969; *NEJM,* 1970).

Gross Anatomy Dissector: A Companion for Atlas of Clinical Anatomy. **Richard S. Snell.** Boston, MA: Little, Brown, 1978.

Guide to human anatomy. Written as a companion to *Atlas of Clinical Anatomy.* Essentially a dissecting manual with instructions keyed back to illustrations in the *Atlas.* Spiral binding and plastic-coated cover will appeal to students.
R: *Lancet* 2: 505 (Sept. 2, 1978).

A Guide to Dissection in Gross Anatomy. 3d ed. **Russell T. Woodburne.** New York: Oxford University Press, 1971.

A concise, logical dissection guide for students.

Medical Terminology and the Body Systems. **Mary A. Collin.** New York: Harper & Row, 1974.

Conveniently organized dictionary of medical terminology. Terms arranged according to body systems and not in usual dictionary format. Includes line drawings, phonetic pronunciations, accent addenda. Helpful to anyone seeking to understand medical terminology, guides the user to correct spelling and definition of terms.

Study Guide and Review Manual of Basic Anatomy and Physiology. **M. H. L. Gibson.** Philadelphia, PA: W. B. Saunders, 1978.

For students of anatomy and physiology, a well-illustrated reference guide. Helpful as a classroom supplement.
R: *Physical Therapy* 59: 801 (June 1979).

ANESTHESIOLOGY AND GENERAL SURGERY

Cosmetic Surgery: A Consumer's Guide. **S. Rosenthal.** New York: Tree Communications, 1977.

Guides the consumer in regard to choice of cosmetic surgeon. Deals with facial operations, nasal surgery, complications of procedures, in order to inform a prospective patient. Detailed, helpful. Recommended for both surgeon and patient.
R: *JAMWA* 32: 11 (Nov. 1977).

Guide to House Surgeons in the Surgical Unit. 6th ed. **G. J. Fraenkel, J. Ludbrook, and H. A. F. Dudley.** London: Heinemann, 1978.

Fifth edition, 1974.
An excellent guide for the resident surgeon. Presents problem situations most likely to be encountered by the house surgeon. Includes diagrams, clear descriptions of treatments. A handy pocket-size guide, highly recommended.
R: *British Journal of Surgery* 63: 84 (Jan. 1976); 66: 371 (May 1979).

Management of Surgical Complications. 3d ed. **Curtis P. Artz and James D. Hardy, eds.** Philadelphia, PA: W. B. Saunders, 1975.
Second edition, 1967.
Discusses current methods of treating patients with surgical complications. Among topics included are thoracic, neurosurgical, pancreatic complications. Numerous references, illustrations, and an index are provided. An excellent reference source recommended for medical libraries and for surgeons at all levels of training.
R: *Annals of Thoracic Surgery* 21: 474 (May 1976); *JAMA* 234: 334 (Oct. 20, 1975); *RSR* 4: 42 (Jan.–Mar. 1976).

Microsurgery: A Practical Guide for Surgeons, Gynecologists, Urologists, Plastic Surgeons, Neurosurgeons, and Orthopaedists. **Sherman J. Silber, ed.** Baltimore, MD: Williams & Wilkins, 1979.
A step-by-step guide to microsurgery. A comprehensive and in-depth review; contains references from the literature; can be useful in all fields of surgery.

The New Physician Surgical Quiz. **Terence S. Carden, Jr.** New York: Appleton-Century-Crofts, 1974.
A study guide for students and residents. Contains quizzes in multiple-choice format.
R: *JAMA* 230: 1204 (Nov. 25, 1974).

BRAIN AND NERVOUS SYSTEM

Clinical Management of Seizures: A Guide for the Physician. **Gail E. Solomon and Fred Plum.** Philadelphia, PA: W. B. Saunders, 1976.
A practical reference for physicians who deal with patients having seizure disorders. Comprehensively covers the management of seizures; contains helpful diagrams and tables and a selective bibliography. A highly recommended reference source for neurologists, psychiatrists, and pediatricians.
R: *American Journal of Diseases of Children* 131: 717 (June 1977); *Annals of Internal Medicine* 85: 838 (Dec. 1976); *Archives of Physical Medicine and Rehabilitation* 59: 50 (Jan. 1978); *Canadian Medical Association Journal* 116: 139 (Jan. 1977); *Journal of Neurosurgery* 46: 405 (Mar. 1977); *JAMA* 236: 2801 (Dec. 13, 1976); *Lancet* 2: 1119 (Nov. 20, 1976).

Neurological Surgery: A Comprehensive Reference Guide to the Diagnosis and Management of Neurosurgical Problems. 3 vols. **Julian R. Youmans, ed.** Philadelphia, PA: W. B. Saunders, 1973.
Three-volume reference source for the diagnosis and management of neurosurgical and allied techniques and problems. Written by 124 international experts and specialists in the areas discussed. Volume I deals primarily with diagnostic procedures; volume II concentrates on vascular disorders, trauma, and spinal tumors; and volume III presents an excellent discussion of brain tumors. The trio of volumes is an outstanding purchase for the lucid chapters on pain alone. Contains exceptional radiological reproductions, diagrams, tables, and photographs. The 112 chapters are well balanced by extensive reference lists. Each volume includes a complete index to the entire set. Highly recom-

mended to neurosurgeons, neurological trainees, and allied specialists.
R: *Archives of Neurology* 30: 272 (Mar. 1974); *Journal of Neurosurgery* 41: 113 (July 1974); *NEJM* 289: 757 (Oct. 4, 1973); Allyn.

Spina Bifida—Problems and Management. **G. T. Stark.** Oxford, England: Blackwell Scientific Publications, 1977.

Encompasses nearly all aspects of the management of spina bifida cases. Stresses the moderate view of treatment rather than the radical surgical procedures previously used. Succinct presentation, excellent bibliography and index.
R: *Brain* 100: 798 (Dec. 1977).

Understanding Aphasia: A Guide for Medical and Paramedical Professionals. **William O. Haynes and Bonita R. Greenberg.** Danville, IL: Interstate, 1976.

CARDIOVASCULAR SYSTEM

Cardiovascular Care Unit: A Guide for Planning and Operation. **Glenn O. Turner.** New York: John Wiley, 1978.

Provides a complete system for improved management of cardiovascular and pulmonary emergencies. Explains how design of the hospital environment can alleviate psychological problems of acute cardiac patients. Also outlines methods for speeding arrival of patients into the cardiovascular unit once they have reached the hospital.

Cardiovascular Diseases: Guidelines for Prevention and Care. **I. S. Wright and D. T. Frederickson, eds.** New York: Inter-Society Commission for Heart Disease Resources, 1973.

A valuable resource on cardiovascular systems and disease, containing information not easily acquired in other standard texts. Discusses hospital facilities and care of coronary patients. Recommended for physicians and hospital administrators.
R: *NEJM* 291: 742 (Oct. 3, 1974).

Cardiovascular Therapy: A Systematic Approach. 2d ed. 2 vols. **Raymond E. Phillips.** Philadelphia, PA: W. B. Saunders, 1979.

Useful guide to diagnosis and treatment of cardiovascular diseases. Emphasis on drug therapy, but clearly defines alternative medical approaches to management of the cardiovascular patient, including diet, blood transfusion, administration of fluid and electrolyte solutions, etc.

Heartbook: A Guide to Prevention and Treatment of Cardiovascular Disease. **American Heart Association.** New York: Dutton, 1980.

Comprehensive guide intended specifically for the layman. Includes 24 chapters written by noted authorities. Emphasis on heart disease prevention. Some chapters devoted to specific disease states, pregnancy, and cardiovascular drugs. Nontechnical treatment of subject matter. Essential for public library reference collections.
R: *LJ* 105: 626 (Mar. 1, 1980).

Hypertension: A Practitioner's Guide to Therapy. **James C. Hutchinson.** Flushing, NY: Medical Examination Publishing, 1975.

Modern Concepts of Cerebrovascular Disease. **John S. Meyer, ed.** New York: Halsted Press, 1975.

Features the important advances in the area of cerebrovascular disease. Concentrates on etiology, diagnosis, and management. The illustrations, particularly the X-rays, are superb. Written by authorities active in the field of cardiovascular disease. Geared toward first-contact physicans, primarily the general practitioner, the internist, and the neurologist.
R: *American Family Physician* 14: 198 (Oct. 1976).

Noninvasive Techniques in Cardiology for the Nurse and Technician. **A. Benchimol.** New York: John Wiley, 1978.

Presents basic guidelines of the technical aspects of noninvasive diagnosis in cardiology. Provides discussion of anatomy and physiology. Includes illustrations.

Practical Pediatric Electrocardiography. **Arthur J. Moss and George C. Emmanouilides.** Philadelphia, PA: J. B. Lippincott, 1973.

A guide to electrocardiography in infants and children. Initial chapters contain handy information on normal values, technical errors, and guidelines for performing electrocardiograms. Remaining sections devoted to electrocardiographic tracings illustrating each disorder. Diagrams support the text. Geared toward family physician, pediatrician, house officer, and intensive care nurses.
R: *Annals of Internal Medicine* 79: 929 (Dec. 1973); Allyn.

A Primer of Cardiac Diagnosis: The Physical and Technical Study of the Cardiac Patient. **Aldo A. Luisada and Gurmukh S. Sainani.** St. Louis, MO: Warren H. Green, 1968.

Focuses on examination of the cardiac patient. Summarizes the procedures, normal findings, and finally, abnormal conditions obtained in common cardiovascular cases. Although limited to a few illustrations, they are clear and original. Recommended for physicians, residents, interns, and medical students.

Treatment of Heart Disease in the Adult. 2d ed. **Ira L. Rubin et al.** Philadelphia, PA: Lea & Febiger, 1972.

Comprehensive coverage of the treatment of adult heart diseases. Systematic guide to bedside, hospital, and office management of cardiac patients. Includes pertinent drug information. Electrocardiograms and diagrams complement the text. Valuable addition to a cardiac collection of the family physician or internist.
R: *American Family Physician* 8: 277 (Oct. 1973).

DENTISTRY

Accepted Dental Therapeutics. Vols. 1–. **American Dental Association.** Chicago, IL: American Dental Association, 1934–. Biennial.

This volume replaces *Accepted Dental Remedies* (with consistent numbering). Guides dentists to appropriate drugs and treatment of oral disease. Index in-

cludes product information and professional reports.
R: Win (EK149; 3EJ18).

Group Practice of Dentistry, DHEW Pub. no. (HRA) 77-8. **US Department of Health, Education, and Welfare.** Washington, DC: US Government Printing Office, 1977.
A guide for dentists forming group practices. Discusses practical aspects; provides an extensive bibliography.
R: *Journal of Oral Surgery* 36: 487 (June 1978).

A Guide to Dental Radiography. **Rita A. Mason.** Chicago, IL: Year Book Medical Publishers, 1978.

An Illustrated Guide to Dental Morphology. **G. C. Downer.** Chicago, IL: Year Book Medical Publishers, 1975.

DERMATOLOGY

Current Concepts in the Management of Skin Cancer. **Perry Robbins and Richard G. Bennett.** New York: Masson, 1978.
A practical guide to diagnosis and treatment of cutaneous malignancies.

Dermatology: An Illustrated Guide. 2d ed. **Lionel Fry.** Fort Lee, NJ: Update Publishing International, 1978.
First edition, 1973.
A basic introductory guide to dermatology which contains succinct, reliable information. Provides numerous photographs. For medical students, dermatologists, and general practitioners.
R: *Archives of Dermatology* 115: 115 (Jan. 1979); *Lancet* 2: 78 (July 14, 1973).

A Guide to Dermatohistopathology. 2d ed. **Hermann Pinkus and Amir H. Mehregan.** New York: Appleton-Century-Crofts, 1976.
First edition, 1969.
Expanded and updated edition; discusses new processes in the field, anatomy of the skin, histology techniques, morphological and pathological changes in the skin. Includes photomicrographs. A handy guide for dermal pathologists of all levels.
R: *Annals of Internal Medicine* 84: 515 (Apr. 1976); *JAMA* 236: 1512 (Sept. 27, 1976).

ENDOCRINOLOGY

Diabetes and its Management. **W. G. Oakley, D. A. Pyke, and K. W. Taylor.** Philadelphia, PA: F. A. Davis, 1973.
A short guide with a clinical orientation. Contains concise information of the disease's etiology, metabolic complications, biochemical relationships to other hormonal functions. Well-written, informative guide for physicians, students, paramedics.
R: *Annals of Internal Medicine* 79: 296 (1973); *Gastroenterology* 66: 330 (Feb. 1974); *Lancet* 1: 919 (Apr. 28, 1973).

Diabetes Guidebook, Diet Section. 2d ed. **John K. Davidson and Mary Goldsmith.** Columbus, GA: Litho-Krome Co., 1972.

Conveys the basic needs of a diabetic diet through the use of color photographs and tables. Emphasizes accurate and precise measurement in food service. Worthwhile for physicians, nurses, dietitians, families with diabetic members.
R: *Diabetes* 25: 470 (May 1976).

Diabetes: Its Physiological and Biochemical Basis. **J. Vallance-Owen, ed.** Baltimore, MD: University Park Press, 1975.

A multi-authored compendium of the biochemistry of diabetes. Subjects arranged by chapters which are well referenced. A handy guide which covers a wide range of topics.
R: *Annals of Internal Medicine* 85: 415 (Sept. 1976); *BMJ* 1: 531 (Feb. 28, 1976); *NEJM* 295: 790 (1976); *Quarterly Review of Biology* 51: 566 (1976).

GASTROINTESTINAL SYSTEM

Gastroenterology. 3d ed. 4 vols. **Henry L. Bockus et al., eds.** Philadelphia, PA: W. B. Saunders, 1974-1976.

First edition, 1944; second edition, 1964.
Volume 1, *Examination of the Patient, The Esophagus, The Stomach,* 1974; volume 2, *The Small Intestine and Colon,* 1976; volume 3, *The Liver, Gallbladder, Bile Ducts, Pancreas,* 1976; volume 4, *The Peritoneum, Parasitic Diseases: System Interrelationships, and Relevant Miscellany,* 1976.
Four volumes form comprehensive work on practical clinical gastroenterology. Physiology of organs, morphological techniques, information about liver and pancreas, and relationships of gastrointestinal tract of other organ systems are among topics covered. Large number of X-rays and color plates, complete references and good index. Definitve source reference for gastroenterologists and physicians.
R: *American Journal of Digestive Diseases* 22: 173 (Feb. 1977); *Annals of Internal Medicine* 85: 835 (Dec. 1976); *Gastroenterology* 68: 623 (Mar. 1975); *JAMA* 232: 856 (May 26, 1975); 236: 1065 (Aug. 30, 1976); 238: 349 (July 25, 1977); Allyn; Brandon; Stearns & Ratcliff (*NEJM,* 1969; *NEJM,* 1970).

Techniques of Clinical Gastroenterology. **Henry W. Boyce, Jr., and Eddy D. Palmer.** Springfield, IL: Charles C. Thomas, 1975.

Depicts various techniques used in the assessment of gastrointestinal conditions. Good reference source for training programs in gastroenterology.
R: *Gastroenterology* 70: 630 (Apr. 1977); *Gastrointestinal Endoscopy* 22: 107 (Nov. 1975); *Proceedings of the Royal Society of Medicine* 69: 462 (June 1976); *Surgery, Gynecology and Obstetrics* 142: 255 (Feb. 1976); *TBRI* 42: 95 (Mar. 1976); 42: 136 (Apr. 1976); 42: 301 (Oct. 1976).

GENETICS

Methods for the Analysis of Human Chromosome Aberrations. **K. E. Buckton and H. J. Evans, eds.** Geneva: World Health Organization, 1973.

A bench reference guide for genetic laboratories, illustrating methods of meas-

uring chromosomal aberrations and their classification. Prepared under auspices of the WHO. Useful and highly recommended.
R: *British Journal of Radiology* 47: 342 (1974); *International Journal of Radiation Biology* 25: 421 (Apr. 1974).

Rare Genetic Diseases: A Guidebook. **T. F. Thurmon, III.** Cleveland, OH: Chemical Rubber Company, 1974.

Comprehensive guide to rare genetic diseases. Introductory matter on basic concepts and genetic counseling. Bulk of book contained in three chapters. Divides genetic disorders into three major categories (chronic, congenital, infantile) and indexes them alphabetically according to major organ system affected. Preferred nomenclature and synonyms listed along with catalog numbers from McKusick's 1971 edition of *Mendelian Inheritance in Man* and code numbers from the eighth edition of *International Classification of Diseases*. Contains lengthy index of diseases.
R: *Annals of Internal Medicine* 82: 444 (Mar. 1975).

GERONTOLOGY

Essentials of Geriatric Medicine. **George Adams.** New York: Oxford University Press, 1978.

Concise and informative guide to essentials of geriatrics. Describes process of aging, special problems in medical care for the elderly, and use of drugs in geriatric medicine.

Homburger and Bonner's Medical Care and Rehabilitation of the Aged and Chronically Ill. 3d ed. **Charles D. Bonner.** Boston, MA: Little, Brown, 1974.

Revised and updated, including a section of physician patient relationships. Also contains much practical information for those who work with the elderly such as choice of crutches, problem of lower extremity amputation. A beneficial guide for physicians and allied health care professionals.
R: *Hospital Administration* 20: 87 (Spr. 1975); *JAMA* 231: 982 (Mar. 3, 1975); *NEJM* 292: 816 (Apr. 10, 1975); *TBRI* 41: 180 (May 1975); Brandon.

HEALTH SERVICES ADMINISTRATION

Blueprint for Medical Care. **David D. Rutstein.** Cambridge, MA: MIT Press, 1974.

A collection of proposals designed by the author to meet the needs of changing health care. Emphasizes trends in medical education, emergency care, and health services. Explores complications of an integrated national health policy. Lacks adequate bibliographic references.
R: *Plastic & Reconstructive Surgery* 55: 486 (1975); *Quarterly Review of Biology* 50: 228 (1975).

Concise Guide to Biomedical Polymers: Their Design, Fabrication, and Molding. **John W. Boretos.** Springfield, IL: Charles C. Thomas, 1973.

Describes rubbers and plastics which are most suitable for use within the body. Techniques and formulations are described in context of their suitability to the development of artificial hearts, vascular grafts, pacemakers, etc.

Developing Policies and Procedures for Long-Term Care Institutions. **American Hospital Association.** Chicago, IL: American Hospital Association, 1975.
A guide for establishing policy procedures in long-term health care institutions.

Governing Hospitals: Trustees and the New Accountabilities. **Robert M. Cunningham.** Chicago, IL: American Hospital Association, 1976.
A guide to hospital administration. Helpful to trustees, planners, physicians, government officials for discussion of management, governance.
R: *Hospitals* 50: 40 (June 16, 1976).

Health and Safety Guide for Hospitals, DHEW Pub. no. (NIOSH) 78-150. **National Institute for Occupational Safety and Health.** Washington, DC: US Government Printing Office, 1978.

Health Maintenance Organizations: A Guide to Planning and Development. Vol. 7. **Roger W. Birnbaum.** New York: Spectrum Publications, 1976.
A prime source for anyone seeking information on health maintenance organizations. Deals particularly with the management, development, and government role in HMOs as they are evolving in this country.
R: *Quarterly Review of Biology* 52: 342 (1977).

Intensive Care Instrumentation. **D. W. Hill and A. M. Dolan.** New York: Academic Press, 1976.
Illustrates techniques associated with intensive care instrumentation such as equipment maintenance and monitoring. Contains many practical guidelines, helpful line diagrams, and bibliographies. Recommended for all ICU departments.
R: *Biomedical Engineering* 11: 286 (1976).

Intensive Care Units: Minimal Criteria and Guidelines. **Michigan Bureau of Health Facilities.** Lansing, MI: Michigan Bureau of Health Facilities, 1972.

Library Practice in Hospitals: A Basic Guide. **Harold Bloomquist et al., eds.** Cleveland, OH: Case Western Reserve University Press, 1972.
Discusses the administration of hospital libraries, including such topics as acquisition policies, medical staff association, information networks. Contains much practical information for medical librarians.
R: *Annals of Internal Medicine* 78: 316 (Feb. 1973); *NEJM* 288: 977 (May 3, 1973).

Management by Objectives for Hospitals. **Arthur X. Deegan.** Germantown, MD: Aspen Systems Corp., 1977.
Systematically outlines procedures for management by objectives in hospital terminology. Provides instructive information for managers at every level in the hospital. A good source of ready reference.

Management of Hospitals. **Rockwell Schulz and Alton C. Johnson.** New York: McGraw-Hill, 1976.
Readable presentation of foundations upon which hospitals are administered.

Complete name index and 25 pages of bibliographic references. Especially appropriate for use in courses in hospital administration.
R: *Hospital and Health Services Administration* 22: 83 (1977); Brandon.

Medical Information Systems: A Resource for Hospitals. **Melville H. Hodge.** Germantown, MD: Aspen Systems Corp., 1977.

A guide which outlines computerized medical information systems for hospitals. Details theoretical and actual guidelines. A valuable tool for any medical organization installing computerized information resources.
R: *American Journal of Psychiatry* 135: 1134 (Sept. 1978).

Medical Records Departments in Hospitals: Guide to Organization. **American Hospital Association.** Chicago, IL: American Hospital Association, 1972.

Presents basic principles of medical record management.

Medicolegal Aspects of Hospital Records. 2d ed. **Emanuel Hayt.** Berwyn, IL: Physicians' Record Co., 1977.

Illustrates how medical and legal matters can be interpreted from medical records. Systematic presentation provides guide to courtroom procedures, hospital record-keeping. Presents actual cases. Helpful to medical record librarians, hospital administrators, and physicians.
R: *American Journal of Psychiatry* 135: 886 (July 1978).

Multilingual Guide for Medical Personnel. **Bernard E. Finch.** Flushing, NY: Medical Examination Publishing, 1967.

Lists questions, expressions, and directions in six languages: English, French, Italian, German, Spanish, and Russian. Intended for medical personnel.
R: Win (EK84).

Physician's Guide to Negotiations. **S. J. Burrows.** Chicago, IL: American Medical Association, 1976.

Surveys the special skills required by health professionals in this area of communication. Emphasis on preparation, negotiation, and consummation. Booklet is beneficial to consumer, provider, and community.
R: *Journal of Oral Surgery* 36: 323 (Apr. 1978).

Practical Medicine: A Guide to Outpatient Management. **P. R. Daggett and D. M. Geddes.** London: Lloyd-Luke, 1976.

Contains relevant information about diagnosis, investigation, and treatment of common medical conditions. Written for newly certified doctors with little or no experience in outpatient management.
R: *Lancet* 1: 570 (Mar. 13, 1976); *New Zealand Medical Journal* 83: 450 (June 23, 1976); *TBRI* 42: 343 (Nov. 1976).

Practical Spanish for Medical and Hospital Personnel. **Marguerite D. Bomse and Julian H. Alfaro.** New York: Pergamon Oxford Spanish Texts, 1974.
R: *MRW* S3, p. 40.

Quality by Objectives: A Practical Method for Quality of Care Assessment and Assurance for Ambulatory Health Centers. **Norbert Hirschhorn et al.** Boston, MA: G. K. Hall, 1978.

Provides practical guidelines for the planning and evaluation of ambulatory health care by health center personnel. A cooperative effort by some 30 urban and rural health centers around the country.

The Rights of Hospital Patients. **George J. Annas.** New York: Avon Books, 1975.

Focuses on the legal rights of the hospital patient. Prepared by the American Civil Liberties Union. Follows a question and answer format and subtly suggests methods by which the consumer may become an advocate for his rights. Helpful information source for both consumers and health care providers.
R: *Journal of Nervous and Mental Disease* 163: 67 (1976).

Safety Guide For Health Care Institutions. **American Hospital Association.** Chicago, IL: American Hospital Association, 1972.

Presents guidelines which help to control accidents and injuries, including fire emergencies. Provides checklists for safety in various situations.

HEMATOLOGY

Diagnosis and Treatment of Hemophilia: A Practical Guide. 3d ed. **Herbert S. Strauss.** Albany, NY: Albany Medical College, 1972.

Concise and well-written compilation of recent advances in the area of hemophilia. Diagnostic approaches and treatment information are explored in depth and are clearly presented. Highly recommended for physicians and others who see hemophiliacs on a consultative basis. Its extensive descriptions of blood coagulation systems warrant reading by medical students.
R: *Annals of Internal Medicine* 78: 464 (Mar. 1973).

INFECTIOUS DISEASES

Clinical Tropical Diseases. 6th ed. **Brian Maegraith.** Oxford, England: Blackwell Scientific Publications, 1976.

Fifth edition, 1971.
Sixth edition of this book concisely describes the diseases of the tropics. Includes accounts of diseases arranged in alphabetical order with attached appendix on vaccination. Useful guide to physicians dealing with these diseases whether they practice in tropical or temperate countries.
R: *Annals of Internal Medicine* 86: 123 (Jan. 1977).

Diagnostic Methods in Clinical Virology. 2d ed. **N. R. Grist, Constance A. C. Ross, and Eleanor J. Bell.** Philadelphia, PA: J. B. Lippincott, 1974.

Practical guide for those who wish to understand well-established methods of diagnostic virology. This second edition has been brought completely up to date through the conclusion of advances in the field since publication of the first edition.

Guide to the Collection and Transport of Virological Specimens. **C. R. Madeley.** Geneva: World Health Organization, 1977.

Discusses aspects of diagnostic virology such as clinical syndromes, epidemiological information, collection and transport of specimens. Details all necessary information concerning laboratory practice in transport of virological specimens.
R: *IBID* 5: 152 (June 1977).

Infectious Diseases: A Modern Treatise of Infectious Processes. 2d ed. **Paul D. Hoeprich, ed.** Hagerstown, MD: Harper & Row, 1977.

First edition, 1972.
A basic and classic source concerning all aspects of infectious disease. Comprehensively illustrates epidemiology, occurrence and manifestations of infectious disease. Contains over 300 figures and illustrations, references, and index.
R: *Annals of Internal Medicine* 78: 800 (1973); 88: 582 (Apr. 1978); *BMJ* 2: 429 (May 19, 1973); *RSR* 2: 122 (Apr.–June 1974); Allyn; Brandon.

Practical Guide to Medicine and Veterinarian Mycology. **R. Vanbreuseghem.** New York: Masson Publishing, 1978.

Complete coverage of diseases caused by yeasts and fungi.
R: *Archives of Dermatology* 115: 781 (June 1979); *Nature* 270: 120 (Nov. 10, 1977).

Travelers to the Tropics—Guidelines for Physicians. **R. Dupuis.** New York: International Development Research Centre, 1978.

An aid to physicians and health workers who deal with patients contemplating a trip to tropical areas or returning from such areas. Various aspects of parasitic diseases and immunizations are included. National immunization requirements listed in appendixes.
R: *IBID* 6: 426 (Dec. 1978).

INTERNAL MEDICINE

Diagnostic Procedures: A Reference for Health Practitioners and a Guide for Patient Counseling. **Barbara Skydell and Anne S. Crowder.** Boston, MA: Little, Brown, 1975.

A manual which elucidates the before and after care of hospital patients undergoing diagnostic procedures. Describes preparation, examination techniques, sensations felt by patients. Intended as a general ready reference for nurses and other health care professionals.
R: *American Journal of Nursing* 76: 1512 (Sept. 1976); *Annals of Internal Medicine* 86: 249 (Feb. 1977); *Canadian Nurse* 73: 50 (Feb. 1977).

Emergency Medical Guide. 4th ed. **John Henderson.** New York: McGraw-Hill, 1978.

Second edition, 1969; third edition, 1973.
Revised and enlarged edition. Includes emergency guide to the treatment of acute heart disease, drug abuse, childbirth, and childhood emergencies, etc. Contains a helpful appendix which has a poison control center directory, a list for immunization records, as well as helpful illustrations and a glossary.
R: *Annals of Internal Medicine* 80: 126 (Jan. 1974); *Archives of Internal Medicine*

134: 185 (July 1974); *RSR* 2: 119 (July–Sept. 1974); *WLB* 48: 419 (Jan. 1974); *ARBA* (1970, p. 134; 1974, p. 631).

Emergency Treatment and Management. 5th ed. **T. J. Flint and H. D. Cain.** Philadelphia, PA: W. B. Saunders, 1975.

A handy ready reference guide for emergency situations; covers a variety of situations. A useful, portable compendium of information for the physician.
R: *Plastic and Reconstructive Surgery* 58: 96 (1976).

Guide to Diagnostic Procedures. 4th ed. **Ruth M. French.** New York: McGraw-Hill, 1975.

A ready reference to diagnostic procedures and services for health care professionals. Concisely discusses laboratory examinations by type (urine, biochemical, immunologic, etc.), with the aid of charts and tables. There is also a helpful index and glossary.
R: *Canadian Nurse* 72: 48 (Mar. 1976); *ARBA* (1976, p. 730).

Immediate Care of the Acutely Ill and Injured. **Hugh E. Stephenson, Jr., ed.** St. Louis, MO: C. V. Mosby, 1974.

A concise book on emergency care; contains a detailed index for quick information retrieval. For medical school and hospital libraries.
R: *RSR* 3: 33 (Apr.–June 1975); Allyn.

Laboratory Guide to Clinical Diagnosis. 4th ed. **R. D. Eastham.** Bristol, England: John Wright, 1976.

Second edition, 1970; third edition, 1973.
A pocket-size manual which presents the results of laboratory diagnosis of diseases. Covers a wide range of topics. Useful to clinicians and medical students. Concise, comprehensive reference.
R: *British Journal of Haematology* 34: 345 (1976); *ABL* 38: entry 425 (Aug. 1973); 41: entry 366 (Sept. 1976).

Management of Neglected Trauma. **J. Francis Silva.** Springfield, IL: Charles C. Thomas, 1972.

A well-written and well-illustrated "how-to" guide for orthopedists who deal with neglected injuries. Allows physicians and therapists to be aware of complications arising from neglected trauma, particularly nerve and joint related areas. Text is arranged by anatomic region.
R: *Archives of Physical Medicine and Rehabilitation* 54: 242 (May 1973).

Medication Guide for Patient Counseling **Dorothy L. Smith.** Philadelphia, PA: Lea & Febiger, 1977.

Provides a concise guide to educate patients taking commonly prescribed drugs. Written in easily understood language, helpful to those who prescribe and dispense drugs.
R: *Journal of Oral Surgery* 36: 734 (Sept. 1978); *ARBA* (1978, p. 733).

Microtechniques for the Clinical Laboratory: Concepts and Applications. **Mario Werner, ed.** New York: John Wiley, 1976.

A multi-authored, though uniformly written guide presenting recent developments in laboratory techniques. Helpful to pathologists, chemists, medical technologists.
R: *Analytical Chemistry* 49: 439A (Apr. 1977); *Archives of Pathology & Laboratory Medicine* 101: 393 (July 1977); *TBRI* 43: 225 (June 1977).

Normal Values in Clinical Chemistry: A Guide to Statistical Analysis of Laboratory Data. **Horace F. Martin, Benjamin J. Gudzinowicz, and Herbert Fanger.** New York: Marcel Dekker, 1975.

Summarizes much of the literature prior to 1972 about the theory of normal values and similar topics. Requires some knowledge of the following disciplines: clinical chemistry, biochemistry, mathematics, statistics, and computer science. Quotations from papers written during the previous decade comprise the bulk of the book. Material could be excessively tedious for the nonspecialist. Despite these flaws, presently the most important reference on normal range methodology.
R: *NEJM* 294: 287 (Jan. 29, 1976).

Pocket Guide to Health Assessment. **Karen J. Berger and Willa L. Fields.** New York: Appleton-Century-Crofts, 1979.

A practical handbook of health assessment. Outlines normal physical conditions as well as common abnormalities. Lists routine examination procedures and their recommended order of performance. Seventy-five anatomical illustrations enhance the text. Good definitions of all medical terms, abbreviations, and symbols.

Rypins' Medical Licensure Examinations. 12th ed. **Arthur W. Wright.** Philadelphia, PA: J. B. Lippincott, 1975.

Concise survey of medicine for students and doctors anticipating the board and licensure examinations. Thoroughly updated twelfth edition. Part I deals with the basic sciences; part II discusses the clinical sciences. Each summary followed by questions. New material includes sections on behavioral science, anatomy, biochemistry and pharmacology. Greater emphasis on genetics and cell biology.

School Health: A Guide for Health Professionals. **Committee on School Health, American Academy of Pediatrics.** Evanston, IL: American Academy of Pediatrics, 1977.

For all who are involved in school health problems. Defines roles of all personnel involved, such as school physician and nurse. Includes vision, hearing, and speech screening tests, immunization schedules, etc. Well written, valuable reference.
R: *American Family Physician* 18: 253 (Sept. 1978).

Stress Testing: Principles and Practice. **Myrvin H. Ellestad.** Philadelphia, PA: F. A. Davis, 1975.

Serves as a guide and reference source for stress testing. Includes numerous, valuable tables, graphs, and illustrations.
R: *Annals of Internal Medicine* 83: 917 (Dec. 1975); *TBRI* 42: 60 (Feb. 1976); Allyn.

Take Care of Yourself: A Consumer's Guide to Medical Care. **Donald M. Vickery and James F. Fries.** Reading, MA: Addison-Wesley, 1976.
Provides a programmed sequence of questions which allow the medical consumer to determine extent of malady and whether or not a doctor needs to be consulted. Questions are grouped in such categories as common inquiries, skin problems, eye problems. Provides information on choosing the right physician and reducing medical costs. Contains flow charts and extensive index. Helpful in asssisting the consumer to make wise medical decisions.
R: *Annals of Internal Medicine* 86: 680 (May 1977); *BMJ* 2: 199 (Feb. 21, 1979); *Journal of School Health* 47: 493 (Oct. 1977); *ARBA* (1978, p. 726).

Todd-Sanford Clinical Diagnosis by Laboratory Methods. 16th ed. **Israel Davidsohn and John B. Henry, eds.** Philadelphia, PA: W. B. Saunders, 1979.
First edition, 1908; fifteenth edition, 1974.
Collection of methodologies and special topics in laboratory medicine. Interprets laboratory findings and discusses quality control and drug interaction. Useful to residents and laboratory directors.
R: *JAMA* 230: 1587 (Dec. 16, 1974); Allyn; Stearns & Ratcliff (*NEJM,* 1970).

Treatment of Shock: Principles and Practice. **William Schumer and Lloyd M. Nyhus.** Philadelphia, PA: Lea & Febiger, 1974.
Practical reference source to the understanding and care of shock patients. Indispensable tool for intensive care units and hospital libraries. Handy guide for all doctors treating seriously ill patients.
R: *Lancet* 2: 261 (Aug. 9, 1975).

The Underwater Handbook: A Guide to Physiology and Performance for the Engineer. **Charles W. Shilling, Margaret F. Werts, and Nancy R. Schandelmeier, eds.** New York: John Wiley, 1977.
Not only intended as a guide for engineers, physiologists and medical practitioners associated with diving and offshore activites also will find useful data in this reference book.
R: *Lancet* 2: 536 (Sept. 10, 1977).

NURSING

Back to Nursing: A Guide to Current Practice for Active and Inactive Nurses. 2d ed. **Ruth P. Stryker.** Philadelphia, PA: W. B. Saunders, 1971.

Basic Steps in Planning Nursing Research: from Question to Proposal. **Pamela J. Brink and Marilyn J. Wood.** North Scituate, MA: Duxbury Press, 1978.
Defines research, outlines levels and methods of approach. Lists suggested readings, research proposals and their developments. Useful for master's students in nursing.
R: *American Journal of Nursing* p. 2150 (Dec. 1978); *Nursing Research* 28: 15 (Jan.–Feb. 1979).

Gastroenterological Nursing. **Helen E. Gribble.** Baltimore, MD: Williams & Wilkins, 1977.

A handy guide to gastrointestinal conditions. Provides clear, concise explanations of abnormalities and treatment. Contains line drawings. Highly recommended.
R: *American Journal of Digestive Diseases* 23: 670 (July 1978).

Geriatric Nursing. **Alison Storrs.** London: Balliere, Tindall, 1976.

Discusses nursing care of the elderly in various settings (hospitals, nursing homes, etc.). Goes into details of geriatric nursing procedures. Maintains British influence throughout. Usual for ready reference.
R: *The Canadian Nurse* 73: 55 (Nov. 1977).

A Guide for Nurse Managers. **Elizabeth Raybould, ed.** Oxford, England: Blackwell Scientific Publications, 1977.

A Guide to Nursing Management of Psychiatric Patents. 2d ed. **Sharon Dreyer et al.** St. Louis, MO: C. V. Mosby, 1979.

Illustrated Guide to Orthopedic Nursing. **Jane Farrell.** Philadelphia, PA: J. B. Lippincott, 1977.

Highlights the management and treatment of orthopedic patients. Lavishly illustrated with photographs, charts, and figures. Concentrates on the rationale behind certain nursing procedures. Text geared toward spot referencing. Handy tool for students and professionals.
R: *American Journal of Nursing* 77: 498 (Mar. 1978); Brandon (*NO*).

Law Every Nurse Should Know. 3d ed. **Helen Creighton.** Philadelphia, PA: W. B. Saunders, 1975.
Second edition, 1970.
R: Brandon (*NO*).

The New Nurse in Industry: A Guide For the Newly Employed Occupational Health Nurse, DHEW Pub. no. (NIOSH) 78-143. **Jane A. Lee.** Bethesda, MD: National Institute for Occupational Safety and Health, 1978.

Nurses' Drug Reference. **Stewart M. Brooks, ed.** Boston, MA: Little, Brown, 1978.

A ready reference which lists alphabetically more than 500 drugs. Includes drug reaction, dosage, administration, glossary of terms, legal information. Well organized. A standard source for nurse practitioners.
R: Brandon (*NO*).

Nurses Guide to Cardiac Monitoring. 2d ed. **P. J. B. Hubner.** London: Bailliere Tindall, 1975.

Based on nursing lecture notes on cardiac arrythmias; tries to convey understanding of cardiac monitoring; reviews anatomy techniques of ECG and cardiac pacing. Provides a brief description of problems in cardiac nursing.
R: *The Canadian Nurse* 72: 48 (Oct. 1976).

The Nurse's Guide to Health Services For Patients. **May D. Futrell and Marie J. Kelleher.** Boston, MA: Little, Brown, 1973.

Outlines the basic function of various health services for nurses and students. Aimed at matching the correct service with the right individual or family. Uses case studies to strengthen objectives.
R: *American Journal of Nursing* 74: 758 (Apr. 1974); 74: 1358 (July 1974).

A Nurse's Guide to the X-Ray Department. 2d ed. **Myer Goldman.** Edinburgh, Scotland: Churchill Livingstone. Distr. Baltimore, MD: Williams & Wilkins, 1972.

Completely updated manual; provides recent information on radiological techniques. Accurate, a helpful guide for nurses.
R: *ARBA* (1974, p. 630).

Nursing Research: A Learning Guide. **Natalie Pavlovich.** St. Louis, MO: C. V. Mosby, 1978.

A workbook which completely outlines all aspects of nursing research. A helpful supplement to research texts. Provides basic concepts and references.

Patient Assessment Series. **American Journal of Nursing.** New York: American Journal of Nursing Co., 1979.

Sixteen comprehensive units of instructive and examination materials for nurses in assessing major common problems in patient care. Uses photographs, how-to discussions and practical techniques to convey information. The sixteen units include "Examinations of the Female Pelvis," two parts; "Taking a Patient's History"; "The Ear"; "The Eye," two parts.

The Patient in Surgery: A Guide for Nurses. 3d ed. **George D. LeMaitre and Janet A. Finnegan.** Philadelphia, PA: W. B. Saunders, 1975.

An in-depth guide to care of surgical patients. Written in clear, concise style. Deals with potential surgical hazards and patients' fears. Includes case histories and illustrations.
R: *American Journal of Nursing* 76: 1339 (Aug. 1976); Stearns & Ratcliff (*AJN*).

The Pediatric Nurse Practitioner: Guidelines For Practice. 2d ed. **Fernando DeCastro et al.** St. Louis, MO: C. V. Mosby, 1976.

First edition, 1972.
Second edition features new chapters and updated information. Consists of four main sections: introduction, health appraisal, clinical problems, and the family and child in society. Includes comments by authorities in their fields and basic black-and-white diagrams. Each chapter concludes with a copious bibliography. Comprehensive reference source for practitioners, nursing students, and veterans in the area of pediatrics.
R: *Canadian Nurse* 73: 54 (Nov. 1977).

Physical Assessment Examinations. **City University of New York, Herbert H. Lehman College, Department of Nursing.** New York: City University of New York, 1975.

Professional Nursing: Foundations, Perspectives and Relationships. 9th ed. **Lucille E. Notter and Eugenia K. Spalding.** New York: J. B. Lippincott, 1976.
Presents an overview of the foundations of professional nursing, including history, employment opportunities, legal aspects, reference materials, and organizations. A valuable reference in the field.
R: Brandon (*NO*).

Staffing For Patient Care: A Guide For Nursing Service, Based on a Research Report. **Elmina M. Price.** New York: Springer Publishing, 1970.
Consists of two sections: a practical guide to improving staff situations and a detailed report of a sample staffing research project. Guide evaluates staffing methods, organization, decisions and standard patterns in institutions. Aimed at nursing service administrators.
R: *ARBA* (1971, p. 538).

Understanding Research in Nursing. **Shirley Chater.** Geneva: World Health Organization, 1975.
Guide to nursing research projects. Follows a step-by-step approach from initial decision to implementation. Includes useful references and suggestions. Valuable addition to hospital and nursing school libraries.
R: *RSR* 4: 43 (Jan.–Mar. 1976).

VD: A Guide for Nurses and Counselors. **Barbara M. Morton.** Boston, MA: Little, Brown, 1976.
Provides concise overview of the prevention and treatment of sexually transmitted diseases. Also highlights the social and psychological implications of VD. Outlines basic interviewing techniques and counseling approaches. Useful glossary of standard and slang terms. Geared toward all levels of nurses in clinical and community settings.
R: *American Journal of Nursing* 77: 499 (Mar. 1977).

NUTRITION

Dietary Nutrient Guide. **Jean A. Pennington.** Westport, CT: AVI Publishing, 1976.
Correlates essential nutrients in commonly eaten foods where they are found. Lists 49 nutrients and their calculated requirements. Also includes a review of the basic four food groups. A valuable tool for dietitians and for the evaluation of menu planning.
R: *American Journal of Clinical Nutrition* 30: 285 (Feb. 1977); *Nutrition Reviews* 35: 28 (Jan. 1977).

Everyone's Guide to Better Food and Nutrition. **Barbara B. Deskins.** Middle Village, NY: David, 1975.
Intended for the layman, written by an experienced nutrition educator.
R: *ARBA* (1976, p. 747); Chen (p. 192).

The Management of Nutritional Emergencies in Large Populations. **C. de Ville**

de Goyet, J. Seaman, and U. Geijer. Geneva: World Health Organization, 1978.

For use by those who deal with malnutrition. Covers major deficiency diseases, food distribution, supplementary feeding, transportation of food, normal and emergency situations. Useful to those concerned with nutritional problems in large populations.
R: *IBID* 6: 408 (Dec. 1978).

Nutrition and Diet Therapy: A Learning Guide for Students. 3d ed. **Sue R. Williams.** St. Louis, MO: C. V. Mosby, 1977.

Discusses basic nutrition as it relates to public health and nursing specialties. Emphasizes the role of nutrition and disease. Provides a complementary guide for instructors.
R: Stearns & Ratcliff (*NEJM,* 1970).

Nutrition Programs for the Elderly—A Guide to Menu Planning, Buying, and the Care of Food for Community Programs. **US Agricultural Research Service.** Washington, DC: US Government Printing Office, 1972.

Provides pertinent information on menu planning and the nutritional value, preservation, and packaging of the foods involved. Aimed at community workers who provide nutritious meals for the elderly.
R: *ARBA* (1973, p. 624).

Obesity, Anorexia Nervosa, and the Person Within. **Hilde Bruch.** London: Routledge & Kegan Paul, 1974.

Comprehensive guide to the understanding of these nutritional disorders.
R: *Lancet* 1: 604 (Apr. 6, 1974).

Selected Guide to Food, Dieting, and Beverage Books. New ed. **Susan Nueckel, ed.** Fleet Press, 1975.

R: Chen (p. 192).

We Want You to Know about Labels on Foods. Washington, DC: US Food and Drug Administration, 1973.

R: Chen (p. 191).

ONCOLOGY AND NUCLEAR MEDICINE

The Cytologic Diagnosis of Cancer. 4th ed. **Ruth M. Graham.** Philadelphia, PA: W. B. Saunders, 1972.

Includes information on the process of cellular diagnosis. Describes cell changes during and after radiation and provides color plates showing normal against abnormal cells. New chapter on effects of oral contraceptives on cellular malformations.
R: *New Zealand Medical Journal* 77: 383 (Nov. 1972); *TBRI* 39: 116 (Mar. 1973); Brandon.

Management of the Patient With Cancer. 2d ed. **Thomas F. Nealon, Jr., ed.** Philadelphia, PA: W. B. Saunders, 1976.

First edition, 1965.
A comprehensive book which presents information pertinent to the management of cancer. Deals with all sites where cancer occurs and so is helpful to general physicians and surgeons. Discusses treatment and therapy. An excellent ready reference.
R: *Annals of Internal Medicine* 86: 837 (June 1977); *JAMA* 238: 896 (Aug. 22, 1977).

OPHTHALMOLOGY

Eye Surgery. 5th ed. **H. B. Stallard.** Baltimore, MD: Williams & Wilkins, 1973.
First edition, 1948.
Serves as a basic reference to techniques in eye surgery covering a wide range of topics. Quality of illustrations suffers a bit, though the guide can be relied on for accurate information.
R: *Archives of Ophthalmology* 92: 181 (Aug. 1974).

Fitting Guide for Hard and Soft Contact Lenses: A Practical Approach. **Harold A. Stein and Bernard J. Slatt.** St. Louis, MO: C. V. Mosby, 1977.
A practical guide for ophthalmologists helping to improve efficiency in the fitting of contact lenses. Outlines procedures, potential difficulties wearer may experience. Close to 500 illustrations and photographs. A valuable book.
R: *American Journal of Ophthalmology* 85: 577 (Apr. 1978); *Archives of Ophthalmology* 96: 920 (May 1978).

Glaucoma Guidebook. **G. L. Portney.** Philadelphia, PA: Lea & Febiger, 1977.
Descriptions of glaucoma examination and aspects of the disease's theory and practice. Contains data not found elsewhere and an annotated bibliography. An informative guide.
R: *Archives of Ophthalmology* 96: 730 (Apr. 1978).

Ocular Examination—Basis and Technique. **Arthur H. Keeney.** St. Louis, MO: C. V. Mosby, 1976.
Assumes a basic knowledge of ophthalmic techniques. Functional topics (motility, ocular tension, photography) receive the best coverage. Includes good discussion and illustrations of ocular instruments. Superb guide for the resident already familiar with the ocular examination but desiring more knowledge. Also includes specialized techniques for the subspecialist.
R: *American Journal of Ophthalmology* 83: 601 (Apr. 1977).

Ophthalmology Study Guide for Medical Students. **Association of University Professors of Ophthalmology.** Rochester, MN: American Academy of Ophthalmology and Otolaryngology, 1975.
A companion study guide to textbooks, useful to both students and physicians. Concise, well written, includes tables, diagrams and question-answer series helpful in commonly encountered diseases of ophthalmology.
R: *American Journal of Ophthalmology* 81: 114 (Jan. 1976).

Parsons' Diseases of the Eye. 16th ed. **S. J. H. Miller.** London: Churchill Livingstone, 1978.

Fourteenth edition, 1964; fifteenth edition, 1970.
Eight sections devoted to common eye diseases; includes some rare conditions. Well-illustrated. Useful tool for students, general practitioners, and surgeons.
R: *ARBA* (1971, p. 531).

ORTHOPEDICS

Anatomic Guide for the Electromyographer: The Limbs. **E. F. Delagi et al., eds.** Springfield, IL: Charles C. Thomas, 1975.

This guide diagrams 100 muscles of the upper and lower limbs and illustrates the site for electromyographical studies. The diagrams clearly show anatomic landmarks and place of electrode insertion. Text is brief. Valuable guide for electrodiagnosis and clinical electromyographers.
R: *Archives of Physical Medicine and Rehabilitation* 57: 492 (Oct. 1976); *Brain* 99: 168 (Mar. 1976); *Rheumatology and Rehabilitation* xv: 56 (Feb. 1976).

Orthopaedic Neurology: A Diagnostic Guide to Neurologic Levels. **Stanley Hoppenfeld.** Philadelphia, PA: J. B. Lippincott, 1977.

A ready reference source on the anatomy of the peripheral central nervous system (spinal cord). The strength of this guide is the clear illustrations which help visualize neurological structures. Also includes neurological testing procedures essential to examinations. A valuable book for neurologists at all levels of training.
R: *Annals of Internal Medicine* 88: 274 (Feb. 1978); *Archives of Physical Medicine and Rehabilitation* 59: 297 (June 1978); *Journal of Neurosurgery* 48: 1048 (June 1978).

Plaster Casting. **Philip I. Salib.** New York: Appleton-Century-Crofts, 1975.

Guidebook on the technique of plaster casting. Begins with introductory material on the history of plaster of paris and routine application techniques. Proceeds to discuss more complicated applications (spicas, patella tendon bearing casts, etc.). Includes excellent chapter on the application of cast braces. Fills a void in the literature for orthopedic technicians and residents. Handy reference source for specialists using plaster.
R: *Archives of Physical Medicine and Rehabilitation* 57: 303 (June 1976); *Journal of Bone and Joint Surgery* 57A: 286 (1975).

Standard Orthopaedic Operations: A Guide for the Junior Surgeon. **John C. Adams.** New York: Churchill Livingstone, 1976.

A personal guide to the technical aspects of orthopedic surgery. Reflects the author's personal procedures. Includes information on proper positioning, selection of surgical instruments, and correct application of bandages. Also reviews postoperative management. Almost 267 drawings enhance the text. Strongly recommended for orthopedists in training, junior hospital doctors, and general surgeons. No surgical library or orthopedic department should be without this volume.

R: *Journal of Bone and Joint Surgery* 58B: 393 (Aug. 1976); *NEJM* 295: 965 (Oct. 21, 1976).

OTORHINOLARYNGOLOGY

Ear, Nose and Throat Disorders: A Practitioner's Guide. **John R. Ausband.** Garden City, NY: Medical Examination Publishing, 1974.

PATHOLOGY

Mediocolegal Investigation of Death: Guidelines for the Application of Pathology to Crime Investigation. **Werner U. Spitz and Russell S. Fisher.** Springfield, IL: Charles C. Thomas, 1973.

Second printing, 1977.
An up-to-date guide of forensic pathology. Establishes procedures that can be directly applied to criminal investigation. Contains useful illustrations and diagrams and can be drawn upon as either a ready reference or textbook. Recommended to pathologists and criminal investigators.
R: *Archives of Pathology & Laboratory Medicine* 97: 190 (Mar. 1974).

PEDIATRICS

Baby and Child Care. 4th ed. **Benjamin Spock.** New York: Hawthorn Books, 1976.

The revised edition of this classic book attempts to eliminate prevailing biases against women and girls. It places a greater emphasis on the role of the father and presents reflections on changing patterns of the family. This will be a useful guide to prospective and young parents.
R: *ARBA* (1977, p. 722).

Management of High-Risk Pregnancy and Intensive Care of the Neonate. 3d ed. **S. Gorham Babson et al.** St. Louis, MO: C. V. Mosby, 1975.

A comprehensive and practical guide to care of the newborn. Deals with complications of pregnancy, fetal heart rate, nutritional standards, among other pertinent topics. Succinctly written, meeting its intended purpose clearly and practically.
R: *American Journal of Diseases of Children* 130: 1039 (Sept. 1976).

The Newborn: A Practical Guide. **J. B. J. McKendry and J. D. Bailey.** Don Mills, Ontario, Canada: Longman Canada Limited, 1977.

A thorough review of neonate medicine; discusses management, feeding, respiratory distress, jaundice, etc., of the newborn. Well indexed, up-to-date. Helpful to physicians who work with the newborn.
R: *Canadian Medical Association Journal* 119: 428 (Sept. 9, 1978).

A Practical Approach to Pediatric Endocrinology. **George E. Bacon, Martha L. Spencer and Robert P. Kelch.** Chicago, IL: Year Book Medical Publishers, 1975.

A handy paperback guide for practicing pediatricians, house officers, and medical students.

R: *Clinical Pediatrics* 16: 451 (May 1977).

Pregnancy, Birth and the Newborn Baby: A Complete Guide for Parents and Parents-To-Be. **The Children's Hospital Medical Center.** Boston, MA: Delacorte Press, 1971.

A guide for parents. This comprehensive book deals with the implications of parenting. Written by experts in the field. The book is of high quality and offers much practical advice. Considered valuable for parent education.
R: *Clinical Pediatrics* 12: 11A (Dec. 1973).

Taking Care of Your Children—A Parents' Guide to Medical Care. **R. H. Pantell, J. F. Fries, and D. M. Vickery.** Reading, MA: Addison-Wesley, 1977.

A concise, well-organized, self-help manual for medical consumers. Discusses problems central to children and young adults. Emphasizes preventive aspects of medicine, offers advice on common complaints, and provides growth charts. Written by three physicians, this succinct book should be useful to parents with children through the age of adolescence.
R: *Journal of School Health* 49: 50 (Jan. 1979).

Visible and Palpable Lesions in Children. **C. Everett Koop.** New York: Grune & Stratton, 1976.

Highlights valuable knowledge on visible and palpable lesions of children. Useful for pediatricians required to explain to and advise parents. Also serves as a helpful guide for deciding when to refer a patient to the pediatric surgeon and explaining expected results. Some minor typographical errors; guide enhanced with black-and-white illustrations. Valuable to all pediatricians.
R: *American Journal of Diseases of Children* 132: 641 (June 1978).

PHARMACY AND PHARMACOLOGY

A Chemist's Guide to Regulatory Drug Analysis. **Daniel Banes.** Washington, DC: Association of Official Analytical Chemists, 1974.

The guide has three parts: a guide to drug control laws and regulations, a guide to literature resources, and a guide to the structure of regulatory drug-analytical methods.
R: ARBA (1975, p. 651); Chen (p. 189).

Clinical Guide to Undesirable Drug Ineractions. **Solomon Garb.** New York: Springer Publishing, 1971.

A guide to the interactions of drugs, with entries arranged alphabetically. Provides drug names, code numbers of interactions, and appropriate reference source also by code, so that information is easily cross-referenced. For physicians and pharmacists, a useful tool.
R: *ARBA* (1972, p. 630); *MRW* S2, pp. 34, 35, 36.

Drug Effects in Hospitalized Patients. **R. R. Miller and D. L. Greenblatt.** New York: John Wiley, 1976.

Drug Information for Patients. **H. Winter Griffith.** Philadelphia, PA: W. B. Saunders, 1978.

Written for medical doctors, helpful in assisting physicians to guide their patients taking therapeutic drugs. Provides general instructions, precautions, possible side-effects, storage, dosage, refill information. Well organized by trade and generic name. Contains much helpful information.

The Essential Guide to Prescription Drugs: What You Need to Know For Safe Drug Use. **James W. Long.** New York: Harper & Row, 1977.

All drug information listed under generic drug names. Includes dosage, side effects, adverse reactions, etc. Useful cross-index from some 1,500 brand names to generic names. Emphasis on commonly used drugs.
R: Sheehy (EK38).

The Family Prescription and Medication Guide. **Albert Pawlina.** Englewood Cliffs, NJ: Prentice-Hall, 1979.

Consumer guide to common, frequently prescribed medications. Dictionary format outlines uses, side effects, and cautions. Basically arranged in four sections: general information, alphabetical encyclopedia of drugs, pharmaceutical definitions, and extensive lists and tables. Also includes information on administration of drops, ointments, and lotions, basic first aid, required immunizations for travelers, and similar handy data. Applicable to community nursing, clinical pharmacy, and medical nutrition programs.

Guidelines for the Preparation of Radiopharmaceuticals in Hospitals. **British Institute of Radiology.** London: British Institute of Radiology, 1975.

Focuses on practical solutions regarding laboratory facilities, work schedules, and quality control. Includes legal information on the Medicine Act, the Radioactive Substances Act, and the Code of Practice. Particularly useful to those who prepare radiopharmaceuticals and those involved with work organization.
R: *Physics in Medicine & Biology* 21: 457 (May 1976).

A Guide to Drug Eruptions. **W. Bruinsma.** Amsterdam: Excerpta Medica, 1973.

A concise listing of drugs that cause cutaneous eruptions, arranged by reaction of skin (i.e. acne, lupus, pigmentary lesions, etc.); also cross-references from drug to reactions. Includes close to 200 references from the literature. A brief, ready reference.
R: *Archives of Dermatology* 108: 442 (Sept. 1973); 111: 1223 (Sept. 1975); *Journal of Pharmaceutical Sciences* 62: 1909 (Nov. 1973); *JAMA* 232: 545 (May 5, 1975); *Lancet* 1: 752 (Apr. 17, 1973).

A Guide to Drug Interactions. **John D. James et al.** New York: McGraw-Hill, 1978.

A computer-derived file of 3,000 generic drugs and their interactions. Includes bibliographic references; provides product and brand names and serves as a quick, ready reference for doctors, nurses, and pharmacists.

Medication Guide For Patient Counseling. **Dorothy L. Smith.** Philadelphia, PA: Lea & Febiger, 1977.

Provides a succinct set of patient-oriented medication instructions. Reviews individual instructions associated with frequently prescribed drugs. Intended as a patient-educational tool for health professionals involved in prescribing, dispensing, and administering of drugs.

150 Commonly Prescribed Durgs. A Guide to Their Uses and Side Effects. Chicago, IL: World Book, 1979.

Lists brand names, generic names, and manufacturers. Describes conditions requiring drug treatment, precautions, possible side effects and drug interactions. Features a chart arranged by drug type and a complete index. Intended for the lay person.

Pharmacy Law and Ethics. **J. R. Dale and G. E. Appelbe.** London: Pharmaceutical Press, 1976.

Outlines laws and statutes governing the pharmaceutical industry. Also lists professional obligations of registered pharmacists. Covers the sale of new remedies and medicines. Emphasizes British law.
R: *ABL* 41: entry 489 (Dec. 1976).

PharmIndex. Portland, OR: Skyline Publishers, 1959–. Semimonthly.

Strategy of Drug Design: A Molecular Guide to Biological Activity. **W. P. Purcell, G. E. Bass, and J. M. Clayton.** New York: John Wiley, 1973.

Describes mathematical models of drug design. Correlates biological activities, presents step-by-step approach, and explains various molecular and metabolic changes. A useful reference on drug structure-activity relationships.
R: *Journal of Pharmaceutical Sciences* 64: 715 (Apr. 1975).

Unlisted Drugs. Vols. 1–. Chatham, NJ: Pharmaco-Medical Documentation, 1949–. Monthly.

Index/Guide II. Chatham, NJ, 1980.
Each monthly issue contains descriptions of 180 to 200 new drugs which are not yet recorded in standard sources. Describes new experimental research compounds and commercial products as they are reported in the journal literature. Entries include composition and chemical structure. Name and number indexes are published annually.
R: Win (EK209).

PHYSICAL MEDICINE AND REHABILITATION

Aids for the Severely Handicapped. **Keith Copeland, ed.** New York: Grune & Stratton, 1974.

A guide for those who work with the severely handicapped; presents informative, practical advice concerning the use of aids. Contains three appendixes which have helpful directories and references.

International Guide to Aids and Appliances for Blind and Visually Impaired

Persons. 2d rev. ed. **American Foundation for the Blind.** New York: American Foundation for the Blind, 1977.

First edition, *International Catalog, Aids and Appliances for Blind and Visually Impaired Persons,* 1973.
Standard reference source in the area of blindness and visual impairment. Title of new edition changed to reflect its nature as a "guide." Comprehensive and up-to-date coverage of some 1,500 devices offered by 270 distributors in 28 countries. Primarily a subject arrangement by aids and appliances, followed by an alphabetical geographic section. Entries include distributor's address, model number, price, and a succinct description of the device. Includes two indexes: devices and International Catalog number (IC). Recommended to visually handicapped people, vision professionals, and all libraries.
R: *American Journal of Nursing* 74: 757 (Apr. 1974); *American Journal of Ophthalmology* 76: 1030 (Dec. 1973); *ARBA* (1975, p. 743; 1978, p. 715); *MRW* S3, p. 48.

Physical Therapy Procedures: Selected Techniques. 2d ed. **Ann H. Downer.** Springfield, IL: Charles C. Thomas, 1974.

An instructive teaching and reference manual; discusses treatment procedures in physical therapy. Emphasizes communication between therapist and patient. A well written, timely book.
R: *Archives of Physical Medicine and Rehabilitation* 56: 48 (Jan. 1975).

Rehabilitation Services in Hospitals and Related Facilities: A Guide to Planning, Organization, and Management. **American Hospital Association.** Chicago, IL: American Hospital Association, 1966.

A practical guide to organization and planning in hospitals.

Upper Extremities Orthotics. 3d printing. **Miles H. Anderson, ed.** Springfield, IL: Charles C. Thomas, 1974.

A revision of the 1958 classic. An excellent guide to a field which lacks comprehensive literature. Of working value to physical therapists.
R: *Physical Therapy* 55: 1385 (Dec. 1975).

PSYCHIATRY AND PSYCHOLOGY

Clinical Guide to Behavior Therapy. **Susan R. Walen, Norma M. Hauserman, and Paul J. Lavin.** New York: Oxford University Press, 1977.

Covers the applications of behavioral technology. Describes numerous behavioral problems and treatments. Contains numerous references, charts, tables, and figures.

A Guide For Beginning Psychotherapists. **Joan St. al Zaro et al.** New York: Cambridge University Press, 1977.

For students and beginning therapists. Offers advice on interviewing, record keeping, treatment of common psychological problems.

Guide for Mental Health Workers. **A. R. Favazzo et al.** Ann Arbor, MI: University of Michigan, 1970.

A guide for the beginning mental health worker; briefly outlines concepts of

mental disease and its treatment. Does not cover specialized material but is excellent for the novice.
R: *ARBA* (1971, p. 535).

A Guide to Alcohol and Drug Dependence. **J. S. Madden.** Bristol, England: John Wright, 1979.
Summarizes some 50 significant research reports on alcoholism and drug dependence. Introductory matter outlines pertinent definitions, incidences, and causes. Section on alcoholism stresses dependence factors, social aspects, and physical and psychological manifestations. Chapters on drug dependence explore the opioids, general sedatives, stimulants, and treatments for drug abuse. Clearly a useful reference tool, prepared for all areas of medical practice today.
R: *BMJ* 1: 1205 (May 5, 1979); *Lancet* 1: 704 (Mar. 31, 1979).

The Harvard Guide to Modern Psychiatry. **Armand M. Nicholi, Jr., ed.** Cambridge, MA: Harvard University Press, 1978.
Synthesizes biological, sociological, and psychological aspects of mental disorder as a result of collaboration by some of world's foremost clinicians and investigators. Scientific in approach, this report of major research developments focuses on the patient as a person, not an object of research. Basic text for medical students, psychiatric nurses and residents, and social workers.
R: *American Journal of Psychiatry* 135: 512 (Apr. 1978); *Annals of Internal Medicine* 89: 433 (Sept. 1978); *Canadian Medical Association Journal* 120: 133 (Jan. 20, 1979); *Inquiry* 15: 202 (June 1978); *Journal of Nervous and Mental Disease* 167: 453 (July 1979); *Lancet* 1: 908 (Apr. 28, 1979).

Help For Your Child: A Parent's Guide to Mental Health Services. **Sharon S. Brehm.** Englewood Cliffs, NJ: Prentice-Hall, 1978.
A guide to mental health facilities for children, covering ages from birth through adolescence. Advises parents as to extent of problems and explains what different facilities have to offer. Maintains a step-by-step, helpful approach.

The Hospitalized Adolescent: A Guide to Managing the Ill and Injured Youth. **Adele Hofmann, R. D. Becler, and H. Paul Gabriel.** New York: Spectrum Publications, 1976.
Deals mainly with the psychosocial attitudes of ill and injured adolescents and the organizational processes of an inpatient unit. Good descriptions of the value of milieu therapy and the legalities involving the mature minor. A useful and successful handbook for the physician who feels unsure when delivering health care to adolescents without parental consent.
R: *Annals of Internal Medicine* 87: 130 (July 1977); *Clinical Pediatrics* 17: 899 (Dec. 1978).

The Maltreated Child: The Maltreatment Syndrome in Children—A Medical, Legal and Social Guide. 3d ed. **Vincent J. Fontana and Douglas J. Besharov.** Springfield, IL: Charles C. Thomas, 1977.
Revised and updated, an indispensable guide to the treatment of the abused and neglected child. Concisely presents nature of neglect, role of the law, statistical

outline of child abuse. Recommended to social workers, medical students, and lawyers as an outstanding, timely source of information.

Mental Handicap: A Brief Guide. **Brian Kirman.** London: Crosby Lockwood Staples, 1975.

A succinct guide to major elements concerning the care of the mentally handicapped. Contains helpful references and a directory as well as information on legal statutes. Highly recommended to teachers, social workers, nurses, therapists.
R: *BMJ* 2: 398 (May 17, 1975); *Lancet* 1: 311 (Feb. 8, 1975).

The MMPI: A Practical Guide. **John R. Graham.** New York: Oxford University Press, 1977.

This is a thorough guide containing information on the Minnesota Multiphasic Personality Inventory. Includes information on how to interpret data and the founding of the basic structure of the MMPI. Very helpful, primarily for psychologists.

Practical Psychiatry for the Primary Physician. **James R. Hodge.** Chicago, IL: Nelson-Hall, 1975.

A concise outline of psychiatry in family practice. Discusses attitudes toward psychiatric diseases. Includes simple explanation of symptoms, nature, diagnosis, and treatment. Definitely a "how-to-do-it" reference source for the practicing family physician and medical student who do not specialize in psychiatry. All psychiatric personnel (social workers, nurses, and residents) will also benefit from this practical guide.
R: *American Family Physician* 12: 147 (Dec. 1975).

Psychiatry and the Criminal: A Guide to Psychiatric Examinations for the Criminal Courts. 3d ed. **John M. Macdonald.** Springfield, IL: Charles C. Thomas, 1976.

Emphasizes forensic psychiatry. New material on homicide, assault, robbery, burglary, kidnapping, and tests of competency to stand trial. Written primarily for psychiatrists and psychologists with little knowledge of forensic psychiatry or experience with criminal offenders.

Psychotropic Drugs: A Guide for the Practitioner. **H. M. Van Praag.** New York: Brunner/Mazel, 1978.

Comprehensively deals with psychotropic drugs. Classifies behavior and related drugs.
R: *American Journal of Psychiatry* 136: 470 (Apr. 1979); *Journal of Psychiatric Nursing and Mental Health Services* 17: 42 (May 1979).

A Selective Guide to Materials For Mental Health and Family Life Education. 3d ed. **Mental Health Materials Center, comp.** Detroit, MI: Gale Research, 1976.

Second edition, 1972.
Describes educational materials including books, films, pamphlets, and hand-

books. Materials included reflect current trends in mental health education. Well arranged, easy to read.
R: *BL* 69: 870 (1973).

Understanding Piaget. **R. Droz and M. Rahmy. Joyce Diamanti, trans.** New York: International Universities Press, 1976.

A practical summary of Piaget's theory. Designed to familiarize the reader with Piagetian thought by providing guidelines for selecting appropriate readings for a particular interest. Provides a basic introduction to major themes, ideas, terminology, and vital cross-references to original French work and/or translations in English. Includes an annotated bibliography of Piaget and his critics. Recommended to the beginning and advanced student of Piaget.
R: *American Journal of Psychiatry* 134: 100 (Jan. 1977); *Journal of Nervous and Mental Disease* 165: 144 (1977).

PUBLIC HEALTH

Community, Culture, and Care: A Cross-Culture Guide for Health Workers. **Ann T. Brownlee.** St. Louis, MO: C. V. Mosby, 1978.

A guide for cross-cultural communication relevant to health care workers. In three parts: community sociology, education, and family. Among groups examined are Black, Native American, Chicano, and Chinese American. Includes bibliography and appendix.

Drug Abuse: A Guide for the Clinician. **Joseph D. Sapira and Charles E. Cherubin.** New York: American Elsevier, 1975.

An encyclopedic review of drug abuse and its complications. An excellent reference on the somatic complications of drug abuse.
R: *Lancet* 1: 1056 (May 15, 1976).

Dying and Death: A Clinical Guide for the Caregiver. **David Barton, ed.** Baltimore, MD: Williams & Wilkins, 1977.

Compassionate study of the emotional struggles of the dying. Contributors include two dying patients, a nurse, a clergyman, an ethicist, and a geriatric specialist.

Environmental and Industrial Health Hazards. **R. A. Trevethick.** London: Heinemann, 1973.

A high-quality presentation of data concerning hazards of toxic substances; hazards are listed in alphabetical order and are cross-referenced to synonyms. A succinct guide, giving hazard threshold-limit values of the Factories Act and Regulations. Useful for factory managers, physicians, and nurses.
R: *Lancet* 2: 242 (Aug. 4, 1973).

A Guide to Radiation Protection. **J. Craig Robertson.** London: Macmillan, 1976.

A sequential guide to radiation protection, written in nontechnical terms and based on courses for firemen, policemen. Summarizes principal points. British

orientation. A basic guide for training in radiation protection.
R: *Physics in Medicine & Biology* 22: 783 (July 1977).

Guide to Simple Sanitary Measures for the Control of Enteric Diseases. **S. Rajagopalan and M. A. Shiffman.** Geneva: World Health Organization, 1974.

Details methods of sanitizing urban and rural water supplies such as use of hypochlorate, chlorine, sewage treatments, as they relate to enteric disease control. Also discusses food hygiene programs, course training programs for disease prevention.
R: *IBID* 3: 186 (Sept. 1975).

Occupational Diseases: A Guide to Their Recognition, DHEW Pub. no. (NIOSH) 77-181. Rev. ed. **Marcus M. Key et al., eds.** Washington, DC: US Department of Health, Education, and Welfare, National Institute for Occupational Safety and Health, 1978.

Completely revised edition due to the impact of OSHA. Concentrates on epidemiologic, toxicologic, and clinical data relating to occupational diseases. Divided into three major sections of hazard: biological, chemical, and physical. Geared toward occupational professionals interested in health.
R: *American Journal of Public Health* 68: 417 (Apr. 1978).

Occupational Diseases: A Syllabus of Signs and Symptoms. **E. R. Plunkett.** Stamford, CT: Barrett Book, 1977.

A concise review of symptoms related to occupational diseases. Designed as a quick reference for the occupational physician. Symptoms presented alphabetically. Also has list of toxins and a glossary.
R: *Occupational Health Nursing* 26: 44 (Apr. 1976).

Occupational Safety and Health: A Guide to Information Sources. **Theodore P. Peck, ed.** Detroit, MI: Gale Research, 1974.

Guide to occupational safety and health information sources. Explores federal and state agencies, training opportunities, media resources, legislation, research institutions, and safety equipment suppliers. Indexed.
R: *Choice* 12: 50 (Mar. 1975); *RSR* 2: 35 (Oct.–Dec. 1974); 2: 129 (Oct.–Dec. 1974); 3: 91 (Apr.–June 1975).

Official Methods of Analysis. 12th ed. **William Horwitz, ed.** Washington, DC: Association of Official Analytical Chemists, 1975.

Classic reference work contains analytical methods for a wide variety of items, including agricultural materials, foods, beverages, and cosmetics with potential for affecting public health. Methods are tested in collaborative studies throughout the world. Volume uses new indexing system by section number.
R: *Journal of the American Dietetic Association* 66: 552 (May 1975).

Patty's Industrial Hygiene and Toxicology. 3d ed. **G. D. Clayton and F. E. Clayton, eds.** New York: John Wiley, 1978.

First edition, 1958.

Volume 1, *General Principles.*
The classic reference on industrial hygiene, in three volumes. Scope of material is vast and includes new developments and legislation as well as historical background. Volumes are 1) *General Principles,* 2) *Toxicology,* 3) *Theory and Rationale of Industrial Hygiene Practice.*
R: *Nature* 274: 724 (Aug. 17, 1978).

A Primer on Chemical Dependency: A Clinical Guide to Alcohol and Drug Problems. **Joseph Westermeyer.** Baltimore, MD: Williams & Wilkins, 1976.
Concentrates on chemical dependency problems and their recognition. Intended for the busy practitioner with little or no knowledge of these serious situations.

Respiratory Protection—OSHA and the Small Businessman. **Walter E. Ruch and Bruce J. Held.** Ann Arbor, MI: Ann Arbor Science Publishers, 1975.
A guide to the organization and management of a respiratory protection program. Closely follows OSHA requirements. Defines respiratory hazards. Evaluates potential dangers and illustrates sampling devices and their proper use. Geared toward industrial situations.
R: *Occupational Health Nursing* 23: 44 (Aug. 1975).

RADIOLOGY

Alphabetical Index of Roentgen Diagnoses and Procedures, with Code Numbers of the American College of Radiology. **Gerhart S. Schwarz and Henry J. Powsner.** Springfield, IL: Charles C. Thomas, 1966.
Alphabetically cross-indexed for a variety of filing systems.
R: *MRW* S1, p. 28.

A Guide for Automatic Radiographic Processing and Film Quality Control. **Cynthia C. Kirby, William E. J. McKinney, and Thomas T. Thompson.** Chicago, IL: American Society of Radiologic Technologists, 1975.
This book is accompanied by sixteen video tapes which together offer a thorough explanation of automatic processing in radiography. Designed to be used as a teaching aid, this book is recommended for inclusion in radiological technology programs.
R: *American Journal of Roentgenology* 131: 1128 (Dec. 1978).

Illustrated Guide to X-Ray Technics. **John E. Cullinan.** Philadelphia, PA: J. B. Lippincott, 1972.
An informative book of radiation techniques. Explains practical use of equipment covering a wide range of procedures. Contains excellent illustrations and drawings.

Mammography: Technique, Diagnosis, Differential Diagnosis. **Walther Hoeffken and Marton Lanyi.** Philadelphia, PA: W. B. Saunders, 1977.
An English translation of a comprehensive German guide to mammography. Contains information on differential diagnosis, interpretation of mammograms. Illustrations are excellent as is the presentation of breast anatomy. Employs ter-

minology used in the United States; recommended as a knowledgeable source.
R: *JAMA* 238: 1767 (Oct. 17, 1977); *Radiology* 126: 372 (1978).

Radiation Protection: A Guide for Scientists and Physicians. **Jacob Shapiro.** Cambridge, MA: Harvard University Press, 1972.

Written for the radiation user in the field of medicine who requires some knowledge of radiation protection. The initial two-thirds of the volume deal with protection principles, radiation dose calculations and measurements. The final sections present practical information on the use of radionuclides and the formulation of radiation protection standards. Definite bias toward U.S. regulations based on NCRP publications. Includes elementary numerical examples.
R: *Health Physics* 27: 235 (Aug. 1974); *Physics in Medicine & Biology* 19: 268 (Mar. 1974).

Radiology of Syndromes. **Hooshang Taybi.** Chicago, IL: Year Book Medical Publishers, 1975.

An alphabetical compilation of 541 syndromes. Lists synonyms, modes of inheritance, and clinical and radiological manifestations. Text enhanced by numerous radiological reproductions. References to additional readings follow each syndrome. Most unique and indispensable feature is the gamut index. Allows for quick correlation between syndromes and specific diagnosis. Index divided into 15 anatomic systems. Handy guide to recognition and classification of syndromes for the pediatric radiologist and primary physician.
R: *American Journal of Roentgenology* 125: 272 (Sept. 1975); *Clinical Pediatrics* 15: 353 (Apr. 1976).

Technologist Guide to Mammography. 2d ed. **Robert L. Egan.** Baltimore, MD: Williams & Wilkins, 1977

First edition, 1968.
Revision of the 1968 edition. Essentially a guide to "the Egan technique" of film mammography. Topics include a history of mammography, a description of equipment, positioning of patients, and mammographic changes due to breast diseases. New chapter devoted to breast self-examination and the role of the technologist. A short questionnaire follows each chapter. Includes glossary and index.
R: *American Journal of Roentgenology* 131: 191 (July 1978).

RESPIRATORY SYSTEM

Applied Physiology of Respiratory Care. **John Hedley-Whyte et al.** Boston, MA: Little, Brown, 1976.

A guide for personnel who treat critically ill patients. Divided into six parts: management of respiratory failure, consequences of surgical problems, respiratory trauma, management of organ failure, physiology, and practical management problems. A high-quality guide with helpful illustrations, graphs, and bibliography.
R: *Anaesthesia* 32: 295 (Mar. 1977); *NEJM* 296: 122 (1977).

Chest Injuries: A Guide for the Accident Department. **G. Keen.** Bristol, England: John Wright, 1975.

A comprehensive guide to the management of chest injuries. Succinctly explains diagnostic procedures, resuscitative surgical techniques, and management fundamentals. Includes helpful case studies and selected references. A ready reference for anesthesiologists and surgeons.
R: *Anaesthesia* 31: 310 (Mar. 1976); *Chest* 70: 30 (1976).

Guide to Pulmonary Medicine. **Donald P. Tashkin and Stanley M. Cassan, ed.** New York: Grune & Stratton, 1978.

A concise guide to advances made in pulmonary medicine in the past ten years. Among topics included are chronic obstructive disease, neoplasms, sarcoidosis, environmental disease, respiratory failure.

RHEUMATOLOGY

Arthritis: A Comprehensive Guide. **James F. Fries.** Reading, MA: Addison-Wesley, 1979.

In three parts: part 1 describes in nontechnical terms symptoms of different types of arthritis; part 2 discusses management and prevention; part 3 deals with day-to-day problems of arthritis patients; lists additional reading. Intended for the arthritis patient. An informative, understandable work.
R: *LJ* 104: 1473 (July 1979).

Arthritis and Allied Conditions: A Textbook of Rheumatology. 9th ed. **Daniel J. McCarty, Jr., ed.** Philadelphia, PA: Lea & Febiger, 1979.

Eighth edition, 1972.
A guide to the diagnosis and treatment of arthritis; contains helpful illustrations.
R: *JAMA* 224: 133 (Apr. 2, 1973); *TBRI* 39: 241 (June 1973); Allyn; Stearns & Ratcliff (*NEJM*, 1969; *NEJM*, 1970).

Understanding Arthritis and Rheumatism: A Complete Guide to the Problems and Treatment. **I. V. Malcolm, M. D. Jayson, and Allan S. J. Dixon.** New York: Pantheon Books, 1975.

Written to provide patient with an understanding of his illness so that he can cooperate with his physician in his treatment program. Twelve chapters provide review of rheumatism in a very readable style. Illustrations are expertly done and a resource directory lists information to assist reader in finding help through agencies. For the general public.
R: *Arthritis and Rheumatism* 19: 271 (Mar.–Apr. 1976).

UROGENITAL SYSTEM

Ambulatory Obstetrics: A Clinical Guide. **R. S. Gibbs and C. E. Gibbs.** New York: Wiley Medical, 1979.

Essential reference information contained in numerous flow sheets, tables, and charts. Working handbook for family physicians, certified nurse midwives, nurse practitioners, and students.

Everywoman, A Gynecological Guide For Life. 2d ed. **D. Llewellyn-Jones.** Boston, MA: Faber & Faber, 1978.

A comprehensive reference text for the general public, includes information on obstetrics, gynecology, male and female anatomy and physiology, and psychology. Offers frank information, presented in a clear yet sophisticated style. Contains pen and ink drawings. Helpful in keeping patients informed.
R: *JAMWA* 34: 48 (Jan. 1979).

Female Sterilization: Guidelines for the Development of Services, WHO Offset Publications, 26. **World Health Organization.** Geneva: World Health Organization, 1976.
Up-to-date techniques on female sterilization. Discusses advantages and disadvantages, equipment, and training needs.
R: *IBID* 4: 239 (Sept. 1976).

The I. U. D.: A Practical Guide. **Robert Snowden, Margaret Williams, and Denis Hawkins,** London: Croom Helm, 1977.
Comprehensive collection of data analysis concerning the use of the IUD. A helpful guide for doctors involved in family planning.
R: *Lancet* 1: 130 (Jan. 21, 1978).

Kidney Biopsy Interpretation. **Edwin H. Jenis and David T. Lowenthal.** Netherlands: European Bookservice, 1977.
A guide to interpretation and classification of kidney biopsy. Discusses light, immunofluorescent, and electron microscope findings. A concise ready source.
R: *British Journal of Surgery* 64: 904 (Dec. 1977).

Managing Contraceptive Pill Patients. **Richard P. Dickey.** Aspen, CO: Creative Informatics, 1977.
In four sections. A guide to the management of oral contraceptive side effects. Discusses composition, potency, identification, and prescription of oral contraceptives. Contains tables and an index.
R: *Nation's Health* 9: 13 (Feb. 1979).

The Menopause: A Guide to Current Research and Practice. **Robert J. Beard, ed.** Lancaster, England: Medical and Technical Publishing, 1976.
A recent guide recommended to gynecologists. This book is considered to be an authoritative guide to menopause.
R: *British Journal of Obstetrics & Gynaecology* 84: 397 (May 1977); *BMJ* 6055: 240 (Jan. 22, 1977); *TBRI* 43: 142 (Apr. 1977).

My Body, My Health: The Concerned Woman's Guide to Gynecology. **Felicia H. Stewart et al.** New York: Wiley Medical, 1979.
R: *LJ* 104: 1348 (June 15, 1979).

The Teaching of Human Sexuality in Schools for Health Professionals, WHO Public Health Papers, no. 57. **D. R. Mace, R. H. O. Bannerman, and J. Burton, eds.** Geneva: World Health Organization, 1974.

VETERINARY MEDICINE

Biological Research Method: A Practical Guide. 2d ed. **H. H. Holman.** New York: Hafner, 1969.

Intended for use by researchers who work with animals. Includes sections on data collections, statistical methods, preparation of scientific papers, etc.
R: Chen (p. 190); Mal (9-25, 9-176); Wal (p. 196).

Practical Guide to Medicine and Veterinary Mycology. **R. Vanbreuseghem.** New York: Masson, 1978.

Pictorial guide to the identification of tropical mycoses particularly prevalent in veterinary medicine.

Veterinarians' Product and Therapeutic Reference. 4th ed. Caldwell, NJ: Therapeutic Communications, 1979. Annual.

First edition, 1972.
Covers virtually all veterinary pharmaceutical and biological product information. Also contains a comprehensive listing of manufacturers and distributors. Ideal reference for veterinarians and hospital, medical, and pharmacy libraries.

CHAPTER 10 ATLASES

ANATOMY

Anatomical Correlates of Clinical Electromyography. **J. Goodgold.** Baltimore, MD: Williams & Wilkins, 1974.

Reference handbook of gross anatomy which illustrates sites which electromyographer must stimulate. Text is photographic atlas with clear pictures and brief but accurate text. Valuable addition to EMG laboratory and for electromyographers.
R: *Electroencephalography & Clinical Neurophysiology* 39: 223 (Aug. 1975).

Anatomy: A Regional Atlas of the Human Body. **Carmine D. Clemente.** Philadelphia, PA: Lea & Febiger, 1975.

Based on Sobotta's *Atlas of Anatomy*. A compilation of the best and most useful plates in one volume. Includes many original Sobotta illustrations and also some new, high-quality pictures. Arrangement by region rather than system. All terminology listed in English and follows that found in *Gray's Anatomy,* 29th ed. Features a comprehensive index. Useful tool for students.
R: *Physical Therapy* 55: 1386 (1975).

Atlas and Dissection Guide for Comparative Anatomy. 3d ed. **Saul Wischnitzer.** San Francisco, CA: W. H. Freeman, 1978.

Second edition, 1972.
Expanded edition; covers anatomy of protochordates, lamprey, dogfish shark, mud puppy, and cat. Systematically presented, three-dimensional drawings. Includes glossary and references. For the undergraduate library.

An Atlas of Anatomy Basic to Radiology. **Isadore Meschan.** Philadelphia, PA: W. B. Saunders, 1975.

An encyclopedic atlas which covers anatomy basic to radiologic interpretation. Textual material is accompanied by close to 1,000 illustrations, both of which precisely describe the full spectrum of anatomic structures. Cross-references and helpful indexes make information retrieval easy. A classic atlas recommended to medical students, radiologists, and medical libraries.
R: *JAMA* 235: 2436 (May 31, 1976); *NEJM* 294: 792 (Apr. 1, 1976); *Radiology* 121: 348 (Nov. 1976); *RSR* 4: 106 (July–Sept. 1976).

Atlas of Anatomy of the Hand. **Johan M. F. Landsmeer.** New York: Churchill Livingstone, 1976.

Illustrates comprehensively the anatomy of the hand through the use of drawings and photographs. Discusses microdissection, functional anatomy. Both text and illustrations are of excellent quality. Recommended to orthopedists and surgeons.
R: *Archives of Surgery* 111: 1043 (Sept. 1976); *Journal of Bone and Joint Surgery* 58A: 1182 (Dec. 1976); *NEJM* 295: 1020 (Oct. 28, 1976); *Plastic and Reconstructive Surgery* 61: 900 (1978).

Atlas of Brain Anatomy for EMI Scans. **Fred C. Shipps et al.** Springfield, IL: Charles C. Thomas, 1975.

A brief atlas of computerized brain scans containing ten brain sections. All major structures are labeled; helpful charts are included. Valuable as a ready reference for beginning EMI interpretation.
R: *Brain* 99: 167 (Mar. 1976); *Electroencephalography & Clinical Neurophysiology* 40: 671 (June 1976); *Journal of Neurosurgery* 44: 399 (Mar. 1976); *Radiology* 118: 96 (1976).

Atlas of Clinical Anatomy. **Richard S. Snell.** Boston, MA: Little, Brown, 1978.

A sequential presentation of anatomy with over 300 color illustrations organized by region of the body. Provides the student with clear, detailed instructions. Illustrations are accompanied by clinical information, enabling the atlas to be used as a ready reference source.
R: *Lancet* 2: 505 (Sept. 2, 1978); *Plastic and Reconstructive Surgery* 63: 561 (1979).

An Atlas of Cross-Sectional Anatomy. **Stephen A. Kieffer and E. Robert Heitzman, eds.** New York: Harper & Row, 1978.

Correlates computed tomographic images with ultrasound images, utilizing full color plates and systematic presentations of anatomy. Clearly identifies important structures on anatomical, radiographical, ultrasound, and computed tomographical levels.

Atlas of Human Anatomy. 3 vols. **Frank H. J. Figge and Walther J. Hild, eds.** Baltimore, MD: Urban and Schwarzenberg, 1977.

Volume 1, *Regions, Bones, Ligaments, Joints and Muscles*; volume 2, *Visceral Anatomy (Cardiovascular, Lymphatic, Digestive, Respiratory and Urogenital Systems)*; volume 3, *Central Nervous System, Autonomic Nervous System, Sense Organs and Skin, Peripheral Nerves and Vessels.*
A popular atlas with high-quality plates of anatomical dissections. Volume I concentrates on the locomotor system; volume II deals with visceral anatomy; and volume III illustrates the nervous system, skin, etc. X-ray reproductions are commendable. Recommended to radiologists.
R: *British Journal of Surgery* 62: 501 (June 1975); *Radiology* 128: 594 (1978).

Atlas of Human Embryos. **Raymond F. Gasser.** New York: Harper & Row, 1975.

Features the cross-sectional anatomy of human embryos during the first eight weeks of life. Contains eight chapters, each one representing a week of embryonic development. High-quality photomicrographs illustrate the transverse sections of the embryo. Captions are informative and precise. Includes comprehensive index. Aimed at medical students, embryologists, and human anatomists.
R: *Journal of Anatomy* 120: 607 (Dec. 1975); *Yale Journal of Biology and Medicine* 49: 99 (1976); *RSR* 3:31 (Apr.–June 1975).

Atlas of Medical Anatomy. **Jan Langman and M. W. Woerdeman.** Philadelphia, PA: W. B. Saunders, 1978.

Splendid collection of photographs, radiographs, and schematic drawings. Bridges gap from cadaver to human patients. Includes embryological illustra-

tions for purposes of comparison with adults. Text is readable and contains in-depth dissection notes. Good anatomical reference source for students and physicians.
R: *Lancet* 2: 456 (Aug. 26, 1978).

An Atlas of Primate Gross Anatomy: Baboon, Chimpanzee, and Man. **Daris R. Swindler and Charles D. Wood.** Seattle, WA: University of Washington Press, 1973.
Highlights the comparative gross anatomy of the baboon, chimpanzee, and man. Text arranged by regional anatomy. Textual material is detailed and complete. The 149 plates occupy double pages; additional drawings are exceptional. Highly recommended to anthropologists, anatomists, and students of human evolution.
R: *Journal of Anatomy* 116: 458 (Dec. 1973); *NEJM* 290: 171 (Jan. 17, 1974); *Science* 183: 192 (Jan. 18, 1974); *ARBA* (1974, p. 635).

An Atlas of the Anatomy of the Ear. **Branislav Vidic and Ronan O'Rahilly.** Philadelphia, PA: W. B. Saunders, 1971.
Fifty drawings and slides cover all aspects of the ear. Each illustration is accompanied by a good description and relevant references. Designed for the specialist.
R: *ARBA* (1972, p. 625).

A Brief Atlas of Histology. **Thomas S. Leeson and C. Roland Leeson.** Philadelphia, PA: W. B. Saunders, 1979.
An atlas which serves as a companion volume to histology textbooks. Clear illustrations, full coverage of all major organ systems.

Color Atlas and Textbook of Human Anatomy. 3 vols. Chicago, IL: Year Book Medical Publishers, 1978.
Volume 1, *Locomotor System,* Werner Platzer; volume 2, *Internal Organs*; volume 3, *Central Nervous System & Sensory Organs.*
R: *Journal of Allied Health* 8: 185 (Aug. 1979); *Physical Therapy* 59: 1037 (Aug. 1979).

A Colour Atlas of Human Anatomy. **R. M. H. McMinn and R. T. Hutchings.** Chicago, IL: Year Book Medical Publishers, 1977.
Over 700 photographs of dissected parts of the body. Photographs are actual size and well produced. Helpful to students.
R: *Lancet* 2: 745 (Oct. 8, 1977).

Cross-Sectional Anatomy: An Atlas for Computerized Tomography. **Robert S. Ledley, H. K. Huang, and John C. Mazziotta.** Baltimore, MD: Williams & Wilkins, 1977.
Computerized tomographic scans of normal cross-sectional anatomy. Presentation consists of location of cross section from a diagram and X-ray, diagram which corresponds to CT, color and black-and-white photographs of actual CT scan of normal anatomy. An atlas which guides the user to human anatomy through the use of up-to-date diagnostic methods.
R: *American Journal of Roentgenology* 131: 764 (Oct. 1978); *British Journal of Radiol-*

ogy 52: 155 (1979); *Journal of Neurosurgery* 48: 153 (Jan. 1978); *Lancet* 1: 1076 (May 20, 1978).

Grant's Atlas of Anatomy. 7th ed. **James E. Anderson, ed.** Baltimore, MD: Williams & Wilkins, 1978.

First edition, 1943; fifth edition, 1962; sixth edition, 1972.
Intended as a companion to textbooks, this atlas is a helpful guide for gross anatomy students. Seventh edition now incorporates color photographs, explanatory diagrams, and radiographs. A classic atlas, recommended to medical students and their professors.
R: *Canadian Medical Association Journal* 119: 1284 (Dec. 9, 1978); *Journal of Anatomy* 128: 409 (Mar. 1979); *ARBA* (1973, p. 616).

The Hand Atlas. **Moulton K. Johnson and Myles J. Cohen.** Springfield, IL: Charles C. Thomas, 1975.

Deals primarily with the anatomy of the hand. Addresses this extremity, layer by layer. The text is clear but the bibliography is meager. Most of the illustrations are black-and-white photographs; some color. However, illustrations do not possess crisp detail. Should appeal to hand surgeons.
R: *JAMA* 234: 1186 (Dec. 15, 1975).

The Johns Hopkins Atlas of Human Functional Anatomy. **George D. Zuidema, ed.** Baltimore, MD: Johns Hopkins University Press, 1977.

A publication of The Johns Hopkins Medical Institution. Concentrates on functional anatomy. Includes 148 color illustrations on 44 plates. The foremost medical illustrator, Leon Schlossberg, is responsible for illustrations. Faculty members of The Johns Hopkins University School of Medicine contributed to the text. Contains helpful glossary of anatomical, physiological, and clinical terms. Despite some discrepancies about the atlas's usefulness, it is intended expecially for students in medicine and allied health professions.
R: *Archives of Physical Medicine and Rehabilitation* 59: 49 (Jan. 1978); *Canadian Medical Association Journal* 117: 338 (Aug. 20, 1977); *Choice* 14: 658 (July–Aug. 1977); *ARBA* (1978, p. 705).

Photographic Atlas of Fetal Anatomy. **Wesley W. Parke.** Baltimore, MD: University Park Press, 1975.

Specialized atlas of the gross anatomy of the late fetus. Specimens fall between the 26- and 30-week gestation period. Illustrations involve 35 mm black-and-white film. Acts as a standard reference source for pathologists and professional anatomists.
R: *JAMA* 234: 1186 (Dec. 15, 1975).

Pocket Atlas of Human Anatomy. **Heinz Feneis.** Stuttgart: Georg Thieme Verlag, 1976.

An English translation of an excellent German anatomical atlas. Consists of beautiful line drawings with corresponding English and Latin anatomical terms. Systematic and comprehensive approach. Includes useful appendixes and index. Well recommended.
R: *Journal of Anatomy* 127: 637 (Dec. 1978).

Review of Gross Anatomy. 3d ed. **Ben Pansky and Earl L. House.** New York: Macmillan, 1975.

Expanded edition contains over 1,000 illustrations. Atlas emphasizes clinical applications of gross anatomy. Functional guide to visual comprehension.

Tissues and Organs: A Text-Atlas of Scanning Electron Microscopy. **Richard G. Kessel and Randy H. Kardon.** San Francisco, CA: W. H. Freeman, 1979.

Well illustrated with diagrams, light photomicrographs, and electron micrographs. Essential reference for professionals in medicine, biology, and pharmacology.
R: *LJ* 105: 570 (March 1, 1980).

ANESTHESIOLOGY AND GENERAL SURGERY

Atlas of Aesthetic Plastic Surgery. **John R. Lewis, Jr.** Boston, MA: Little, Brown, 1973.

Step-by-step explanations of plastic surgery techniques accompanied by drawings. Includes references. Helpful to plastic surgeons of all levels.
R: *Archives of Surgery* 109: 590 (Oct. 1974); *JAMA* 228: 506 (Apr. 22, 1974); *NEJM* 291: 157 (July 18, 1974).

An Atlas of Head and Neck Surgery. 2d ed. 2 vols. **John M. Lore, Jr.** Philadelphia, PA: W. B. Saunders, 1973.

First edition, 1963.
Monumental atlas of head and neck surgery. Two volumes provide a comprehensive outline of surgical procedures and techniques. Contains superb black-and-white drawings by Dr. Robert Wabnitz and 375 splendid plates. Text material found adjacent to pertinent illustration. Extensive bibliographies follow each section. Highly recommended to head and neck surgeons, otolaryngologists, and oncologists.
R: *Annals of Otology, Rhinology and Laryngology* 83: 8341 (1974); *Archives of Surgery* 108: 752 (May 1974); *Journal of Oral Surgery* 32: 312 (Apr. 1974); *JAMA* 228: 1592 (June 17, 1974); *NEJM* 290: 638 (Mar. 14, 1974); *Plastic and Reconstructive Surgery* 54: 94 (1974); *ARBA* (1975, p. 746).

Atlas of Radical Pelvic Surgery. 2d ed. **James H. Nelson, Jr.** New York: Appleton-Century-Crofts, 1977.

More of a manual on management of surgical patient. Clearly outlines steps necessary in preoperative stages. Includes detailed discussion of postoperative care of patients with colostomies and urinary conduits. Features outstanding sections on surgical procedures and possible complications. Anatomical illustrations are of the highest quality. All references are up to date. A "must" for physicians practicing gynecologic oncology or residents considering this subspecialty.
R: *JAMWA* 33: 446 (Oct. 1978).

Atlas of Surgery. 2d ed. **Horst-Eberhard Grewe and Karl Kremer. H. J. Hirsch, trans.** Philadelphia, PA: W. B. Saunders, 1979.

Extensively revised edition; retains the two-volume format. Chapters on vascular surgery and surgery of the extremities contain the most up-to-date information. Completely new illustrations. Geared toward the practicing general surgeon.

Atlas of Surgical Operations. 4th ed. **Robert M. Zollinger and Robert M. Zollinger, Jr.** New York: Macmillan, 1975.

First edition, 1939; second edition, 1952; third edition, 1967.
Outstanding text of surgical techniques. Fourth edition returns to the original format of one volume. Successfully outlines the most commonly performed abdominal surgical procedures. Approximately half the volume devoted to gastrointestinal details. Urology and neurosurgery excluded. Descriptions of operations appear opposite excellent drawings. Heartily recommended to surgical residents. Described as a living classic.
R: *Archives of Surgery* 111: 207 (Feb. 1976); *British Journal of Surgery* 63: 838 (Oct. 1976); *Gastroenterology* 70: 462 (Mar. 1976); *JAMA* 234: 977 (1975); *NEJM* 294: 791 (Apr. 1, 1976); *Surgery, Gynecology and Obstetrics* 143: 110 (1976); *RSR* 4: 49 (Jan.–Mar. 1976).

Atlas of Technics in Surgery. 2d ed. 2 vols. **John L. Madden.** New York: Appleton-Century-Crofts, 1964.

Volume 1, *General and Abdominal Surgery*; volume 2, *Thoracic and Cardiovascular Surgery.*
A two-volume atlas that covers general, abdominal, thoracic, and cardiovascular surgery. Systematic presentation; over 2,400 illustrations accompanied by detailed discussion. Contributions from more than 140 authorities.
R: Stearns & Ratcliff (*NEJM*, 1969; *NEJM*, 1970).

Color Atlas of General Surgical Diagnosis. **William F. Walker, ed.** Chicago, IL: Year Book Medical Publishers, 1976.

Four-color illustrations which describe general surgical procedures, accompanied by concise discussion of etiology and treatment of disease. Organized by chapters which present specific organ systems. Helpful to general practitioners and nurses.
R: *Canadian Medical Association Journal* 116: 139 (Jan. 1977); *Lahey Clinic Foundation Bulletin* 26: 48 (Jan.–Mar. 1977); *Plastic and Reconstructive Surgery* 59: 846 (1977).

Color Atlas of Surgery. **Rainer F. Lick.** Philadelphia, PA: W. B. Saunders, 1979.

Over 1,000 illustrations which depict surgical pathologies and their diagnosis. Corresponding text provides relevant surgical and clinical introduction.

Laproscopy in Gynecology, Surgery and Pediatrics: Textbook and Atlas. 3d ed. **Hans G. Frangenheim.** Chicago, IL: Year Book Medical Publishers, 1978.

Profusely illustrated text of laproscopic techniques.

The Plastic Surgery Atlas. 3 vols. **Frantisek Burian.** New York: Macmillan, 1968.

Volume 1, *General Concepts*; volume 2, *The Head*; volume 3, *Trunk and Extremities.*

BRAIN AND NERVOUS SYSTEM

Atlas of Cerebrospinal Fluid Cells. 2d ed. **Hans Wolfgang Kölmel.** New York: Springer-Verlag, 1977.

First edition, 1976.
Recommended tool for interpreting histology of the subject. Describes cell preparation, staining techniques, and interpretation of CSF. Includes color illustrations. Recommended to those involved with CSF cytodiagnosis.
R: *Journal of Neurosurgery* 47: 129 (July 1977); 49: 470 (Sept. 1978).

Atlas of Cerebrovascular Disease. **William F. McCormick and Sydney S. Schochet, Jr.** Philadelphia, PA: W. B. Saunders, 1976.

Mainly an atlas of pathology of the central nervous system. Contains clearly presented text and black-and-white photographs. Consists of six chapters which deal with such topics as hemorrhagic disorders, occlusive disorders, aneurysms and vascular anatomy. Presents helpful case studies. A valuable reference recommended for inclusion in all library collections.
R: *Annals of Internal Medicine* 87: 259 (Aug. 1977); *BMJ* 1: 1592 (June 18, 1977); *Journal of Neurosurgery* 46: 403 (Mar. 1977); *JAMA* 236: 2801 (Dec. 13, 1976); *Physical Therapy* 57: 1215 (1977).

An Atlas of Clinical Neurology. 2d ed. **John D. Spillane.** New York: Oxford University Press, 1976.

First edition, 1968.
An atlas comprised of high-quality photographs of neuropathology which are grouped according to both anatomical region and disease. Illustrations are of high quality; scope is encyclopedic. Notably helpful is the section on the optic fundi and the accompanying color plates. Recommended to all medical students and physicians in diverse fields of medicine.
R: *American Family Physician* 15: 237 (Feb. 1977); *American Journal of Psychiatry* 133: 1359 (Nov. 1976); *Annals of Internal Medicine* 86: 373 (Mar. 1977); *Brain* 99: 605 (Sept. 1976); *Journal of Neurology, Neurosurgery & Psychiatry* 39: 1137 (1976); *Journal of Neurosurgery* 46: 261 (Feb. 1977); *Lancet* 1: 128 (Jan. 17, 1976).

Atlas of Cross Section Anatomy of the Brain: Guide to the Study of the Morphology and Fiber Tracts of the Human Brain. 14th rev. ed. **Emil Villiger.** New York: McGraw-Hill, 1951.

Atlas of Electroencephalography in Coma and Cerebral Death. **Donald R. Bennett et al.** New York: Raven Press, 1976.

A by-product of a collaborative research study of cerebral death undertaken by the National Institute of Neurological Diseases and Stroke from 1971–1973. Consists of 2,000 EEGs recorded on 503 patients who met the required specifications. Illustrates the various EEG abnormalities associated with comatose patients. No pediatric recordings included. EEG reproductions are excellent. Standard reference source for electroencephalographers, EEG technicians, and medical personnel.
R: *Anesthesiology* 45: 373 (Sept. 1976); *Electroencephalography & Clinical Neurophysiology* 42: 147 (Jan. 1977); *Journal of Neurosurgery* 46: 264 (Feb. 1977).

Atlas of Neuropathology. 2d ed. **Nathan Malamud and Asao Hirano.** Berkeley, CA: University of California Press, 1974.

First edition, 1957.

Focuses on central nervous system pathology, particularly the brain. Each section deals with a specific disease or pathological process. Utilizes 12,000 case studies to explain the excellent black-and-white photographs. Electron micrographs are an added feature. Text and illustrations arranged side by side. Index is complete. The lack of a comprehensive bibliography detracts from the atlas's usefulness. Intended for neuropathologists and neurological clinicians.
R: *Journal of Neurosurgery* 43: 642 (Nov. 1975); *Neuropsychology* 14: 398 (1976); *RSR* 3: 113 (Jan.–Mar. 1975).

Atlas of Neuropathology. **Sumner I. Zacks.** New York: Harper & Row, 1971.

Surveys the wide spectrum of neurologic diseases with 300 photographs, photomicrographs, and electron micrographs. Good presentation of vascular, infectious, and degenerative diseases. One critical observation is the large amount of wasted space. Excellent visual reference source for pathologists, neurosurgeons, and students of neuropathology.
R: *Growth* 38: 248 (June 1974).

Atlas of the Arteries of the Human Brain. 2d ed. **Georges Salamon.** Paris: Sandoz, 1973.

First edition, 1971.

Second edition has undergone very little change from the successful first edition. Accurately describes the anatomy of the cerebral arteries and their branches. Text written in both French and English and divided into three sections. Photographs are essentially in color. Also includes transparencies. Loose-leaf format is very practical for students of anatomy and neurosciences.
R: *American Journal of Roentgenology* 124: 335 (June 1975); *British Journal of Radiology* 49: 280 (1976); *Journal of Neurosurgery* 39: 677 (Nov. 1973).

An Atlas of Tumours Involving the Central Nervous System. **Robin O. Barnard, Valentine Logue, and Patterson S. Reaves.** Baltimore, MD: Williams & Wilkins, 1976.

A beautifully illustrated atlas of all types of CNS tumors. Composed of 52 brief case studies. Most of the space devoted to neuroepithelial tumors of the brain. Features 200 color photomicrographs which lack sharpness of detail. The clinical details appear on the left-hand page while the accompanying illustrations are on the opposite page. A brief bibliography concludes each section. A beneficial volume for clinicians and trainees in pathology and neuropathology.
R: *Brain* 100: 390 (June 1977); *BMJ* 1: 884 (Sept. 10, 1976); *Electroencephalography & Clinical Neurophysiology* 44: 411 (Mar. 1978); *Journal of Neurosurgery* 46: 841 (June 1977); *Lancet* 2: 940 (Oct. 30, 1976).

A Basic Atlas of the Human Nervous System. **Gary B. Dunkerley.** Philadelphia, PA: F. A. Davis, 1975.

Complementary photographs and drawings of the human brain and spinal cord which help to visualize their complex anatomy. Illustrations are accompanied by

succinct text, making this a handy reference for doctors and scientists.
R: *Brain* 99: 605 (Sept. 1976); *Journal of Neurosurgery* 44: 398 (Mar. 1976); *Physical Therapy* 56: 504 (1976); 58: 810 (1978).

Basic Human Neuroanatomy: An Introductory Atlas. 2d ed. **Craig Watson.** Boston, MA: Little, Brown, 1977.

First edition, 1974.
In three parts, reviews organization, pathways, and computerized tomography of the brain. Concise and clear reference to neurology; helpful to medical students and neurologists. Photographs are of good quality and are helpful.
R: *Journal of Anatomy* 126: 394 (June 1978); *Neurology* 26: 98 (Jan. 1976).

A Colour Atlas of Neuropathology. **C. S. Treip.** Chicago, IL: Year Book Medical Publishers, 1978.

An atlas of broad scope which serves as an introduction to neuropathologic diagnosis. Contains over 300 photographs of histological sections; clearly presents basic anatomy and manifestations of disease. Well recommended to pathologists; includes bibliographies.
R: *Journal of Clinical Pathology* 31: 703 (1978); *Journal of Neurosurgery* 50: 398 (Mar. 1979); *Lancet* 1: 640 (Mar. 25, 1978).

Neuropathology of Vision: An Atlas. **Richard Lindenberg, Frank B. Walsh, and Joel G. Sacks.** Philadelphia, PA: Lea & Febiger, 1973.

A reference gem dealing with the sensory aspects of neuro-ophthalmology. Correlates clinical symptoms with the anatomic location of visual lesions. Side-by-side arrangement of text and illustrations. Text consists mainly of case studies and captions. Illustrations number about 752 and consist of gross pathology, photomicrographs, and anatomical drawings. All illustrations exhibit excellent quality. Outstanding subject index, references, and cross-references establish this volume as a source book. No neurologist, neurosurgeon, neuropathologist, or ophthalmologist should be unaware of its existence.
R: *American Journal of Ophthalmology* 78: 351 (Aug. 1974); *Archives of Neurology* 31: 71 (July 1974); *Archives of Ophthalmology* 92: 270 (Sept. 1974); *Brain* 97: 610 (Sept. 1974); *JAMA* 228: 401 (Apr. 15, 1974); *NEJM* 291: 684 (Sept. 26, 1974).

Radiologic Anatomy of the Brain. **George Salamon and Yun Peng Huang.** New York: Springer-Verlag, 1976.

An atlas in three parts, covering cerebral hemispheres, the mesencephalic and diencephalic region and basal ganglia, and the posterior fossa. Anatomic descriptions are excellent and are accompanied by over 450 illustrations which include photographs, radiographs, and drawings. Considered an essential reference for neuro-anatomists and radiologists.
R: *American Journal of Roentgenology* 130: 416 (Feb. 1978); *Brain* 101: 378 (June 1978); *Journal of Neurosurgery* 47: 640 (Oct. 1977); *Radiology* 128: 108 (1978).

The Spine: A Radiological Text and Atlas. 4th ed. **Bernard S. Epstein.** Philadelphia, PA: Lea & Febiger, 1976.

First edition, 1955; second edition, 1962; third edition, 1969.
Up-to-date fourth edition of a classic atlas; emphasizes clinical approach to study

of diseases of the spine. Includes 500 illustrations of consistent high quality and many new advances in radiologic study of the vertebral column. Chapter format provides quick ready reference to an encyclopedic amount of information. Recommended to orthopedic surgeons, neurologists, pathologists, and radiologists for thoroughness. Contains a bibliography and numerous references.
R: *British Journal of Radiology* 50: 100 (1977); *Journal of Bone and Joint Surgery* 59B: 259 (May 1977); *Journal of Neurosurgery* 45: 721 (Dec. 1976); *JAMA* 236: 2553 (Nov. 29, 1976); *Lahey Clinic Foundation Bulletin* 27: 130 (July–Sept. 1978); *Neurology* 27: 802 (Aug. 1977); *Radiology* 125: 668 (1977). Also reviewed in *Group Practice* & *New Physician*.

Stereotaxic Atlas of the Human Brainstem and Cerebellar Nuclei: A Variability Study. **F. Afshar, E. S. Watkins, and J. C. Yap.** New York: Raven Press, 1977.
A unique atlas which synthesizes the variability study of 30 brains, concerning the location and variability of structures. Includes statistics and meticulously presented facts.
R: *Lancet* 1: 1062 (May 19, 1979).

Structure of the Human Brain. 2d ed. **Stephen J. DeArmond, Madeline M. Fusco, and Maynard M. Dewey.** New York: Oxford University Press, 1976.
First edition, 1974.
An atlas of photographs, line drawings, and light micrographs which serve to illustrate the anatomy of the brain. Also includes information on vascular structure and cytoarchitecture. Excellent illustrations, helpful in teaching neuroanatomy. For beginners in the field.
R: *Journal of Anatomy* 119: 627 (July 1975); *Journal of Neurosurgery* 46: 840 (June 1977); *Yale Journal of Biology and Medicine* 50: 692 (1977). Also reviewed in *Neuroscience*.

CARDIOVASCULAR SYSTEM

Atlas of Adult Echocardiography. **Robert Kraus and Howard N. Allen.** Philadelphia, PA: J. B. Lippincott, 1979.
A profusely illustrated atlas of echocardiograms which is geared toward acquiring evaluation skills. Presents common and uncommon examples, some straightforward, some varying in interpretation. Recommended to those learning to evaluate echocardiograms.

An Atlas of Cardiology: Electrocardiograms and Chest X-Rays. **Neville Conway.** Chicago, IL: Year Book Medical Publishers, 1977.
A ready reference containing both illustrations and electrocardiograms.

Atlas of Carotid Angiography. **Mutsumasa Takahashi.** New York: Igaku-Shoin Medical Publishers, 1977.
Ties together basic concepts of angiography with recent developments. Reviews anatomy of arterial and venous systems and pathology of each angiographic system. Illustrations are of high quality and accompanied by helpful arrows and

legends. A recommended guide to the interpretation of angiograms.
R: *Annals of Internal Medicine* 89: 585 (Oct. 1978); *NEJM* 299: 1140 (Nov. 16, 1978); *Radiology* 126: 660 (1978).

Atlas of Echocardiography. **Ernesto E. Salcedo.** Philadelphia, PA: W. B. Saunders, 1978.

Up-to-date illustrations of echocardiograms, both normal and abnormal. Overall presentation is excellent, as is the helpful bibliography. Pictorial presentation contributes to good format. An atlas valuable to echocardiologists.
R: *American Heart Journal* 98: 139 (July 1979); *Annals of Internal Medicine* 89: 437 (Sept. 1978); *Physics in Medicine & Biology* 24: 655 (May 1979).

Color Atlas of Cardiac Pathology. **Geoffrey Farrer-Brown.** Chicago, IL: Year Book Medical Publishers, 1977.

Over 400 illustrations; a comprehensive atlas of the heart, detailing normal and pathologic anatomy. Contains a good index; recommended to residents, pathologists, and all medical libraries.
R: *Canadian Medical Association Journal* 118: 904 (Apr. 22, 1978); *Lancet* 2: 386 (Aug. 20, 1977); *NEJM* 299: 1085 (Nov. 9, 1978).

Coronary Heart Disease: Clinical, Angiographic, and Pathologic Profiles. **Zeev Vlodaver et al.** New York: Springer-Verlag, 1976.

A large format atlas replete with radiographs, electrocardiograms, pathological sections, photomicrographs, which illustrate aspects of coronary heart disease. Reproduction is excellent, as is brief but authoritative text. Includes helpful legends. Recommended to radiologists.
R: *American Heart Journal* 94: 395 (Sept. 1977); *JAMA* 237: 1623 (Apr. 11, 1977); *Radiology* 125: 316 (1977).

Echocardiography: A Teaching Atlas. **Joel M. Felner and Robert C. Schlant.** New York: Grune & Stratton, 1976.

A compilation of echocardiographs of normal and diseased cardiac conditions. Contains an extensive bibliography. An excellent reference for echocardiographers.
R: *Annals of Internal Medicine* 88: 273 (Feb. 1978).

Heart and Coronary Arteries: An Anatomical Atlas for Clinical Diagnosis, Radiological Investigation, and Surgical Treatment. **Wallace A. McAlpine.** New York: Springer-Verlag, 1975.

An impressive collection of photographs and illustrations of cardiac anatomy. Divided into two main sections: the normal heart and the coronary arteries. Features 800 dissection views and 300 detailed diagrams, mostly in color. Illustrations are truly superb due to the special lighting and angular effects. Text and illustrations are located on two opposing pages. A work of art of extreme value to surgeons, coronary angiographers, cardiologists, and cardiology trainees.
R: *American Heart Journal* 92: 545 (1976); *British Journal of Radiology* 50: 76 (1977); *Lahey Clinic Foundation Bulletin* 26: 151 (July–Sept. 1977); *Radiology* 122: 116 (1977).

DENTISTRY

Atlas of Diseases of the Jaws. **Jens J. Pindborg and E. Horting-Hansen.** Philadelphia, PA: W. B. Saunders, 1974.

A compilation of radiographs and color photomicrographs of diseases of the mandible and maxilla; briefly discusses major features of each jaw disease. High-quality illustrations and presentations. Table of contents classified according to the World Health Organization format. A good, ready-reference source.
R: *Archives of Pathology & Laboratory Medicine* 100: 111 (Feb. 1976); *Journal of Oral Surgery* 33: 630 (Aug. 1975).

A Color Atlas and Textbook of Oral Anatomy. **B. K. B. Berkovitz et al.** Chicago, IL: Year Book Medical Publishers, 1978.

A photographic survey of tooth morphology.

Color Atlas of Oral Pathology. 3d ed. **Robert A. Colby, Donald A. Kerr, and Hamilton B. G. Robinson.** Philadelphia, PA: J. B. Lippincott, 1971.

A ready-reference source for dentists. Contains clear descriptions and illustrations. Divided into five sections: histology and embryology, diseases of teeth, diseases of oral mucosa and jaws, neoplasms, and developmental disorders.
R: *American Journal of Clinical Pathology, Journal of Prosthetic Dentistry.*

Development of the Human Dentition: An Atlas. **Frans P. G. M. van der Linden and Herman S. Duterloo.** New York: Harper & Row, 1976.

A visual presentation of the development of human dentition; includes over 300 photographs and 28 line drawings which span developmental stages from prenatal to old age. Depicts normal and some less common anatomy. Illustrations are clearly presented.

Oral Disease. **C. E. Renson, ed.** Fort Lee, NJ: Update Publications, 1978.

An atlas which acquaints the general practitioner with oral disease. Color photographs, well referenced.
R: *Journal of Oral Surgery* 37: 451 (1979).

Oral Roentgenographic Diagnosis. 4th ed. **Edward C. Stafne and J. A. Gilbilisco.** Philadelphia, PA: W. B. Saunders, 1975.

First edition, 1958; third edition, 1969.
Magnificent contribution to the literature of roentgenology. First edition (1958) was considered a classic; fourth edition worthy of same praise. Features outstanding roentgenograms and seven additional chapters. Chapter on oral roentgenographic manifestations of systemic disease remains a jewel in this volume. Reliable guide for students of dentistry and radiology, oral surgeons, and roentgenologists.
R: *American Journal of Roentgenology* 127: 882 (Nov. 1976); *Radiology* 122: 314 (Feb. 1977).

Orban's Oral Histology & Embryology. 8th ed. **S. N. Bhasker and Harry Sicher, eds.** St. Louis, MO: C. V. Mosby, 1976.

Seventh edition, 1972.

A much expanded atlas covering major aspects of dental embryology and histology. Profusely illustrated and well indexed.

Principles and Practice of Periodontics: With an Atlas of Treatment. **Frank M. Wentz, ed.** Springfield, IL: Charles C. Thomas, 1978.

A therapy planning guide for dental students and practitioners. Includes illustrations of procedures, surgery, etiology of disease, and advances in immunologic research.

R: *Journal of Oral Surgery* 36: 822 (Oct. 1978).

DERMATOLOGY

Atlas of Aquatic Dermatology. **Alexander A. Fisher.** New York: Grune & Stratton, 1978.

Acquaints practicing physician with dermatitis caused by sea creatures and related aquatic objects. Features succinct descriptions, excellent photographs, and useful tabular data. Includes current references. Standard reference source for all physicians.

R: *Archives of Dermatology* 115: 902 (July 1979).

Atlas of Dermatology. **Gernot Rassner. Guinter Kahn, ed. & trans.** Munich, Germany: Urban and Schwarzenberg, 1978.

A translation of the German edition. Arranges some 200 color photographs of dermatologic diseases according to principal sites and structures affected. Diagrammatic black-and-white illustrations are keyed to photographs. Succint captions outline noteworthy features. Fine color reproduction and unusually large format contribute to the outstanding quality of this atlas.

R: *Archives of Dermatology* 115: 781 (June 1979)

An Atlas of the Ultrastructure of Human Skin: Development, Differentiation, and Post-natal Features. **A. S. Breathnach.** London: Churchill Livingstone, 1971.

Useful compendium of submicroscopic anatomy of human skin. Fine scientific prose attests to the author's scholarship. Electron micrographs are of good quality; additional illustrations are well reproduced. Illustrations of retinal melanosome and human hair cortex are classic. Geared toward biologists, embryologists, anatomists, pathologists, and research dermatologists.

R: *Journal of Histochemistry and Cytochemistry* 21: 504 (May 1973).

Atlas of Tumors of the Skin. **Alfred W. Kopf, Robert S. Bart, and Rafael Andrade.** Philadelphia, PA: W. B. Saunders, 1978.

Companion atlas to *Cancer of the Skin*. Consists entirely of 900 color photographs devoted to skin tumors. Photographs culled from the files of the Oncology Section of the Skin and Cancer Unit, New York University Medical Center. Alphabetical arrangement of pictures by diagnosis. Features high-quality photographs, adequate index. Lacks extensive cross-references. Billed as an "encyclopedic collection of benign and malignant cutaneous tumors" and geared toward student and physician.

R: *Archives of Dermatology* 115: 782 (June 1979); *Plastic and Reconstructive Surgery* 64: 93 (July 1979).

Color Atlas of Dermatology. **G. M. Levene and C. D. Calnan.** Chicago, IL: Year Book Medical Publishers, 1974.

An excellent color atlas which helps to assist diagnosis in dermatology. Well organized; recommended to all departments of dermatology.
R: *Archives of Dermatology* 110: 480 (Sept. 1974).

Color Atlas of Pediatric Dermatology. **Samuel Weinberg, Lewis Shapiro, and Morris Leider.** New York: McGraw-Hill, 1975.

Over 770 pictures of skin diseases. Illustrations are of high quality and are accompanied by brief text which explains elements of skin anatomy, physiology, diagnosis, and treatment of disease. Well indexed; highly recommended to hospital and medical school libraries.
R: *Annals of Internal Medicine* 83: 924 (Dec. 1975); *Archives of Dermatology* 112: 265 (Feb. 1976); *ARBA* (1976, p. 735).

Diseases of the Skin in Children and Adolescents: A Colour Atlas. 3d ed. **G. W. Korting. Translated and adapted by William Curth and Helen O. Curth.** Philadelphia, PA: W. B. Saunders, 1978.

English translation of a fine German text. Comprehensive coverage of diseases with special emphasis on rarities. Includes 398 illustrations, ranging in quality from good to excellent. Greatest appeal to dermatologists, pediatricians, and physicians.
R: *Lancet* 2: 191 (July 25, 1970); *NEJM* 301: 280 (Aug. 5, 1979).

Pocket Color Atlas of Dermatology. **Joseph Kimmig and Michel Janner. Translated and revised by Herbert Goldschmidt.** Chicago, IL: Year Book Medical Publishers, 1975.

Attempts to illustrate skin diseases through the use of 302 color photographs which are of good quality. Accompanying text is succinct. Also includes references, helpful index. A handy ready reference.
R: *Archives of Dermatology* 112: 573 (Apr. 1976).

GASTROINTESTINAL SYSTEM

Abdominal Operations. 6th ed. 2 vols. **Rodney Maingot, ed.** New York: Appleton-Century-Crofts, 1974.

A classic work on abdominal surgery. Outlines all approved techniques related to abdominal operations practiced in hospitals and surgical clinics in Great Britain and the United States. Intended primarily for surgeons.
R: *JAMA* 230: 135 (Oct. 7, 1974).

Abdominal Surgery: An Atlas of Operative Techniques. **Pietro Valdoni. Translated and adapted by George Nardi.** Philadelphia, PA: W. B. Saunders, 1976.

Presents a thorough review of gastrointestinal surgery. Applies basic surgical principles to relevant operations. Magnificent color illustrations serve as step-by-

step guides. Reflects the personal preference of one experienced surgeon which may cause some disagreement within the profession. Gold mine of information for the experienced surgeon; medical students and residents should be mindful of the atlas's limitations.
R: *JAMA* 237: 692 (Feb. 14, 1977); *Lahey Clinic Foundation Bulletin* 26: 151 (July–Sept. 1977); *NEJM* 296: 120 (Jan. 13, 1977).

Atlas der Rectoskopie und Coloskopie. **Peter Otto and Klaus Ewe.** Berlin: Springer-Verlag, 1976.

In German; illustrates diseases of the rectum and colon through use of color photographs. High quality; recommended to physicians able to read German.
R: *Annals of Internal Medicine* 85: 413 (Sept. 1976).

Atlas of Coloscopy. **F. P. Rossini.** Padua, Italy: Piccin, 1975.

Emphasizes the preparation of a patient for coloscopy. Numerous illustrations familiarize reader with the normal and diseased appearances of the colon. Carefully details the methods and techniques of passing an instrument to the caecum.
R: *British Journal of Surgery* 63: 836 (Oct. 1976).

Atlas of Colposcopy. 2d ed. **Per Kolstad and Adolf Stafl.** Baltimore, MD: University Park Press, 1977.

First edition, 1971.
Comprehensively illustrates colposcopic techniques through use of photographs. Succinctly presents diagnostic techniques, terminology, and histopathologic correlations. Second edition discusses exposure to stilboestrol. Recommended to pathologists and gynecologists.
R: *BMJ* 2: 1342 (Nov. 19, 1977); *Obstetrics and Gynecology* 41: 481 (Mar. 1973).

Atlas of Enteroscopy. **L. Demling, M. Classen, and P. Fruhmorgen.** Berlin: Springer-Verlag, 1975.

Endoscopy limited to diseases of the intestines and pancreas. Translated from German; contains superb illustrations and color photographs. Particularly useful to gastroenterologists.
R: *Annals of Internal Medicine* 85: 413 (Sept. 1976).

Atlas of Gastrointestinal Surgery. **Komei Nakayama.** Philadelphia, PA: J. B. Lippincott, 1969.

Nearly one-third of atlas devoted to esophageal surgery. Systematic presentation of author's surgical methods. Gastrointestinal surgical techniques comprise the remaining two-thirds. Includes photographs of and instructions for the use of Dr. Nakayama's surgical instruments. Excellent reference source for surgeons of all English-speaking countries interested in gastrointestinal surgery.

An Atlas of Gastrointestinal Surgery. **Ward D. O'Sullivan.** Philadelphia, PA: F. A. Davis, 1974.

Contains 150 color slides accompanied by 60 pages of descriptive text. Devoted to common GI surgical problems. Conditions arranged by anatomical region of the GI tract. High-quality photographs and reproductions compliment text. Ref-

erences conclude each chapter. Superb teaching aid for medical students, interns, and residents.
R: *American Journal of Digestive Diseases* 26: 899 (Sept. 1975).

Atlas of Liver Biopsies. **Hemming Poulson and Per Christoffersen.** Copenhagen: Munksgaard, 1979.
An up-to-date atlas which aids in the interpretation of liver biopsies. Describes and illustrates morphological changes through 185 color and black-and-white illustrations. Contains an appendix of staining techniques. Helpful for histologists.
R: *BMJ* 2: 38 (July 7, 1979); *Lancet* 1: 1007 (May 5, 1979).

Atlas of Practical Proctology. **Alexander Neiger.** Baltimore, MD: Williams & Wilkins, 1974.
Illustrates a wide variety of perianal and rectal disorders. Hemorrhoids are granted considerable space. Includes many photomicrographs and diagrams of these diseases. Useful information on equipment and techniques necessary to perform proctoscopy, rectal biopsy, and polypectomy. No histological correlation given. Brief section on venereal diseases concludes the text. Practical atlas for students and house officers.
R: *Archives of Internal Medicine* 136: 375 (Mar. 1976).

The Color Atlas of Intestinal Parasites. 7th printing. **Francis M. Spencer and Lee S. Monroe.** Springfield, IL: Charles C. Thomas, 1977.
Revised sixth printing, 1975.
Aids laboratory technicians in the identification of intestinal parasites. Contains over 200 color photomicrographs, descriptions of laboratory techniques and a new section on amebic disease. Helpful in illustrating parasites as they appear in body excretions. A good ready reference for gastroenterologists and internists.
R: *Annals of Internal Medicine* 84: 514 (Apr. 1976); *Gastroenterology* 70: 820 (May 1976).

A Colour Atlas of Liver Disease. **Dame S. Sherlock and John A. Summerfield.** London: Wolfe, 1979.
Illustrates clinical manifestations, radiology, anatomy, and histology of liver diseases. Excellent photomicrographs convey the physical symptoms as the disease progresses. Should be used in conjunction with a standard textbook. Geared toward medical students and postgraduates.
R: *BMJ* 1: 1273 (May 12, 1979).

The Digestive System: An Ultrastructural Atlas and Review. **P. G. Toner, K. E. Carr, and G. M. Wyburn.** New York: Appleton-Century-Crofts, 1971.
Electron photomicrographs of cell ultrastructure, covering the esophagus, stomach, intestine, accessory digestive organs, and nonepithelial components of digestive organs. Deals mainly with normal cell structure. High quality illustrations; a useful reference manual for gastroenterologists and electron microscopists.
R: *Archives of Internal Medicine* 131: 612 (Apr. 1973).

Endoscopy and Biopsy of the Esophagus and Stomach: A Color Atlas. **L. Dem-**

ling, R. Ottenjann, and K. Elster.** Philadelphia, PA: W. B. Saunders, 1973.
A brief, up-to-date color atlas of endoscopy. Contains over 200 high-quality photographs which represent what is seen through the instrument. Has helpful accompanying text and references. Well organized; recommended to gastroenterologists on all levels.
R: *Archives of Internal Medicine* 133: 322 (Feb. 1974); *Archives of Surgery* 107: 817 (Nov. 1973); *Gastroenterology* 64: 1196 (June 1973).

Radiological Atlas of Biliary and Pancreatic Disease. **Hiram Baddely, Daniel J. Nolan, and Paul R. Salmon.** Aylesbury, Bucks, England: Harvey, Miller, & Medcalf, 1978.
A handy volume of plain and contrast radiographs. Covers anatomy of biliary system and pancreas as well as various diseases. Text is concise, radiographs are comprehensive in their coverage. Beautifully printed, helpful reference for physicians, endoscopists.
R: *Lancet* 2: 1184 (Dec. 2, 1978).

Radiology of the Abdomen: Anatomic Basis. **Joseph P. Whalen.** Philadelphia, PA: Lea & Febiger, 1976.
A comprehensive atlas helpful in understanding the relationship between anatomy and disease processes of the abdomen. Contains cross-sectional illustrations from frozen cadaver sections which correspond to radiographs, line drawings, and ultrasound scans. Includes a wealth of detailed information; a valuable reference for radiologists.
R: *JAMA* 238: 896 (Aug. 22, 1977); *Radiology* 125: 34 (1977).

GENETICS

An Atlas of Mammalian Chromosomes. **T. C. Hsu and Kurt Benirschke.** New York: Springer-Verlag. (Unbound).
Volume 7, 1973; volume 8, 1974.
Comprehensive treatment of many mammalian chromosomes worldwide. Consists of loose-leaf sheets for easy insertion into binders. Description of chromosomes based on size and shape. Includes list of references for each animal. Quality of chromosomal reproduction is not of the highest standard. However, no other source gathers so much information about chromosomes of so many species. Valuable to cytogeneticist in the field of taxonomy or evolution.
R: *American Journal of Veterinary Research* 35: 865 (June 1974); *Social Biology* 23: 181 (1976).

Atlas of Men: A Guide for Somatotyping the Adult Male at All Ages. **William H. Sheldon.** New York: Harper & Row, 1954. Repr. New York: Hafner, 1970.
A standard reference file of somatotype variations based on 46,000 adult men subjects. Contains 1,175 sets of photographs, displaying front, side, and rear views. Each somatotype is assigned a number which corresponds to the endomorphy, mesomorphy, and ectomorphy. Valuable reference source for use in

the classification of the human body by somatotyping.
R: *Choice* 7: 1646 (Feb. 1971); *ARBA* (1972, p. 624).

Atlas of Protein Sequence & Structure, 1967–68. **M. O. Dayhoff and R. V. Eck.** Silver Spring, MD: The National Biomedical Research Foundation, 1968.
R: *American Scientist* 57: 36A (Spring 1969).

Atlas of the Face in Genetic Disorders. 2d ed. **Richard M. Goodman and Robert J. Gorlin.** St. Louis, MO: C. V. Mosby, 1977.
Lists more than 225 genetic syndromes, accompanied by over 1,000 illustrations. Disorders arranged by mode of transmission. Two glossaries of medical and genetic terminology and various diagnostic tables make up the appendix.
R: *American Journal of Diseases of Children* 131: 1411 (Dec. 1977); *Plastic and Reconstructive Surgery* 62: 110 (1978).

Birth Defects Compendium. 2d ed. **Daniel Bergsma, ed.** New York: Alan R. Liss, 1979.
First edition entitled *Birth Defects Atlas and Compendium*, 1973.
A comprehensive atlas of both text and photographs which aid in the diagnosis of birth defects.

Clinical Atlas of Human Chromosomes. **Jean deGrouchy and Catherine Turleau.** New York: John Wiley, 1977.
Sequentially organized atlas of the 24 human chromosomes. Contains pertinent morphological information, pathways of pathology which indicate different syndromes for each chromosome. Originally published in French, this is an extremely useful atlas.
R: *American Journal of Diseases of Children* 133: 226 (Feb. 1979); *American Scientist* 66: 501 (July–Aug. 1978); *Canadian Medical Association Journal* 119: 698 (Oct. 7, 1978); *Heredity* 42: 122 (Feb. 1979).

An Electron Micrographic Atlas of Viruses. **Robley C. Williams and Harold W. Fisher.** Springfield, IL: Charles C. Thomas, 1974.
Visual compendium of the structure of 31 viruses. Electron micrographs of each virus accompanied by a brief description of their history, biology, chemistry, and physical aspects. Text is less impressive than illustrations. References conclude each account. Includes an index. Useful addition to college, medical, and special libraries.
R: *American Journal of Tropical Medicine and Hygiene* 24: 1045 (Nov. 1975); *American Scientist* 63: 583 (Sept.–Oct. 1975); *RSR* 3: 46 (Jan.–Mar. 1975).

Mental Retardation: An Atlas of Diseases with Associated Physical Abnormalities. **Lewis B. Holmes et al.** New York: Macmillan, 1972.
A most comprehensive encyclopedic atlas of the physical abnormalities associated with mental retardation. Side-by-side illustration and full description of 173 diseases are provided. Well-organized format; includes information on physiological, neurological, pathological, and genetic characteristics of disease syndromes of mental retardation. Well indexed; clearly printed. Recommended to clinicians

who deal with mentally retarded patients.
R: *American Journal of Human Genetics* 26: 530 (July 1974); *American Journal of Psychiatry* 130: 1166 (Oct. 1973); *Archives of Internal Medicine* 132: 626 (Oct. 1973); 132: 775 (Nov. 1973); *Clinical Pediatrics* 12: 14A (Apr. 1973); *Teratology* 8: 78 (Aug. 1973); *Yale Journal of Biology and Medicine* 47: 66 (1974).

HEMATOLOGY

Atlas of Haematology. 4th ed. **George A. McDonald, T. C. Dodds, and Bruce Cruickshank.** Edinburgh: Churchill Livingstone, 1978.

Fourth edition of a superb atlas. Features a new section on the ultrastructure of blood cells, complete wtih electron microphotographs. Excellent presentation on parasites and lymphomas; well illustrated with 408 figures. Valuable addition to hematological and pathological laboratories.
R: *British Journal of Haematology* 40: 294 (1979); *Journal of Clinical Pathology* 32: 199 (1979).

An Atlas of the Blood and Bone Marrow. 2d ed. **R. Philip Custer.** Philadelphia, PA: W. B. Saunders, 1974.

First edition, 1949.
Few changes made from the first edition. A fine collection of photomicrographs depicting various hematologic diseases in fixed tissue. Large format illustrations are in black and white. Section on infection contains some unique photographs and information. Second edition contains four additional chapters written by authorities in the field.
R: *Annals of Internal Medicine* 82: 440 (Mar. 1975); *Archives of Internal Medicine* 135: 1406 (Oct. 1975); *JAMA* 232: 76 (Apr. 7, 1975).

Atlas of Vascular Surgery. 3d ed. **Falls B. Hershey and Carl H. Calman.** St. Louis, MO: C. V. Mosby, 1973.

A first-class reference book on the technics of vascular surgery. About 700 illustrations. Primarily for surgical residents.
R: *Annals of Surgery* 181: 12A (Apr. 1975); *JAMA* 228: 1435 (June 10, 1974); *NEJM* 291: 854 (Oct. 17, 1974).

Atlas of Vascular Surgery. **Robert R. Linton.** Philadelphia, PA: W. B. Saunders, 1973.

Written by the "master" of vascular surgery. Contains some 220 plates complemented by detailed, accurate descriptions. Includes excellent references. A "must" for every surgical resident and vascular surgeon.
R: *Archives of Surgery* 108: 881 (June 1974).

Bone Marrow and Bone Tissue: Color Atlas of Clinical Histopathology. **Rolf Burkhardt, ed.** New York: Springer-Verlag, 1971.

A German translation; atlas contains over 700 color photomicrographs of bone marrow biopsies which are of exceptionally high quality. Describes biopsy methods and histological techniques. Highly recommended.
R: *Annals of Internal Medicine* 78: 804 (May 1973); *Pediatrics* 51: 164 (Jan. 1973).

Bone Marrow Interpretation. **Lawrence Kass.** Springfield, IL: Charles C. Thomas, 1973.

An atlas of bone marrow morphology; contains over 200 black-and-white photographs of high quality. Discusses disease of bone marrow. Helpful in every hematology and medical library.
R: *Annals of Internal Medicine* 78: 990 (June 1973).

Corpuscles: Atlas of Red Blood Cell Shapes. **Marcel Bessis.** New York: Springer-Verlag, 1974.

Three-dimensional topography of red blood cells obtained from scanning electron micrographs. Pictorial reproduction is of the highest quality; provides practical classification of differently shaped erythrocytes. Important atlas for all hematologists and cell biologists.
R: *Annals of Internal Medicine* 82: 129 (Jan. 1975); *Archives of Internal Medicine* 135: 1406 (Oct. 1975); *Blood* 45: 892 (1974); *Journal of Histochemistry and Cytochemistry* 23: 392 (May 1975); *JAMA* 230; 1704 (Dec. 1974); *NEJM* 292: 377 (Feb. 13, 1975).

Living Blood Cells and Their Ultrastructure. **Marcel Bessis. Robert Weed, trans.** New York: Springer-Verlag, 1973.

Encyclopedic atlas of blood cell morphology. Carefully blends phase microscopy, scanning electron microscopy (SEM), electron microscopy, and superb line drawings. Except for two color plates, all illustrations are in black and white. Excellent subject index; nearly 5,000 references conclude the volume. Valuable standard reference source for cell biologists, histochemists, and hematologists.
R: *Annals of Internal Medicine* 81: 420 (Sept. 1974); *Archives of Internal Medicine* 135: 1406 (Oct. 1975); *Journal of Histochemistry and Cytochemistry* 22: 1068 (Nov. 1974); *JAMA* 230: 134 (Oct. 7, 1974); Allyn.

Procedures in Vascular Surgery. 2d ed. **Chilton Crane and Richard Warren.** Boston, MA: Little, Brown, 1976.

First edition, 1960.
An excellent atlas which reviews standard vascular operations as well as some more complicated and controversial ones. Explanations are clear and succinct; references are complete. Highly recommended for surgeons and medical libraries.
R: *Annals of Surgery* 184: 531 (Oct. 1976); *Archives of Surgery* 111: 1311 (Nov. 1976); *British Journal of Surgery* 63: 838 (Oct. 1976); *JAMA* 236: 1629 (Oct. 4, 1976); *NEJM* 295: 178 (July 15, 1976).

Sandoz Atlas of Haematology. 2d ed. **Erik Undritz.** Hanover, NJ: Sandoz Pharmaceuticals, 1973.

The expanded edition of this atlas contains many color plates which focus on hematologic morphology. Deals with normal and abnormal structure. Morphologies are cross-referenced. Also includes clearly labeled diagrams and well-written text. Useful reference for classroom, laboratory, and office.
R: *Annals of Internal Medicine* 79: 930 (Dec. 1973); *JAMA* 227: 1065 (Mar. 14, 1974); *NEJM* 289: 1316 (Dec. 13, 1973); *Postgraduate Medicine* 56: 66 (1974).

Text-Atlas of Hematology. **Matthew H. Block.** Philadelphia, PA: Lea & Febiger, 1976.
Pathophysiological and morphological correlations of hematology through illustrations of tissue sections and smears. Among subjects covered are biopsy techniques, red and white blood cells, diseases of the blood. Thoroughly indexed. As an atlas and text, should become a standard reference for pathologists, oncologists, and hematologists.
R: *Archives of Internal Medicine* 137: 1737 (Dec. 1977); *JAMA* 238: 429 (Aug. 1, 1977); *Lahey Clinic Foundation Bulletin* 27: 34 (Jan.–Mar. 1978); *ARBA* (1977, p. 704); Brandon.

Ultrastructure of Haemic Cells: A Cytological Atlas of Normal and Leukaemic Blood and Bone Marrow. **J. C. Cawley and F. G. J. Hayhoe.** Philadelphia, PA: W. B. Saunders, 1973.
Descriptive atlas of normal and abnormal blood and marrow cells. There are electron micrographs of each cell type and sequential illustration of cell changes in disease. Illustrations are clearly labeled. Contains bibliography. A helpful reference for hematologists.
R: *Annals of Internal Medicine* 81: 420 (Sept. 1974); *Blood* 45: 597 (1975); *BMJ* 1: 332 (Feb. 23, 1974); *JAMA* 228: 1433 (June 10, 1974).

INFECTIOUS DISEASES

Atlas of Diagnostic Microbiology. **S. Stanley Schneierson, ed.** North Chicago, IL: Abbott Laboratories, 1974.
For laboratory use, an atlas of microbiology which covers bacteriology, mycology, and parasitology. Concise, introductory work which covers all pertinent main points.
R: *Archives of Pathology & Laboratory Medicine* 101: 109 (Feb. 1977).

Atlas of Medical Helminthology and Protozoology. 2d ed. **H. C. Jeffrey and R. M. Leach.** New York: Churchill Livingstone, 1975.
A product of the Royal Army Medical College. Visually highlights tropical medicine. Well illustrated with concise drawings of the life cycles, pathology, and diagnostic features of all known parasites. Particularly helpful with diseases such as malaria, trypanosomiasis, a whole host of parasitic diseases, etc. Atlas audience includes medical students and practitioners.
R: *BMJ* 1: 49 (Jan. 3, 1976).

An Atlas of Medical Microbiology: Common Human Pathogens. **B. C. Stratford.** Philadelphia, PA: J. B. Lippincott, 1977.
Covers all topics in microbiology. Excellent color illustrations enhance the text. Recommended as a reference source to medical students, nurses, medical technologists, and biology students.

Atlas of Medical Parasitology. **Viqar Zaman.** Philadelphia, PA: Lea & Febiger, 1979.
A color atlas visually displays the morphology, life cycle, and clinical aspects of important parasites. High-quality color illustrations. For microbiologists, public

health workers, and parasitologists.
R: *BMJ* 1: 1619 (June 16, 1979).

Bacteriology Illustrated. 3d ed. **R. R. Gillies and T. C. Dodds.** Edinburgh: Churchill Livingstone, 1973.

An atlas of bacteriology; clear illustrations and text. Third edition includes sections on mycology and protozoology; however, lacks some information on mycology. A valuable aid to medical students.
R: *Laboratory Practice* 23: 73 (Feb. 1974).

Color Atlas and Textbook of Diagnostic Microbiology. **Elmer W. Koneman.** Philadelphia, PA: J. B. Lippincott, 1979.

Identifies bacteria commonly tested in laboratories. Contains 40 color plates, test procedure charts, and material on antimicrobial testing. Recent, up-to-date procedures.

Color Atlas of Medical Mycology. **Jean Delacrétaz, Dodé Grigoriu, and Georges Ducel, eds.** Bern, Switzerland: Hans Huber, 1976.

An English translation of a French atlas of clinical disease caused by fungi. Concisely outlines biology, classification, and identification, accompanied by over 400 photographs. Describes a wide variety of fungi accurately and completely. Highly recommended to mycologists and physicians.
R: *BMJ* 1: 718 (Mar. 12, 1977); *Canadian Medical Association Journal* 117: 738 (Oct. 8, 1977); *JAMA* 238: 2075 (Nov. 7, 1977).

Color Atlas of Microbiology. **R. J. Olds.** Chicago, IL: Year Book Medical Publishers, 1975.

Latest volume in the Wolfe series of color atlases. A high-quality collection of 398 color photographs, illustrating common bacteria, fungi, and microbiological tests. Magnification, variety, and quality of photographs add up to an excellent reference source for laboratory and clinical workers.
R: *Journal of Allied Health* 4: 49 (Summer 1975); *Laboratory Practice* 24: 101 (Feb. 1975); *RSR* 3: 32 (Apr.–June 1975).

A Colour Atlas of Tropical Medicine and Parasitology. **Wallace Peters and Herbert M. Gilles.** London: Wolfe, 1976.

Over 760 illustrations of parasitic disorders common to tropical areas. Also includes fifteen tables which describe parasites and their vectors. Valuable to doctors, parasitologists, medical students. Also available in Spanish.
R: *Lancet* 1: 518 (March 5, 1977).

INTERNAL MEDICINE

A Color Atlas of Histological Staining Techniques. **Arthur Smith and J. W. Bruton.** Chicago, IL: Year Book Medical Publishers, 1978.

An illustrated reference on techniques and standards in histology. Available also in Spanish.

ONCOLOGY AND NUCLEAR MEDICINE

Atlas of Cancer Mortality for U.S. Counties: 1950–1969, DHEW Pub. no. (NIH) 75-780. **Thomas J. Mason et al.** Bethesda, MD: US Department of Health, Education, and Welfare, US National Institutes of Health, 1975.

Presents cancer mortality rates by geographic location and age through the use of color-keyed maps and tables. Maps can be read concurrently with tables, giving a clear understanding of subject matter. Helpful to cancer researchers and epidemiologists.

R: *Annals of Internal Medicine* 83: 914 (Dec. 1975).

Atlas of Nuclear Medicine. 4 vols. **Pablo E. Dibos and Henry N. Wagner, Jr.** Philadelphia, PA: W. B. Saunders, 1969–1978.

Volume 1, *Brain,* 1969; volume 2, *Lung,* 1970; volume 3, *Reticuloendothelial System, Liver, Spleen, and Thyroid,* 1972; volume 4, *Bone,* 1978.

A new, four-volume atlas of nuclear medicine. Displays excellent organization of typical cases, editorial content, quality of photographic reproductions of scan, and clear, well-drawn illustrations. Valuable addition to hospital libraries which service nuclear medicine departments. A reference atlas for physicians involved in the interpretations of various scanning procedures.

R: *American Journal of Roentgenology* 133: 369 (Aug. 1979); *Archives of Internal Medicine* 132: 624 (Oct. 1973); *Canadian Medical Association Journal* 102: 767 (Apr. 11, 1970); *Journal of Bone & Joint Surgery* 61A: 798 (July 1979); *Lancet* 1: 1007 (May 12, 1979); *Radiology* 132: 168 (July 1979); *ARBA* (1973, p. 675).

Atlas of Tumor Pathology. **Armed Forces Institute of Pathology.** Washington, DC: Armed Forces Institute of Pathology, 1949–

Second series published in the 1970s in several fascicles, such as Fascicle 6, *Tumors of the Central Nervous System,* by L. J. Rubinstein, 1972; Fascicle 7, *Tumors of the Esophagus and Stomach,* by S'-Chun Ming, 1973; Fascicle 8, *Tumors of the Male Genital System,* by F. K. Mostofi and E. B. Price, 1973; Fascicle 9, *Tumors of the Extra-Adrenal Paraganglion System (Including Chemoreceptors),* by G. G. Glenner and P. M. Grimley, 1974; Fascicle 10, *Tumors of the Major Salivary Glands,* by A. C. Thackray and R. B. Lucas, 1974; Fascicle 13, *Tumors of the Thymus,* by J. Rosai and G. D. Levine, 1976.

A series of fascicles published under the auspices of the Armed Forces Institute of Pathology in conjunction with the National Cancer Institute and the American Cancer Society. Atlas designed to set standards of diagnosis and terminology. Characterized by excellent illustrations, most of which are naked-eye photographs of tumors or light micrographs of structures, and a lucid writing style. Publication continues the high level of excellence of previous volumes.

R: *Annals of Internal Medicine* 79: 931 (Dec. 1973); 81: 285 (Aug. 1974); *Archives of Pathology & Laboratory Medicine* 99: 68 (Jan. 1975); 102: 332 (1978); *Brain* 96: 647 (Sept. 1973); *Chest* 72: 20 (July 1977); *Journal of Clinical Pathology* 27: 85 (1974); 32: 311 (Mar. 1979); *Neurology* 23: 895 (Aug. 1973); *NEJM* 296: 400 (Feb. 17, 1977).

Radiological Atlas of Bone Tumors. Vol. 2. **Netherlands Committee on Bone Tumours.** Baltimore, MD: Williams & Wilkins, 1973.

Comprehensive documentation of benign tumors and tumorlike lesions on bone; illustrated through the use of radiographs which are well reproduced. Tumors classified in accordance with general pathologic practice; includes descriptions of salient clinical and pathologic features. This second companion volume contains a wealth of information, useful data, and is highly recommended for medical libraries.
R: *JAMA* 227: 945 (Feb. 25, 1974); *NEJM* 289: 1318 (Dec. 13, 1973); *Radiology* 110: 276 (1974).

OPHTHALMOLOGY

Atlas of Cataract Surgery. **William H. Havener and Sallie L. Gloeckner.** St. Louis, MO: C. V. Mosby, 1972.

A highly detailed account of the authors' cataract surgical procedures which include use of an operating microscope. Includes valuable illustrations; recommended to cataract surgeons.
R: *American Journal of Ophthalmology* 76: 167 (July 1973); *Archives of Ophthalmology* 90: 424 (Nov. 1973).

An Atlas of Diseases of the Eye. 2d ed. **E. S. Perkins and Peter Hansell.** Baltimore, MD: Williams & Wilkins, 1971.

First edition, 1957.
Organized for ready access to information on problems in ophthalmology. Illustrates most common diseases with the help of color and black-and-white photographs, drawings, and diagrams. Valuable to the student and general practitioner. Indexed.
R: *American Family Physician* 7: 203 (Feb. 1973); *American Journal of Ophthalmology* 75: 737 (Apr. 1973); *Archives of Ophthalmology* 90: 86 (July 1973).

Atlas of External Diseases of the Eye. **David D. Donaldson.** St. Louis, MO: C. V. Mosby, 1973.

Volume 4, *Anterior Chamber, Iris, and Ciliary Body.*
Emphasizes external ocular diseases, including the anterior segment of the eye minus the lens. Main feature is the sixteen reels of stereoscopic color transparencies and attached stereo viewer. Black-and-white photographs, accompanied by text, enhance the atlas's usefulness. Includes some well-documented case histories. Primarily a teaching atlas. A must for ophthalmologists and students of ophthalmology.
R: *American Journal of Ophthalmology* 77: 928 (June 1974); *Archives of Ophthalmology* 91: 428 (May 1974); *JAMA* 228: 1302 (June 3, 1974).

Atlas of Eye Surgery and Related Anatomy. **Frederick H. Davidorf and Donald A. Keller, eds.** Columbus, OH: Ophthalmology Illustrated, 1979.

Illustrates anatomy and surgery of the eye. Emphasizes use of operating microscope. Clear, up-to-date discussions. Useful for eye surgeons.
R: *Lancet* 1: 1379 (June 30, 1979).

Differential Diagnosis of Eye Diseases. **Hans Pau. Gerhard W. Cibis, trans.** Philadelphia, PA: W. B. Saunders, 1978.

Atlas depicts all aspects of many ophthalmic afflictions. Text enhanced by hundreds of black-and-white illustrations and 32 full-color plates.

Ocular Pathology: A Text and Atlas. **Myron Yanoff and Ben S. Fine.** Hagerstown, MD: Harper & Row, 1975.
Significant contribution to the literature of ophthalmic pathology. Consists of 700 pages in an outline format. Over 1,600 illustrations present an equal balance between clinical, pathological, and schematic material. Includes an extensive index and hundreds of references (many of classical importance). Up-to-date guide for residents in ophthalmology and pathology. Valuable reference for advanced pathologists and ophthalmologists.
R: *American Journal of Ophthalmology* 81: 542 (Apr. 1976); *Archives of Ophthalmology* 94: 1054 (June 1976); *JAMA* 234: 762 (Nov. 17, 1975).

ORTHOPEDICS

An Atlas of Examination, Standard Measurements and Diagnosis in Orthopedics and Traumatology. **Otto Russe, ed.** Baltimore, MD: Williams & Wilkins, 1972.
Focuses on established knowledge about examination of the vertebral column and extremities from a musculoskeletal, neurologic, and vascular viewpoint. Richly illustrated with diagrams and photographs. Includes standardized, international terminology. Highly recommended for physiatrists, orthopedists, and medical students. Basic reference source for rehabilitation department library, casualty insurance adjudication, and the law.
R: *Archives of Physical Medicine and Rehabilitation* 58: 142 (Mar. 1977); 58: 186 (Apr. 1977); *Journal of Bone and Joint Surgery* 55A: 1330 (1973); *JAMA* 227: 1183 (Mar. 11, 1974); *NEJM* 289: 928 (Oct. 25, 1973).

Atlas of Hand Radiographs. **Philip Jacobs.** Baltimore, MD: University Park Press, 1973.
Four volumes devoted to 147 diseases manifesting radiographic changes in the hands and wrists. Beautifully illustrated with 300 life-size reproductions of hand roentgenograms. Captions supply the only text. Major drawback is the lack of a bibliography. Geared toward radiologists and trainees. An aid to diagnosis for the rheumatologist, nephrologist, and general practitioner.
R: *American Journal of Roentgenology* 126: 913 (Apr. 1976); *British Journal of Radiology* 47: 178 (1974); *Lancet* 2: 86 (July 13, 1974); *NEJM* 289: 928 (Oct. 25, 1973).

Atlas of Hand Surgery. **Robert A. Chase.** Philadelphia, PA: W. B. Saunders, 1973.
Surverys surgical operations of the hand. Proceeds in a logical manner from basic principles to reconstructive surgery. Reflects the personal experience of the author as noted in the many case studies. Each section generously illustrated with excellent line drawings, roentgenograms, and clinical photographs. Powerful presentation on nerve, vascular, and tendon trauma. Classic atlas for physical therapists and surgeons.
R: *Archives of Surgery* 110: 132 (Jan. 1975); *Journal of Bone and Joint Surgery* 56A:

652 (Mar. 1974); *Physical Therapy* 54: 1042 (1974); *Plastic and Reconstructive Surgery* 53: 586 (1974).

Atlas of Hand Surgery. **Marc Iselin et al. John C. Colwill, trans.** New York: McGraw-Hill, 1964.

Atlas of Orthopaedic Surgery. 2 vols. **Louis A. Goldstein and Robert C. Dickerson.** St. Louis, MO: C. V. Mosby, 1974.

Two-volume atlas of over 200 selected orthopedic, surgical procedures. Arranged by anatomical region. Features 1,674 elegant illustrations with supplemental line drawings. Text is located on the left with corresponding illustrations on the right. Sixteen chapters are fully referenced with classical and up-to-date citations. The subject and author indexes are comprehensive. Obvious weakness is the lack of diversity and personal preference of surgical procedures. Highly recommended to practicing surgeons, orthopedic residents, interns, and students of medicine.

R: *British Journal of Surgery* 62: 756 (Sept. 1975); *Journal of Bone and Joint Surgery* 58B: 148 (Feb. 1976); *Journal of Neurosurgery* 42: 241 (Feb. 1975); *JAMA* 230: 906 (Nov. 11, 1974); *NEJM* 292: 375 (Feb. 13, 1975); *RSR* 2: 118 (July–Sept. 1974); 3: 42 (Jan.–Mar. 1975).

Atlas of Orthotics: Biomechanical Principles and Application. **American Academy of Orthopaedic Surgeons.** St. Louis, MO: C. V. Mosby, 1975.

Approved by the Committee on Prosthetics and Orthotics of the American Academy of Orthopaedic Surgeons. Reflects the most up-to-date information on orthotic devices and appliances from a biomechanical standpoint. Text divided into six parts; employs case studies to handle each condition. More than 800 illustrations complement the text. All 35 contributors are specialists in the field of orthotics. Belongs on the reading list of all physical therapists, physicians, and biomedical engineers.

R: *Journal of Bone and Joint Surgery* 58A: 293 (Mar. 1976); *Physical Therapy* 56: 1080 (1976); 57: 970 (1977).

Fairbank's Atlas of General Affections of the Skeleton. 2d ed. **Ruth Wynne-Davies and T. J. Fairbank.** New York: Churchill Livingstone, 1976.

First edition, 1951.

The second edition of this classic atlas which deals with disorders of the skeletal system includes a wealth of new information such as the identification of new disorders. Disease descriptions are clearly and concisely organized. The atlas is profusely illustrated, containing some 460 radiographs. Comprehensive coverage of skeletal disease. A well-recommended atlas for libraries, orthopedists, physical therapists. Includes helpful index and tables.

R: *American Journal of Diseases of Children* 132: 100 (Jan. 1978); *Archives of Physical Medicine and Rehabilitation* 58: 378 (Aug. 1977); *BMJ* 2: 39 (July 7, 1977); *Clinical Pediatrics* 17: 658 (Aug. 1978); *JAMA* 237: 2757 (June 20, 1977); *Physical Therapy* 57: 1223 (1977); *Radiology* 126: 66 (1978).

Muscle and Its Innervation: An Atlas of Fine Structure. **Y. Ufhara, G. R. Campbell, and G. Burnstock.** London: Edward Arnold, 1976.

Covers characteristics of muscle. Features illustrative plates of high quality. La-

beling of plates unsatisfactory. Text characterized by simple lucid statements. Several useful references follow the nine chapters.
R: *Journal of Anatomy* 127: 194 (Sept. 1978).

OTORHINOLARYNGOLOGY

An Atlas of Otolaryngologic Radiology. **Judith Zizmor and Arnold M. Noyek.** Philadelphia, PA: W. B. Saunders, 1978.
A well-illustrated diagnostic aid.

Color Atlas of Ear, Nose and Throat. **T. R. Bull.** Chicago, IL: Year Book Medical Publishers, 1974.

Human Larynx-Coronal Section Atlas. **Gabriel F. Tucker, Jr.** Washington, DC: Armed Forces Institute of Pathology, 1971.
Deals primarily with the field of laryngology. Presents 37 different levels of the normal human larynx. Black-and-white photographs are of high quality. Valuable as a teaching aid for residents in otolaryngology and as a reference source for otolaryngologists and pathologists.
R: *Annals of Otology, Rhinology and Laryngology* 83: 416 (1975); *Archives of Otolaryngology* 98: 434 (Dec. 1973).

PATHOLOGY

An Advanced Atlas of Histology. **W. H. Freeman and Brian Bracegirdle.** London: Heinemann Educational, 1976.
Not an advanced atlas. Illustrations and tables comprise the bulk of this book. Illustrations are at the light microscope level and consist of black-and-white photomicrographs accompanied by well-labeled line drawings. Also includes sixteen excellent color plates. Most material illustrated derived from mammals other than humans. Very serviceable introduction to histology for technicians and undergraduate biology majors.
R: *BMJ* 1: 1350 (May 29, 1976); *Lancet* 2: 720 (Oct. 2, 1976).

Atlas of Arterial Histology. **Donald F. M. Bunce II.** St. Louis, MO: Warren H. Green, 1975.
Aims to illustrate the structure of 82 named arteries, providing a ready reference source to normal morphology through the use of photomicrographs. Contains two differently stained sections of each artery in its collapsed state. Detailed, clear presentation.

An Atlas of Artifacts: Encountered in the Preparation of Microscopic Tissue Sections. **Samuel W. Thompson II and Lee G. Luna.** Springfield, IL: Charles C. Thomas, 1978.
Illustrates, with the aid of 500 photographs, how faulty histological preparation can interfere with interpretation. Gives examples of most commonly encountered problems. Helpful to pathologists, morphologists, and histotechnicians.

Atlas of Cell Biology. **Jean-Claude Roland, Annette Szöllösi, and Daniel Szöllösi.** Boston, MA: Little, Brown, 1977.

Electron micrographs of cell ultrastructure which are accompanied by corresponding line drawings, both of excellent quality. Text is brief. Useful as an introductory source to cell biology.
R: *Journal of Neurosurgery* 49: 154 (July 1978).

Atlas of Diagnostic Cytology. **Claude Gompel.** Chichester, Sussex, England: John Wiley, 1978.

An atlas of over 360 color plates which deal with diagnostic and clinical aspects of cytological morphology. An up-to-date, worthy reference for medical students and cytologists.
R: *Journal of Clinical Pathology* 32: 94 (1979); *Nature* 274: 96 (July 6, 1978). Also reviewed in *Human Pathology* (Sept. 1978) and *Journal of the Royal Society of Medicine* (Jan. 1979).

Atlas of Gross Neurosurgical Pathology. **Klaus J. Zülch.** New York: Springer-Verlag, 1975.

Written as a companion volume to *Atlas of the Histology of Brain Tumors* (1971) by the same author. Devoted entirely to gross pathology. Initially discusses the structural effects of increased intracranial pressure. Remainder of volume concentrates on various types of brain neoplasms. Text is short; references limited. Features 379 excellent illustrations (photographs and diagrams). Minor criticism in the use of older nomenclature. High-quality atlas, should be of value to neuroradiologists, neurologists, and neurosurgeons.
R: *Annals of Internal Medicine* 83: 593 (Oct. 1975); *Archives of Neurology* 33: 665 (Sept. 1976); *Archives of Surgery* 111: 95 (Jan. 1976); *Journal of Neurosurgery* 43: 779 (Dec. 1975); *RSR* 3: 34 (Apr.–June 1975).

An Atlas of Histology. **Johannes A. G. Rhodin.** London: Oxford University Press, 1975.

A complete reproduction of the atlas section of *Histology: A Text and Atlas.*

Atlas of Human Histology. 3d ed. **Mariano S. H. di Fiore.** Philadelphia, PA: Lea & Febiger, 1974.

Reviews three basic histological fields: histochemistry, morphology, and ultrastructure. Detailed description of histochemical reactions accompany color micrographs. Over 100 fine color reproductions complement the morphological and ultrastructural presentations. Includes brief explanation of standard histological techniques.
R: *ARBA* (1974, p. 633).

Atlas of Microscopic Anatomy: A Companion to Histology and Neuroanatomy. **Ronald A. Bergman and Adel K. Afifi.** Philadelphia, PA: W. B. Saunders, 1974.

Designed as a companion to the study of histology. Basically a collection of 300 colored plates of histological preparations of cells, tissues, and organs. Contains helpful appendixes on the preparation of microscopic slides and comments on different techniques of staining and fixation. Not intended to replace standard histology textbook. Planned as an aid to the student; useful reference source in physiology, biochemistry, and pathology departments.

R: *American Scientist* 63: 469 (July–Aug. 1975); *Journal of Anatomy* 123: 227 (Feb. 1977); *Lancet* 1: 1200 (June 15, 1974); *NEJM* 291: 584 (Sept. 12, 1974).

Atlas of Neonatal Histopathology. **Augusto Moragas, Angel Ballabriga, and Maria T. Vidal.** Philadelphia, PA: W. B. Saunders, 1977.

An atlas provides sketches of neonatal pathology through use of color photomicrographs. Generally well produced. Recommended for clinical pathologists.
R: *Archives of Pathology & Laboratory Medicine* 103: 490 (Aug. 1979); *NEJM* 299: 204 (July 27, 1978).

Atlas of Pathologic Anatomy. **Wilheim Doerr, Gerhild Schumann, and Günter Ule.** Littleton, MA: Publishing Sciences Group, 1978.

Arranged systematically, considered a fine atlas of gross and microscopic pathology. Translated from the German edition, the volume includes excellent photomicrographs. Intended for pathologists.
R: *Archives of Pathology & Laboratory Medicine* 103: 548 (Sept. 1979).

Atlas of Scanning Electron Microscopy in Medicine. **Tsuneo Fujita et al.** New York: American Elsevier, 1971.

R: *Transactions of the American Microscopial Society* 91: 76 (Jan. 1972); *TBRI* 38: 57 (Mar. 1972).

Atlas of the Ultrastructure of Human Breast Diseases. **Ali Ahmed.** New York: Churchill Livingstone, 1978.

Electron micrographs which help to illustrate breast pathology. Covers all common as well as some less common breast lesions. Useful for electron histopathologists.
R: *Journal of Clinical Pathology* 32: 310 (Mar. 1979).

A Brief Atlas of Histology. **T. S. Leeson and C. R. Leeson.** Philadelphia, PA: W. B. Saunders, 1979.

Illustrates all body structures as histological sections. Utilizes 40 different stains to attain the high standard of preparation. Chapters are systems oriented. Features over 450 color pictures including electronmicrographs, detailed diagrams, and pictures of freeze-itch preparations. Atlas neglects to relate function to structure. Despite this shortcoming, valuable atlas for physiologists, pathologists, and clinicians.
R: *Lancet* 1: 1169 (June 2, 1979).

Cell Fine Structure: An Atlas of Drawings of Whole-Cell Structure. **Thomas L. Lentz.** Philadelphia, PA: W. B. Saunders, 1971.

Consists of close to 200 full page line drawings accompanied by cytologic, structural, functional description. Clearly presented information; a helpful reference for students and researchers.
R: *Archives of Internal Medicine* 131: 310 (Feb. 1973).

Color Atlas and Textbook of Macropathology. 2d ed. **Walter Sandritter and C. Thomas Sandritter.** Chicago, IL: Year Book Medical Publishers, 1976.

First edition, 1972.
Second edition contains high-quality color photographs accompanied by concise legends; serves to illustrate pathology of disease. Helpful in diagnosis. Contains useful index and references.
R: *Journal of Clinical Pathology* 30: 393 (Apr. 1977); *Lancet* 1: 408 (Feb. 24, 1973); *Medical Journal of Australia* 1: 827 (May 28, 1977); *NEJM* 289: 164 (July 19, 1973); *ARBA* (1974, p. 635).

Color Atlas of Histopathology. Rev. ed. **R. C. Curran.** New York: Oxford University Press, 1972.

Original edition, 1966; republished each year to 1970.
A standard atlas of histopathology; photo reproduction in atlas is excellent. A good source for illustrations of histologic lesions. Recommended to pathologists.
R: *Annals of Internal Medicine* 78: 323 (Feb. 1973); *Archives of Internal Medicine* 133: 160 (Jan. 1974).

Color Atlas of Pathology. 3 vols. **US Naval Medical School of the National Naval Medical Center.** Philadelphia, PA: J. B. Lippincott, 1950–1963.

Volume 1, 1950; volume 2, out of print; volume 3, *Central Nervous System*, 1963.
A comprehensive source. Photographs and photomicrographs are of excellent quality and are in color.

A Colour Atlas of Forensic Pathology. **Geoffrey A. Gresham.** London: Wolfe, 1975.

A color photographic atlas of forensic pathology. Recommended to police surgeons, pathology residents. Contains a good bibliography.
R: *Lancet* 1: 958 (Apr. 26, 1975); *Medical Journal of Australia* 2: 776 (Nov. 15, 1975); *TBRI* 42: 99 (Mar. 1976).

A Colour Atlas of Histology. **M. B. L. Craigmyle.** London: Wolfe, 1975.

Over 500 color photomicrographs of normal histology. Gives brief description of structure of organs illustrated. Helpful as a supplement to textbooks. Students and residents of pathology will profit most from this book.
R: *BMJ* 2: 473 (Nov. 22, 1975); *Laboratory Practice* 25: 322 (May 1976); *Lancet* 1: 180 (Jan. 24, 1976).

Gross Pathology: A Color Atlas. **R. C. Curran and E. L. Jones.** New York: Oxford University Press, 1974.

Companion volume to R. C. Curran's *Color Atlas of Histopathology*. Illustrates common and unknown lesions of general and organ pathology. Over 750 color photographs of high quality, complemented by a concise text. Contains comprehensive index. Valuable investment for the teaching budget or medical school library. Good review for the pathology resident or student preparing for medical school examinations.
R: *Annals of Internal Medicine* 83: 298 (Aug. 1975); *Archives of Pathology & Laboratory Medicine* 100: 59 (Jan. 1976); *Archives of Surgery* 110: 850 (July 1975); *JAMA* 231: 1395 (Mar. 31, 1975); *Lancet* 2: 1182 (Nov. 16, 1974); *RSR* 3: 42 (Jan.–Mar. 1975).

Gynecologic Cytopathology: A Color Atlas of Differential Diagnosis. **Marie Louise Schneider and Hans-Joachim Staemmler. Volker Schneider, trans.** Philadelphia, PA: W. B. Saunders, 1978.
Illustrates cytopathology of gynecological diseases using full-color illustrations and helpful text. Covers a variety of diseases.

Microanatomy of Cell and Tissue Surfaces: An Atlas of Scanning Electron Microscopy. **Pietro Motta, Peter M. Andrews, and Keith R. Porter.** Philadelphia, PA: Lea & Febiger, 1977.
An outstanding atlas for histologists, biologists. Clear depictions of cell surface and microanatomy.

PEDIATRICS

Atlas of Abdominal Ultrasonography in Children. **Gary F. Gates.** London: Churchill Livingstone, 1978.
Clinical orientation. Offers practical hints on the use of ultrasonography in the pediatric examination. Good correspondence between text and illustration. Written in an easy-to-read style.
R: *Journal of Nuclear Medicine* 20: 175 (Feb. 1979).

An Atlas of Children's Surgery. **Robert E. Gross.** Philadelphia, PA: W. B. Saunders, 1970.
Based on the author's immense experience at Boston's Children's Hospital. Carefully outlines standard techniques and procedures of operative surgery. Illustrations include brief descriptive captions. Includes outstanding bibliography and index.
R: *BMJ* 4: 417 (Nov. 14, 1970).

Atlas of Pediatric Echocardiography. **Howard P. Gutgesell and Marc Paquet.** New York: Harper & Row, 1978.
A one-volume collection of echocardiograms with accompanying clear and precise legends. Illustrations are of high quality. For pediatricians, cardiologists, and ultrasound technologists.
R: *American Heart Journal* 97: 819 (June 1979); *Canadian Medical Association Journal* 119: 124 (July 22, 1978).

Atlas of Pediatric Surgery. 2d ed. **Robert P. White, ed.** New York: McGraw-Hill, 1978.
Comprehensive coverage of pediatric surgery. Describes in detail operative procedures and major surgical complications. Second edition features 28 new chapters. Combines illustrations with practical discussions. Numerous contributions from specialists in the pediatric field.

Atlas of Roentgen Anatomy of the Newborn and Infant Skull: Including Illustrations of Some Pathologic Changes and Congenital Variations with Emphasis on Fetal Radiology. **Charles N. Chasler.** St. Louis, MO: Warren H. Green, 1972.
Authoritative presentation of abnormalities in the newborn skull. Beautifully il-

lustrated atlas is composed of seven sections; newborn skull fractures receive particular attention. Illustrations drawn from over 100,000 roentgenograms. Includes good index and bibliography. This collection of skull roentgenograms makes a useful atlas for obstetricians, pediatricians, and radiologists.
R: *Pediatrics* 51: 166 (Jan. 1973); *Teratology* 8: 75 (Aug. 1973); *ARBA* (1973, p. 675).

Atlas of Surgery in the First Six Months of Life. **S. Frank Redo.** New York/Hagerstown, MD: Harper & Row, 1978.
Covers the surgical techniques commonly used in operative procedures to correct problems of the abdomen, head and neck, and chest encountered in the first six months of life. Format is concise, well organized. Illustrations are clear, well labeled. Shows standard as well as alternative surgical methods.
R: *Archives of Surgery* 114: 642 (May 1979); *British Journal of Surgery* 66: 218 (Mar. 1979).

Atlas of the Newborn. **Neil O'Doherty.** Lancaster, England: MTP, 1979.
Over 500 color photographs which help to familiarize the user with conditions of the newborn. Illustrations are well labeled. Recommended to all those who work with newborns.
R: *Lancet* 1: 958 (May 5, 1979).

The Cranium of the Newborn Infant: An Atlas of Tomography and Anatomical Sections, DHEW Pub. no. (NIH) 78-788. **Robert H. Pierce, Michael W. Mainen, and James F. Bosma.** Bethesda, MD: US Department of Health, Education, and Welfare, 1978.
A tomographic atlas with accompanying anatomical illustrations, well organized and referenced. For radiologists and pediatricians.
R: *American Journal of Radiology* 133: 177 (July 1979).

Surgery of the Neonate. **Arnold C. Coran et al.** Boston, MA: Little, Brown, 1978.
A well-illustrated atlas of neonatal surgery, which includes all basic techniques. Clear and easy to follow. Recommended for both beginning and advanced pediatric surgeons.
R: *BMJ* 1: 1481 (June 2, 1979); *Lancet* 2: 128 (July 21, 1979).

PHYSICAL MEDICINE AND REHABILITATION

Atlas of Plaster Cast Techniques. 2d ed. **Eugene E. Bleck et al.** Chicago, IL: Year Book Medical Publishers, 1974.

Physically Handicapped Children: A Medical Atlas for Teachers. **Eugene E. Bleck and Donald A. Nagel, eds.** New York: Grune & Stratton, 1975.
Written specifically for special education students and teachers. Covers anatomy, nervous, muscular, and skeletal systems and is geared toward problems and needs of physically handicapped children. Subjects arranged alphabetically for quick reference. A timely book, written in nontechnical terms with helpful glossary.

R: *Archives of Physical Medicine and Rehabilitation* 58: 189 (Apr. 1977); *Physical Therapy* 56: 508 (1976).

PUBLIC HEALTH

Atlas of Diagnostic and Therapeutic Procedures for Emergency Personnel. **James H. Cosgriff, Jr.** Philadelphia, PA: J. B. Lippincott, 1978.

Profusely illustrated, detailed descriptions of diagnostic and therapeutic procedures in emergency situations. Contains well-presented, wide-ranging information. Procedures are in alphabetical order. An up-to-date reference source.
R: Brandon (*NO*).

National Atlas of Disease Mortality in the United Kingdom. 2d ed. **G. Melvyn Howe.** London: Nelson, 1970.

Limited to fourteen major killing diseases. Concentrates on material from 1959 to 1963. Visual effect achieved by maps and transparent overlays. Maps contain about 9,000 tidbits of information in the form of standard mortality ratios (SMR) for every administrative area in the United Kingdom. Mentions possible related factors like water hardness, smoking, air pollution.
R: *Lancet* 1: 702 (Mar. 28, 1970).

RADIOLOGY

Atlas of Computed Body Tomography: Normal and Abnormal Anatomy. **Lee C. Chiu and Rolf L. Schapiro.** Baltimore, MD: University Park Press, 1980.

Correlates gross anatomy as shown by cross-sectional computed tomography, with meticulous line drawings and radiographs of cadavers. Features 650 high-quality illustrations. Ideal reference for radiologists, ultrasonographers, nuclear imaging specialists, and anatomists.

Atlas of Gray Scale Ultrasonography. **Kenneth J. W. Taylor.** New York: Churchill-Livingstone, 1978.

Imparts an overview of ultrasound imaging and diagnostic capabilities. Characterized by excellent images and line drawings. Covers various anatomical features: abdomen, thyroid, thorax, etc. Useful introduction for beginning ultrasonographer and reference text for clinician.
R: *American Journal of Roentgenology* 131: 947 (Nov. 1978); *Physics in Medicine and Biology* 24: 200 (Jan. 1979); *Radiology* 132: 420 (Aug. 1979).

An Atlas of Non-Invasive Techniques: Sound and Pulse Tracings—Echograms. **Aldo A. Luisada, Gloria L. Perez, and Pachalla K. Bhat.** Springfield, IL: Charles C. Thomas, 1976.

Two hundred fifty-one illustrations of noninvasive recordings in cardiology highlight this atlas. Most recordings include tracings of common cardiac problems. Interpretations and discussions of these tracings are excellent. Useful atlas for residents and fellows training in cardiology.
R: *American Heart Journal* 94: 541 (Oct. 1977); *Annals of Internal Medicine* 87: 385 (Sept. 1977); *Chest* 72: 27 (Sept. 1977).

An Atlas of Normal Roentgen Variants That May Simulate Disease. **Theodore E. Keates.** Chicago, IL: Year Book Medical Publishers, 1973–1975.

Emphasizes the recognition of normal variants in diagnostic radiology. Half of atlas devoted to normal variants in the skeletal system. High-quality illustrations accompanied by succinct captions. Does not include an index. However, table of contents is very complete. Recommended to resident and practicing radiologists and trauma and emergency room physicians.

R: *BMJ* 4: 597 (Dec. 7, 1974); *Lancet* 2: 760 (Sept. 28, 1974); *Lahey Clinic Foundation Bulletin* 25: 195 (Oct.–Dec. 1976); *Radiology* 120: 704 (Sept. 1976).

An Atlas of Radiation Histopathology, TID-26676. **David C. White.** Oak Ridge, TN: US Energy Research and Development Administration Technical Information Center, 1975.

Based on the wealth of information gathered at the US Armed Forces Institute of Pathology. The text is divided into two basic parts: a complete description of the effects of whole-body irradiation and radiation effects on special tissues and organs. Two hundred photomicrographs and 30 excellent drawings enhance the volume. Weakness lies in the abundance of pre-1970 references. Paperback edition will be an excellent addition to the libraries of all radiation biologists.

R: *British Journal of Radiology* 49: 285 (1976); *Health Physics* 31: 83 (July 1976); *JAMA* 235: 2436 (May 31, 1976).

An Atlas of Radiological Anatomy. **Jamie Weir and Peter Abrahams.** Chicago, IL: Year Book Medical Publishers, 1978.

Includes a full range of radiological examinations. Provides comparisons for all clinical problems. A useful source for evaluating roentgenographic images.

R: *American Journal of Radiology* 133: 370 (Aug. 1979); *Journal of Bone & Joint Surgery* 61A: 638 (June 1979).

Atlas of Roentgenographic Measurement. 4th ed. **Lee B. Lusted and Theodore E. Keats.** Chicago, IL: Year Book Medical Publishers, 1978.

First edition, 1959; third edition, 1972.

Fourth edition reflects the recent changes in imaging techniques and procedures. Handy reference tool for the doubtful physician faced with the interpretation of roentgenograms. Features many tables and statistical material. All data is extensively referenced. Arrangement of material according to organ system. New edition highlights the international interest in roentgenographic measurements. Designed primarily for the radiologist, but other specialists (orthopedic surgeons) will realize its value.

R: *American Journal of Roentgenology* 119: 214 (Sept. 1973); *Journal of Bone & Joint Surgery* 61A: 317 (Mar. 1979); *ARBA* (1974, p. 633).

Atlas of Roentgenographic Positions and Standard Radiologic Procedures. 4th ed. 3 vols. **Vinita Merrill.** St. Louis, MO: C. V. Mosby, 1975.

Third edition, 1967.

Completely revised fourth edition. Classic reference source in the area of roentgenographic positioning and procedures. Volume I deals extensively with the anatomy and radiography of the skeletal system. Contains improved illustrations and a new section on pediatric radiography. Volume II describes head anatomy

and radiography; no considerable changes. Volume III introduces new material on ultrasonography, thermography, and nuclear medicine. Over 1,500 illustrations complement the text. Extensive bibliography and glossary listed. Ideal quick reference source for X-ray technologists.
R: *Radiology* 117: 466 (1975); Stearns & Ratcliff (*NEJM,* 1970).

Atlas of the Human Brain and the Orbit for Computed Tomography. **William R. Scott, Joseph Hanaway, and Charles M. Strother.** St. Louis, MO: Warren H. Green, 1977.

Written by experienced authors in radiology, anatomy, and neurology. Presents cross-sectional views of the brain and orbit in the planes most commonly used in computed tomography. Anatomic sections of the head are matched with corresponding normal computed tomographic section. Includes complete cross-index of anatomic terms.

An Atlas of the Human Brain for Computerized Tomography. **Takayoshi Matsui.** New York: Igaku-Shoin Medical Publishers, 1978.

Concentrates on the cross-sectional anatomy of the brain at several planes and degrees of angulation. Excellent photographs and labeled drawings of normal anatomical structures enhance the atlas. Computerized, tomographic scans are of lesser quality. Weakness lies in the scattering of related photographs. Scans are labeled drawings throughout the text. Useful addition to medical school and radiology department libraries.
R: *Annals of Internal Medicine* 89: 733 (Nov. 1978); *Radiology* 132: 106 (July 1979).

Atlas of Tumor Radiology. 14 vols. **Philip J. Hodes, ed.** Chicago, IL: Year Book Medical Publishers, 1968–.

The Head & Neck, edited by Gilbert H. Fletcher and Bao-Shan Jing, 1968; *The Breast,* edited by David M. Witten, 1969; *The Endocrines,* edited by Howard L. Steinbach and Hideyo Minagi, 1969; *The Bones & Joints,* edited by Gwilym S. Lodwick, 1971; *The Female Reproductive System,* edited by G. Melvin Stevens, 1971; *The Kidney,* edited by John A. Evans and Morton A. Bosniak, 1971; *The Chest,* edited by Roy R. Greening and J. Haynes Heslep, 1973; *The Gastrointestinal Tract,* edited by George N. Stein and Arthur K. Finkelstein, 2 volumes, 1973; *The Vertebral Column,* edited by Bernard S. Epstein, 1974; *The Accessory Digestive Organs,* edited by Robert E. Wise and Austin P. O'Keeffe, 1975; *The Brain & the Eye,* edited by Ernest H. Wood et al., 1975; *The Adrenal, Retroperitoneum & Lower Urinary Tract,* edited by Morton A. Bosniak et al., 1976; *The Hemopoietic & Lymphatic Systems,* in preparation.

A multivolume tumor atlas series depicting radiographic changes resulting from various neoplasms. It describes radiologic features of tumors in all major organs. Plain radiographs, angiograms, and air studies illustrate the manifestations of different neoplasms. Series sponsored by the American College of Radiology under the editorship of Dr. Philip J. Hodes.
R: *American Journal of Roentgenology* 128: 542 (Mar. 1977); *BMJ* 2: 147 (Apr. 19, 1975); *NEJM* 291: 745 (Oct. 3, 1974); *Radiology* 116: 616 (1975); 121: 398 (1976).

Cerebral Computed Tomography: A Text-Atlas. **Leon A. Weisberg, Charles Nice, and Myron Katz.** Philadelphia, PA: W. B. Saunders, 1978.
Introductory textbook of tomography. Deals exclusively with the Mark I EMI scanner. Outlines data collection, resolution of data, detectors, means of projection, etc. Aimed at clinicians in a radiology department employing a CT scanner.
R: *Physics in Medicine and Biology* 24: 655 (May 1979).

Computed Brain and Orbital Tomography: Technique and Interpretation. **Carlos F. Gonzalez, Charles B. Grossman, and Enrique Palacios.** New York: John Wiley, 1976.
Helpful in correlating computed tomography to radiographic and pathologic specimens for diagnoses; brings together much basic information for teaching purposes. Deals with anatomy of the orbit and brain. Useful for neuroradiologists.
R: *Archives of Neurology* 34: 452 (July 1977); *Brain* 100: 796 (Dec. 1977).

Normal Radiologic Patterns and Variances of the Human Skeleton: An X-Ray Atlas of Adults and Children. **Rudolf Birkner.** Baltimore, MD: Urban and Schwarzenberg, 1978.
A translation of the German edition. Consists of three main sections: summary of fundamentals of image formation; examination of the normal adult skeleton, complete with excellent quality radiographs; and skeletal development in children and adolescents. Additional photographs and diagrams keyed to radiographs. Includes comprehensive index and list of references, mainly to German literature. Particularly useful reference source for medical students, radiologists, and technologists.
R: *American Journal of Radiology* 133: 370 (Aug. 1979); *Radiology* 132: 42 (July 1979).

Radiologic Transverse Anatomy of the Human Thorax, Abdomen, and Pelvis: An Atlas of Anatomic, Radiologic, Computed Tomographic, and Ultrasonic Correlation. **Alvin C. Wyman, Thomas L. Lawson, and Lawrence R. Goodman.** Boston, MA: Little, Brown, 1978.
An atlas of computerized tomography and ultrasound which correlates approaches to regional anatomy. High-quality illustrations, clinically oriented.
R: *Lancet* 1: 1119 (May 26, 1979).

Radiology of Trauma: Textbook and Atlas. **Hermann Birzle, Rudolf Bergleiter, and Eugen H. Kuner. H. J. Kaufmann, trans.** Philadelphia, PA: W. B. Saunders, 1978.
A brief introductory atlas of traumatology; helpful to radiology residents, traumatologists, orthopedic surgeons, and neurosurgeons. Contains approximately 1,000 excellent drawings which guide the user to correct interpretation of injury, along with helpful text. Recommended.
R: *American Journal of Roentgenology* 132: 699 (Apr. 1979).

RHEUMATOLOGY

Color Atlas of Rheumatology. **A. C. Boyle.** Chicago, IL: Year Book Medical Publishers, 1974.

Demonstrates clinical and radiographic features of rheumatologic arthritis. Disease characteristics are clearly expressed through the use of 150 illustrations. A helpful, ready reference for family physicians and libraries.
R: *Annals of Internal Medicine* 82: 861 (June 1975).

UROGENITAL SYSTEM

An Atlas of Gynecologic and Obstetric Pathology. **James L. Breen and William J. Jaffurs.** Philadelphia, PA: F. A. Davis, 1973.

Comprised of 197 pages of text followed by 200 color illustrations. Spiral-bound format.

Atlas of Infertility Surgery. **Robert W. Kistner and Grant W. Patton, Jr.** Boston, MA: Little, Brown, 1975.

Comprehensive presentation of infertility surgery in women. Outlines the classic and conservative surgical procedures involved in the management of infertile patients. Analyzes the merits of all mentioned procedures. Based on author's personal clinical experience. Includes 300 up-to-date references. Clear illustrations and comprehensive index round out this volume. A sensible guide for gynecologists, obstetricians, and general surgeons.
R: *BMJ* 1: 1541 (June 19, 1976); *JAMA* 236: 880 (Aug. 16, 1976); *Lahey Clinic Foundation Bulletin* 26: 51 (Jan.–Mar. 1977); *Lancet* 1: 1276 (June 12, 1976).

Atlas of Vaginal Surgery. **C. Sani and L. Kos.** New York: John Wiley, 1977.

Systematically illustrates vaginal operations through photographs and diagrams. Provides an excellent review of prolactin physiology and pathology and of bromoscriptine treatment. A must for surgeons, research workers, and clinicians.
R: *European Journal of Obstetrics, Gynecology & Reproductive Biology* 8: 237 (1978); *International Surgery* 63: 93 (May–June 1978); *Postgraduate Medicine* 64: 162 (1978).

Atlas of Vaginal Surgery: Surgical Anatomy and Technique. 2 vols. **E. A. Friedman, ed.** Philadelphia, PA: W. B. Saunders, 1975.

A fine presentation of anatomic concepts and operative techniques. Two-volume English translation of the well-written German text. Color plates complement the text. Side-by-side arrangement of illustrations and text allows for ease in visualizing each procedure. Each chapter ends with a "Technical Problems" section, which contains many hints, fine points, and special comments. Although not intended as an exhaustive volume, one good procedure for every vaginal surgery situation is presented. No references included. Worthy of inclusion in every medical library.
R: *British Journal of Obstetrics & Gynaecology* 84: 559 (July 1977); *Lahey Clinic Foundation Bulletin* 27: 36 (Jan.–Mar. 1978).

Clinical Urography: An Atlas and Textbook of Roentgenologic Diagnosis. 3d ed.

3 vols. **John L. Emmett and David M. Witten.** Philadelphia, PA: W. B. Saunders, 1971.
First edition, 1951; second edition, 1964.
Considerably updated; extensively covers radiologic studies of genitourinary disease. Contains over 2,500 illustrations which are well reproduced. Also includes fine text and bibliographers. Regarded as a necessary reference source for medical libraries.
R: *ARBA* (1972, p. 622); Allyn.

Color Atlas of Cytodiagnosis of the Prostate. **W. Staehler et al.** Chicago, IL: Year Book Medical Publishers, 1977.

A Color Atlas of Gynecological Surgery. 6 vols. **David H. Lees and Albert Singer.** Chicago, IL: Year Book Medical Publishers, 1978–1979.
Volume 1, *Vaginal Procedures*; volume 2, *Abdominal Procedures*; volume 3, *Cervical, Uterine and Ovarian Procedures*; volume 4, *Vulva*; volume 5, *Procedures for Infertility*; volume 6, *Complications of Pregnancy*.
Over 3,000 color photographs illustrating surgical procedures.

Color Atlas of Laparoscopy. **K. Beck et al.** New York: F. K. Schattauer-Verlag, 1970.
An English translation from a German atlas which reviews the peritoneum and liver systems. Contains 385 photographs of extreme clarity in addition to numerous references. Recommended to gastroenterologists and surgeons of all levels.
R: *Archives of Internal Medicine* 131: 756 (May 1973).

Color Atlas of Renal Diseases. **George Williams.** Chicago, IL: Year Book Medical Publishers, 1973.

Emmett's Clinical Urography: An Atlas and Textbook of Roentgenologic Diagnosis. 4th ed. 3 vols. **David M. Witten, George H. Myers, and David C. Utz, eds.** Philadelphia, PA: W. B. Saunders, 1977.
First edition, 1951; second edition, 1964; third edition, 1971.
A classic atlas of radiographic diagnosis of urology; consists of over 3,000 illustrations; encyclopedic in scope. Thoroughly updated, including new information on various aspects of renal disease. A handy reference for students, clinicians, and practitioners.
R: *American Journal of Roentgenology* 131: 763 (Oct. 1978); *NEJM* 299: 1139 (Nov. 16, 1978).

The Human Female Reproductive Tract: A Scanning Electron Microscopic Atlas. **H. Ludwig and H. Metzger.** New York: Springer-Verlag, 1976.
Emphasizes the microanatomy of the female genital tract. Superb illustrations cover the surface appearance of the epithelium from vagina to ovary. The placenta is described in detail. A minimum amount of text appears on pages facing the illustrations. An aid to students and house officers in obstetrics and gynecology.
R: *British Journal of Obstetrics & Gynaecology* 84: 399 (May 1977); *JAMA* 237: 904

(Feb. 28, 1977); *Obstetrics and Gynecology* 52: 380 (Sept. 1978); *Surgery, Gynecology and Obstetrics* 145: 94 (July 1977).

Operative Surgery; Fundamental International Techniques: Urology. 3d ed. **D. Innes Williams, ed.** Woburn, MA: Butterworths, 1977.

An atlas for both students and practitioners of urology.
R: *JAMA* 239: 865 (Feb. 25, 1978).

Te Linde's Operative Gynecology. 5th ed. **Richard F. Mattingly.** Philadelphia, PA: J. B. Lippincott, 1977.

Fifth edition of a surgical atlas of gynecology. Information on pelvic anatomy, urology, gynecologic malignancy, fallopian tubes, etc, presented from pathological, physiological, embryological, and epidemiological standpoints. Also covers medical-legal aspects of pelvic surgery. Recommended for gynecologists.

Ultrasonoscopic Differential Diagnosis in Obstetrics and Gynecology. **R. O. Neudt and M. Hinselmann.** New York: Springer-Verlag, 1975.

An atlas of obstetrical diagnosis. Authoritative information on fetal growth, vaginal bleeding in pregnancy, site of placenta, and other basic problems in pregnancy. Illustrates and discusses gynecological tumors. A practical guide for clinicians and gynecologists.
R: *Growth* 39: 401 (Sept. 1975).

Urologic Surgery: Diagnosis, Techniques and Postoperative Treatment. **Georges Mayor and Ernst J. Zingg.** Stuttgart: Georg Thieme Verlag, 1976.

An English translation of a German atlas. Illustrates step-by-step procedures in urological surgery. Major sections cover kidney, bladder, seminal vesical, urethra, prostate. A well-illustrated and useful reference source for urologic surgeons.
R: *JAMA* 236: 2675 (Dec. 6, 1976); *NEJM* 295: 1146 (Nov. 11, 1976).

VETERINARY MEDICINE

Atlas of Small Animal Surgery; Thoracic, Abdominal and Soft Tissue Techniques. 2d ed. **Richard E. Hoffer.** St. Louis, MO: C. V. Mosby, 1977.

Follows a systematic approach to surgical technique. Concentrates mainly on dogs and cats. Includes alternate techniques where applicable. Superb drawings complement text.
R: *Veterinary Medicine & Small Animal Clinician* 72: 1893 (Dec. 1977).

Atlas of Topographical Anatomy of the Domestic Animals. 2d ed. 3 vols. **Peter Popesko.** Philadelphia, PA: W. B. Saunders, 1978.

Up-to-date, covers topographic anatomy of cattle, horses, dogs, cats, and rabbits.
R: *Journal of the American Veterinary Medical Association* 175: 214 (July 15, 1979).

Color Atlas of Neoplasia in the Cat, Dog and Horse. **D. E. Bostock and L. N. Owen.** Chicago, IL: Year Book Medical Publishers, 1975.

CHAPTER 11 DIRECTORIES, YEARBOOKS, BIOGRAPHICAL SOURCES

DIRECTORIES

BIBLIOGRAPHICAL SOURCES

Directory of Scientific Directories: A World Guide to Scientific Directories Including Medicine, Agriculture, Engineering, Manufacturing and Industrial Directories. **Anthony P. Harvey, comp.** Guernsey, England: Hodgson. Distr. New York: International Publications, 1972.

Earlier edition, 1969.
A world guide to over 1,800 directories published since 1950. Includes publications issued both separately and in periodicals.
R: *LJ* 94: 3431 (Oct. 1, 1969); *ARBA* (1970, p. 102; 1971, p. 477); Chen (p. 232); Mal (3-57); Wal (p. 40); Win (3EA20).

Guide to American Scientific and Technical Directories. **B. Klein, ed.** Rye, NY: Klein Publications, 1972.
R: Chen (p. 232).

International Bibliography of Directories of Economics, Science and Technique. 4th ed. Munchen-Pullach and Berlin: Verlag Documentation. Distr. New York: Bowker, 1970.

First edition, 1962.
Titles arranged under 50 main subject categories.
R: *ARBA* (1971, p. 477); Chen (p. 232).

GENERAL

Annual Register of Grant Support. **Alvin Renetzky, ed.** Los Angeles, CA: Academic Media, 1969–. Annual.

Focuses on grant support programs sponsored by government agencies, foundations, businesses and professional organizations. Entries arranged under headings: General, Humanities, Social Sciences, and Sciences. Features information on eligibility, application information, address, purpose, duration, and deadlines. Geographical index.
R: *MRW* S2, p. 92.

Awards, Honors, and Prizes: A Source Book and Directory. 3d ed. **Paul Wasserman, ed.** Detroit: Gale Research, 1975.

Second edition, 1969.
Volume 1, *United States and Canada*; volume 2, *International and Foreign*.
Emphasizes some 2,300 prizes and awards bestowed on Americans and Canadians for outstanding achievement. Coverage of 28 broad fields, including science

and medicine. Name and address of organization capture main listing. Complete with awards and subject indexes.
R: *Choice* (Mar. 1973); *Catholic Library World* (Feb. 1970); *RQ* (Fall 1973); *ARBA* p. 123 (1970, p. 123); *MRW* S2, p. 9; Chen (p. 232).

ChemBuyDirect, the International Chemical Buyers Directory. 3 vols. New York: W. de Gruyter, 1974–1976.

Chem Sources Europe. Mountain Lakes, NJ: Chemical Sources Europe, 1973–. Annual.

Annual listing of chemicals produced by over 420 companies in western Europe. Arranged alphabetically by chemical, includes statistical information and addresses of each manufacturer.
R: *MRW* S3, p. 9.

Chem Sources U. S. A. 19th ed. Flemington, NJ: Directories Publishing, 1978.

Fifteenth edition, 1974.
Annual edition of a well-known directory of chemical products manufactured by over 650 companies in the United States. Includes statistical data, addresses, and sales information on each company.
R: *MRW* S3, p. 9.

Consultants and Consulting Organizations Directory. 4th ed. **Paul Wasserman and Janice McLean, eds.** Detroit, MI: Gale Research, 1979.

Third edition, 1976.
Lists over 6,000 consultants and consulting organizations in 135 major areas of activities. The areas of specific interests to medical professionals are listed under headings such as dental and medicine, health administration, pharmaceutical industry, psychology-industrial, sanitation, urban and social problems, etc.
R: *Choice* (Nov. 1973); *Consultants News* (May 1973); *Engineering Societies Library Book Review* (May 1976); *Industrial Bookshelf* (Sept. 1973); *Management Review* (Apr. 1974); *WLB* (Oct. 1973).

Consumer Sourcebook: A Directory and Guide to Government Organizations, Associations, Centers, and Institutes; Media Services; Company and Trademark Information; and Bibliographic Material Relating to Consumer Topics, Sources of Recourse, and Advisory Information. 2d ed. 2 vols. **Paul Wasserman, ed.** Detroit, MI: Gale Research, 1978.

First edition, 1974.
A consolidated and comprehensive source book on many different types of consumer information sources. The new edition is nearly three times the size of the first. A helpful tool for every library.
R: *Business Literature* (Nov./Dec. 1977); *Catholic Library World* (Apr. 1975); *Choice* (Mar. 1975); *LJ* (Jan. 15, 1975); *RQ* (Spring 1975); *RSR* (Oct./Dec. 1974).

Directory of Agencies: U.S. Voluntary, International Voluntary, Intergovernmental. **National Association of Social Workers.** Washington, DC: National Association of Social Workers, 1973.

Directory of some 300 social work agencies, exclusive of national government agencies. Entries list directory-type data: name, address, membership, director, activities, etc.
R: *MRW* S3, p. 50.

Directory of Federal Health/Medicine Grants and Contracts Programs. 2d ed. Bethesda, MD: National Health Directory, 1980.

Updates all 223 federal grants and contract programs in 11 federal agencies dealing with health or medicine. Includes for every program: title, congressional authorization, eligibility requirements, application considerations, regulations, audits, guidelines, deadlines, etc. Current as of December 1979.

A Directory of Information Resources in the United States: Biological Sciences. **US National Referral Center, Science and Technology Division, US Library of Congress.** Washington, DC: US Government Printing Office, 1972.

Lists some 2,230 organizations, government agencies, research insitutites, libraries, and museums. Covers the fields of education, recreation, and business. Alphabetical arrangement by name. Includes subject index.
R: *MRW* S3, p. 7, 30, 50.

A Directory of Information Resources in the United States: Physical Sciences, Engineering. **US National Referral Center for Science and Technology, US Library of Congress.** Washington, DC: US Government Printing Office, 1971.

Describes 2,891 resources alphabetically arranged by organization name. Entries include standard directory-type information: publications, areas of interest, and holdings. Subject index.
R: *MRW* S2, p. 95.

Directory of Scientific Directories: A World Guide to Scientific Directories, Including Medicine, Agriculture, Engineering, Manufacturing and Industrial Directories. 2d ed. **Anthony P. Harvey.** Guernsey, England: Hodgson, 1972.

First edition, 1969.
Books and journal articles from 1945 to 1971 provide the nearly 2,210 annotated citations. Geographical, followed by broad subject, arrangement. Includes original title, author, and KWIC index.
R: *MRW* S2, pp. 32, 94, 101; *MRW* S3, pp. 48, 53.

Directory of Special Libraries and Information Centers. 5th ed. 3 vols. **Margaret L. Young and Harold C. Young, eds.** Detroit, MI: Gale Research, 1979.

Fourth edition, 1977.
Volume 1, *Special Libraries and Information Centers in the United States and Canada*; volume 2, *Geographic and Personnel Indexes*; volume 3, *New Special Libraries.*
A key to the holdings, services, and personnel of over 14,000 special libraries, information centers, documentation centers, and similar units in the United States and Canada, and 600 networks and consortia. Health sciences libraries and information centers are included.

R: *Choice* (Dec. 1974); *Sci-Tech News* (Oct. 1977); *WLB* (Nov. 1974); *ARBA* (1970–1976).

Encyclopedia of Associations. 14th ed. 3 vols. **Nancy Yakes and Denise Akey, eds.** Detroit, MI: Gale Research, 1980.

Volume 1, *National Organizations of the U.S.*; volume 2, *Geographic and Executive Index*; volume 3, *New Associations and Projects.*
A key to "inside" information of 13,589 national organizations of the United States. Organizations are arranged in seventeen subject categories. Information given in each entry includes the organization's name, address, chief executive, telephone number, purpose and activities, membership, publications, convention schedule, and other pertinent information. Further indexed by geographic area and the executives mentioned. A major directory of organizations.
R: *Food Technology* (Sept. 1977); *Medical Meetings* (Oct. 1977); *American Libraries* (Dec. 1970); *ASLIB Proceedings* (June 1975); *Choice* (1976); *Herald of Library Science* (Oct. 1974); *BL* (Oct. 15, 1975); *LJ* (Dec. 15, 1956); *RQ* (Spring 1973); *SL* (July 1975); *ARBA* (1971, 1977); Chen (p. 421).

Encyclopedia of Governmental Advisory Organizations: A Reference Guide to Presidential Advisory Committees, Public Advisory Committees, Interagency Committees and Other Government-Related Boards, Panels, Task Forces, Commissions, Conferences, and Other Similar Bodies of Serving in a Consultative, Coordinating, Advisory, Research, or Investigative Capacity. 2d ed. **Linda E. Sullivan and Anthony P. Kruzas, eds.** Detroit: Gale Research, 1975.

Index to organization names and keywords. Supplemented by *New Governmental Advisory Organizations* between editions.
R: *RSR* (Oct.–Dec. 1974); *WLR* (Mar. 1972); *ARBA* (1971); Chen (p. 239).

European Research Index. 3d ed. 2 vols. Guernsey, England: Hodgson. Distr. New York: International Publications, 1973.

Second edition, 1969.
Provides information on government and private establishments throughout Europe that conduct or promote scientific research. Includes organizations in eastern Europe. Keyword cross-referenced.
R: *CRL* 28: 66 (1967); *ARBA* (1970, p. 102); Chen (p. 233); Jenkins (A115); Mal (3-53); *MRW* S2, pp. 4, 41, 90, 97, 98, 101; Wal (p. 45); Win (1EA23).

Federal Regulatory Directory 1979–80. Washington, DC: Congressional Quarterly, 1979–. Quarterly.

Indexed by agency and subject. Provides information concerning federal regulatory agencies. Comprehensive cross-indexing. Covers such subjects as housing, nutrition, product safety.

The Foundation Directory. 6th ed. **Marianna O. Lewis, ed.** New York: The Foundation Center. Distr. New York: Columbia University Press, 1977.

Fifth edition, 1975.
Lists over 2,500 foundations. Describes foundations possessing assets of 1 million dollars or more. Includes foundations devoted to science and technology, engi-

neering, and medical research. Foundation, field-of-interest, donor, trustee, and administrator indexes.
R: Chen (p. 234); Mal (3-60).

Funk and Scott Index of Corporations and Industries. Cleveland: Predicasts, 1973.
Information on new products and technological developments.
R: Chen (p. 234).

ISI's Who is Publishing in Science: An International Directory of Research & Development Scientists. Philadelphia, PA: Institute for Scientific Information, 1967–. Annual.
Author and address directory of initial authors of papers published in journals covered by *Current Contents*. Arranged in three sections: author, organization, and geographical. Includes list of journals covered by *Current Contents*.
R: *MRW* S1, p. 31; *MRW* S2, pp. 91, 94; *LCIB* 32: 348 (Oct. 5, 1973).

International Foundation Directory. 2d ed. **H. V. Hodson, ed.** Detroit, MI: Gale Research, 1979.
First edition, 1974.
Comprehensive directory of some 1,000 foundations active in science, technology, medicine, etc. Geographically arranged.
R: *Choice* (May 1975); *RQ* (Summer 1975); Chen (p. 234).

MacRae's Blue Book. 5 vols. Hinsdale, IL: MacRae's, 1974.
National directory of manufacturers and products. Corporate, product, catalog, and trade name indexes.
R: Chen (p. 234).

National Directory of State Agencies 1976–77. **Matthew J. Vellucci et al., comps.** Washington, DC: Information Resources Press, 1976. Annual.
R: Chen (p. 234).

NSF Factbook: Guide to National Science Foundation Programs and Activities. **US National Science Foundation.** Chicago, IL: Marquis Academic Media, 1971 + updates.
Information about US National Science Foundation grants, personnel, support programs, legislation and career opportunities. Includes subject index.
R: *MRW* S2, pp. 92, 95, 104.

1980–1981 National Directory of Health/Medicine Organizations. Bethesda, MD: National Health Directory, 1980.
Describes some 1,300 national health/medicine organizations. Listed in alphabetical order in six categories (i.e. professional societies, medical specialty organizations, voluntary health organizations, etc.). Includes directory-type information: name, address, elected official, paid staff, etc.

1980–1981 National News Media Directory; Medicine/Health. Bethesda, MD: National Health Directory, 1980.

Fills a major gap in the communication structure of the medicine/health field. Lists key contact people for health/medicine matters for newspapers, magazines, television stations, radio stations, and newsletters. Invaluable source for finding documents, news releases, and news outlets.

Research Centers Directory: A Guide to University-Related and Other Nonprofit Research Organizations. 6th ed. **Archie M. Palmer, ed.** Detroit, MI: Gale Research, 1978.

Fourth edition, 1972; fifth edition, 1975.
Features over 6,000 information packed entries concentrating on nonprofit research activities in universities, colleges, technological institutes, and professional schools in the United States and Canada. Arrangement by subject. Entries reflect nearly sixteen valuable pieces of information, from mailing address to seminars and conferences given. Indexed by institutions, research center names, and subject. Handy reference tool for all but the smallest library.
R: *MRW* S2, pp. 90, 91; *Catholic Library World* (Feb. 1973); *Choice* (Jan. 1973); *ARBA* (1973); Chen (p. 234).

Scientific Directory and Annual Bibliography. **US National Institutes of Health.** Washington, DC: US Government Printing Office, 1959–. Annual.

1979 edition, DHEW Pub. no. (NIH) 79-4. Known as the *NIH Directory.*
Outlines the structure of NIH. Serves as a directory to NIH professional staff and a guide to NIH scientific and technical publications. Intended for use by research workers in the biomedical field.
R: *RSR* 4: 109 (Oct.–Dec. 1976).

Services & Organization Guide. **Personnel Department, American Medical Association.** Chicago, IL: American Medical Association, 1971.

Handbook of services and administrative structure of the American Medical Association. Provides locations and brief descriptions of persons and departments as well as summary information of their responsibilities.
R: *MRW* S3, p. 50.

Subject Directory of Special Libraries and Information Centers. 5th ed. 5 vols. **Margaret L. Young and Harold C. Young, eds.** Detroit, MI: Gale Research, 1979.

Volume 1, *Business and Law Libraries, Including Military and Transportation Libraries*; Volume 2, *Education and Information Science Libraries, Including Picture, Audiovisual, Publishing, Rare Book, and Recreational Libraries*; volume 3, *Health Sciences Libraries, Including all Aspects of Basic and Applied Medical Sciences*; volume 4, *Social Sciences and Humanities Libraries, Including Area/Ethnic, Art, Geography/Map, History, Music, Religion/Theology, Theater, and Urban/Regional Planning Libraries*; volume 5, *Science and Technology Libraries, Including Agricultural, Energy, Environmental/ Conservation, and Food Science Libraries.*
R: *BL* (June 15, 1978); *Catholical Library World* (Oct. 1975); *NTB* (Feb. 1978); *ARBA* (1976).

Subject Index of Current Research Grants Administered by the National Cancer Institute, DHEW Pub. no. (NIH) 74-541, etc. **US National Institutes of**

Health. Bethesda, MD: US National Institutes of Health, US Department of Health, Education, and Welfare, 1973.

Lists essential aspects of research grants including grant number, research topic, and primary investigator. Well cross-referenced with various indexes.
R: *MRW* S3, pp. 36, 45.

Summary of Grants and Contracts Administered by the National Center for Health Services Research and Development. **US National Center for Health Services Research and Development.** Washington, DC: US Government Printing Office, 1969.

A document of the US National Center for Health Services. Lists studies and programs, arranged according to area. Indexes of institutions, investigators, states, and grant numbers.
R: *MRW* S3, pp. 27, 45.

Thomas' Register of American Manufacturers and Thomas' Register Catalog File. 11 vols. New York: Thomas, 1980. Annual.

Volumes 1–6, comprehensive list of products and services; volume 7, list of companies; volume 8, brand name index; volumes 9–11, company catalogs.
R: Chen (p. 234).

United States Government Manual. **US General Services Administration. National Archives and Records Service. Office of the Federal Register.** Washington, DC: US Government Printing Office, 1973/1974–. Annual.

Voluntary Social Services: A Handbook of Information and Directory of Organizations. Rev. ed. **National Council of Social Service.** London: National Council of Social Service, 1970.

Alphabetical list of about 314 voluntary social service and health agencies located in Great Britain. Entry includes address, telephone, secretary, and descriptive data. Contains index by organization.
R: *MRW* S2, p. 108.

Washington Information Directory. Washington, DC: Congressional Quarterly Inc., 1975/1976–. Annual.

Some 5,000 information sources in Congress, the Executive Branch, and independent private organizations arranged by subject. Includes valuable sections on health and consumer affairs and natural resources, environment, and agriculture. Contains detailed subject and agency and organization indexes.

World Guide to Abbreviations of Organizations 5th ed. **F. A. Buttress.** Detroit: Gale Research, 1975.

Lists approximately 18,000 abbreviations, 5,000 of which relate to the European economic community.
R: Chen (p. 234); Mal (3-27).

World Guide to Technical Information and Documentation Services: Guide Mondial des Centres de Documentation et d'Information Techniques. **UNESCO.** Paris: UNESCO, 1969.

A companion to *World Guide to Science Information and Documentation Services*. Bilingual description: French/English. Lists 273 centers in 75 countries and territories. Emphasis on developing countries. Separate section on international centers. Also, lists international, regional, and national directories. Includes subject index.
R: *MRW* S2, pp. 57, 62, 94, 101; Chen (p. 234); Wal (p. 2).

GENERAL—MEDICINE

American Medical Association Directory of National Voluntary Health Organizations. **Council on Voluntary Health Agencies, American Medical Association, comps.** Chicago, IL: American Medical Association, 1964–. Irregular.
R: *MRW* S1, p. 5.

American Medical Directory. 1st ed.–. **American Medical Association.** Chicago, IL: American Medical Association, 1906–.
Twenty-fifth edition, 1969, 3 volumes; twenty-sixth edition, 1974, 4 volumes; 27th edition, 1979.
A register of physicians in the United States and US territories who possess a degree from an AMA certified school. Also includes doctors of osteopathy. A necessary reference tool.
R: Win (EK107).

Bio-Energy Directory. **The Bio-Energy Council.** Washington, DC: The Bio-Energy Council, 1978.
A directory of over 200 energy programs in both governmental and private sectors. Includes information on alternative energy sources. Provides full information on organizations and sponsors of bio-energy programs.

Canadian Medical Directory. Toronto, Canada: Seccombe House, 1954–. Annual.
An alphabetical listing of Canadian physicians. Also provides a geographic list of physicians and general lists of medical and nursing schools, hospitals, and medical journals.
R: Win (EK111).

Directory of Federal Health/Medicine Grant and Contract Programs. **US Department of Health, Education, and Welfare and Office of Management and Budget Documents.** Washington, DC: US Government Printing Office, 1979.
Explains over 200 grant programs in entries that include title, congressional authorization, objectives, eligibility requirements, application considerations, formula and matching requirements, guidelines, etc.

Directory of Health Sciences Libraries in the United States, 1973. 2d ed. **Susan Crawford and Gary Dandurand, comps. and eds.** Chicago, IL: American Medical Association, 1974.
First edition, 1970.

Comprehensive list of 2,984 entries arranged by state, then city, and by name of library. Information for each library includes address, telephone number, identification, size of collection, staff, and type of user. Also discusses methods used to gather data; tables accompany text. Index of names of libraries. Important library reference tool. Third edition is being prepared.
R: *BMLA* 63: 238 (Apr. 1975); *LJ* 96: 452 (Feb. 1, 1971); *SL* 66: 12A (Apr. 1975); *ARBA* (1976, p. 733); Win (EK110; 3EJ13).

Directory of Medical Specialists. 1st ed.–. 3 vols. Chicago, IL: Marquis Who's Who, 1940–.

Sixteenth edition, 1974; nineteenth edition, 1979–1980.
Lists over 221,000 biographies of specialists authorized by the 22 boards that constitute the American Board of Medical Specialists. Arrangement by specialty and geogvaphic location. Includes cross-references and alphabetical index. A standard reference tool.
R: *BL* 70: 954 (May 1, 1974); *ARBA* (1975, p. 743); Stearns & Ratcliff (*NEJM*); Win (EK134).

Directory of Self-Assessment Programs for Physicians. 3d ed. Chicago, IL: American Medical Association, 1974.

Eurohealth Handbook. 6th ed. New York: Robert S. First, 1980.

General Clinical Research Centers: A Research Resources Directory. DHEW Pub. no. (NIH) 78-1433. **Research Resources Information Center, prep.** Bethesda, MD: National Institutes of Health, US Public Health Service, US Department of Health, Education, and Welfare, 1978.
Lists 80 research centers funded by Division of Research Resources. Describes facilities which investigate human disorders. Entries are arranged geographically by state and give areas of investigation, personnel, and center resources. Geographical index.
R: *Hospitals* 52: 32 (Sept. 1978).

Health: A Multimedia Source Guide. **Joan Ash and Michael Stevenson.** New York: Bowker, 1976.
An annotated directory which guides the user to organizations concerned with health care. Lists about 700 sources. Three indexes: source, subject, material. Intended for librarians, professionals as a practical ready reference.
R: *Occupational Health Nursing* 24: 43 (Nov. 1976); *SL* 68: 102 (Feb. 1977); *WLB* 51: 539 (Feb. 1977); *ARBA* (1977, p. 704).

The Health Care Directory, 77–78. **Craig T. Norback and Peter G. Norback, eds.** Oradell, NJ: Medical Economics Co., 1977.
Contains 40,000 listings in 60 categories. First section lists companies alphabetically by city and state while the second part is an alphabetical list of products and services of supplying companies.
R: *Modern Healthcare* 7: 87 (July 1977); Sheehy (EK20).

Health Organizations of the United States, Canada and Internationally: A Directory of Voluntary Associations, Professional Societies and Other Groups Con-

cerned With Health and Related Fields. 4th ed. **Paul Wasserman and Jane K. Bussart, eds.** Ann Arbor, MI: Anthony T. Kruzas, 1977.

First edition, 1961; second edition, 1965; third edition, 1974.
Expanded fourth edition of directory which lists about 1,300 societies, foundations, associations, and other nongovernmental organizations in health field. Each entry provides address, telephone number, founding date, principal official, and information on finances, meetings, purposes, activities, and publications. Subject index of 29 pages lists organizations by field, interest, or form of association.
R: *American Journal of Public Health* 64: 921 (1974); *BL* 72: 925 (May 1, 1975); *Choice* 3: 19 (Mar. 1966); *RSR* 6: 67 (1978); *WLB* 45: 854 (June 1974); 52: 348 (Dec. 1977); *ARBA* (1976, p. 734); Win (EJ140; EK218; 1EJ26).

International Directory of Population Information and Library Resources. 1st ed.–. **C. Fogle, K. Gleiter, and M. McIntyre.** Chapel Hill, NC: Carolina Population Center, Technical Information Service, 1972–.

International directory of organizations and libraries that collect and publish literature about population and family planning. Entries, arranged geographically, provide names, addresses, chiefs of personnel, and descriptions. Contains indexes of periodicals, names of organizations, abbreviations, and special collections.
R: *MRW* S2, pp. 45, 57, 80.

Medical and Health Information Directory: A Guide to State, National and International Organizations, Government Agencies, Educational Institutions, Hospitals, Grant-Award Sources, Health Care Delivery Agencies, Journals, Newsletters, Review Serials, Abstracting Services, Publishers, Research Centers, Computerized Data Banks, Audiovisual Services, and Libraries and Information Centers. 2d ed. **Anthony T. Kruzas, ed.** Detroit, MI: Gale Research, 1980.

First edition, 1977.
Reference source contains over 12,000 entries providing basic data on agencies, institutions, companies, and associations concerned with medicine and health care at state and national level. Material is arranged in 32 subject sections and includes biomedical journals, abstracts, books, and computerized information services. Introduction outlines scope and selection criteria for each section. Indexes and references are given. Recommended for public, academic, and medical libraries.
R: *Radiology* 128: 600 (1978); *LJ* 102: 2421 (Dec. 1, 1977); 103: 510 (Mar. 1, 1978); *WLB* 52: 649 (Apr. 1978); *ARBA* (1978, p. 716); Sheehy (EK21).

National Health Directory, 1980. Rev. ed. **John T. Grupenhoff.** Washington, DC: Science and Health Publications, 1980.

Earlier edition, 1977.
Includes name, title, address, and telephone number of key information sources on health programs and legislation. Eight sections, beginning with names of congressional senators and representatives. Following are lists of key persons involved in health programs, short biographies of some: federal regional officials, governors, and top health officials of each state. Two indexes, one for congress-

men and the other for names appearing throughout directory. Useful in medical, public, or academic libraries.
R: *American Journal of Public Health* 67: 639 (1977); 67: 693 (July 1977); *Hospitals* 51: 48 (1977); *WLB* 52: 266 (Nov. 1977); *ARBA* (1978, p. 716); Sheehy (EK22).

NIH Factbook: Guide to National Institutes of Health Programs and Activities. Chicago, IL: Marquis Academic Media, 1976.
Brings together in one volume information about the National Institutes of Health: history, organization, statistics, advisory groups, research, grants, and indexes. Logical and readable format. Contains both subject and personnel indexes. Recommended for any library faced with questions relating to NIH.
R: *Choice* 13: 798 (Sept. 1976); *LJ* 101: 1105 (May 1, 1976); *RSR* 4: 86 (Jan.–Mar. 1976); *ARBA* (1977, p. 715).

National Institutes of Health Scientific Directory and Annual Bibliography. **US National Institutes of Health.** Washington, DC: Government Printing Office. Annual.
Outlines organizational structure of the National Institutes of Health, their staff, and their scientific and technical publications. Includes names of scientific staff personnel.
R: *ARBA* (1972, p. 627).

U.S. Medical Directory. 3d ed. **US Directory Service.** Miami, FL: US Directory Service, 1975.
Alphabetical arrangement of medical doctors, hospitals, nursing facilities, laboratories, and medical information centers in the United States. Medical doctor's listing features additional languages spoken by the physician. Incredibly helpful for patients whose native language is not English.
R: *Occupational Health Nursing* 23: 44 (Aug. 1975).

Washington Information Workbook. Washington, DC: Washington Researchers, 1979.
A complete guide to government information available in special reports. Includes statistical sources, scientific and technical information.

GENERAL—MEDICAL EDUCATION AND CARE

Admission Requirements of U.S. and Canadian Dental Schools, 1977–1978. 14th rev. ed. Washington, DC: American Association of Dental Schools, 1976.
Provides detailed information on United States and Canadian dental schools. Includes general information, size of program and degree awarded, requirements for admissions, expenses, financial aid information, addresses, etc. Arranged alphabetically by state or province. Frequently updated; thorough directory.
R: *ARBA* (1977, p. 714); Sheehy (EK26).

Allied Medical Education Directory. **Council on Medical Education, American Medical Association.** Chicago, IL: American Medical Association, 1971–. Annual.

A directory indispensable to the medical profession. In two sections: geographical listing of educational programs (AMA approved) and separate listing by type of program. Provides complete information, bibliography, statistical information, list of pertinent organizations. A valuable tool for all libraries and professionals of all strata in the medical field.
R: *RSR* 4: 42 (Jan.–Mar. 1976); *ARBA* (1973, p. 614); Win (EK105).

AAMC Curriculum Directory. **Association of American Medical Colleges.** Evanston, IL: Association of American Medical Colleges, 1972/1973–. Annual.

Gives information on required courses, conferences, laboratory periods, electives, opportunities for early specialization, etc.
R: Win (EK108).

AAMC Directory of American Medical Education. **Association of American Medical Colleges.** Evanston, IL: Association of American Medical Colleges. Annual.

Title varies.
Lists member institutions with information on their administration and facilities.
R: Win (EK108).

Directory of Accredited Allied Medical Educational Programs 1969/70. **Council on Medical Education, American Medical Association.** Chicago, IL: American Medical Association, 1971.

Listing of 2,524 programs approved as of July 1, 1971, described under eighteen allied occupations. Entries, alphabetically by state, provide information on entrance requirements, tuition, and degree granted. Includes selected list of national organizations concerned with allied medical education.
R: *MRW* S2, p. 52.

Directory of Accredited Institutions With Programs in Biocommunications. 3d ed. **HeSCA Committee on Education, comp.** Wauwatosa, WI: Health Sciences Communications Association, 1979.

Directory of Approved Internships and Residencies. **American Medical Association. Council on Medical Education and Hospitals.** Chicago, IL: American Medical Association, 1961–. Annual.

Geographic listing of hospital programs which accept interns and residents. Supplies detailed statistics of performance and essentials of each program. Also provides information on the National Intern and Resident Matching Program. An essential reference tool for every medical library.
R: Win (EK109).

Directory of Graduate Research: Faculties, Publications, and Doctoral Theses in Departments or Divisions of Chemistry, Chemical Engineering, Biochemistry, and Pharmaceutical and/or Medicinal Chemistry at Universities in the United States and Canada. **Committee on Professional Training, American Chemical Society.** Columbus, OH: American Chemical Society, 1958–.

Latest edition, 1977.
Comprehensive listing of graduate programs which lead to doctoral degrees. Arranged alphabetically by subject. Includes information on programs, specialization, biographical information of instructors. Includes statistical summary.
R: *MRW* S2, pp. 17, 32, 90, 91.

Directory of Universities and Colleges Offering Graduate Programs in the Medical Laboratory Sciences. **National Committee for Careers in the Medical Laboratory.** Rockville, MD: National Committee for Careers in the Medical Laboratory, 1971.

Alphabetical arrangement of US graduate programs specializing in clinical laboratory sciences (microbiology, medical technology) and educational programs for laboratory administrators and educators. Includes directory information: names, address, and area of concentration.
R: *MRW* S2, pp. 39, 102.

FIND: Financial Information National Directory: Health Careers. **American Medical Association.** Chicago, IL: American Medical Association, 1972.

Lists sources of financial aid for students in health-related fields. The 350 entries are arranged by federal, national, state, and minority funding. Provides full information.
R: *MRW* S2, pp. 52, 103.

Foreign Medical School Catalogue. Bay Shore, NY: Foreign Medical Schools Information Center, 1971–. Annual.

Relates data on medical schools in 65 foreign countries. Lists statistics on the following topics: admissions, graduates, and performance on the ECFMG exams.
R: Sheehy (EK19).

Guide to Foreign Medical Schools. 3d ed. **Daniel Marien.** New York: Queens College Press/Institute of International Education, 1973.

Alphabetically arranged by country, this directory provides information on foreign medical schools admitting American students. Includes some information on transferring to American schools.
R: *MRW* S3, p. 46.

Health Careers Guidebook. **US Department of Labor.** Washington, DC: US Government Printing Office, 1973.

Provides descriptions of over 150 health-related occupations. Outlines aptitudes, skills, training, duties, and advancement opportunities. Also lists organizations and available financial support.
R: *ARBA* (1974, p. 632).

Medical School Admission Requirements U.S.A. and Canada. **Association of American Medical Colleges.** Evanston, IL: Association of American Medical Colleges, 1951–. Annual.

Includes premedical planning, choosing a medical school, admission process, financial information, nature of medical education and information for foreign

and minority group students. Also discussed are foreign medical schools, alternatives open to rejected applicants, and information on medical schools.
R: Win (EK108).

Medical School Alumni. **American Medical Association.** Chicago, IL: American Medical Association, 1975.

A helpful directory providing tabulations and statistics on over 350,000 practicing physicians by specialty, professional activity, geographical location, sex, etc., graduated from 98 active US medical schools and selected Canadian and foreign schools.

Peterson's Annual Guides to Graduate Study. 1979 ed. **Karen C. Hegener, ed.** Princeton, NJ: Peterson's Guides, 1978.

Book 1, *Graduate Institutions in the United States and Canada/ An Overview*; book 2, *Humanities and Social Sciences*; book 3, *Biological, Agricultural, and Health Sciences*; book 4, *Physical Sciences*; book 5, *Engineering and Applied Sciences*.
R: *MRW* S2, pp. 13, 39, 52.

Physician's Medical Book Reference 1978. Fort Lee, NJ: Medi-Facts Publishing, 1979. Annual.

Lists both books and audiovisual materials for continuing education of physicians. Arranged by specialty. Entries are annotated and include cataloging information. Author index.
R: *RSR* 3: 113 (Jan.–Mar. 1975); *MRW* S3, pp. 4, 6.

ANATOMY

Directory: Departments of Anatomy of the United States and Canada: Schools of Medicine, Dentistry, Osteopathic Medicine, Veterinary Medicine. **American Association of Anatomists.** Philadelphia, PA: American Association of Anatomists, 1968.
R: *MRW* S1, p. 6.

BRAIN AND NERVOUS SYSTEM

Parkinson's Disease & Related Disorders: International Directory of Scientists, 1970. **Parkinson Information Center, US National Institute of Neurological Disease and Stroke.** Washington, DC: US Government Printing Office, 1970.

A directory of researchers who work on Parkinson's disease and related neurological disorders. Arranged by geographic area, personal name, and institution. Information provided includes name, entry, address, department, and subject interest of researchers.
R: *MRW* S2, pp. 76, 90.

DENTISTRY

American Dental Directory. Vols. 1–. **American Dental Association.** Chicago, IL: American Dental Association, 1947–. Annual.

Annual geographic listing of dental organizations, educational institutions, and dentists. A useful tool for libraries, dental students, and practitioners.
R: Win (EK151).

The Dentists Register. **General Dental Council.** London: General Dental Council, 1879–. Annual.

Annual register lists directory information of dental practitioners. Includes three lists: United Kingdom list, Commonwealth list, and foreign list.
R: Win (EK152).

Orthodontic Directory of the World. 27th ed. **William H. Oliver.** Nashville, TN: American Association of Orthodontists, 1974.

Twenty-sixth edition, 1972.
Listing of orthodontic societies of the world and principal officers, alphabetically by state and country.

GENETICS

International Directory of Genetic Services. 4th ed. **Daniel Bergsma and H. T. Lynch, eds.** New York: National Foundation for the March of Dimes, 1974.
R: Chen (p. 242).

GERONTOLOGY

A National Guide to Government and Foundation Funding Sources in the Field of Aging. **Lilly Cohen and Marie Oppedisano-Reich, comps. and eds.** Garden City, NY: Adelphi University Press, 1977.

Lists comprehensive information for more than 85 federal funding programs.
R: *Modern Healthcare* 7: 83 (Mar. 1977).

HEALTH SERVICES ADMINISTRATION

American Hospital Association Guide to the Health Care Field; 1979 edition. **American Hospital Association.** Chicago, IL: American Hospital Association, 1979. Annual.

An annual and indispensable directory listing alphabetically by state health care institutions, organizations, educational programs, American Hospital Association memberships. A detailed directory of 7,000 hospitals. A valuable tool for all hospital libraries, educational institutions, and health care professionals.
R: *RSR* 2: 130 (Oct.–Dec. 1974); *ARBA* (1978, p. 713); Win (EK106).

Biomedical Electronics: Marketing Guide and Company Directory for Patient Care Systems and Laboratory Equipment. **Technomic Research Staff.** Westport, CT: Technomic Publishing, 1972.

Gives broad perspective of available equipment in biomedical electronics. Valuable photographs and index.

British Health Centres Directory. **Brian Brookes, comp.** London: King Edward's Hospital Fund for London, 1973.

Provides information on health centers in the British Isles, England, Scotland, Ireland. Information includes address, personnel, and services offered. Also includes statistical information, maps, index.
R: *MRW* S3, p. 11.

Directory of Architects For Health Facilities. Chicago, IL: American Hospital Association, 1979.
Alphabetical and geographical directory.

Directory of Medicare Providers and Suppliers of Services, Hospitals, Extended Care Facilities, Outpatient Physical Therapy, Independent Laboratories, Portable X-Ray Units. **Social Securities Administration, US Department of Health, Education, and Welfare.** Washington, DC: US Government Printing Office, 1972.

Health Services in the United States. **Florence A. Wilson and Duncan Neuhauser.** Cambridge, MA: Ballinger, 1974.
Originally designed for the Harvard School of Public Health, this directory provides descriptive and statistical information on health services. Appendixes include chronology of legislation. For public health and medical libraries.
R: *American Journal of Public Health* 65: 187 (Feb. 1975); *RSR* 3: 33 (Apr.–June 1975).

Hospital Year-Book: An Annual Record of the Hospitals of Great Britain and Ireland Incorporating "Burdett's Hospitals and Charities" Founded 1889. Vols. 1–. London: British Hospital Association, 1931–. Annual.
Directory information for government departments, hospitals, local health authorities, hospital suppliers, etc. Includes technical and general reference information such as bed and patient statistics and blood transfusion services.
R: Win (EK112).

List of Approved Hospitals and Recognized House Officer Posts; England, Wales, Scotland, Northern Ireland, and the Republic of Ireland. 5th ed. **Great Britain. General Medical Council.** London: General Medical Council, 1967.
First edition, 1952.
Lists approved hospitals in Great Britain and the British Isles. Arranged geographically. Includes index of hospitals, statistical tables.
R: *MRW* S1, p. 13; *MRW* S3, p. 29.

The Medical and Healthcare Marketplace Guide. 2d ed. Acton, MA: International Bio-Medical Information Service, 1977.
First edition, 1975.
Updated, authoritative directory to the United States health care system. Covers all major providers of equipment, service organizations. Geographical index of firms, personnel index. Also provides information on foreign-based companies.

Medical Disposables: Marketing Guide and Company Directory. Stamford, CT: Technomic Publishing, 1971.

Provides information on 200 manufacturers and about 2,000 distributors. Trade publication aimed at hospital purchasers.
R: *ARBA* (1972, p. 626).

The Worldwide Guide to Medical Electronics Marketing Representation. Acton, MA: International Bio-Medical Information Service, 1977.
Handy pocket-size directory of international medical electronics firms. Includes all pertinent information, demographic data of hospitals. Over 400 entries from Central and South America, Africa, the Middle East, Asia, western Europe, Canada, and Mexico. Indexes: geographical, classified, and management.

HEMATOLOGY

Directory for the National Clearinghouse Program of the American Association of Blood Banks. 8th ed. **National Clearinghouse Program, American Association of Blood Banks.** San Francisco, CA: American Association of Blood Banks, 1972.
Geographical arrangement of blood banks and related services. Special mention of five regional clearinghouses. Given information includes name, address, and helpful comments.
R: *MRW* S3, p. 7.

INFECTIOUS DISEASES

American Society for Microbiology: Directory and Constitution. Ann Arbor, MI: American Society for Microbiology, 1906–.
Latest edition, 1979.

American Society of Parasitologists Directory of Members. Lawrence, KS: American Society of Parasitologists. Annual.

World Directory of Collections of Cultures of Microorganisms. **S. M. Martin et al.** New York: Wiley-Interscience, 1972.
Sponsored by WHO and Unesco. Microorganisms included: algae, bacteria, fungi, lichens, protozoa, tissue cultures, animal viruses, bacterial viruses, insect viruses, plant viruses, and yeasts.
R: *ARBA* (1973, p. 554); Chen (p. 242); Mal (9-35).

INTERNAL MEDICINE

Acupuncture Directory: Yellow Pages. Los Angeles, CA: Chans Books, 1974.
Directory provides publications, research clinics, journals. Lists research and acupuncture treatment centers in the United States and abroad.
R: *MRW* S3, p. 1.

American College of Physicians Directory. **American College of Physicians.** Philadelphia, PA: American College of Physicians, 1929–. Biennial.

Directory of Osteopathic Specialists. 1st ed.–. Chicago, IL: Marquis Who's Who, 1974–. (Published for the American Osteopathic Association).

Lists certified osteopaths with some biographical information, arranged by speciality and geographic area. Includes information on certification requirements.
R: *ARBA* (1976, p. 733); *MRW* S3, p. 39.

Index of Opportunity in the Paramedical Fields: A Directory of Career Opportunities for Mental Health and Social Workers; Public Welfare Workers; Dental, Medical, and Laboratory Technicians; Physical Therapists; and Other Allied Paramedical Specialists. Princeton, NJ: Resource Publications, 1970.

For paramedics; describes career opportunities in hospitals. Alphabetically arranged, geographic index.
R: *MRW* S2, pp. 41, 52, 55.

NURSING

In addition to the following directories, *The American Journal of Nursing* (April issues) and *Nursing Outlook* (March and September issues) publish official directories of nursing and related organizations, including voluntary organizations and government bureaus.

Directory of Certified Nurses. **American Nurses Association. Divisions on Nursing Practice.** Kansas City, MO: American Nurses Association, 1979.

Directory of Schools of Nursing in the European Region. **Regional Office for Europe, World Health Organization.** Copenhagen: Regional Office for Europe, World Health Organization, 1971.

Provides general descriptions of schools of nursing. Includes name, address, number of students, administrative information. Entries include western and eastern European countries. Covers private, public, and religious institutions. Alphabetically arranged by geographic region.
R: *MRW* S2, p. 93.

Doctoral Programs in Nursing: Nurse Scientist Graduate Training Grants Program. **Department of Baccalaureate and Higher Degree Programs, National League for Nursing.** New York: National League for Nursing, 1974.

Nursing Job Guide. Weston, MA: Prime National Publishing, 1979.

Directory includes hospital employment information for more than 7,000 hospitals in the United States. Guide lists type and size of hospital, sample resumes, state licensing procedures, specialties offered, benefits, and educational opportunities.
R: *Modern Health Care* 9: 73 (Feb. 1979).

Preparing Registered Nurses for Expanded Roles: A Directory of Programs, DHEW Pub. no. (NIH) 74-31. **American Nurses Association.** Washington, DC: US Government Printing Office, 1974.

A directory which lists approximately 140 programs which lead to nursing certificates or master's degrees. Entries include length of program, financial aid information, and area of concentration.

R: *MRW* S3, p. 21.

State-Approved Schools of Nursing—L.P.N./L.V.N. State Approved Schools of Nursing—R.N. New York: National League for Nursing. Annual.

These two directories contain the most complete and up-to-date information on schools of nursing.

NUTRITION

Food Ingredients Directory. Hasting-on-Hudson, NY: Food Ingredients Directory. Annual.

Guide to several-thousand natural and synthetic ingredients in all types of food.
R: Chen (p. 246).

ONCOLOGY AND NUCLEAR MEDICINE

Directory of Cancer Research Information Resources, NTIS Pub. no. 77-16275. Item no. 507-G-10. **National Cancer Institute, US Department of Health, Education, and Welfare.** Springfield, VA: National Technical Information Service, 1977.

International list of sources of information on cancer provides sufficient detail for postal access and covers journals, registries, libraries, and information retrieval services. Clearly indexed; valuable addition to medical library.
R: *British Journal of Radiology* 52: 133 (1979).

International Directory of Specialized Cancer Research and Treatment Establishments, UICC Technical Report Series, Volume 33. 2d ed. **International Union Against Cancer/Union Internationale Centre le Cancer.** Geneva: International Union Against Cancer, 1978.

Revised and expanded, contains results of an international study conducted by the UICC. Provides data on over 670 cancer research institutes. Geographically arranged with alphabetical indexes.

Strike Back at Cancer: What You Can Do and Where You Can Go For the Best Medical Care. **Stephen A. Rapaport.** Englewood Cliffs, NJ: Prentice-Hall, 1978.

Geographical and alphabetical listing of cancer care and research centers throughout the world. Geared toward the lay person, the book describes warning signals for early cancer detection and describes current treatments, including immunotherapy and chemotherapy. An extensive directory for public and medical libraries.

OPHTHALMOLOGY

American Academy of Ophthalmology and Otolaryngology Directory. **William F. Hughes, ed.** Rochester, MN: American Academy of Ophthalmology and Otolaryngology, 1941–. Annual.

Alphabetical and geographical listing of members of American Academy of Ophthalmology and Otolaryngology.

American Optometric Association Directory. St. Louis, MO: American Optometric Association, 1972–.

Arranged alphabetically and geographically, lists names of colleges granting degrees, membership publications, addresses, telephone numbers. Also includes association information, such as ethical code, constitution.
R: *MRW* S3, p. 39.

Blue Book of Optometrists: A Directory of Legally Registered Optometrists of the U.S. 1st ed.–. Chicago, IL: Professional Press, 1912–.

Thirty-third edition, 1976.
Lists legally registered optometrists in the United States, Canada, Mexico, etc. Entries are arranged alphabetically by states and provinces and provide address, telephone number, personal information, professional membership, and specialty. Indexed.
R: *Journal of the American Optometric Association* 44: 548 (May 1973); *RSR* 2: 130 (Oct.–Dec. 1974).

Optical Society of America Directory. **Optical Society of America.** New York: American Institute of Physics. Annual.

Directory of membership as of March 15 each year which provides alphabetical and geographical listings. Entries for individual and corporate members in alphabetical section give names, addresses, and areas of interest by code.
R: *MRW* S2, p. 74.

Pathology

World List of Forensic Science Laboratories. 2d ed. **Forensic Science Society.** London: Forensic Science Society, 1971.

First edition, 1963.
Lists over 750 laboratories dealing in 58 diverse fields of investigation. Arrangement by geographical area under 83 countries. Each entry states laboratory name, address, director, and fields of investigation.
R: *MRW* S2, pp. 47, 60.

Pediatrics

Directory for Exceptional Children. 8th ed. **Porter Sargent Staff et al.** Boston, MA: Porter Sargent, 1978.

Sixth edition, 1969; seventh edition, 1972.
Lists educational and training facilities classified by special needs.

Pharmacy and Pharmacology

American Druggist Blue Book. 1st ed.–. New York: American Druggist, 1928–. Annual.

Annually published listing of drug product information, including prices. Alphabetical listing, includes index.
R: Win (EK202).

Colleges of Pharmacy, Accredited Programs. Chicago, IL: American Council on Pharmaceutical Information, 1979. Annual.

Directory of accredited programs in US colleges of pharmacy. Arranged alphabetically by state. Revised annually.

Compendium of Pharmaceuticals and Specialties. Toronto, Ont.: Canadian Pharmaceutical Association. Annual.

Continuing Pharmaceutical Education, Approved Providers. Chicago, IL: American Council on Pharmaceutical Information, 1979. Annual.

Directory of continuing education programs in pharmacy in the United States, arranged alphabetically by state. Revised annually.

Directory of Drug Information and Treatment Organizations. **Student Association for the Study of Hallucinogens (STASH).** Madison, WI: STASH Press, 1972.

A directory of drug education, treatment, and counseling centers in the United States and Canada. Arranged geographically. Entries include address, services, clientele, administrative personnel.
R: *MRW* S3, pp. 11, 18, 19.

Drug and Cosmetic Catalog. New York: Drug and Cosmetic Industry. Annual.

Hayes Druggist Directory. 67th ed. Newport Beach, CA: E. N. Hayes, 1978.

Provides a complete and accurate list of all retail drug stores in the United States.

Hospital Purchasing Guide 1978. **Calvin Probst, ed.** Ambler, PA: Medical Business Services, 1978.

Contains three sections: products by category, products by manufacturer, and business directory. Excellent guide for hospital purchasing department.

JAPTA List 1973; Japanese Drug Directory. 2d ed. Tokyo, Japan: Japan Pharmaceutical Traders' Association, 1973.

First edition, 1968.
Entries describe over 17,000 drugs produced by Japanese pharmaceutical companies. Information includes composition, use, mode of supply, international proprietary name.
R: *MRW* S3, pp. 8, 19–20.

Pharmaceutical Directory. **American Pharmaceutical Association.** Washington, DC: American Pharmaceutical Association, 1900–. Annual.

Most recent edition is 1977.

Pharmaceutical Manufacturers of the United States. Park Ridge, NJ: Noyes Data, 1977.

Lists over 300 references to US pharmaceutical and health product manufacturers. Alphabetical arrangement by business title. Outlines directory and descriptive information: address, number of employees, product area, annual sales,

location of subsidiaries, and names of executives. Comprehensive index provides company, division, and subsidiary names. Limited interest for health sciences and special libraries.
R: *ARBA* (1978, p. 732).

Pharmaceutical Marketers Directory. Clifton, NJ: Pharmaceutical Marketers Directory, 1979.
A directory to pharmaceutical companies, advertising agencies, medical publications. Also contains a classified section which is a guide to employment agencies, art services, market research.

PMD: Pharmaceutical Marketers Directory. Clifton, NJ: Fisher-Stevens Publications, 1977.
Extensive information on accredited pharmacy programs in the United States, including description of curriculum, residence and entrance requirements, timetable of application and acceptance, financial aid, fees, etc.

Pharmacy School Admission Requirements, Actual 1977–78, Projected 1978–79. 4th ed. Bethesda, MD: American Association of Colleges of Pharmacy, 1978.

World Pharmaceutical Directory. Chatham, NJ: Unlisted Drugs, 1980.
Lists some 120,000 entries in two sections: producers profile and corporate names and addresses.

PHYSICAL MEDICINE AND REHABILITATION

Directory of Agencies Serving the Visually Handicapped in the United States. 20th ed. **American Foundation for the Blind.** New York: American Foundation for the Blind, 1978.
Seventeenth edition, 1971; eighteenth edition, 1973; nineteenth edition, 1975. Comprehensive listing of nonprofit state and local agencies which provide financial, educational, and rehabilitation assistance to the visually handicapped. Provides directory type information: address, telephone number, director, services provided and membership associations. Supplementary lists outline specialized agencies. Useful addition to college, public, and institutional libraries.
R: *Physical Therapy* 54: 1146 (1974); *RSR* 2: 129 (Oct.–Dec. 1974); *MRW* S2, p. 14; *ARBA* (1977, p. 714).

Directory of Catholic Special Facilities and Programs in the US for Handicapped Children and Adults. 5th ed. **Elmer H. Behrmann and Ann D. Moll, eds.** Washington, DC: National Catholic Educational Association, 1971.
A directory of Catholic sponsored facilities arranged geographically by state, under categories of facilities. Provides descriptive information, telephone numbers, addresses. Indexes: catholic schools, hospitals, institutions.
R: *MRW* S2, pp. 40, 89.

Library Resources for the Blind and Physically Handicapped: A Directory of NLS Network Libraries and Machine-Lending Agencies, 1978. **National Li-**

brary Service for the Blind and Physically Handicapped, US Library of Congress. Washington, DC: National Library Service for the Blind and Physically Handicapped, US Library of Congress, 1978.
R: *LCIB* 37: 777 (Dec. 22, 1978).

National Directory of Rehabilitation Facilities. 10 vols. **US Rehabilitation Services Administration. Division of Rehabilitation Facilities.** Washington, DC: US Rehabilitation Services Administration, 1971–.

Rehabilitation facilities are arranged geographically by ten DHEW regions. Each entry provides name of facility, address, and coded data.
R: *MRW* S3, pp. 45, 49.

Volunteers Who Produce Books: Braille, Large Type, Tape. Rev. ed. **Division for the Blind and Physically Handicapped, US Library of Congress.** Washington, DC: US Government Printing Office, 1974.

Intended as a guide to services provided by volunteer groups interested in handling the reading needs of blind and handicapped people. Entries are arranged alphabetically by state and city. Annotations describing the types of material produced complement each entry. Features succinct reviews of public and private sources of reading materials and braille equipment.
R: *LCIB* 34: 131 (Apr. 4, 1975).

Psychiatry and Psychology

Directory of Outpatient Psychiatric Clinics and Other Mental Health Resources in the United States, Public Health Service No. 1129. Bethesda, MD: US Department of Health, Education, and Welfare, 1963–.

Latest edition, 1977.
Continues the *Directory of Psychiatric Clinics.*

Directory of Social and Health Agencies of New York City. New York: Columbia University Press, 1883–. Biennial.

A directory which lists over 1,200 social, welfare, and health agencies in New York City. Agencies are listed alphabetically and by function. Entries include concise description of services offered, those eligible, and information about fees, hours, and personnel. Cross-referenced. Personnel and subject indexes.
R: *RSR* 3: 71 (July–Dec. 1975); *ARBA* 1970, p. 140).

A Directory of World Psychiatry. **John Gunn, comp.** Basel, Switzerland: World Psychiatric Association, 1971.

Lists psychiatric facilities in 89 countries. Covers hospitals, universities, journals, organizations, and associations. Provides diagrammatic maps.
R: *MRW* S2, p. 82.

International Directory of Mental Retardation Resources. **Rosemary F. Dybwad.** Washington, DC: President's Committee on Mental Retardation, 1971.

Two-part directory of organizations and services in over 60 countries. Part 1

contains names, addresses, and information about international organizations. Part 2 presents reports by country of the mental retardation picture, including general description, government agencies, organizations, research, and publications.
R: *MRW* S2, p. 67.

Mental Health Directory, DHEW Pub. no. (ADM) 77–266. **US National Institute of Mental Health.** Washington, DC: US Government Printing Office, 1977.
Earlier edition, 1971.
Directory of state mental health facilities which provide direct mental health services to mentally ill and emotionally disturbed. Information is given to geographic area served, type of operating agency, and services provided. Useful for mental health planners, administrators, practitioners, and persons in need of services.
R: *ARBA* (1971, p. 536; 1972, p. 629).

National Directory of Mental Health: A Guide to Adult Outpatient Mental Health Facilities and Services Throughout the United States. **Neal-Schuman Publishers, Inc., eds.** New York: John Wiley, 1980.
A comprehensive guide to over 5,000 mental health services and facilities that treat adults (16 years and over) on an outpatient basis. Geographical arrangement of entries, with a name and type of service index.

PUBLIC HEALTH

Consumer Protection Directory: A Comprehensive Guide to Environmental Organizations in the United States and Canada. 2d ed. **Thaddeus C. Trzyna and Sally R. Osberg eds.** Chicago, IL: Marquis Academic Media, 1975.
First edition, *Directory of Consumer Protection and Environmental Agencies,* 1973; second edition in two sections. See also *Environmental Protection Directory: A Comprehensive Guide to Environmental Organizations in the United States and Canada,* 1975. Source of information on 2,664 government and private organizations in the United States and Canada. In two sections: consumer protection and environmental protection. Entries include address, telephone number, personnel, functions, purposes, and activities. Organization, personnel, publications, and subject indexes.
R: *MRW* S3, pp. 12, 23, 26.

Directory of Environmental Information Sources. **M. M. Kessler and G. V. Soccolich, eds.** Boston, MA: National Foundation for Environmental Control, 1971.
Sources are listed by type: educational, governmental, etc. Also lists bibliographies, serials, documents, periodicals. Telephone numbers, addresses are provided.
R: *MRW* S2, pp. 43, 57.

A Directory of Information Resources in the United States: General Toxicology. **National Referral Center for Science and Technology, US Library of**

Congress. Washington, DC: US Government Printing Office, 1969.

Directory of toxicological information centers. Alphabetical arrangement by name. Appendixes labeled: A. Poison Control Centers; B. US Professional Toxicological Organizations; and C. US Periodicals Related to Toxicology. Includes geographic and subject indexes.
R: *ARBA* (1970, p. 109); Chen (p. 241); *MRW* S2, pp. 57, 103; Win (EK226; 3EJ38).

Directory of Poison Control Centers. Rev. ed. **US Food and Drug Administration.** Washington, DC: US Government Printing Office, 1971.

Lists round-the-clock (24-hour) poison control centers. Arrangement is alphabetical by state, and entries cover directory-type information.
R: *ARBA* (1972, p. 626).

Directory of Selected Training Facilities in Family Planning and Allied Subjects. **International Planned Parenthood Federation.** London: International Planned Parenthood Federation, 1967.

Facilities which provide training in reproductive biology, population studies, and demography are also included in the goegraphically arranged directory.
R: *MRW* S1, p. 29.

Directory of State and Local Alcoholism Services. **US National Institute on Alcohol Abuse and Alcoholism.** Rockville, MD: US National Institute of Mental Health, 1972.

A directory of alcohol rehabilitation centers in the United States, arranged geographically. Provides address, telephone number, information on administrative personnel, extent of program, etc. No index.
R: *MRW* S3, pp. 2–3; 29, 34, 45.

Directory of State, Territorial, and Regional Health Authorities, Public Health Service no. 75. **US Public Health Service.** Washington, DC: US Government Printing Office, 1976.

Includes information about principal health authorities, with contents covering state and territorial health offices, designated state agencies for comprehensive planning, regional medical programs and rehabilitation services. Useful to those administering grant programs of Health Services and Mental Health Administration.
R: *ARBA* (1970, p. 140).

Environmental Protection Directory: A Comprehensive Guide to Environmental Organizations in the United States and Canada. 2d ed. **Thaddeus C. Trzyna and Sally R. Osberg, eds.** Chicago, IL: Marquis Academic Media, 1975.

First edition, *Directory of Consumer Protection and Environmental Agencies,* 1973; second edition in two publications. See also *Consumer Protection Directory: A Comprehensive Guide to Environmental Organizations in the United States and Canada,* 1975. Source of information on 2,664 government and private organizations in the United States and Canada. In two sections: consumer protection and environmental protection. Entries include address, telephone number, personnel, func-

tions, purposes, and activities. Organization, personnel, publications, and subject indexes.
R: *MRW* S3, pp. 12, 23, 26.

International Directory of Occupational Safety and Health Services and Institutions, Occupational Health and Safety Series, 16. 3d ed. **International Labour Office.** Washington, DC: International Labour Office, 1977.

A listing of occupational safety and health institutions in 79 countries. Provides address, function, and activities of each institution. In English, alphabetically arranged.
R: *IBID* 6: 194 (June 1978).

NRC Switchboard: Selected Information Resources on Industrial Safety and Occupational Health. **US National Referral Center, Science and Technology Division.** Washington, DC: US Government Printing Office, 1976.

Lists 72 organizations which will provide information relating to industrial safety or occupational health. Entries provide name, address, telephone number, and description of information services. They are arranged under the following headings: general resources, occupational health, mining, explosives, hazardous materials, construction, toxicology, radiation, transportation, and other occupations.
R: *LCIB* 35: 277 (May 14, 1976).

Occupational Safety and Health: A Guide to Information Sources. **Theodore P. Peck, ed.** Detroit, MI: Gale Research, 1974.

Emphasizes organizations, agencies, and libraries that record and initiate developments in the field. Includes full bibliographic information on publications, addresses, and descriptions of purpose for all groups.

Pollution Control Companies, U.S.A., 1972. **Noyes Data Corporation.** Park Ridge, NJ: Noyes Data Corporation, 1972.

Entry emphasis is on companies active in environmental control and pollution prevention. Arranged alphabetically, entries include around 2,000 companies which either market useful products or provide professional services.
R: *MRW* S2, pp. 5, 16, 93, 109.

Public Welfare Directory, 1940–. Washington, DC: American Public Welfare Association, 1940–. Annual.

Latest edition, 1979/1980.
Annual publication which lists federal, state, and local public assistance agencies with their directors. Included for each state is an introductory statement on its administration of public welfare and the place to write for information on assistance, birth and death records, marriage and divorce records, mental health and correctional institutions.
R: Sheehy (CC39).

State and Local Environmental Libraries: A Directory. **Library Systems Branch, US Environmental Protection Agency.** Washington, DC: US Government Printing Office, 1973.

Geographical listing of state and local libraries throughout the United States concerned primarily with environmental literature. Entries include name of library, address, telephone number, and name of librarian when available.
R: *MRW* S3, pp. 20, 23, 31.

World Directory of Environmental Research Centers. 2d ed. **William K. Wilson, Morgan D. Dowd, and Phyllis Sholtys, eds.** New York: Oryx Press, 1974.

First edition, 1970.
Identifies some 4,800 international research centers. Outlines resources and researchers devoted to environmental studies. Entries include center name, address, and a succinct description of activities. Arranged by subject. Includes a geographical index.
R: *BL* 70: 197 (Oct. 1, 1974); *Choice* 11: 1288 (Nov. 1974); *LJ* 99: 1796 (July 1974); *WLB* 49: 186 (Oct. 1974); *ARBA* (1975, p. 703); Chen (p. 256); *MRW* S3, pp. 22, 45, 50.

World Directory of Schools of Public Health 1971. 2d ed. **World Health Organization.** Geneva: World Health Organization, 1972.

First edition, 1968.
Focuses on 121 public health schools in 44 countries relating to the academic year 1970/1971. Summarizes curricula, admissions requirements, examinations, year of initial public health course, student enrollment, and faculty. Emphasizes the differences between countries.
R: *Lancet* 1: 468 (Mar. 3, 1973); *IBID* 1: 116 (June 1973).

World Environmental Directory, Volume 2, 1975. Silver Spring, MD: Business, 1975.

This is actually the second edition of this directory devoted to product manufacturers, consulting agencies, and educational facilities concerned with various aspects of pollution.
R: *ARBA* (1976, p. 702); Chen (p. 256).

RADIOLOGY

Directory of High-Energy Radiotherapy Centres, 1976 Edition. 3d ed. **International Atomic Energy Agency.** Vienna: International Atomic Energy Agency, 1976.

Computer printout listing of radioisotope and other high-energy teletherapy installations throughout the world. Entries include address, radiotherapists, physicists, manufacturers, output rate, and X-ray generating potential. Addresses are presented alphabetically by country, province, and city.
R: *IBID* 4: 349 (Dec. 1976); *ARBA* (1978, p. 714).

Membership Directory. **American College of Radiology.** Chicago, IL: American College of Radiology, 1957–. Annual.

UROGENITAL SYSTEM

Directory of Contraceptives. Directoire de Contraceptifs. Directorio de Anticoncep-

tivos. **N. Hardy and P. Kestelman, eds.** London: Medical Department, International Planned Parenthood Federation, 1971.

Reports on availability of all types of contraceptives, by brand name and country. Separate listing of chemical compounds of oral contraceptives. Addresses of International Planned Parenthood Federation regional offices as well as addresses of principal manufacturers and distributors.
R: *MRW* S2, pp. 23, 59.

Kidney Disease Services, Facilities, and Programs in the United States. **Kidney Disease Control Program.** Washington, DC: US Government Printing Office, 1969–. (Vol. for 1969 issued as Public Health Service Pub. no. 1942).
Issued 1971– by the National Kidney Foundation.

VETERINARY MEDICINE

Animals for Research: A Directory of Sources of Laboratory Animals, Equipment and Materials. 9th ed. **Institute for Laboratory Animal Resources, US National Research Council.** Washington, DC: US National Research Council, US National Academy of Sciences, 1975.

A directory of sources that provide animals, equipment, and materials for laboratory research.

YEARBOOKS

In this section, all publications with titles starting "yearbook" are listed, although many of them are published serially and are similar in nature to "Advances," "Progress In," and other series, which are included in chapter 13, "Important Series."

GENERAL

Legal Medicine Annual. New York: Appleton-Century-Crofts, 1969–. Annual.

Latest edition, 1979.
Up-to-date reference tool of medical-legal subjects contains papers of forensic interest written by experts. Articles are concise and supported by excellent list of references. Illustrative material includes photographs, tables, and graphs. Complete index. Of interest to forensic pathologists, physicians, and attorneys.
R: *Archives of Pathology* 102: 111 (1978); *JAMA* 238: 630 (Aug. 15, 1977); *JAMWA* 33: 527 (Dec. 1978); *ARBA* (1978, p. 718).

McGraw-Hill Yearbook of Science and Technology. **Staff of McGraw-Hill Encyclopedia of Science and Technology, comp.** New York: McGraw-Hill, 1972–. Annual.

An A–Z listing of authoritative articles on the advances and developments in science and technology during the preceding year. Includes maps, charts, illustrations, etc.
R: *American Scientist* 59: 479 (July/Aug. 1971); 61: 476 (July/Aug. 1973); *BL* 71:

1020 (June 1975); *LJ* 92: 2146 (1967); *RQ* 11: 177 (Winter 1971); *ARBA* (1976, p. 635; 1973, p. 535; 1971, p. 476); Chen (p. 257); Jenkins (A50); Mal (3-16); Wal (p. 17).

Science News Yearbook. **Prepared by Science Service.** New York: Scribner's, 1969–. Annual.

A popular-language account of recent developments in science and technology. Based primarily on material published in *Science News*.
R: *Choice* 6: 1374 (Dec. 1969); *LJ* (Sept. 1969); *Saturday Review* (Dec. 6, 1969); *ARBA* (1970, p. 103); Chen (p. 257).

Science Year; the World Book Science Annual. Chicago: Field Enterprises 1965–. Annual.

An issue may be devoted to one significant scientific topic, through a series of articles written by specialists. Shorter articles will summarize advances covering a wide range of topics.
R: *Science* 152: 917 (1966); *BL* 62: 725–727 (Apr. 1, 1966); *LJ* 92: 1577 (Apr. 15, 1967); *ARBA* (1971, p. 476); Chen (p. 257); Jenkins (A53); Wal (p. 17); Win (1EA12).

Yearbook of Family Practice. Vol. 1–. Chicago, IL: Year Book Medical Publishers, 1977–. Annual.

ANESTHESIOLOGY AND GENERAL SURGERY

Surgery Annual. Vols. 1–. **Lloyd M. Nyhus, ed.** New York: Appleton-Century-Crofts, 1969–. Annual.
Volume 11, 1979.
Analyzes in depth selected subjects important in surgery. Newer concepts in fields of general, cardiac, orthopedic, and pediatric surgery are explored. Abundant illustrative material includes tables, figures, line drawings, and X-ray photographs. Citations accompany articles; detailed index. Written primarily for general surgeons.
R: *JAMA* 228: 767 (May 6, 1974); *Lancet* 2: 399 (Aug. 22, 1970); *Plastic and Reconstructive Surgery* 59: 569 (1977); *ARBA* (1977, p. 718).

Year Book of Anesthesia. **James E. Eckenhoff et al., eds.** Chicago, IL: Year Book Medical Publishers, 1961–. Annual.

Compiles abstracts of articles, taken mostly from English-language medical journals, of interest to anesthesiologists. Abstracts, with short editorial comments, references, extracts, are grouped according to topic. Well written and edited, serves as a reference to advances and developments in anesthesiology.
R: *Anesthesiology* 43: 138 (July 1975); 47: 482 (Nov. 1977); 49: 65 (July 1978); *Lahey Clinic Foundation Bulletin* 25: 199 (Oct.–Dec. 1976).

Year Book of Plastic and Reconstructive Surgery. Chicago, IL: Year Book Medical Publishers, 1970–. Annual.

Based on literature selected from wide range of international medical journals. Presented in condensed form, articles are referenced and conclude with editorial

comments. Reference source which lists significant articles as well as provides synopsis of content. Useful addition to libraries in plastic surgery departments.
R: *British Journal of Surgery* 62: 419 (May 1975); 63: 168 (Feb. 1976); 63: 837 (Oct. 1976); *Plastic and Reconstructive Surgery* 55: 355 (1975); 61: 438 (1978); 63: 117 (1979).

Year Book of Surgery. **Seymour I. Schwartz et al., eds.** Chicago, IL: Year Book Medical Publishers, 1900–. Annual.

Annual and up-to-date collection and critical summaries of important American and British journal articles in the field of general and cardiothoracic surgery. Of value to general surgeons as well as those who are in academic positions.
R: *British Journal of Surgery* 62: 753 (Sept. 1975); 63: 502 (June 1976); 65: 67 (Jan. 1978); 66: 144 (Feb. 1979); 66: 446 (June 1979); *Lahey Clinic Foundation Bulletin* 26: 149 (July–Sept. 1977).

Brain and Nervous System

Year Book of Neurology and Neurosurgery. Chicago, IL: Year Book Medical Publishers, 1969–. Annual.

Continues in part *Year Book of Neurology, Psychiatry and Neurosurgery*.
R: *Brain* 96: 650 (Sept. 1973); 98: 729 (Dec. 1975); 99: 615 (Sept. 1976); *Journal of Neurosurgery* 43: 780 (Dec. 1975).

Cardiovascular System

Year Book of Cardiology. **W. P. Harvey et al., eds.** Chicago, IL: Year Book Medical Publishers, 1968–. Annual.

Presents abstracts of articles appearing in variety of journals with comments on their importance. Serves as a useful guide to the literature on normal and altered cardiovascular functional diseases. A must to all clinicians interested in cardiology.
R: *JAMWA* 33: 491 (Nov. 1978).

Year Book of Cardiovascular Medicine and Surgery. Chicago, IL: Year Book Medical Publishers, 1968–. Annual.

Considered an important annual publication in the field; comprises a collection of excellently edited articles. A helpful tool for all cardiovascular surgeons and cardiologists, useful as a review of all current information.
R: *British Journal of Surgery* 60: 81 (Jan. 1973); 61: 927 (Nov. 1974); 63: 334 (Mar. 1976); 63: 567 (July 1976).

Dentistry

Yearbook of Dentistry. Chicago, IL: Year Book Medical Publishers, 1936–. Annual.

Part of the series *Practical Medicine Year Books*.

Dermatology

Year Book of Dermatology. Chicago, IL: Year Book Medical Publishers,

1902–. Annual.
Formerly *Yearbook of Dermatology and Syphilogy.*
Includes critical editorial comments, grouping of related manuscripts, and full reviews rather than abstracts. Features current material and is of great importance to practicing dermatologists.
R: *Archives of Dermatology* 110: 648 (Oct. 1974).

ENDOCRINOLOGY

Contemporary Endocrinology. Vol. 1–. New York: Plenum, 1979–.
Supersedes *Year in Endocrinology.*

Contemporary Metabolism. Vol. 1–. New York: Plenum, 1979–.
Supersedes *Year in Metabolism.*

Year Book of Endocrinology. Vols. 1–. Chicago, IL: Year Book Medical Publishers, 1950–. Annual.
Continues *Year Book of Endocrinology, Metabolism & Nutrition.*
R: *Annals of Internal Medicine* 89: 1022 (Dec. 1978).

HEALTH SERVICES ADMINISTRATION

Selected Studies in Medical Care and Medical Economics: Annual Report. Chicago, IL: Blue Cross Association and the National Association of Blue Shield Plans, 1969–. Annual.
Contains abstracts of health care studies. Entries arranged by topics; include objectives of study, content, methodology, principal findings, other appropriate data. Continues the *Annual Report of the National Association of Insurance Commissioners.*
R: *MRW* S2, pp. 38, 58.

HEMATOLOGY

The Year in Hematology. Vol. 1–. New York: Plenum, 1977–. Annual.

INFECTIOUS DISEASES

Microbiology. **David Schlessinger, ed.** Washington, DC: American Society for Microbiology, 1974–. Annual.
R: *American Journal of Clinical Nutrition* 29: 492 (Apr. 1976); *American Journal of Tropical Medicine & Hygiene* 24: 1046 (Nov. 1975); *Immunology* 32: 372 (Mar. 1977); *Journal of Allied Health* 6: 67 (Winter 1977); *Journal of Pharmaceutical Sciences* 66: 612 (Apr. 1977); 67: 592 (Apr. 1978).

INTERNAL MEDICINE

Current Medical Diagnosis and Treatment. Vol. 1–. Los Altos, CA: Lange Medical Publications, 1974–. Annual.
R: *British Journal of Surgery* 66: 144 (Feb. 1979).

Medical and Health Annual. **Douglas C. Benson et al., eds.** Chicago, IL: Encyclopaedia Britannica, 1977–. Annual.

Brings together topical information on a variety of subjects in health and medicine. Contains many illustrations, a first aid handbook. Intended for the lay public.
R: *JAMA* 239: 2489 (June 9, 1978); *WLB* 52: 266 (Nov. 1977).

Medicine. New York: John Wiley, 1977–. Annual.
R: *Canadian Medical Association Journal* 118: 1372 (June 10, 1978).

Year Book of Medicine. **David E. Rogers et al., eds.** Chicago, IL: Year Book Medical Publishers, 1949–. Annual.

Reviews of international literature are presented in abstract form with concise editorial comments. About 100 pages for each of the seven major sections: infections, chest, blood and blood forming organs, heart and blood vessels, digestive system, metabolism and kidney, and water and electrolytes. Recommended for physicians and students who wish to keep abreast of recent development in medicine.
R: *American Journal of Digestive Diseases* 23: 575 (June 1978); *Gastroenterology* 70: 628 (Apr. 1976); 72: 1365 (June 1977); 75: 159 (July 1978); *Lancet* 1: 1237 (June 10, 1978).

NURSING

Nursing Digest 1975 Review of Medicine & Surgery. **Eileen C. Hodgman, ed.** Wakefield, MA: Contemporary Publishing, 1975.

ONCOLOGY AND NUCLEAR MEDICINE

International Agency for Research on Cancer: Annual Report. **International Agency for Research on Cancer.** Lyon, France: World Health Organization, 1968–. Annual.

Outlines IARC prospects for long-term prevention of cancer and provides field reports and references. Helpful to physicians.
R: *British Journal of Radiology* 48: 953 (1975).

Year Book of Cancer. **Randolph L. Clark and Russell W. Cumley, eds.** Chicago, IL: Year Book Medical Publishers, 1957–. Annual.

An extensive collection of abstracts of major articles in oncology which includes summaries and criticism of each article. Comprises a multidisciplinary approach to the treatment and management of cancer. Beneficial tool to surgeons and oncologists.
R: *American Journal of Roentgenology* 133: 575 (Sept. 1979); *Lahey Clinic Foundation Bulletin* 26: 149 (July–Sept. 1977).

Year Book of Nuclear Medicine. Chicago, IL: Year Book Medical Publishers, 1966–. Annual.
R: *American Journal of Roentgenology* 130: 813 (Apr. 1978); *British Journal of Ra-*

diology 47: 15 (1974); 49: 49 (1976); 50: 204 (1977); *Physics in Medicine & Biology* 20: 150 (Jan. 1975); 21: 320 (Mar. 1976); 21: 997 (Nov. 1976); *Radiology* 122: 162 (1977).

OPHTHALMOLOGY

Year Book of Ophthalmology. **William F. Hughes, ed.** Chicago, IL: Year Book Medical Publishers, 1901–. Annual.

Abstracts most important ophthalmological publications of world literature. Chapters are introduced by statement written by an expert in the field which highlights important aspects in that subspecialty. Recommended as a useful reference for all ophthalmologists.

R: *American Journal of Ophthalmology* 75: 903 (May 1973); 77: 929 (June 1974); 79: 527 (Mar. 1975); 81: 368 (Mar. 1976); 85: 128 (Jan. 1978); *Archives of Ophthalmology* 91: 521 (June 1974); 93: 470 (June 1975); 94: 1427 (Aug. 1976); 95: 529 (Mar. 1977); 96: 730 (Apr. 1978); 97: 564 (Mar. 1979).

ORTHOPEDICS

Year Book of Orthopedics and Traumatic Surgery. Chicago, IL: Year Book Medical Publishers, 1969–. Annual.

R: *Archives of Physical Medicine and Rehabilitation* 58: 378 (Aug. 1977); *British Journal of Surgery* 63: 729 (Sept. 1976).

OTORHINOLARYNGOLOGY

Year Book of Otolaryngology. Chicago, IL: Year Book Medical Publishers, 1976–. Annual.

Continues the *Year Book of the Ear, Nose and Throat.*
R: *Plastic and Reconstructive Surgery* 60: 274 (1977).

PATHOLOGY

Pathobiology Annual. Vols. 1–. New York: Appleton-Century-Crofts, 1971–. Annual.

Volume 9, 1979.
R: *JAMA* 227: 944 (Feb. 25, 1974).

Pathology Annual. Vols. 1–. **Sheldon C. Sommers, ed.** New York: Appleton-Century-Crofts, 1966–. Annual.

Volume 14, 1979.
Anthology of review articles of interest to pathologists. Carefully written and includes extensive references. Straightforward treatment of current concepts. Considered a high-quality annual, recommended to all pathologists as a succinct reference source.

R: *Annals of Internal Medicine* 78: 476 (Mar. 1973); 85: 145 (July 1976); *Archives of Internal Medicine* 132: 777 (Nov. 1973); *Archives of Pathology & Laboratory Medicine* 103: 369 (July 1979); *JAMA* 231: 766 (May 6, 1974); 235: 96 (Jan. 5, 1976); 237: 1011 (Mar. 7, 1977); *Lancet* 2: 1068 (Nov. 21, 1970).

Year Book of Pathology and Clinical Pathology. Chicago, IL: Year Book Medical Publishers, 1940–. Annual.
R: *Canadian Medical Association Journal* 118: 245 (Feb. 4, 1978); *Journal of Clinical Pathology* 32: 413 (Apr. 1979).

PEDIATRICS

Year Book of Pediatrics. Chicago, IL: Year Book Medical Publishers, 1933–. Annual.

PHARMACY AND PHARMACOLOGY

Year Book of Drug Therapy. Vols. 1–. Chicago, IL: Year Book Medical Publishers, 1949–. Annual.
Continues *Year Book of General Therapeutics.*
R: *American Family Physician* 17: 301 (Apr. 1978).

PSYCHIATRY AND PSYCHOLOGY

The Annual of Psychoanalysis. Vols. 1–. **Chicago Institute for Psychoanalysis.** New York: International Universities Press, 1973–. Irregular.
Volume 5, 1977.
This series aims to publish outstanding theoretical and clinical contributions to psychoanalysis. Each volume covers history, developmental psychology, clinical studies, psychoanalytic education, etc. An important annual for students of psychoanalysis.
R: *American Journal of Psychiatry* 135: 1261 (Oct. 1978); *Journal of Nervous and Mental Disease* 161: 280 (1975); 165: 147 (1977); *RQ* 13: 349 (Summer 1974).

Year Book of Psychiatry and Applied Mental Health. Chicago, IL: Year Book Medical Publishers, 1970–. Annual.
Continues in part the *Year Book of Neurology, Psychiatry, Neurosurgery.*
R: *American Family Physician* 15: 237 (Feb. 1977); *American Journal of Psychiatry* 133: 1099 (Sept. 1976); *RSR* 3: 38 (July–Dec. 1975).

PUBLIC HEALTH

Environmental Quality—1976, 7th Annual Report. **US Council on Environmental Quality, 1976.** Washington, DC: US Government Printing Office. Annual.
R: Chen (p. 260).

Toxicology Annual. **C. L. Winek, ed.** New York: Marcel Dekker, 1975–1977.
Selects articles of significant interest in toxicology such as the hazards of household chemicals, saccharin, etc. Useful to pathologists, toxicologists as a concise reference to recent developments in the field.
R: *Archives of Pathology & Laboratory Medicine* 100: 288 (May 1976); *Journal of Pharmaceutical Sciences* 65: 1416 (Sept. 1976).

Radiology

Yearbook of Diagnostic Radiology. Chicago, IL: Year Book Medical Publishers, 1975–. Annual.

Continues *Yearbook of Radiology,* 1932–1975.
Serves as both a yearbook and a review source for radiologists. Contains abstracts of recent developments in diagnosis and therapy, high-quality illustrations and photographs. Author and subject indexes.
R: *American Journal of Roentgenology* 122: 200 (Sept. 1974); 124: 519 (July 1975); 130: 812 (Apr. 1978); *British Journal of Radiology* 49: 649 (1976); 50: 22 (1977).

Urogenital System

Obstetrics and Gynecology Annual. Vols. 1–. **Ralph M. Wynn, ed.** New York: Appleton-Century-Crofts, 1972–. Annual.
Volume 8, 1979.
R: *JAMA* 234: 103 (Oct. 6, 1975); 237: 1011 (Mar. 7, 1977); *JAMWA* 32: 236 (June 1977); *ARBA* (1977, p. 718).

Year Book of Obstetrics and Gynecology. Vols. 1–. Chicago, IL: Year Book Medical Publishers, 1933–. Annual.
Continues in part *Practical Medicine Series.*

Yearbook of Urology. Vol. 1–. Chicago, IL: Year Book Medical Publishers, 1933–. Annual.

Veterinary Medicine

Animal Health Yearbook: Annuaire de la Sante Animale: Anuario de Sanidad Animal. **Food and Agriculture Organization of the United Nations.** Rome: Food and Agriculture Organization of the United Nations, 1957–. Annual.

An annual publication of world animal diseases arranged in coded tabular form. Provides information for all major animal groups including bees and fish.
R: *ARBA* (1971, p. 543; 1974, p. 645).

The Veterinary Annual. Vol. 1–. Chicago, IL: Year Book Medical Publishers, 1960–. Annual.

BIOGRAPHICAL SOURCES

General

American Men and Women of Science. 13th ed. 7 vols. New York: Bowker, Nov. 1976.
Twelfth edition, 1971–1973.
With this edition, all volumes have appeared simultaneously. The most comprehensive, up-to-date source of its kind. Alphabetically arranged profiles on some 110,000 US and Canadian scientists engaged in activities in 1,000 areas of physical, biological, and selected social sciences. The six biographical volumes provide

pertinent information on personnel from the fields of economics, veterinary sciences, medical sciences, etc. Includes a geographic and discipline index. In keeping with the pattern of earlier editions, supplementary material may be anticipated.
R: *Choice* 11: 1730 (Feb. 1975); *CRL* 28: 68 (1967); *LJ* 92: 2751 (1967); *RQ* (Fall 1970); *WLB* 48: 340 (Dec. 1973); *ARBA* (1974, p. 550; 1971, p. 478); Chen (p. 261); Jenkins (A87); Mal (3-49); Wal (p. 57); Win (EA183, 1EA34, 1EA35, 2EA35).

American Men and Women of Science: Medical and Health Sciences 1977. **Jaques Cattell Press, ed.** New York: Bowker, 1977.
Over 26,000 entries alphabetically arranged, covering the fields of medicine, pharmacology, and veterinary science. Also includes scientists whose work is related to the medical and health sciences. Provides full biographic information.

American Men and Women of Science: The Medical Sciences 1975. **Jaques Cattell Press, ed.** New York: Bowker, 1975.
Biographies of all medical scientists and professionals in the twelfth edition of *American Men and Women of Science* are included. Also lists additional 2,000 biographies.
R: *RSR* 3: 71 (July–Dec. 1975); *ARBA* (1976, p. 735).

Asimov's Biographical Encyclopedia of Science and Technology: The Lives and Achievements of 1,195 Great Scientists from Ancient Times to the Present Chronologically Arranged. New rev. ed. **Isaac Asimov.** Garden City, NY: Doubleday, 1972.
First edition, 1964.
Contains 1,195 readable biographical sketches intended for students and laymen. More a popular reference than a scholarly undertaking.
R: *ARBA* (1973, p. 536); Chen (p. 261).

BIO-BASE. **Dennis La Beau, ed.** Detroit, MI: Gale Research, 1980.
A master index to approximately 500 biographical dictionaries in microfiche format.

A Biographical Dictionary of Scientists. 2d ed. **Trevor I. Williams, ed.** New York: John Wiley, 1974.
First edition, 1969.
Handy volume provides brief accounts of over 1,000 scientists, no longer living, who have been prominent in medicine, biology, etc. Initialed biographies usually range from 200 to 400 words and are arranged alphabetically by names. Appendix is a list of scientists whose names occur in book but for whom no full biographies are given.
R: *JAMA* 233: 89 (July 7, 1975); *Science* 167: 363 (Jan. 23, 1970); *Choice* 12: 516 (June 1975); *LJ* 94: 2774 (Aug. 1969); *WLB* 50: 126 (Oct. 1975); *ARBA* (1976, p. 642); Chen (p. 261); *MRW* S2, p. 94; Wal (p. 54); Win (3EA33).

A Biographical History of Medicine: Excerpts and Essays on the Men and Their Work. **John H. Talbott.** New York: Grune & Stratton, 1970.

A ready source of historical/biographical data of over 550 contributors to the medical sciences dating from 2250 B.C. through the first half of the twentieth century: includes information not found in other tools and pictures of biographical subject. Indexed by name.
R: *LJ* 96: 1354 (Apr. 15, 1971); *ARBA* (1972, p. 628).

Biographical Memoirs. Vols. 1–. **US National Academy of Sciences.** New York: Columbia University Press, 1877–.

Index to volumes 1–40, 1877–1969, in volume 40.
Volume 50, 1979.

Catalog of Biographies. **New York Academy of Medicine Library.** Boston, MA: G. K. Hall, 1960.

Represents a photographic reproduction of the library's shelflist. Consists of biographies of physicians and scientists, interspersed with some autobiographies and family histories.
R: Win (EK129).

Dictionary of Scientific Biography. 15 vols. **Charles C. Gillespie, ed.** New York: Charles Scribners, 1970–78.

The most scholarly and comprehensive reference on scientific biography for the scientist and science historian. International in scope, it will provide well-documented biographies of deceased scientists of major importance.
R: *American Scientist* 61: 353 (May/June 1973); *ISIS* (Sept. 1971); *Physics Today* 18: 86 (1965); *Science* 170: 615 (Nov. 27, 1970); *BL* 67: 201 (1971); *CRL* 32: 38 (1971); *LJ* (July 1970); *WLB* 45: 185 (Oct. 1970); *ARBA* (1976, p. 642; 1971, p. 478); Jenkins (A88); Wal (p. 53); Win (3EA30).

Disease and Destiny: A Bibliography of Medical References to the Famous. **Judson B. Gilbert.** London: Dawson, 1962.

A medical biographical bibliography which details birth and death facts about famous people. Entries alphabetically arranged are drawn from *Index-Catalogue of the Surgeon General's Office* and *Index Medicus.*
R: Win (EK10).

Great Women of Medicine. **Ruth F. Hume.** New York: Random House, 1964.

International Directory of Research and Development Scientists. Philadelphia: Institute for Scientific Information, 1967–. Annual.

Best single source for names and addresses of scientists throughout the world.
R: *BMLA* 57: 94 (1969); *LJ* 93: 2790 (1968); Chen (p. 262); Jenkins (A117); Mal (3-48); Wal (p. 40); Win (3EA22).

Jewish Physicians: A Biographical Index. **Nathan Koren.** Jerusalem: Israel Universities Press, 1973.

Some 9,000 entries divided into 2 parts: all known Jewish physicians from earliest times through the eighteenth century and prominent Jewish physicians of the nineteenth and twentieth centuries. Lists noteworthy teachers, clinicians, practitioners, and medical researchers. Pertinent data included in entry: name, dates, brief annotation, and coded reference to source.

LC Science Tracer Bullet: Biographical Sources in the Sciences, TB 77-14. **Janet Terner, comp.** US Library of Congress, Science and Technology Division, Reference Section. Washington, DC: US Government Printing Office, 1978.

Concentrates on American men and women of science. Covers both historical and contemporary scientists in a systematic approach. Useful reference tool.
R: *LCIB* 37: 456 (Aug. 4, 1978).

McGraw-Hill Modern Men of Science. 2 vols. New York: McGraw-Hill, 1966–1968.

Some 900 biographies of scientists not included in the *McGraw-Hill Encyclopedia of Science and Technology.*
R: *Science* 153: 731 (1966); *Choice* 5: 1418; *Subscription Books Bulletin* 64: 793 (1968); Chen (p. 262); Jenkins (A91); Wal (p. 54); Win (1EA36; 2EA36).

Minorities in Science: The Challenge for Change in Biomedicine. **Melnick and Hamilton.** New York: Plenum, 1977.

Nobel Prize Winners in Medicine and Physiology, 1901–1965. Rev. ed. **Theodore L. Sourkes.** New York: Abelard-Schuman, 1967.

First edition, 1953.
Outlines biographical details of prize winners. Special mention of individual prize discovery with a brief explanation of the contribution. Includes revised and updated early biographies. Chronological arrangement.
R: Win (EK131).

A Select Bibliography of Medical Biography: With an Introductory Essay on Medical Biography. 2nd ed. **John L. Thornton.** London: Library Association, 1970.

First edition, 1961.
A bibliography of more than 400 medical biographies, some with several entries. Almost 100 collective biographies are listed separately.
R: Win (EK125).

Who's Who in Health Care. New York: Hanover Publications, 1977.
R: Sheehy (EK23).

Women in Medicine: A Bibliography of the Literature of Women Physicians. **Sandra L. Chaff et al., comps. and eds.** Metuchen, NJ: Scarecrow Press, 1977.

Annotated descriptions of over 4,000 articles and books on women physicians spanning the period from 1750 to 1975. Citations are divided into fourteen broad subject categories covering aspects of women physicians' experiences, subdivided by geographic locations and finally by alphabetical listings of authors. Thorough indexing of authors, subjects, and personal names. Important reference tool for medical, university, and large public libraries.

R: *JAMWA* 33: 527 (Dec. 1978); *ARBA* (1978, p. 707).

Anesthesiology and General Surgery

Yearbook—American College of Surgeons. Chicago, IL: American College of Surgeons, 1913–1950/1952; 1974–.

Issued 1953–1971 as *Directory—American College of Surgeons*, with supplements in between edition.
Listing of Fellows of the American College of Surgeons in two parts: biographical and geographical. Provides both historical and current information. Includes fellows from the United States and Canada.
R: *MRW* S3, p. 52.

Dentistry

Oral Maxillo-Facial Surgeons of the World. 5th ed. **W. Harry Archer, ed.** Pittsburg, PA: Oral Maxillo-Facial Surgeons of the World, 1976.

First edition, 1957; second edition, 1961; third edition, 1966; fourth edition, 1971. Earlier editions under the title *Oral Surgery Directory of the World*.
Provides biographical information for oral surgeons in the United States and names and addresses for those in foreign countries. State dental laws relating to oral surgery, dental societies and schools are included. Chapters on history of oral surgery and name index are included.
R: *MRW* S2, pp. 26, 100; Win (EK154; 1EJ20).

Internal Medicine

Biographical Directory of the American College of Physicians. **Jaques Cattell Press, ed.** Ann Arbor, MI: Bowker, 1979.

Lists over 26,000 qualified internists and allied specialists who are members of the College. Geographically arranged, each entry provides the basic background and professional information on each biographee. A helpful tool.

Biographical Memoirs of Fellows of the Royal Society. Vols. 1–. London: Royal Society, 1955–. Annual.

Presents biographical sketches of Fellows of the Royal Society deceased within the previous year. Copious descriptions of personal and educational backgrounds and scientific work. Data listed in concise tabular form. Each memoir concludes with honors, memberships, honorary degrees, references, and bibliography. Complete biography written by contemporaries in the Royal Society.
R: *BMJ* 1: 1341 (May 19, 1979).

Dictionary of American Medical Biography. **Howard A. Kelly and Walter L. Burrage.** New York: Appleton, 1928. Repr. Boston, MA: Milford House, 1971.

Published in 1912 as *Cyclopedia of American Medical Biography*, and in 1920 as *American Medical Biography*.
Biographies of 2,049 deceased American physicians and surgeons from colonial days to 1927. Includes bibliographies.
R: Win (EK135).

Directory of Women Physicians in the US. **American Medical Association.** Chicago, IL: American Medical Association, 1973–.

Supplement to the *American Medical Directory,* 1973–.
A comprehensive listing of women physicians, arranged geographically and alphabetically. Includes all women belonging to the American Medical Association. Lists medical schools around the world.
R: *MRW* S3, pp. 41, 55.

Lives of the Fellows of the Royal College of Surgeons of England, 1930–1951. **Sir D'Arcy Power and William Richard Le Fanu.** London: Royal College of Surgeons, 1953.

Lists biographies of fellows of the College deceased during the time span from 1930 to 1951. Includes fellows' publications.
R: Win (EK139).

Notable Names in Medicine and Surgery. 3d ed. **Hamilton Bailey and W. J. Bishop.** London: H. K. Lewis, 1959.

Lists biographical material on 79 men whose medical discoveries bear their names (e.g. Potter's disease). Provides additional biographies for further study.
R: Win (EK126).

The Roll of the Royal College of Physicians of London. 2d rev. ed. **William Munk, ed.** London: Royal College of Physicians of London, 1878.

Volume 1, 1518–1700; volume 2, 1701–1800; volume 3, 1801–1825. Continued by *Lives of the Fellows of the Royal College of Physicians of London,* 1826–1925, edited by G. H. Brown, 1955; *Lives of the Fellows of the Royal College of Physicians of London,* continued to 1965, edited by R. R. Trail, 1968.
Volumes 1–3 list more than 1,700 names, arranged chronologically, with name indexes in each volume. A subject index to all three volumes and a brief history of the College are included in volume 3. Two later volumes list additional 1,296 fellows.
R: Win (EK136, EK137, EK137a); Sheehy (p. 813).

PHYSICAL MEDICINE AND REHABILITATION

Yearbook of the American Occupational Therapy Association. New York: American Occupational Therapy Association, 1972–. Annual.

Continues the *Registry of the American Occupational Therapy Association.*
Annual publication which includes alphabetically arranged biographical listings of registered occupational therapists and certified occupational therapy assistants. Accredited programs in the United States and the world are also included.
R: *MRW* S2, p. 74.

PSYCHIATRY AND PSYCHOLOGY

Biographical Directory of the American Psychological Association. **American Psychological Association.** Washington, DC: American Psychological Association, 1970–. Annual.

Issued alternately with the association's membership register. Alphabetically lists

members, with biographical information. Includes bylaws, statement of ethics, etc.
R: *MRW* S2, p. 83.

Biographical Directory of the Fellows and Members of the American Psychiatric Association. 7th ed. **Jaques Cattell Press, comps.** American Psychiatric Association. New York: Bowker, 1977.
First edition, 1941; fifth edition, 1968; sixth edition, 1973.
Over 23,000 biographical entries of fellows and members in the United States and the world, alphabetically arranged by name. Entries include such information as birthdate, education, publications, address, and telephone number. Geographic index.
R: *MRW* S3, p. 42.

Names in the History of Psychology: A Biographical Sourcebook. **Leonard Zusne.** New York: John Wiley, 1975.
Over 500 biographies of prominent but deceased psychologists comprise this valuable reference tool. Biographical information includes birth and death dates, education level, positions, and honors. Portraits enhance the text. Cross-references and a comprehensive index contribute to its reference value in school, public, and special libraries.
R: *RSR* 4: 49 (Jan.–Mar. 1976).

The Psychologists. Vol. 2. **T. S. Krawiec, ed.** New York: Oxford University Press, 1974.
Volume 1, 1972.
This volume is the second in a series of autobiographies of prominent psychologists. Eleven contributors to the field of psychology are included, each about 50 pages in length and accompanied by a list of selected references. Interesting reading and a valuable reference tool for students and professionals.
R: *American Journal of Psychiatry* 132: 884 (Aug. 1975).

Public Health

Biographical Directory of the American Public Health Association. **Jaques Cattell Press, ed.** New York: Bowker, 1979.
Alphabetically arranged biographical information concerning 26,000 members of the American Public Health Association. Geographical and subject (social work, environment, engineers, industrial hygiene, etc.) indexes.

Veterinary Medicine

American Men and Women in Science: Agricultural, Animal and Veterinary Sciences 1974. **Jaques Cattell Press, ed.** New York: Bowker, 1974.
Lists 14,200 men and women whose biographies were included in the twelfth edition of *American Men and Women of Science.*
R: *RQ* 15: 169 (Winter 1975); *ARBA* (1975, p. 752).

CHAPTER 12   HISTORY

GENERAL

Adventures in Medical Research: A Century of Discovery at Johns Hopkins. **A. McGehee Harvey.** Baltimore, MD: Johns Hopkins University Press, 1976.

This book details the history of the Johns Hopkins Medical School, one of the most eminent schools in this country. Its interesting format includes portraits of individual physicans and bibliographic references. Despite limited focus, the book should be useful and interesting to a wide audience.
R: *Annals of Internal Medicine* 85: 549 (Oct. 1976).

American Medical Bibliography, 1639–1783. **Francisco Guerra.** New York: Lathrop C. Harper, 1962.

A chronological catalog of medical literature. Includes books, journals, pamphlets, and broadsides. Covers medicine, surgery, pharmacy, veterinary medicine, and dentistry. Divided into three sections according to printed media.
R: Win (EK120).

American Medical Education: The Formative Years, 1765–1910. **Martin Kaufman.** Westport, CT: Greenwood Press, 1976.

This book presents the development of medical education, drawing upon the perspective of various institutions. Divided into chapters, each with a complete subject bibliography. Contains a good deal of useful information.
R: *Journal of Medical Education* 52: 697 (Aug. 1977).

American Physicians in the Nineteenth Century: From Sects to Science. **William G. Rothstein.** Baltimore, MD: Johns Hopkins University Press, 1972.

This is an historical analysis of the medical profession in the United States covering the time period of the nineteenth century. Examines licensing laws, scientific developments, changing therapies, and education. Also discusses the formation of the AMA in 1901. Considered a significant work, useful to sociologists, historians, and medical educators.
R: *Annals of Internal Medicine* 78: 159 (Jan. 1973); *Choice* 9: 1462 (Jan. 1973).

Bibliography of the History of Medicine. Vols. 1–. **US National Library of Medicine.** Bethesda, MD: US National Library of Medicine, 1965–.
Volume 12, *1976*, 1978. Cumulates annual volumes at intervals.
Annual bibliography of the history of medicine and its related sciences, professions, and institutions. Covers all chronological periods and geographical areas. Includes journal articles, monographs, historical chapters in general monographs, and entries for symposia, congresses, and similar publications. Bibliography consists of three additional sections: biographies, subjects, and authors. A list of reprints currently received at the National Library of Medicine completes the volume.
R: *RSR* 2: 118 (July–Sept. 1974); 3: 101 (July–Dec. 1975); *ARBA* (1970, p. 132; 1974, p. 625); Sheehy (EK24); Win (EA178; EK117; 1EJ16).

Bibliography of the History of Medicine of the United States and Canada, 1939–1960. **Genevieve Miller, ed.** Baltimore, MD: Johns Hopkins University Press, 1964.
R: Win (EK116).

Biological Abstracts/BIOSIS: The First Fifty Years: The Evolution of a Major Science Information Service. **William C. Steere, ed.** New York: Plenum, 1976.

Biology: Its Historical Development. **Howard Baumel.** New York: Philosophical Library, 1978.
A brief account of the history of biology which covers a broad spectrum of events. Well written. Recommended to students and teachers of biology.
R: *Journal of Anatomy* 128: 409 (Mar. 1979).

A Catalogue of Incunabula and Manuscripts in the Army Medical Library, by Dorothy M. Schullian and Francis E. Sommer. **US National Library of Medicine.** Bethesda, MD: US National Library of Medicine, 1948.
Divided into two parts, the first section lists 490 incunabula with full bibliographical descriptions and citations to listings in other bibliographies and about 35 early Western manuscripts. Part 2 describes some 137 Oriental manuscripts.
R: Win (EK33).

A Catalogue of Printed Books in the Wellcome Historical Medical Library. 2 vols. **Wellcome Historical Medical Museum Library.** London: Wellcome Historical Medical Library, 1962–1966.
In two volumes: 7,000 titles of books printed before 1641, alphabetical by author; 18,000 titles printed from 1641 to 1850.
R: Win (EK25).

A Catalogue of Sixteenth Century Printed Books in the National Library of Medicine. **Richard J. Durling, comp.** US National Library of Medicine. Washington, DC: US Government Printing Office, 1967.
Includes over 4,800 entries with brief bibliographical notes. Indexed by name of printer and publisher and by geographic region.
R: Win (EK20).

The Cole Library of Early Medicine and Zoology: Catalogue of Books and Pamphlets. Vol. 1. **Nellie B. Eales, comp.** University of Reading Library. Oxford, England: Alden Press, 1969.
Volume 1, *1472–1800.*
Descriptive catalog of a distinguished collection arranged chronologically. Entries contain full bibliographic data with annotations. Author and subject indexes. Valuable source book for historians of medicine and science.
R: *Library Association Record* 75: 105 (May 1973); Win (EK17).

Current Work in the History of Medicine: An International Bibliography. Vols. 1–. **Wellcome Historical Medical Library.** London: Wellcome Historical

Medical Library, 1954–. Quarterly.

Reviews international literature on the history of medicine. Subject arrangement with author index in each issue. A list of new books on the topic published at end of issue. A retrospective cumulative index maintained at the Wellcome Library.
R: Win (EK118).

Development of Biochemical Concepts from Ancient to Modern Times. **Henry M. Leicester.** Cambridge, MA: Harvard University Press, 1974.

Covers the subject of human biochemistry, detailing knowledge of specific body functions from ancient times. Chronological presentation, well referenced and indexed. Recommended to medical school, college, and public libraries.
R: *RSR* 3: 36 (July–Dec. 1975).

The Development of Medical Bibliography. **Estelle Brodman.** Baltimore, MD: Medical Library Association, 1954.

A comprehensive list of medical bibliographies dating from 1500. Bibliographies are in western languages and cover general medicine; indexes and abstracts are also included. Provides brief biography of compilers, two appendixes, one with references, the other listing medical bibliographies not discussed in the text. Material is chronologically arranged by century.
R: Win (EK7).

The Development of Medicine As A Profession. **V. W. Bullough.** Basel: S. Karger, 1966.

This book examines the development of medicine as a profession from ancient times to the end of the medieval period. Includes bibliographical essay.

Doctors Wanted: No Women Need Apply. **Mary Roth Walsh.** New Haven, CT: Yale University Press, 1977.

This is a scholarly account of the roots of women in the medical profession in the United States. Contains classic material and useful statistics. Highly recommended.
R: *NEJM* 297: 66 (July 7, 1977).

Early American Medical Imprints: A Guide to Works Printed in the United States, 1668–1820. **Robert B. Austin.** US National Library of Medicine. Washington, DC: US Government Printing Office, 1961.

Lists over 2,000 separately published items, including books, pamphlets, theses, broadsides, and selected periodicals, arranged alphabetically by author. Includes full bibliographical citations. Indicates holdings for 67 libraries. Contains valuable chronological index and a list of 74 items also cited in Evans's *American Bibliography.*
R: Win (EK22).

Ethics in Medicine: Historical Perspectives and Contemporary Concerns. **Stanley J. Reiser, Arthur J. Dyck, and William J. Curran, eds.** Cambridge, MA: MIT Press, 1977.

A comprehensive anthology which examines medical ethics from the time of Hippocrates. Emphasizes current problems, drawing on over 100 documents from interdisciplinary historical sources. A thorough reference source for medical students and historians.
R: *JAMA* 239: 548 (Feb. 6, 1978); *Physical Therapy* 59: 358 (1979); *Quarterly Review of Biology* 53: 355 (1978).

Explorers of the Body. **Steven Lehrer.** Garden City, NY: Doubleday, 1979.

A survey of significant ideas and individuals in the history of medicine. Includes excellent bibliography.
R: *LJ* 105: 572 (Mar. 1, 1980).

The Flexner Report on Medical Education in the United States and Canada. **Abraham Flexner.** New York: Arno, 1972.

The *Flexner Report* of 1910 is considered the classic study of medical education, revolutionizing the format of medical education in America. This book is an exact reprint of the original study and is indexed.

The Great Medical Bibliographers: A Study in Humanism, The Historical Library, Yale University School of Medicine, Publication No. 26. **John F. Fulton.** Westport, CT: Greenwood Press, 1977.

Reprint of 1951 edition.
Covers medical bibliographers from the second through the twentieth century.

Half a Century of Medical Research. Vol. 2. **A. Landsborough Thomson.** London: Her Majesty's Stationery Office, 1975.

A well-written history of the British Medical Research Council. Contains accounts of the numerous achievements of this institution.
R: *BMJ* 1: 947 (Oct. 16, 1976).

A Half-Century of American Medical Education. **Vernon W. Lippard.** New York: Josiah Macy, Jr. Foundation, 1975.

A critical review of medical education in the United States from 1920 to 1970. Explores such factors as changes in the economy, citizen philanthropists, licensure examinations. A concise and useful reference.
R: *Annals of Internal Medicine* 83: 743 (Nov. 1975); *Journal of Medical Education* 50: 829 (Aug. 1975).

The Healers: The Rise of the Medical Establishment. **John Duffy.** New York: McGraw-Hill, 1976.

This is a comprehensive survey of the history of medicine in America from the sixteenth century to 1975. Focuses on scientific and social aspects. Succinctly presents the most significant events. Well documented. Recommended to a wide audience.
R: *JAMA* 237: 275 (Jan. 17, 1977).

The Healer's Art: The Doctor Through History. **J. Camp.** London: Frederick Muller, 1978.

This history explores the medical profession from primitive times to the twen-

tieth century, citing numerous anecdotes and events.
R: *Pharmaceutical Journal* 222: 16 (1979).

History of General Physiology 600 B.C. to A.D. 1900. 2 vols. **Thomas S. Hall.** Chicago, IL: University of Chicago Press, 1975.

A collection of essays which give an overview of the history of biology. Presents the thoughts of individual scientists, philosophers, and physicians in chronological order. Helpful as an introduction to the history of ideas in biology.
R: *JAMA* 235: 950 (Mar. 1, 1976).

History of Medical Illustration, From Antiquity to 1600 A. D. **Robert Herrlinger.** London: Pitman Medical, 1970.

A History of Medicine. 2d ed. **Arturo Castiglioni.** New York: Alfred Knopf, 1947.

A History of Medicine. **Ralph H. Major.** Springfield, IL: Charles C. Thomas, 1954.

History of Medicine in the United States. 2 vols. **Francis R. Packard.** New York: Hoeber, 1931. Repr. New York: Hafner, 1963.

A valuable reference on American medical history; contains biographical information, illustrations, and bibliographies, including one of pre-Revolutionary War medical publications.
R: Win (EK124).

The History of the Negro in Medicine. **Herbert M. Morais.** New York: Publishers, 1969.

A History of Women in Medicine From Earliest Times to the Beginnings of the Nineteenth Century. **Kate C. H. Mead.** Haddam, CT: Haddam Press, 1938.

Incunabula and Sixteenth Century Printed Books in the National Library of Medicine, Supplement 1. **US National Library of Medicine.** Washington, DC: US Government Printing Office, 1972.

A supplement to *A Catalogue of Sixteenth Century Printed Books in the National Library of Medicine.* Lists 27 incunabula and 272 books added to the NLM collection since 1967.
R: *ARBA* (1973, p. 607).

Incunabula Scientifica et Medica: Short Title List. **Arnold C. Klebs.** Bruges, Belgium: St. Catherine Press, 1938.

History of medicine series sponsored by the New York Academy of Medicine.
R: Win (EK32).

Index Catalogue of the Library of the Surgeon General's Office, United States Army (Army Medical Library), Authors and Subjects. 61 vols. **US National Library of Medicine.** Washington, DC: US Government Printing Office, 1880–1961.

Series 1, A–Z (1880–1895), 16 vols.; series 2, A–Z (1896–1916), 21 vols.; series 3, A–Z (1918–1932), 10 vols.; series 4, A–Mn (1936–1955); series 5, (1959–1961), 3 vols.
A bibliography of selected monographs, imprints, pamphlets, theses, and periodical articles taken from the unpublished files of the *Catalog* of the National Library of Medicine (formerly the Surgeon General's Library and the Army Medical Library). Covers the nineteenth and first half of the twentieth century.
R: Win (EK22).

International Bibliography of the History of Legal Medicine, DHEW Publication no. (NIH) 73-535. **Jaroslav Nemec.** US National Library of Medicine, US Department of Health, Education, and Welfare. Washington, DC: US Government Printing Office, 1974.
Contains 1,615 annotated references which cover published monographic literature journal articles, and dissertations. Entries cover 26 languages and range from sixteenth-century to present-day literature. Concentrates on legal medicine, toxicology, forensic psychiatry and dentistry, war crimes of a medical nature, and international medical law. Entries are alphabetically arranged by author; subject index included.
R: *RSR* 2: 118 (July–Sept. 1974); 3: 101 (July–Dec. 1975); *MRW* S3, p. 25.

An Introduction to the History of Medicine. 4th ed. **Fielding H. Garrison.** Philadelphia, PA: W. B. Saunders, 1929.
First edition, 1913; second edition, 1917; third edition, 1921.
The classic reference source on the history of medicine from prehistoric times until 1928. Includes biographies, bibliographies, special subject histories from all eras. Contains an appendix of important dates; well indexed by subject and name. An invaluable source.
R: *Plastic and Reconstructive Surgery* 57: 510 (1976); Win (EK123).

A Medical Bibliography (Garrison and Morton): An Annotated Check-List of Texts Illustrating the History of Medicine. 3d ed. **Leslie T. Morton.** Philadelphia, PA: J. B. Lippincott, 1970.
First edition, 1943; second edition, 1954.
Chronological bibliography of most important contributions to world literature on medicine. Annotations explain significance of individual contributions to development of medical science. Over 7,500 entries, arranged by medical category, include author, date, title, and citation. Aid to researcher and historian working with medical literature. Complete author and subject indexes are included.
R: *Lancet* 2: 82 (July 11, 1970); *ARBA* (1971, p. 528); *MRW* S2, pp. 11, 54; Win (EJ77; EK119; 3EJ17).

The Medical Profession in Mid-Victorian London. **M. Jeanne Peterson.** Berkeley, CA: University of California Press, 1978.
A vivid account of Victorian medicine during the nineteenth century. Particular emphasis is accorded to the period 1858 to 1886 since these dates reflect the passage of the Medical Registration Act and the Amendment Act, respectively. Reflects the major reorganization in medical care during the nineteenth century.

References are thorough and up-to-date. Well-produced medical history.
R: *Lancet* 2: 1236 (Dec. 9, 1978).

Medicine and Society in America. 1660–1860. **Richard H. Shryock.** Ithaca, NY: Cornell University Press, 1962.

Medieval English Medicine. **Stanley Rubin.** New York: Barnes & Noble, 1975.
Concentrates on the most prevalent afflictions of the average Englishman. Spans the time from Anglo-Saxon folk medicine to the more sophisticated medical practices in the twelfth and thirteenth centuries. Archeological findings, surviving medical records, and the lives of the saints provide most of the evidence. Includes a selected bibliography. Useful to the medical historian but will also appeal to the general reader.
R: *ABL* 40: entry 225 (June 1975); *BL* 72: 984 (July 1975).

Notable American Women, 1607–1950: A Biographical Dictionary. 3 vols. **Edward T. James and Janet W. James.** Cambridge, MA: Harvard University Press, 1971.

Organized Medicine in the Progressive Era: The More Toward Monopoly. **J. O. Burrow.** Baltimore, MD: Johns Hopkins University Press, 1977.
Illustrates the history/evolution of medical practice in the United States.
R: *LJ* 102: 2355 (Nov. 1977).

Origins of the Healing Art. **Irving I. Edgar.** New York: Philosophical Library, 1978.
Traces the evolution of medicine from its primitive origins to its present day importance. Although major sections deal with infections, development of preventive medicine, psychiatry, pharmacology, and surgery, it attempts to integrate all individual topics into a comprehensive volume. An absorbing history for all physicians, nurses, and historians.
R: *American Journal of Gastroenterology* 71: 124 (Jan. 1979).

A Pictorial History of Medicine. **Otto L. Bettman.** Springfield, IL: Charles C. Thomas, 1956.

A Short History of Medicine. Rev. printing. **Erwin H. Ackerknecht.** New York: Ronald Press, 1968.

A Short History of Medicine. 2d ed. **Charles Singer and E. A. Underwood.** Oxford, England: Clarendon Press, 1962.
An excellent brief history of medicine with extensive bibliography. Arranged primarily by subject, accentuating the conceptual developments. Also contains Nobel prize winners.

Speakers and Lecturers: How to Find Them. **Paul Wasserman and Jacqueline R. Bernero, eds.** Detroit, MI: Gale Research, 1978.
A convenient guide to speakers in a wide range of subjects, including alcoholism, dealing with handicaps, death and mourning, drug use, family relationship,

health and medicine, human sexuality, mental health, etc. Well indexed by speaker, lecture titles and key words, geographic location, and subject.

A Syllabus of Medical History. **Fred B. Roger.** Boston, MA: Little, Brown, 1962.

A very brief history, with a listing of Nobel prize winners, Hippocratic and other medical oaths.

Triumphs of Medicine. **H. Keen and J. Jarrett.** London: Elek Books, 1976.

Well illustrated, entertaining yet informative portrayal of the history of medicine. Follows a subject arrangement with individual chapters devoted to outstanding developments in specialized medical topics. The prominence of the contributors guarantees the scholarship of this history.
R: *Nature* 264: 593 (Dec. 9. 1976); *ABL* 41: entry 485 (Dec. 1976); *TBRI* 43: 60 (Feb. 1977).

Two Centuries of American Medicine 1776–1976. **James Bordley III and A. McGehee Harvey.** Philadelphia, PA: W. B. Saunders, 1976.

Provides a sound historical overview of medicine in America over the past two centuries. Focuses on three eras of American medicine: "The First Century: 1776–1876," "Period of Scientific Advance: 1876–1946," and "Period of Explosive Growth: 1946–1976." More than 400 pages devoted to the last three decades. Chapters arranged chronologically; individual chapters devoted to special topics. Its highly selective approach limits its usefulness as the source book of American medical history. Two minor complaints: scanty references and a poor index. Essentially written for interested lay people and physicians. This handsome volume should be on every library shelf.
R: *Annals of Internal Medicine* 86: 512 (Apr. 1977); *Chest* 72: 26 (1977); *JAMA* 237: 1731 (Apr. 18, 1977); *Science* 197: 750 (Aug. 19, 1977).

ALLERGY AND IMMUNOLOGY

A History of Immunization. **Henry J. Parish.** Baltimore, MD: Williams & Wilkins, 1965.

ANESTHESIOLOGY AND GENERAL SURGERY

Great Teachers of Surgery in the Past. **British Journal of Surgery.** Chicago, IL: Year Book Medical Publishers, 1969.

The Rise of Surgery: From Empiric Craft to Scientific Discipline. **Owen H. Wangensteen and Sarah D. Wangensteen.** Minneapolis, MN: University of Minnesota Press, 1979.

Contains profiles of important people and events in medical and surgical history. The history is both factual and interpretive; includes numerous photographs. Provides a clear account in two parts. The first deals with such subjects as amputation and debridement. The next deals with broader applications of institutional developments and the prevention of infection. Considered an authoritative history.

R: *BMJ* 1: 1618 (June 6, 1979); *Lancet* 2: 16 (July 7, 1979); *NEJM* 301: 113 (July 12, 1979); *LJ* 105: 572 (Mar. 1, 1980).

The Scientific Revolution in Victorian Medicine. **A. J. Youngson.** London: Croom Helm, 1979.

An historical introduction to the evolution of antisepsis and anesthesia techniques. Contains numerous references, explores the slow acceptance of new ideas in medicine.
R: *Lancet* 2: 288 (Aug. 11, 1979).

The Source Book of Plastic Surgery. **Frank McDowell, comp. and ed.** Baltimore, MD: Williams & Wilkins, 1977.

Summarizes the history of plastic surgery. The text consists of articles which were first reprinted in the journal *Plastic and Reconstructive Surgery* over the last 20 years. Pertinent commentaries follow most articles. Includes a 50-page section on biographies of seven early pioneers in plastic surgery. Readers interested in surgical history and all surgeons involved in plastic or reconstructive surgery will find this a welcome addition to the library.
R: *American Journal of Ophthalmology* 86: 288 (Aug. 1978); *Canadian Medical Association Journal* 120: 27 (Jan. 6, 1979).

BRAIN AND NERVOUS SYSTEM

Archives of the Internationl Congresses and Society of Neuropathology, 1952–1977. **Matthew T. Moore, ed.** Philadelphia, PA: Lea & Febiger, 1978.

An historical survey of origin, organization, and development of the International Congresses and Society of Neuropathology. Presents photographs, documents, and proceedings. A significant history for neuropathologists.
R: *Archives of Neurology* 36: 389 (June 1979).

Brain Control. **Elliot S. Valenstein.** London: John Wiley, 1974.

Reviews a century of the historical development of neurosurgery. Covers such topics as electrical and chemical stimuli, treatments in psychiatry, and psychosurgery. Contains close to 500 references. Well written. For both the professional and the lay reader.
R: *Brain* 98: 182 (Mar. 1975).

Centennial Anniversary Volume of the American Neurological Association. **Derek Denny-Brown, Augustus S. Rose, and Adolph L. Sahs, eds.** New York: Springer Publishing, 1975.

An encyclopedic review of the history of the American Neurological Association, including excerpts from the semicentennial volume published in 1925. Provides biographical and regional sketches, amasses a great deal of information useful in medical school and university libraries. Lists training centers and members of the American Neurological Association.
R: *Archives of Neurology* 33: 666 (Sept. 1976); *Brain* 99: 791 (Dec. 1976); *Journal of Nervous and Mental Disease* 166: 142 (1978); *Neurology* 26: 499 (May 1976); *RSR* 4: 44 (Jan.–Mar. 1976); *ARBA* (1976, p. 723).

An Illustrated History of Brain Function. **Edwin Clarke and Kenneth Dew-**

hurst. Berkeley, CA: University of California Press, 1972.

Reveals the history of brain function through reproduction of classic medical illustration. Divided into chapters, proceeding chronologically from ancient times until the nineteenth century. The text emphasizes physiology and anatomy. Each chapter has a complete bibliography. A unique, scholarly undertaking, recommended to historians, physiologists, and neurologists.
R: *Annals of Internal Medicine* 79: 771 (Nov. 1973); *Brain* 96: 211 (Jan. 1973); *BMJ* 1: 496 (Feb. 24, 1973); *Electroencephalography & Clinical Neurophysiology* 35: 559 (Nov. 1973); *Neuropsychology* 12: 161 (Jan. 1974); *Yale Journal of Biology and Medicine* 47: 298 (1974).

CARDIOVASCULAR SYSTEM

The History of Cardiac Surgery 1896–1955. **Stephen L. Johnson.** Baltimore, MD: Johns Hopkins University Press, 1970.

The History of Coronary Heart Disease. **J. O. Leibowitz.** London: Wellcome Institute for the History of Medicine, 1970.

A comprehensive account of the historical progression of events relating to the understanding of heart disease. Begins with the landmark paper by Heberden in 1768. Discusses advancement in instrumentation and diagnosis. A scholarly work.
R: *Lancet* 2: 1346 (Dec. 26, 1970).

DENTISTRY

A Bibliography of Dentistry in America, 1790–1840. **M. B. Asbell.** Cherry Hill, NJ: Sussex House, 1973.

A comprehensive listing of books and articles on dentistry, citing location of copies and list of journals searched.
R: Win (EK156).

Dental Education in the United States and Canada. A Report to the Carnegie Foundation. **William J. Gies.** New York: Carnegie Foundation, 1926.

A History of Dentistry from the Most Ancient Times Until the End of the Eighteenth Century. **Vincenzo Guerini.** Philadelphia, PA: Lea & Febiger, 1909. Repr. Atlantic Highlands, NJ: Humanities Press, 1967.

A classic history of dentistry published under the authority of the National Dental Association. Well documented and indexed.
R: Win (EK157).

An Introduction to the History of Dentistry, With Medical and Dental Chronology and Bibliographic Data. 2 vols. **Bernhard W. Weinberger.** St. Louis, MO: C. V. Mosby, 1948.

Volume 2, *An Introduction to the History of Dentistry in America.*
A chronological history of dentistry; includes bibliography.
R: Win (EK158).

Prints Relating to Dentistry. **US National Library of Medicine.** Bethesda, MA: US National Library of Medicine, 1967.

GENETICS

A Century of DNA: A History of the Discovery of the Structure and Function of the Genetic Substance. **Franklin H. Portugal and Jack S. Cohen.** Cambridge, MA: MIT Press, 1977.

An historical survey of DNA from the mid-nineteenth century to the present. Includes over 800 references to DNA research, biographical information, and illustrations. Written for both the scientist and the lay person.
R: *BMJ* 2: 422 (Aug. 5, 1978).

History of Genetics, From Prehistoric Times to the Rediscovery of Mendel's Laws. **Hans Stubbe. T. R. W. Waters, trans.** Cambridge, MA: MIT Press, 1973.

Translated from the German edition. Arranged chronologically. Includes brief biographies of prominent geneticists, with 45 photographs interspersed throughout the text. A supplementary reading list and bibliography of 500 references is particularly useful. Aimed at the advanced student or genetics scholar.
R: *Science* 181: 336 (July 27, 1973); *Choice* 10: 1010 (Sept. 1973); Chen (p. 274).

The Path to the Double Helix. **Robert Olby.** London: Macmillan, 1974.

Historical survey of DNA research focusing on both technical achievements and personality conflicts which sometimes interfered with these. Discusses all major researchers involved with DNA: Watson, Crick, Franklin, Pauling, Chargaff, Astbury. A well-written account; considered an excellent scientific history.
R: *Heredity* 38: 125 (Feb. 1977); *Physics in Medicine & Biology* 20: 504 (May 1975).

Rh: The Intimate History of a Disease and Its Conquest. **David R. Zimmerman.** New York: Macmillan, 1973.

Discusses history and treatment of the disease.
R: *Journal of the Medical Society of New Jersey* 71: 77 (Jan. 1974); *LJ* 98: 878 (Mar. 15, 1973); *TBRI* 40: 124 (Mar. 1974).

HEALTH SERVICES ADMINISTRATION

History of the Royal College of Physicians of Edinburgh. **W. S. Craig.** Oxford, England: Blackwell Scientific Publications, 1976.

This is a definitive study of the three centuries of the Royal College of Physicians. It focuses on individual personalities, but has a wide-ranging scope and is to be considered a thorough history of this influential medical insititution which has had a role in changing such things as the national health service and medical reform.
R: *Lancet* 2: 719 (Oct. 2, 1976).

The Hospital: A Social and Architectural History. **John D. Thompson and Grace Goldin.** New Haven, CT: Yale University Press, 1975.

Provides an historical survey as well as a glimpse of the future of hospitals. Focuses on architecture for the infirm and the repercussions of planning (or lack of) in hospital buildings. Includes illustrations, diagrams, bibliography, and index. A valuable reference source for physicians, medical libraries, and students.

R: *Annals of Internal Medicine* 85: 270 (Aug. 1976); *RSR* 4: 92 (Apr.–June 1976).

Labor-Management Relations in the Health Service Industry. **Norman Metzger and Dennis D. Pointer.** Washington, DC: Science and Health Publications, 1972.

A summary of labor relations in the hospital setting. Correlates federal and state mandates to situtations at hand. Exhibits sample ballots and examples of printed publicity associated with union campaigns. A labor-management text for all nursing directors.
R: *American Journal of Nursing* 74: 93 (Jan. 1974).

University College Hospital and Its Medical School: A History. **W. R. Merrington.** London: Heinemann Medical, 1976.

Contains nuggets of information on the history of University College Hospital and its medical school. Lists delightful biographical tidbits of many renowned persons associated with the institution which will be of interest to the general reader. Offsetting the emphasis on biography are brief sketches of professional units and individual medical departments. Brief section on nursing included.
R: *JAMA* 237: 68 (Jan. 3, 1977); *Lancet* 2: 348 (Aug. 14, 1976).

INFECTIOUS DISEASES

Cholera 1832. **R. J. Morris.** London: Croom Helm, 1976.

This book traces the problems and events of the cholera epidemic of 1832, which spread from Bengal to England. Discusses sanitary engineering, nature of health care, and theories of the epidemic spread of cholera at the time. Well written, contains a complete bibliography; helpful in understanding the natural history of the disease.
R: *BMJ* 1: 586 (Feb. 26, 1977).

A Guide to the History of Bacteriology. **Thomas H. Grainger.** New York: Ronald Press, 1958.

Infectious Diseases: Prevention and Treatment in the Nineteenth and Twentieth Centuries. **Wesley W. Spink.** Folkestone, Kent: William Dawson & Son, 1979.

Chronicles the history of nineteenth- and twentieth-century microbiology and public health as they related to the control of infectious diseases. Discusses such topics as the introduction of penicillin, the use of maggots to induce alkalinity unfavorable to infection, etc. In three sections: outline of early concepts of public health; development of anti-infection therapy; and, specific infections and their diagnosis and treatment. A detailed, fascinating work.
R: *BMJ* 1: 1555 (June 9, 1979); *Lancet* 1: 958 (May 5, 1979).

Influenza in America, 1918–1976; History, Science, and Politics. **June Osborn, ed.** New York: Prodist, 1977.

A history of the 1918 swine flu epidemic and how this influenced federal legislation and immunization programs (1976). Appendixes provide text of the *Congressional Record.*

R: *American Journal of Public Health* 68: 278 (Mar. 1978).

An Introduction to the History of Virology. **A. P. Waterson and Lise Wilkinson.** London: Cambridge University Press, 1978.

A history which details the progressive understanding of the nature of the virus. The work centers around four viruses: rabies, smallpox, fowl-plague, and tobacco-mosaic. Also covers tumors, slow-growing viruses. Includes numerous references, annotations, and pertinent biographies.
R: *Lancet* 2: 556 (Sept. 9, 1978).

Mosquitoes, Malaria and Man: A History of the Hostilities Since 1880. **Gordon Harrison.** London: John Murray, 1978.

Superb history of malaria. Traces the study of the malarial virus from Ronald Ross, a British doctor in the Indian Medical Service, to the concern and intervention by WHO in 1955.
R: *BMJ* 1: 109 (Jan. 13, 1979).

Plagues and Peoples. **William H. McNeill.** New York: Anchor Press/Doubleday, 1976.

Weaves together the prominent aspects of epidemiology and immunology with demography, cultural anthropology, and the progress of civilization. Analyzes historical movements in terms of infectious diseases. Obvious examples given are the plague in the fourteenth century and the sudden fall of the Mexican and Peruvian cultures in the face of weak European adventurers. Well-documented text covering both Eastern and Western literature in history and medicine.
R: *JAMA* 236: 2800 (Dec. 13, 1976); *Pharmaceutical Journal* 220: 531 (1978).

The Swine Flu Affair. **R. E. Neustadt and H. V. Fineberg.** Bethesda, MD: US Department of Health, Education, and Welfare, 1978.

Details the history of the United States Swine Flu vaccine campaign in 1976. Presents statistics and events and discusses the role of the Center for Disease Control.
R: *BMJ* 2: 438 (Aug. 18, 1979).

Three Centuries of Microbiology. **Hubert A. Lechevalier and Morris Solotorovsky.** New York: Dover Publications, 1974.

INTERNAL MEDICINE

Antique Medical Instruments. **Elisabeth Bennion.** London: Sotheby Parke Bernet Publications, 1978.

A first-class presentation dealing with extensive illustrations of surgical, dental, and veterinary instruments. Contains a valuable directory of surgical instrument makers to 1870.
R: *Lancet* 1: 648 (Mar. 24, 1979); *Pharmaceutical Journal* 220: 270 (1979); *LJ* 105: 576 (Mar. 1, 1980).

The Birth of the Clinic—An Archaeology of Medical Perception. **Michel Foucault.** New York: Pantheon Books, 1973.

This history describes the evolution of clinical practice in medicine, concentrating on eighteenth- and nineteenth-century practice in France. Combines medical and theoretical evolution while examining political, social, and economic factors. A book to be studied by medical and historical professionals.
R: *Journal of Medical Education* 49: 1073 (Nov. 1974).

The Colonial Physician and Other Essays. **Whitfield J. Bell, Jr.** New York: Science History Publications, 1975.

A collection of essays concerning people in medicine in seventeenth- and eighteenth-century colonial America. Cohesive and well documented. Recommended for all medical and historical collections.
R: *RSR* 4: 86 (Apr.–June 1976).

The Medicine Show: Physicians and the Perplexities of the Health Revolution in Modern Society. **Patricia Branca, ed.** Folkestone, Kent, England: Science History Publications, 1977.

A series of essays on the social history of medicine in America and continental Europe. Each of the fourteen essays revolves around a central theme: the growth of medicine in the nineteenth century. Unlike most histories, this volume focuses on ordinary practitioners and common beliefs and practices.
R: *BMJ* 1: 1044 (Apr. 22, 1978).

Nobel Lectures in Phyiology—Medicine, 1901–1970. 4 vols. New York: Elsevier, 1967–1973.
Volume 1, *1901–1921,* 1967; volume 2, *1922–1941,* 1965; volume 3, *1942–1962,* 1964; volume 4, *1963–1970,* 1973.

NURSING

The Advance of American Nursing. **Philip A. Kalish and Beatrice J. Kalish.** Boston, MA: Little, Brown, 1978.
R: Brandon (*NO*).

American Nursing; History and Interpretation. **Mary M. Roberts.** New York: Macmillan, 1954.
Out of print, but a classic history.

The Care of the Sick: The Emergence of Modern Nursing. **Vern L. Bullough and Bonnie Bullough.** New York: Neale Watson Academic Publications, 1978.

Comprehensive volume on the history of nursing. Follows trends from primitive times through the mid-1970s. Well documented with footnotes and bibliographies. Lacks illustrations, charts, and diagrams. Geared toward undergraduates and graduate students and professional nurses.
R: *American Journal of Nursing* 79: 1221 (July 1979).

History and Trends of Professional Nursing. 8th ed. **Grace L. Deloughery.** St. Louis, MO: C. V. Mosby, 1977.

The eighth edition of this classic text focuses on the significant historical and

contemporary trends in nursing. Also emphasizes the role of women and minorities in nursing, professionalism, and legal aspects.
R: Brandon (NO).

A History of Nursing. 4 vols. **Adelaide M. Nutting and Lavinia L. Dock.** New York: G. P. Putnam, 1907–1935.
The classic history of nursing.

A History of Nursing From Ancient to Modern Times. 5th ed. **Isabel M. Stewart and Anne L. Austin.** New York: G. P. Putnam, 1962.
First edition, 1920, entitled *A Short History of Nursing.*
Divided into four sections. Covers the historical trends in nursing from primitive to modern era. Uses charts, diagrams, and maps to illustrate the patterns of growth. Good section on international nursing. Each chapter concludes with specialized bibliography. Includes subject and name indexes.
R: Win (EK169).

History of Nursing Source Book. **Anne L. Austin.** New York: G. P. Putnam, 1957.
Out of print but a valuable source of primary sources of nursing history.

Nursing in Society: A Historical Perspective. 14th ed. **Josephine A. Dolan.** Philadelphia, PA: W. B. Saunders, 1978.
First edition, 1916.
A classic book on the history of nursing. Correlates the improvement of nursing education to medical advances.
R: *American Journal of Nursing* 74: 1363 (July 1974); Brandon (NO).

Nursing Opportunities. Oradell, NJ: R. N. Publications, 1970–. Annual.

NUTRITION

Food: The Gift of Osiris. 2 vols. **W. J. Darby, P. Ghalioungui, and L. Grivetti, eds.** New York: Academic Press, 1977.
This is an anecdotal history of nutrition in the Near East, mainly Egypt, from ancient times. Discusses cultural acceptance of foods, folklore, disease, and findings from mummy autopsies. A detailed scholarly account, profusely illustrated. Of interest to medical historians as well as lay people.
R: *BMJ* 1: 1210 (May 7, 1977).

A Good Idea: The History of The Nutrition Foundation. **Charles G. King.** New York: The Nutrition Foundation, 1977.
A chronological history of The Nutrition Foundation and its contributions to nutrition research and education. Includes much significant information on research development and applications to nutrition.
R: *Journal of the American Dietetic Association* 71: 355 (Sept. 1977).

Notes on the History of Nutrition Research. **Clive M. McCay and F. Verzár, eds.** Bern, Switzerland: Huber. Distr. Baltimore: Williams & Wilkins, 1973.

R: *Science* 182: 377 (Oct. 26, 1973); Chen (p. 274).

OPHTHALMOLOGY

The History and Traditions of the Moorfields Eye Hospital. Vol. 2. **Frank W. Law.** London: H. K. Lewis, 1975.

Volume 1, 1929.

This is a history of a prominent British ophthalmological hospital. It contains many useful facts and biographies; covers international influences of the hospital. Useful for medical historians and ophthalmologists.

R: *Archives of Ophthalmology* 94: 875 (May 1976).

The Unseen Minority: A Social History of Blindness in the United States. **Frances A. Koestler.** New York: David McKay, 1976.

Not only traces the story of blindness but also the story of many who conquered their handicap and those who helped them succeed. Twenty-seven chapters discuss all aspects of blindness, from the American Foundation for the Blind to the slow development of Braille. Includes biographical sketches of such personalities as Helen Keller and Ann Sullivan Macy and Peter J. Salmon. Additional chapters are devoted to workshops for the blind and present employment opportunities. Individual chapter notes and a complete index enhance the value of this text. No photos included. This extensive research will be useful to the blind, their families, and all social and rehabilitation workers.

R: *Archives of Physical Medicine and Rehabilitation* 58: 332 (July 1977).

PATHOLOGY

A History of Microtechnique. **B. Bracegirdle.** London: Heinemann, 1978.

A chronology of the development of preparative techniques in microscopy in the eighteenth and nineteenth centuries. Much attention is given to instrumentation, various phases of the microtome, and perfection of mounts. For science historians and histologists; a standard reference in the field.

R: *Nature* 277: 155 (Jan. 11, 1979).

PEDIATRICS

The Father of Child Care—Life of William Cadogan, 1711–1797. **John Rendel-Short.** Chicago, IL: Year Book of Medical Publishers, 1966.

PHARMACY AND PHARMACOLOGY

American Self-Dosage Medicines: An Historical Perspective. **James H. Young.** Lawrence, KS: Coronado, 1974.

A succinct account of the history of self-medication and methods used to control this in the United States. Referenced. Recommended for public libraries.

R: *RSR* 3: 38 (July–Dec. 1975).

Chemical, Medical, and Pharmaceutical Books Printed Before 1800, in the Collection of the University of Wisconsin Libraries. **John Neu, ed.** Madison, WI: University of Wisconsin Press, 1965.

Includes the D. I. Duveen collection in chemistry and alchemy.
R: Chen (p. 273).

Chronicles of Pharmacy. 2 vols. **A. C. Wootton.** London: Macmillan, 1910. Repr. Kennebunkport, ME: Milford House, 1971.

This book illustrates the discovery of medicines and their use. Covers ancient through nineteenth century history. Contains biographies of famous apothecaries.
R: Win (EK211).

Kremer's and Urdang's History of Pharmacy. 4th ed. **Glenn Sonnedecker, rev.** Philadelphia, PA: J. B. Lippincott, 1976.

First edition, 1940.
Classic text traces the growth and development of pharmacy from ancient Egypt to modern America. Comprehensive coverage of pharmacy in the United States. Views the pharmaceutical evolution in the Western world from a sociohistorical perspective. New edition covers some areas of international pharmacy. Numerous illustrations and photographs complement text. The definitive work for pharmacists, students, and medical and social historians.
R: *JAMA* 237: 485 (Jan. 31, 1977); *Pharmaceutical Journal* 219: 145 (1977).

Scientific Contributions from the Laboratories 1866–1966. Parke, Davis & Company, 1966.

Therapeutics From the Primitives to the 20th Century. **Erwin H. Ackerknecht.** New York: Hafner Press, 1973.

PSYCHIATRY AND PSYCHOLOGY

Abstracts of The Standard Edition of the Complete Psychological Works of Sigmund Freud. **Carrie L. Rothgeb, ed.** US National Institute of Mental Health. Washington, DC: US Government Printing Office, 1971.

A chronological list of the works of Sigmund Freud comprising James Strachey's *Standard Edition.* Abstracts are thorough yet concise. Subject index.
R: *JAMA* 228: 1689 (June 24, 1974); *MRW* S2, p. 82.

An Assessment of the Community Mental Health Movement. **Walter E. Barton and Charlotte J. Sanborn, eds.** Lexington, MA: Lexington Books, 1977.

A history of the community mental health movement in the United States. Reviews philosophic trends and operating programs and evaluates the literature of the field. An excellent book covering a wide scope.
R: *American Journal of Psychiatry* 134: 1455 (Dec. 1977).

C. G. Jung: Letters 1906–1961. 2 vols. Princeton, NJ: Princeton University Press, 1974–1976.

Volume 1, *The Freud/Jung Letters 1906–1913.* Ralph Manheim and R. F. C. Hull, eds., 1974; volume 2, *Jung: Letters 1951–1961.* Gerhard Adler with Aniela Jaffe, eds., 1976.
R: *American Journal of Psychiatry* 132: 980 (Sept. 1975); 133: 1476 (Dec. 1976).

The Collected Works of C. G. Jung. Vol. 2. **Herbert Read, Michael Fordham, and Gerhard Adler, eds.** Boston, MA: Routledge & Kegan Paul, 1973.

An historical perspective of the work of C. G. Jung. Details experiments and clinical observations Jung applied to brain function. An important book which underlies the fundaments of Jungian psychology.
R: *BMJ* 3: 358 (Aug. 11, 1973).

Community Mental Health: A General Introduction. **Bernard L. Bloom.** Monterey, CA: Brooks/Cole Publishing, 1977.

A well-written introduction to community mental health in three parts: development of the community mental health movement, mental health in perspective, and mental health in practice. Also includes regulations of the Community Mental Health Centers Act. Contains much information, bibliographies. Useful as a reference source.
R: *American Journal of Psychiatry* 136: 472 (Apr. 1979).

1851 Colney Hatch Asylum: Friern Hospital 1973. A Medical and Social History. **Richard Hunter and Ida Macalpine.** London: Dawson, 1974.

Outlines the evolution of a psychiatric hospital from a Victorian asylum. Well documented, profusely illustrated. Of value to medical and social historians.
R: *Lancet* 2: 560 (Sept. 7, 1974).

The First Century of Experimental Psychology. **E. S. Hearst.** New York: Halstead Press, 1979.

Provides an introduction to the history of the field.

Freud: The Fusion of Science and Humanism: The Intellectual History of Psychoanalysis. **John E. Gedo and George H. Pollock, eds.** New York: International Universities Press, 1976.

Multi-authored collection of papers depicting the development of Freud's theories and methods and their influence on the history of psychoanalysis. Recommended for students and specialists in the field.
R: *American Journal of Psychiatry* 133: 1213 (Oct. 1976).

The History of Childhood. **Lloyd deMause, ed.** New York: Psychohistory Press, 1974.

An international and historical survey of attitudes toward child rearing prepared under the auspices of the Association for Applied Psychoanalysis. Discusses such topics as infanticide, wet-nursing, foster age, parental affection and intimidation. A valuable work recommended for all medical libraries.
R: *American Journal of Psychiatry* 132: 308 (1975).

The History of Mental Retardation: Collected Papers. 2 vols. **Marvin Rosen, Gerald R. Clark, and Marvin S. Kivitz, eds.** Baltimore, MD: University Park Press, 1976.

A comprehensive review of the social and historical advances in mental retardation. Deals with such topics as changing humanitarian feelings, education, and

categorization of the mentally retarded. Time period covered is from mid-nineteenth century through 1944. A useful, relevant work.
R: *JAMA* 237: 584 (Feb. 7, 1977).

The History of Psychiatry: An Evaluation of Psychiatric Thought and Practice from Prehistoric Times to the Present. **Franz G. Alexander and Sheldon T. Selesnick.** New York: New American Library, 1974.

Medical Dissertations of Psychiatric Interest (Printed Before 1750). **Oskar Diethelm.** New York: S. Karger, 1971.

Material culled from over 1,000 student dissertations devoted to psychiatric disorders. Notes the history of Renaissance psychiatry from 1550 to 1750. This historical research will be of particular importance to psychiatrists and historians.
R: *American Journal of Psychiatry* 131: 735 (June 1974). Also reviewed in *British Journal of Psychiatry.*

Mental Health in the United States: A Fifty-Year History. **Nina Ridenour.** Cambridge, MA: Commonwealth Fund, 1961.

Mental Institutions in America. Social Policy to 1875. **Gerald N. Grob.** New York: The Free Press, 1973.

Focuses on mental illness and the fate of the mentally ill from the colonial period to 1875. Also a sensitive portrayal of the dreams and frustrations experienced by advocates of social and medical reform. The section on the growth of psychiatry and the role of the institution is excellent.
R: *Journal of Nervous and Mental Disease* 162: 149 (1976).

Neuropsychiatry in World War II, Publication 0832-00047. Vol 2. **Col. William S. Mullins and Col. Albert J. Glass, eds.** Washington, DC: Office of the Surgeon General, US Department of the Army, 1973.

Historical reference source prepared by the Office of the Surgeon General. Primarily concerned with the emotional problems, treatments, and dispositions of the neuropsychiatric casualties during World War II. Outlines the role of psychiatric personnel in specific campaigns within different theaters of the war. Provides information on "combat exhaustion" and many syndromes unfamiliar to civilians. Illustrations add human and historical importance. Psychiatric, institutional, and personal libraries will benefit greatly.
R: *American Journal of Psychiatry* 132: 1227 (Nov. 1975); *Archives of Physical Medicine and Rehabilitation* 57: 252 (May 1976); *Brain* 98: 729 (Dec. 1975).

Research in the Service of Mental Health: Report of the Research Task Force of the National Institute of Mental Health, DHEW Pub. no. 75-236. **Julius Segal, Donald S. Boomer, and Lorraine Bouthilet, eds.** US National Institute of Mental Health, US Department of Health, Education, and Welfare. Rockville, MD: US National Institute of Mental Health, 1975.

A review of the work of the NIMH since 1948, covering a broad scope of research including biological and psychological processes, cultural processes, mental illness, drug abuse, etc. An impressive overview of the history of this institution and its research activities. Contains much scholarly information. Con-

sidered an informative publication. Recommended to academic institutions and to government officials interested in research projects supported by the U.S. government.
R: *American Journal of Psychiatry* 133: 866 (July 1976).

Rites of Passage: Adolescence in America 1790 to the Present. **Joseph F. Kett.** New York: Basic Books, 1977.

Traces the historical roots and precursors of contemporary adolescence from 1790 to the present. Records society's attitude toward youth rather than the clinical viewpoints. Good background reading for the reflective scholar and the busy practitioner, who requires a fresh perspective amid repetitious problems.
R: *American Journal of Psychiatry* 135: 397 (Mar. 1978).

A Source Book in the History of Psychology. **Richard J. Herrnstein and Edwin G. Boring, eds.** Cambridge, MA: Harvard University Press, 1965.

The Symbolic Life: Miscellaneous Writings: The Collected Works of C. G. Jung. Vol. 18. **C. G. Jung.** Princeton, NJ: Princeton University Press, 1976.

This volume of the work of C. G. Jung includes the Tavistock lectures, theories on symbolism, mental disease, psychology, and religion. An essential part of the 22 volumes of Jung's work. A valuable reference for all major libraries.
R: *American Journal of Psychiatry* 134: 1456 (Dec. 1977).

PUBLIC HEALTH

History and Geography of the Most Important Diseases. **Edwin H. Ackerknecht.** New York: Hafner, 1965.

A History of Public Health. **George Rosen.** New York: M.D. Publications, 1958.

An historical survey of public health from its beginning to the present. Includes biographical sketches, references, list of schools, subject and author indexes.
R: Win (EK219).

Insects and History. **J. L. Cloudsley-Thompson.** London: Weidenfeld & Nicolson, 1976.

An historical collection of references on insect-caused disease and epidemics from classical times to the present; arranged by chapters according to diseases. A useful book, providing diverse, informative topics such as malaria, dysentery, typhus, scurvy, and famine.
R: *BMJ* 1: 849 (Mar. 26, 1977).

Preventive Medicine in the United States, 1900–1975. **George Rosen.** New York: Science History Publications, 1975.

Written as background material for the National Conference on Preventive Medicine held in June 1975. Reviews basic elements in the preventive medicine scene since 1900. Numerous references enable the reader to delve deeper into many subjects. The omission of an index seriously detracts from the volume's usefulness. Valuable addition to public and college library collections.
R: *RSR* 4: 90 (Apr.–June 1976).

Public Health and the State: Changing Views in Massachusetts, 1842–1936. **Barbara G. Rosenkrantz.** Cambridge, MA: Harvard University Press, 1972.

Weaves the story of the birth and growth of the State Board of Health in Massachusetts. Also incorporates social sentiments about health and describes the health-related careers of the advocates of this movement. Since Massachusetts has played a significant role in the history of public health in the United States, this book is intended for all public, college, and medical libraries.
R: *RSR* 3: 45 (Jan–Mar. 1975).

The Scientific Background of the International Sanitary Conferences 1851–1938. **Norman Howard-Jones.** Geneva: World Health Organization, 1975.

Outlines the fascinating history of international health with detailed discussions of the fourteen international health conferences which laid the foundations for the World Health Organization. Photographs of prominent events and brief vignettes of notable scientific personalities compliment the text. This scholarly publication is a valuable contribution to the literature on international health cooperation and communicable disease. Recommended for public, college, and medical libraries.
R: *BMJ* 1: 592 (Sept. 4, 1976); *RSR* 3: 36 (July–Dec. 1975).

A Social History of Medicine. **Frederick F. Cartwright.** New York: Longman, 1977.

Spans the time from early Greek medicine to the recent past. Great emphasis throughout on Great Britain. Contains pertinent information on public health and epidemiology. The National Health Service receives considerable attention. Intended for a general audience.
R: *JAMA* 239: 1553 (Apr. 14, 1978); *Science* 202: 622 (Nov. 10, 1978).

RADIOLOGY

Marie Curie. **Robert Reid.** London: William Collins, 1974.

Fascinating account of the character of Marie Curie which has been written from letters and her own accounts. Text discusses her life as a scientist in a vital, enthralling manner.
R: *British Journal of Radiology* 47: 656 (1974).

RESPIRATORY SYSTEM

The Natural History of Chronic Bronchitis and Emphysema. **Charles Fletcher et al.** London: Oxford University Press, 1976.

Lucid interpretation of the largest prospective study of chronic bronchitis in its preclinical stages. Clearly distinguishes between two forms of chronic bronchitis: the obstructive and hypersecretary. Also establishes the relationship between smoking and bronchitis. Truly a milestone in the bibliography of this and related disorders.
R: *BMJ* 1: 515 (Feb. 19, 1977).

UROGENITAL SYSTEM

Abortion in America: The Origins and Evolution of National Policy, 1800–1900. **James C. Mohr.** New York: Oxford University Press, 1978.

An historical examination of the changing attitudes toward abortion in this country. Considers legal and medical influence on attitudes of society helpful in understanding abortion law and reform. This book documents the historical trends of abortion in this country from the early nineteenth century to the present.
R: *Quarterly Review of Biology* 53: 499 (1978).

The History of Urology. **Leonard J. T. Murphy and Ernest Desnos.** Springfield, IL: Charles C. Thomas, 1972.

A translation of the classic monograph *L'histoire de l'urologie* by Ernest Desnos with additional historical material from the late nineteenth century to the present. Involves the history of the diagnosis and treatment of urological diseases. Basically, a catalog of events in the history of urology written by urologists. Well illustrated. Valuable to the historian.
R: *Archives of Internal Medicine* 132: 462 (Sept. 1973); *British Journal of Surgery* 60: 167 (Feb. 1973); *Choice* 10: 484 (May 1973).

Midwives and Medical Men: A History of Inter-Professional Rivalries and Women's Rights. **Jean Donnison.** New York: Schocken Books, 1977.

A history of midwifery from the sixteenth century to the present. Carefully illustrates the relationship between doctor and midwife.
R: *ABL* 43: entry 201 (Apr. 1978).

VETERINARY MEDICINE

The Veterinarian in America 1625–1975. **J. F. Smithcors.** Wheaton, IL: American Veterinary Publications, 1975.

This history integrates the social and medical aspects of veterinary concerns in this country. Describes such things as the introduction of domestic animals, treatment of disease, relation to public health. A useful science covering 200 years of veterinary medicine.
R: *JAMA* 236: 88 (July 5, 1976).

CHAPTER 13 IMPORTANT SERIES AND OTHER REVIEWS OF PROGRESS

For series with titles beginning "Yearbook," see chapter 11. Many of these publications are of the same nature as "Advances in" and "Progress in" series in this chapter.

GUIDE TO SERIES PUBLICATIONS

Irregular Serials and Annuals; An International Directory. 3d ed. New York: Bowker, 1974–1975.

List of Annual Reviews of Progress in Science and Technology; Liste de "mises au point" annuelles sur les progrès de la science et de la technique. 2d ed. **UNESCO.** Paris: UNESCO, 1969.

First edition, 1965.
A classified listing.
R: Chen (p. 278); Wal (p. 32); Win (3EA11).

Scientific and Technical Series. **E. B. Ocran.** Metuchen, NJ: Scarecrow Press, 1973.

Annotated listings of series publications. Author-and-subject index.
R: *Choice* 10: 949 (Sept. 1973); ARBA (1974, p. 541), Chen (p. 278).

IMPORTANT SERIES

GENERAL

Advances in American Medicine. Vols. 1–. New York: Josiah Macy, Jr. Foundation, 1976–.

Volume 2, 1976.
R: *NEJM* 296: 697 (Mar. 24, 1977).

Advances in Biochemical Engineering. Vols. 1–. New York: Springer-Verlag, 1971–.

Volume 5, 1977.
R: *Journal of Pharmaceutical Sciences* 63: 312 (Feb. 1974).

Advances in Biological and Medical Physics. Vols. 1–. New York: Academic Press, 1948–.

Volume 15, 1974.
R: Chen (p. 281).

Advances in Biomedical Engineering. Vols. 1–. New York: Academic Press, 1971–.

Volume 8, 1979.

R: *American Scientist* 62: 747 (Nov./Dec. 1974); 63: 473 (July/Aug. 1975); *Yale Journal of Biology and Medicine* 50: 223 (1977); Chen (p. 294).

Advances in Biomedical Engineering and Medical Physics. Vols. 1–. New York: John Wiley, 1967–. Annual.

Volume 4, 1971.

Advances in Cell and Molecular Biology. Nos. 1–. New York: Academic Press, 1971–.

Number 3, 1975.

R: *Nature* 234: 283 (Dec. 3, 1971); *Science* 175: 510 (Feb. 2, 1972); Chen (p. 290).

Advances in Cell Biology. Vols. 1–. New York: Plenum, 1970–.

Volume 2, 1971.

R: *American Scientist* 60: 790 (Nov./Dec. 1972); *ARBA* (1971, p. 493); Chen (p. 290).

Advances in Chromatography. Vols. 1–. New York: Marcel Dekker, 1966–.

Volume 16, 1978.

R: *Pharmaceutical Journal* 220: 85 (1978).

Advances in Experimental Medicine and Biology. Vols. 1–. New York: Plenum, 1967–.

Volume 127, 1980.

R: *American Journal of Human Genetics* 29: 412 (July 1977); *American Scientist* 62: 734 (Nov.–Dec. 1974); *Annals of Human Genetics* 42: 262 (Oct. 1978); *Brain* 101: 375 (June 1978); *Electroencephalography & Clinical Neurophysiology* 35: 671 (Dec. 1973); *Journal of Pharmaceutical Sciences* 63: 1496 (Sept. 1974); *Neurology* 27: 597, 598 (June 1977); *New Scientist* (Dec. 9, 1971); Chen (p. 287); Mal (9-11).

Advances in the Biosciences. Vols. 1–. Oxford: Pergamon Press, 1969–.

Volume 16, 1974.

R: Chen (p. 288).

Amino-Acids, Peptides, and Proteins. London: The Chemical Society, 1969–. Annual.

An annual review of the periodical literature in the field of amino acids, peptides, and proteins.

R: *Journal of Pharmaceutical Sciences* 62: 347 (Feb. 1973).

Annual Review of Clinical Biochemistry. Vols. 1–. New York: Wiley Medical, 1980.

Annual Review of Medicine. Palo Alto, CA: Annual Reviews, 1950–. Annual.

Volume 29, 1978.

Provides a year's review of important research being conducted of particular interest to the practicing general internist. Reviews followed by lengthy bibliographies. Includes author and subject indexes. Valuable reference tool.

R: *Archives of Physical Medicine and Rehabilitation* 54: 46 (Jan. 1973); 55: 100 (Feb. 1974); 56: 185 (Apr. 1975); 58: 422 (Sept. 1977); 59: 249 (May 1978); *RSR* 2: 129 (Oct.–Dec. 1974); *ARBA* (1970, p. 131; 1976, p. 730).

Biomembranes. Vols. 1–. New York: Plenum, 1971–.
Volume 10, 1979.

Computers in Chemical and Biochemical Research. Vols. 1–. New York: Academic Press, 1972–.
Volume 2, 1974.
R: Chen (p. 284).

Current Diagnosis. Philadelphia, PA: W. B. Saunders, 1966–. Biennial.
R: Allyn.

Current Topics in Biochemistry. Vols. 1–. New York: Academic Press, 1972–.
Volume 2, 1974.
R: *Archives of Internal Medicine* 132: 460 (Sept. 1973).

Current Topics in Membranes and Transport. Vols. 1–. New York: Academic Press, 1970–.
Volume 12, 1979.
R: *American Scientist* (July/Aug. 1971); Chen (p. 288).

Methods in Cell Biology. Vols. 1–. New York: Academic Press, 1964–.
Volume 20, 1978.
Continues *Methods in Cell Physiology.*
R: *American Scientist* 64: 445, 452 (July/Aug. 1976); Chen (p. 290).

Methods in Membrane Biology. Vols. 1–. New York: Plenum, 1974–.
Volume 1, 1974.
R: *American Scientist* 63: 469 (July/Aug. 1975); Chen (p. 288).

Perspectives in Medicine. Vols. 5–. Basel: S. Karger, 1973–.
Volume 7, 1976.

Review of Allied Health Education. Vols. 1–. **Joseph Hamburg, ed.** Lexington, KY: The University Press of Kentucky, 1974–.
R: *Journal of Allied Health* 4: 42 (Spring 1975).

ALLERGY AND IMMUNOLOGY

Advances in Immunology. Vols. 1–. New York: Academic Press, 1961–.
Volume 28, 1980.
R: *American Scientist* 61: 590 (Sept.–Oct. 1973); *JAMA* 237: 1011 (Mar. 7, 1977); *Quarterly Review of Biology* 50: 126 (1975); 51: 204 (1976); 51: 352 (1976); 51: 469 (1976); *Yale Journal of Biology and Medicine* 49: 99 (1976); *RSR* 4: 86 (Jan.–Mar. 1976); Chen (p. 291); Allyn.

Annual Review of Allergy. Vols. 1–. Flushing, NY: Medical Examination

Publishing, 1972–. Annual.
R: *American Journal of Ophthalmology* 77: 604 (Apr. 1974); 78: 742 (Oct. 1974); 81: 115 (Jan. 1976); *Annals of Otology, Rhinology and Laryngology* 83: 417 (1974); 85: 299 (1976); *Archives of Dermatology* 110: 480 (Sept. 1974); *Archives of Otolaryngology* 100: 247 (1974).

Contemporary Topics in Immunobiology. Vols. 1–. New York: Plenum, 1972–.
Volume 10, 1980.
R: *American Scientist* 62: 491 (July–Aug. 1974); 63: 469 (July/Aug. 1975); *Science* 179: 888 (Mar. 2, 1973); Chen (p. 292).

Contemporary Topics in Molecular Immunology. Vols. 1–. New York: Plenum, 1972–.
Volume 7, 1978.
R: *American Scientist* 62: 491 (July–Aug. 1974); *Quarterly Review of Biology* 51: 469 (Aug. 1976).

Immunological Aspects of Allergy and Allergic Diseases. Vols. 1–. New York: Plenum, 1974–.
Volume 8, 1977.

Progress in Allergy. Vols. 1–. Basel: S. Karger, 1939–.
Volume 27, 1979.
R: *Annals of Internal Medicine* 91: 344 (Aug. 1979); *Archives of Dermatology* 111: 1223 (Sept. 1975); 112: 1624 (Nov. 1976); *Archives of Internal Medicine* 131: 757 (May 1973); 134: 190 (July 1974); *BMJ* 2: 507 (May 31, 1975); *Immunology* 28: 207 (Jan. 1975); 32: 369 (Mar. 1977); 33: 149 (July 1977); 33: 437 (Sept. 1977); 34: 789 (Apr. 1978); Allyn.

Progress in Clinical Immunology. Vols. 1–. New York: Grune & Stratton, 1972–.
Volume 3, 1977.
R: *Annals of Internal Medicine* 78: 627 (Apr. 1973); 83: 590 (Oct. 1975); *Archives of Dermatology* 107: 781 (May 1973).

Progress in Immunology II. Vols. 1–. Amsterdam: North-Holland, 1974–.
Volumes 1–5, 1974.
R: *Immunology* 29: 581 (Sept. 1975).

Recent Advances in Clinical Immunology. Nos. 1–. Edinburgh: Churchill Livingstone, 1977–.
R: *British Journal of Haematology* 39: 288 (1978); *BMJ* 1: 567 (Mar. 4, 1978); *Journal of Clinical Pathology* 31: 1007 (Oct. 1978); *Lancet* 1: 190 (Jan. 28, 1978).

ANATOMY

Advances in Reproductive Physiology. Vols. 1–. London: Science, 1966–.
Volume 6, 1973.
R: Chen (p. 292).

Annual Review of Physiology. Vols. 1–. Palo Alto, CA: Annual Reviews, 1939–. Annual.

Volume 41, 1979.
R: *Archives of Physical Medicine and Rehabilitation* 54: 288 (June 1973); 55: 44 (Jan. 1974); 56: 326 (July 1975); 56: 506 (Nov. 1975); 58: 188 (Apr. 1977); 58: 502 (Nov. 1977); 60: 189 (Apr. 1979); *Physical Therapy* 56: 126 (1976); 58: 226 (1978); *ARBA* (1976, p. 656); Chen (p. 292).

Benchmark Papers in Human Physiology Series. Vols. 1–. New York: Academic Press, 1973–.

Volume 7, *Aging,* 1977; volume 13, *Hypertension,* 1980.

Bibliotheca Anatomica. Nos. 1–. Basel: S. Karger, 1961–.

Number 18, 1979.

Clinical Physiology Series. **American Physiological Society.** Baltimore, MD: Williams & Wilkins, 1977–.

One of the latest volume, *Pulmonary Edema,* 1979.
R: BMJ 2: 326 (Aug. 4, 1979); *Lancet* 2: 179 (July 28, 1979).

Current Topics in Developmental Biology. Vols. 1–. New York: Academic Press, 1966–.

Volume 13, 1979.

ANESTHESIOLOGY AND GENERAL SURGERY

Advances in Pain Research and Therapy. Vols. 1–. New York: Raven Press, 1976–.

Volume 3, 1979.
R: *Journal of Oral Surgery* 35: 601 (July 1977); 36: 323 (Apr. 1978).

Advances in Surgery. Vols. 1–. Chicago, IL: Year Book Medical Publishers, 1966–.

Volume 11, 1977.
R: *British Journal of Surgery* 60: 82 (Jan. 1973); 62: 333 (Apr. 1975); 66: 218 (Mar. 1979).

Current Surgical Practice. Vols. 1–. London: Edward Arnold, 1976–.
R: *BMJ* 1: 1022 (Apr. 16, 1977).

Current Topics in Surgical Research. Vols. 1–. New York: Academic Press, 1969–.

Volume 3, 1971.
R: *Lancet* 2: 1018 (Nov. 14, 1970).

Major Problems in Clinical Surgery. Vols. 1–. Philadelphia, PA: W. B. Saunders, 1964–.

Volume 22, 1977.
R: *NEJM* 291: 803 (Oct. 10, 1974).

Progress in Surgery. Vols. 1–. Basel: S. Karger, 1961–.

Volume 16, 1979.
R: *British Journal of Surgery* 60: 986 (Dec. 1973); *BMJ* 2: 429 (May 19, 1973); 1: 341 (Feb. 8, 1975); *Canadian Medical Association Journal* 116: 730 (Apr. 1977); *Gastroenterology* 66: 483 (Mar. 1974); 68: 1331 (May 1975); 71: 708 (Sept. 1976); 73: 860 (Oct. 1977); *Journal of Bone and Joint Surgery* 57B: 127 (Feb. 1975); *JAMA* 238: 520 (Aug. 8, 1977).

Recent Advances in Plastic Surgery. Vols. 1–. New York: Churchill Livingstone, 1976–.

R: *Lancet* 2: 550 (Sept. 11, 1976); *Plastic and Reconstructive Surgery* 59: 845 (1977).

Recent Advances in Surgery. Nos. 1–. New York: Churchill Livingstone, 1928–.

Number 9, 1977.
R: *BMJ* 1: 1526 (June 11, 1977); *JAMA* 239: 865 (Feb. 27, 1978); *Lahey Clinic Foundation Bulletin* 27: 38 (Jan.–Mar. 1978).

Brain and Nervous System

Advances and Technical Standards in Neurosurgery. Vols. 1–. New York: Springer-Verlag, 1974–.

Volume 5, 1978.
R: *Brain* 99: 398 (June 1976); *Journal of Neurology, Neurosurgery and Psychiatry* 40: 205 (Feb. 1977); *Journal of Neurosurgery* 43: 641 (Nov. 1975); 45: 360 (Sept. 1976); 46: 841 (June 1977); 47: 973 (Dec. 1977); *Lahey Clinic Foundation Bulletin* 26: 190 (Oct.–Dec. 1977).

Advances in Diagnosis and Therapy. Vols. 1–. Berlin: Springer-Verlag, 1975–.

Volume 5, 1978.
R: *Brain* 99: 163 (Mar. 1976); *Journal of Neurosurgery* 44: 265 (Feb. 1976).

Advances in Neurochemistry. Vols. 1–. New York: Plenum, 1975–.

Volume 3, 1978.
R: *Brain* 99: 392 (June 1976), *Neurology* 29: 531 (April 1979).

Advances in Neurology. Vols. 1–. New York: Raven Press, 1973–.

Volume 26, 1979.
R: *Amercian Scientist* 62: 738 (Nov.–Dec. 1974); 62: 739 (Nov.–Dec. 1974); *Anesthesiology* 42: 115 (Jan. 1975); *Archives of Internal Medicine* 134: 191 (July 1974); *Archives of Neurology* 28: 420 (June 1973); 31: 143 (Aug. 1974); 31: 144 (Aug. 1974); 32: 345 (May 1975); *Archives of Pathology & Laboratory Medicine* 96: 287 (Oct. 1973); *Brain* 97: 223 (Mar. 1974); 97: 614 (Sept. 1974); 100: 797 (Dec. 1977); *BMJ* 4: 682 (Dec. 15, 1973); 1: 120 (Jan. 19, 1974); 2: 181 (Apr. 20, 1974); 4: 112 (Oct. 12, 1974); 1: 1021 (Apr. 24, 1976); *Electroencephalography & Clinical Neurophysiology* 36: 445 (Apr. 1974); 38: 112 (Jan. 1975); 38: 221 (Feb. 1975); 38: 223 (Feb. 1975); 40: 440 (Apr. 1976); 40: 557 (May 1976); 40: 558 (May 1976); 40: 559 (May 1976); 41: 108 (July 1976); 41: 223 (Aug. 1976); 45:

131 (July 1978); *Journal of Neurosurgery* 39: 422 (Sept. 1973); 41: 780 (Dec. 1974); 44: 132 (Jan. 1976); 44: 265 (Feb. 1976); 44: 396 (Mar. 1976); 44: 647 (May 1976); 45: 239 (Aug. 1976); 45: 359 (Sept. 1976); 46: 403 (Mar. 1977); 46: 838 (June 1977); 50: 268 (Feb. 1979); *JAMA* 235: 210 (Jan. 12, 1976); 235: 2771 (June 21, 1976); *Lancet* 2: 834 (Oct. 16, 1976); 1: 23 (Jan. 7, 1978); 1: 587 (Mar. 18, 1978); *Neurology* 24: 299 (Mar. 1974); *NEJM* 289: 644 (Sept. 20, 1973); *Physical Therapy* 55: 199 (Feb. 1975); 55: 200 (1975); 57: 1438 (1977); 59: 73 (1979); *Quarterly Review of Biology* 51: 350 (1976); 51: 471 (1976); *Yale Journal of Biology and Medicine* 47: 204 (Sept. 1974).

Advances in Neurosurgery. Vols. 1–. New York: Springer-Verlag, 1973–.
Volume 4, 1977.
R: *Brain* 99: 164 (Mar. 1976); *Journal of Neurosurgery* 41: 648 (Nov. 1974); 44: 530 (Apr. 1976); 45: 723 (Dec. 1976); 48: 310 (Feb. 1978); *Yale Journal of Biology and Medicine* 50: 430 (1977).

Annual Review of Neuroscience. Vols. 1–. Palto Alto, CA: Annual Reviews, 1978–.
Volume 2, 1979.
R: *American Scientist* 66: 757 (Nov.–Dec. 1978); *Archives of Physical Medicine and Rehabilitation* 59: 397 (Aug. 1978).

Contemporary Neurology Series. Vols. 1–. Philadelphia, PA: F. A. Davis, 1966–.
Volume 9, 1971.
R: *American Journal of Psychiatry* 131: 739 (June 1974).

Current Neurology. Vols. 1–. **H. Richard Tyler and David M. Dawson, eds.** Boston, MA: Houghton Mifflin, 1979–.
R: *BMJ* 2: 37 (Feb. 7, 1979); *Lancet* 2: 232 (Aug. 4, 1979); *Neurology* 29: 531 (Apr. 1979).

International Review of Neurobiology. Vols. 1–. New York: Academic Press, 1959–.
Volume 21, 1979.
R: *American Scientist* 63: 585 (Sept.–Oct. 1975); Chen (p. 288).

Major Problems in Neurology. Vols. 1–. Philadelphia, PA: W. B. Saunders, 1973–.
Volume 8, 1978.
R: *Archives of Neurology* 31: 143 (Aug. 1974); 36: 324 (May 1979); *Archives of Pathology & Laboratory Medicine* 99: 291 (May 1975); 102: 110 (Feb. 1978); *Journal of Clinical Pathology* 27: 340 (1974); *NEJM* 292: 377 (Feb. 13, 1975).

Modern Trends in Neurology. Vols. 1–. London: Butterworths, 1951–.
Volume 6, 1975.
R: *Brain* 99: 162 (Mar. 1976).

Neurology Series. Vols. 1–. New York: Springer-Verlag, 1969–.

Volume 20, 1978.

Progress in Brain Research. Vols. 1–. New York: American Elsevier, 1963–.
Volume 49, 1979.
R: *American Heart Journal* 96: 567 (1978); *American Scientist* 61: 589 (Sept.–Oct. 1973); *Archives of Neurology* 28: 420 (June 1973); 30: 424 (May 1974); *Brain* 97: 613 (Sept. 1974); *Journal of Neurosurgery* 38: 672 (May 1973); 43: 645 (Nov. 1975); *Nature* 276: 302 (Nov. 16, 1978); *Neurology* 23: 1349 (Dec. 1973).

Progress in Clinical Neurophysiology. Vols. 1–. Basel: S. Karger, 1978–.
Volume 8, 1980.
R: *Journal of Neurosurgery* 49: 938 (Dec. 1978); 49: 939 (Dec. 1978); *Lancet* 1: 192 (Jan. 27, 1979); *Nature* 274: 296 (July 20, 1978); 274: 517 (Aug. 3, 1978); *Neurology* 29: 532 (Apr. 1979).

Progress in Neurobiology. Vols. 1–. New York: Pergamon, 1973–.
Volume 10, 1979.
R: *Archives of Neurology* 30: 424 (May 1974); *Electroencephalography & Clinical Neurophysiology* 37: 110 (July 1974); *Journal of Histochemistry and Cytochemistry* 21: 933 (Oct. 1973); *Neurology* 23: 1018 (Sept. 1973); 24: 1102 (Nov. 1974); 25: 693 (July 1975); Chen (p. 289).

Progress in Neurological Surgery. Vols. 1–. Basel: S. Karger, 1966–.
Volume 10, 1980.
R: *Brain* 97: 813 (Dec. 1974); 99: 397 (June 1976); *Journal of Neurosurgery* 38: 396 (Mar. 1973); 48: 484 (Mar. 1978); *JAMA* 231: 769 (Feb. 17, 1975); 235: 2657 (June 14, 1976); *Lancet* 2: 1020 (Nov. 22, 1975); 1: 856 (Apr. 21, 1979); *Neurology* 28: 515 (May 1978); *Physical Therapy* 59: 86 (1979); 59: 92 (1979); *MRW* S1, p. 32.

Progress in Neurology and Psychiatry, An Annual Review. Vols. 1–. New York: Grune & Stratton.
Volume 1, 1946; Volume 28, 1973. Ceased.
R: *American Journal of Psychiatry* 130: 233 (1973); *Archives of Internal Medicine* 131: 614 (Apr. 1973); 133: 505 (Mar. 1974); *Journal of Nervous and Mental Disease* 159: 293 (1974); 160: 373 (1975); *Journal of Neurosurgery* 38: 126 (Jan. 1973); 40: 674 (May 1974); 41: 404 (Sept. 1974).

Progress in Neuropathology. Vols. 1–. New York: Grune & Stratton, 1971–.
Volume 3, 1976.
R: *Archives of Internal Medicine* 131: 308 (Feb. 1973); 132: 459 (Sept. 1973); *Archives of Neurology* 34: 322 (May 1977); *BMJ* 4: 788 (Dec. 29, 1978); *Journal of Neurosurgery* 40: 277 (Feb. 1974); 48: 151 (Jan. 1978); *Neurology* 23: 1140 (Oct. 1975); *ARBA* (1974, p. 632).

Progress in Neurophysiology. Vols. 1–. Basel: S. Karger, 1977–.
Volume 3, 1977.
R: *American Journal of Psychiatry* 135: 1122 (Sept. 1978); *Annals of Otology, Rhinology and Laryngology* 87: 883 (1978).

Radiology of the Skull and Brain. Vols. 1–. St. Louis, MO: C. V. Mosby, 1971–.
Volume 3, 1977.
R: *Journal of Neurosurgery* 42: 111 (Jan. 1975).

Recent Advances in Clinical Neurology. Nos. 1–. Edinburgh: Churchill Livingstone, 1975–.
Number 2, 1978.
R: *Brain* 99: 160 (Mar. 1976); *Lancet* 2: 853 (Nov. 1, 1975).

Research and Clinical Studies in Headache: An International Review. Vols. 1–. Basel: S. Karger, 1967–. Annual.

CARDIOVASCULAR SYSTEM

Advances in Cardiology. Vols. 1–. Basel: S. Karger, 1967–.
Volume 27, 1979.
R: *American Heart Journal* 89: 266 (1975); 90: 129 (1975); 91: 828 (1976); 94: 277 (1977); 94: 395 (1977); 95: 677 (1978); *American Journal of Cardiology* 31: 532 (1973); 36: 273 (1975); *Archives of Internal Medicine* 134: 189 (July 1974); *Canadian Medical Association Journal* 118: 240 (Feb. 4, 1978); 118: 136 (June 10, 1978); *Chest* 73: 26 (1978); *Physical Therapy* 58: 657 (1978).

Advances in Cardiopulmonary Diseases. Vols. 1–. Chicago, IL: Year Book Medical Publishers, 1963–. Annual.

Advances in Electrocardiography. Vols. 1–. New York: Grune & Stratton, 1972 .
Volume 2, 1976.
R: *American Family Physician* 7: 203 (Feb. 1973); *American Heart Journal* 94: 267 (Aug. 1977); *Annals of Internal Medicine* 78: 472 (Mar. 1973); 78: 473 (Mar. 1973); *Archives of Internal Medicine* 132: 912 (Dec. 1973); 137: 1738 (Dec. 1977); *Canadian Medical Association Journal* 117: 29 (July 9, 1977); *JAMA* 237: 1010 (Mar. 7, 1977); Allyn.

Advances in Heart Disease. Vols. 1–. New York: Grune & Stratton, 1977–.
Volume 2, 1978.
R: *JAMA* 239: 1912 (May 5, 1978); *Lancet* 2: 746 (Oct. 8, 1977).

Advances in Microcirculation. Vols. 1–. Basel: S. Karger, 1968–.
Volume 9, 1979.
R: *American Journal of Ophthalmology* 75: 736 (Apr. 1973); *Annals of Internal Medicine* 78: 805 (May 1973); *MRW* S1, p. 10.

Advances in Noninvasive Diagnostic Cardiology. Vols. 1–. Thorofare, NJ: Charles B. Slack, 1976–.
R: *Annals of Internal Medicine* 85: 414 (Sept. 1976).

Current Cardiovascular Topics. Vols. 1–. New York: Stratton Interconti-

nental Medical Book Corporation, 1975–.
Volume 4, 1978.
R: *American Heart Journal* 97: 413 (1979); *American Scientist* 64: 92 (Jan.–Feb. 1976).

Progress in Cardiac Rehabilitation. Vols. 1–. New York: Stratton Intercontinental Medical Book Corporation, 1973–.
R: *Archives of Physical Medicine and Rehabilitation* 55: 436 (Sept. 1974).

Progress in Cardiology. Vols. 1–. Philadelphia, PA: Lea & Febiger, 1972–.
Volume 8, 1979.
R: *American Heart Journal* 89: 820 (1975); 89: 890 (1975); *American Journal of Cardiology* 31: 408 (1975); 36: 542 (1975); *Archives of Internal Medicine* 132: 456 (Sept. 1973); 133: 873 (May 1974); *BMJ* 1: 115 (July 10, 1976); 1: 1342 (May 19, 1978); *Chest* 73: 23 (1978); *JAMA* 238: 350 (July 25, 1977); *Lancet* 1: 696 (Apr. 1, 1978); Allyn.

Dentistry

Advances in Oral Surgery. Vols. 1–. Chicago, IL: American Dental Association, 1971–.
Advances in Oral Surgery, 1971–1975.
Update in Oral Surgery, 1977.
R: *Journal of Oral Surgery* 32: 153 (Feb. 1974); 32: 931 (Dec. 1974); 34: 948 (Oct. 1976); *MRW* S2, p. 100.

Current Advances in Oral Surgery. Vols. 1–. St. Louis, MO: C. V. Mosby, 1974–.
Volume 2, 1977.
R: *Journal of Oral Surgery* 33: 470 (June 1975); 36: 323 (Apr. 1978).

Current Therapy in Dentistry. Vols. 1–. St. Louis, MO: C. V. Mosby, 1964–.
Volume 6, 1977.
Extensively covers all aspects of dental practice. Clinically and biologically oriented, multi-authored text.

Dermatology

Advances in Biology of Skin. Vols. 1–. New York: Plenum, 1960–.
Volume 12, 1972.

Current Problems in Dermatology. Vols. 2–. Basel: S. Karger, 1968–.
Volume 9, 1979.
Continues *Aktuelle Probleme der Dermatologie,* volume 1, 1959.

Endocrinology

Advances in Enzymology and Related Areas of Molecular Biology. Vols. 1–. New York: John Wiley, 1941–.

Volume 49, 1979.
R: *American Scientist* 63: 584 (Sept.–Oct. 1975); *Journal of Histochemistry and Cytochemistry* 23: 702 (Sept. 1975); 24: 757 (June 1976); Chen (p. 291); Wal (p. 203).

Clinics in Endocrinology and Metabolism. Vols. 1–. Philadelphia, PA: W. B. Saunders, 1972–.
Volume 7, 1978.
R: *Lancet* 1: 912 (Apr. 29, 1978).

Current Topics in Experimental Endocrinology. Vols. 1–. New York: Academic Press, 1971–.
Volume 3, 1978.
R: *American Scientist* 61: 488 (July–Aug. 1973); 63: 352 (May–June 1975); *Science* 176: 1228 (June 16, 1972); *Yale Journal of Biology and Medicine* 46: 250 (1973); Chen (p. 288).

Diabetes Mellitus: Diagnosis and Treatment. Vols. 1–. New York: American Diabetes Association, 1964–.
Volume 3, 1971.
R: *Annals of Internal Medicine* 77: 665 (1972); *Archives of Internal Medicine* 132: 773 (Nov. 1973); Allyn; Stearns & Ratcliff (*NEJM*, 1969; *NEJM*, 1970).

Frontiers in Neuroendocrinology. Vols. 1–. New York: Oxford University Press, 1969–.
Volume 5, 1978.
R: *Annals of Internal Medicine* 79: 770 (1973); *Lancet* 1: 1145 (June 8, 1974); *Neurology* 24: 100 (Jan. 1974), *Quarterly Review of Biology* 54: 120 (Mar. 1979).

Frontiers of Hormone Research. Vols. 1–. Basel: S. Karger, 1972–.
Volume 5, 1978.

Modern Trends in Endocrinology. Vols. 1–. New York: Appleton-Century-Crofts, 1958–.
Volume 4, 1972.
R: *Annals of Internal Medicine* 78: 322 (1973).

Recent Advances in Endocrinology and Metabolism. Nos. 1–. Edinburgh: Churchill Livingstone, 1978–.
R: *BMJ* 1: 436 (Feb. 18, 1978).

Recent Progress in Hormone Research. Vols. 1–. New York: Academic Press, 1947–.
Volume 35, 1979.
R: *American Scientist* 58: 558 (Sept./Oct. 1970); 60: 630 (Sept./Oct. 1972); *Science* 168: 1335 (June 12, 1970); Chen (p. 289).

Vitamins and Hormones: Advances in Research and Applications. Vol. 1–. New York: Academic Press, 1943–.
Volume 37, 1980.

Gastrointestinal System

Clinical Gastroenterology Monographs. Vols. 1–. New York: John Wiley, 1977–.
R: *Annals of Internal Medicine* 91: 145 (July 1979).

Clinics in Gastroenterology. Vols. 1–. Philadelphia, PA: W. B. Saunders, 1972–.
Volume 8, 1979.
R: *Lancet* 2: 1027 (Nov. 11, 1978); 1: 475 (Mar. 3, 1979); 2: 232 (Aug. 4, 1979).

Progress in Gastroenterology. Vols. 1–. New York: Grune & Stratton, 1968–.
Volume 3, 1978.
R: *BMJ* 4: 667 (Dec. 12, 1970); *JAMA* 239: 2488 (June 9, 1978); *NEJM* 299: 1083 (Nov. 9, 1978); *ARBA* (1972, p. 612); *MRW* S1, p. 13.

Progress in Liver Diseases. Vols. 1–. New York: Grune & Stratton, 1961–.
Volume 6, 1979.
R: *Annals of Internal Medicine* 78: 801 (May 1973); *Archives of Internal Medicine* 133: 503 (Mar. 1974); *BMJ* 4: 543 (Nov. 28, 1970); 1: 749 (Mar. 24, 1973); *Gastroenterology* 72: 188 (Jan. 1977); *NEJM* 290: 171 (Jan. 17, 1974); *ARBA* (1972, p. 613); Allyn.

Genetics

Advances in Genetics. Vols. 1–. New York: Academic Press, 1947–.
Volume 20, 1979.
R: *Nature* 266: viii (Apr. 28, 1977).

Advances in Human Genetics. Vols. 1–. New York: Plenum, 1970–.
Volume 10, 1980.
R: *American Journal of Human Genetics* 29: 213 (Mar. 1977); *American Scientist* 61: 593 (Sept.–Oct. 1973); 64: 219 (Mar.–Apr. 1976); *Clinical Pediatrics* 16: 536 (June 1977); *Heredity* 41: 409 (Dec. 1978); Allyn.

Advances in Teratology. Vols. 1–. New York: Academic Press, 1966–.
Volume 5, 1972.
R: *American Scientist* 61: 95 (Jan.–Feb. 1973); Chen (p. 288).

Annual Review of Genetics. Vols. 1–. Palo Alto, CA: Annual Reviews, 1967–. Annual.
R: *MRW* S1, p. 14.

Benchmark Papers in Genetics. Vols. 1–. Stroudsberg, PA: Dowden, Hutchinson & Ross, 1974–.
Volume 10, 1979.
R: *Annals of Human Genetics* 43: 82 (July 1979).

Chemical Mutagens. Vols. 1–. New York: Plenum, 1971–.

Volume 5, 1978.
R: *Annals of Human Genetics* 41: 391 (Jan. 1978).

Progress in Medical Genetics. Vols. 1–. New York: Grune & Stratton, 1961–.
Volume 10, 1974.
R: *American Scientist* 64: 219 (Mar.–Apr. 1976); *Archives of Internal Medicine* 133: 156 (Jan. 1974); *BMJ* 2: 106 (July 12, 1975); *Quarterly Review of Biology* 49: 66 (1974); *Teratology* 9: 247 (Apr. 1974); *ARBA* (1972, p. 613).

GERONTOLOGY

Interdisciplinary Topics in Gerontology. Vols. 1–. Basel: S. Karger, 1968–.
Volume 16, 1979.

Recent Advances in Geriatric Medicine. Nos. 1–. Edinburgh: Churchill Livingstone, 1978–.
R: *Lancet* 1: 1342 (June 24, 1978).

HEMATOLOGY

Bibliotheca Haematologica. Nos. 1–. Basel: S. Karger, 1955–.
Number 46, 1979.

Clinics in Haematology. Vols. 1–. Philadelphia, PA: W. B. Saunders,1972–.
Volume 8, 1979.
R: *British Journal of Haematology* 38: 4322 (1978); *BMJ* 1: 1206 (May 5, 1979); *Lancet* 1: 535 (Mar. 11, 1978); 1: 476 (Mar. 3, 1979).

Progress in Hematology. Vols. 1–. New York: Grune & Stratton, 1956–.
Volume 10, 1977.
R: *Annals of Internal Medicine* 78: 163 (1973); *Archives of Internal Medicine* 131: 612 (Apr. 1973); *British Journal of Haematology* 38: 579 (1978); *Clinical Pediatrics* 13: 613 (July 1974); *JAMA* 229: 84 (July 1, 1974); 236: 607 (Aug. 9, 1976); *Lancet* 2: 1282 (Dec. 11, 1976); *Quarterly Review of Biology* 49: 383 (1974).

Progress in Hemostasis and Thrombosis. Vols. 1–. New York: Grune & Stratton, 1972–.
Volume 4, 1978.
R: *Annals of Internal Medicine* 78: 321 (Feb. 1973); 91: 148 (July 1979).

Recent Advances in Haematology. Nos. 1–. Edinburgh: Churchill Livingstone, 1971–.
Number 2, 1977.
R: *Archives of Pathology & Laboratory Medicine* 103: 317 (June 1979); *British Journal of Haematology* 38: 152 (1978); *BMJ* 1: 164 (Jan. 21, 1978); *Journal of Clinical Pathology* 31: 297 (Mar. 1978).

Recent Advances in Thrombosis. Vols. 1–. Edinburgh: Churchill Livingstone, 1973–.

R: *Lancet* 2: 540 (Sept. 8, 1973).

Topics in Hematology. Vols. 1–. New York: Plenum, 1978–.
Volume 3, *Trace Elements and Iron in Human Metabolism,* 1978.
R: *Annals of Internal Medicine* 91: 340 (Aug. 1979); *British Journal of Hematology* 42: 491 (July 1979); *Lancet* 1: 647 (Mar. 24, 1979).

INFECTIOUS DISEASES

Advances in Applied Microbiology. Vols. 1–. New York: Academic Press, 1959–.
Volume 25, 1979.
R: *Nature* 266: viii (Apr. 18, 1977); *Yale Journal of Biology and Medicine* 48: 264 (1975).

Advances in Parasitology. Vols. 1–. New York: Academic Press, 1963–.
Volume 15, 1977.
R: *Journal of Parasitology* 60: 292 (Apr. 1974); 60: 612 (Aug. 1974).

Advances in Virus Research. Vols. 1–. New York: Academic Press, 1953–.
Volume 19, 1974.
R: Chen (p. 291).

Annual Review of Microbiology. Vols. 1–. Palo Alto, CA: Annual Reviews, 1947–. Annual.
Volume 30, 1976.
R: *Nature* 190: 662 (May 20, 1961); *ARBA* (1976, p. 656); Chen (p. 291); Jenkins (G171); Wal (p. 199).

Benchmark Papers in Microbiology. Vols. 1–. Stroudsburg, PA: Dowden, Hutchinson & Ross, 1973–.
Volume 6, 1974.

Current Topics in Microbiology and Immunology. Vols. 48–. New York: Springer, 1968–.
Continues *Ergenbisse der Mikrobiologie und Immunitaeforschung.*
Volume 85, 1979.

Developments in Medical Microbiology and Infectious Diseases. New York: John Wiley.
Recent volume in the series *The Gonococcus,* R. B. Roberts, ed., 1977.
R: *Canadian Medical Association Journal* 118: 1370 (June 1978); *Immunological Communications* 7: 477 (1978).

Methods in Microbiology. Vols. 1–. New York: Academic Press, 1969–.
Volume 13, 1980.
R: *American Scientist* 59: 766 (Nov./Dec. 1971); *Chemistry and Industry* 42: 1196 (Oct. 16, 1971); Chen (p. 292).

Progress in Medical Virology. Vols. 1–. New York: S. Karger, 1958–.
Volume 26, 1980.
R: *American Journal of Diseases of Children* 128: 428 (Sept. 1974); *American Scientist* 63: 583 (Sept.–Oct. 1975); *BMJ* 2: 736 (June 29, 1974); 1: 177 (Jan. 15, 1977); *Canadian Medical Association Journal* 119: 430 (Sept. 9, 1978); *Immunology* 26: 230 (Jan. 1974); 28: 1179 (June 1975); 32: 370 (Mar. 1977); 32: 603 (Apr. 1977); 33: 436 (Sept. 1977); *Lancet* 2: 1234 (Nov. 23, 1974); Allyn.

Recent Advances in Clinical Virology. Nos. 1–. Edinburgh: Churchill Livingstone, 1977–.
R: *BMJ* 2: 1016 (Oct. 15, 1977); *Lancet* 1: 457 (Feb. 26, 1977).

INTERNAL MEDICINE

Advances in Clinical Chemistry. Vols. 1–. New York: Academic Press, 1958–.
Volume 20, 1978.

Advances in Internal Medicine. Vols. 1–. Chicago, IL: Year Book Medical Publishers, 1954–.
Volume 25, 1980.
R: *American Family Physician* 19: 225 (Apr. 1979); *Annals of Internal Medicine* 91: 148 (July 1979); *Archives of Internal Medicine* 132: 301 (Aug. 1973); *Lahey Clinic Foundation Bulletin* 26: 45 (Jan.–Mar. 1977).

Advances in Lipid Research. Vols. 1–. New York: Academic Press, 1963–.
Volume 17, 1980.
R: *American Scientist* 59: 269–70 (Mar.–Apr. 1971); 61: 594–595 (Sept.–Oct. 1973); *Yale Journal of Biology and Medicine* 50: 324 (1977); Chen (p. 287).

Major Problems in Internal Medicine. Vols. 1–. Philadelphia, PA: W. B. Saunders, 1971–.
Volume 15, 1978.
R: *Annals of Internal Medicine* 91: 146 (July 1979); *Archives of Pathology & Laboratory Medicine* 103: 371 (July 1979); *JAMA* 237: 903 (Feb. 28, 1977).

Medicine and Sport. Vols. 1–. **E. Jokl, ed.** Basel: S. Karger, 1966–.
Irregular.
Volume 12, *Health Aspects of Endurance Training,* 1978.
Text in English.

Progress in Clinical and Biological Research. Vols. 1–. New York: Alan R. Liss, 1975–.
Volume 23, 1978.
R: *American Journal of Human Genetics* 30: 449 (July 1978); *Archives of Pathology & Laboratory Medicine* 103: 549 (Sept. 1979); *Electroencephalography & Clinical Neurophysiology* 45: 307 (Aug. 1978); *Journal of Clinical Pathology* 32: 742 (July 1979); *Journal of Neurosurgery* 49: 624 (Oct. 1978); *Yale Journal of Biology & Medicine* 52: 240 (Mar./Apr. 1979).

Recent Advances in Clinical Biochemistry. Nos. 1–. Edinburgh: Churchill Livingstone, 1978–.
Number 1, 1978.
R: *BMJ* 1: 568 (Mar. 4, 1978).

Recent Advances in Intensive Therapy. Nos. 1–. Edinburgh: Churchill Livingstone, 1977–.
R: *BMJ* 1: 707 (Mar. 18, 1978), *Lancet* 1: 363 (Feb. 18, 1978).

The Science and Practice of Clinical Medicine. Vols. 1–. New York: Grune & Stratton, 1976–.
Volume 1, *Disorders of the Gastrointestinal Tract; Disorders of the Liver; Nutritional Disorders,* 1976; volume 2, *Disorders of the Respiratory System,* 1976; volume 3, *Clinical Cardiology,* 1977; volume 4, *Rheumatology and Immunology,* 1979.
R: *JAMA* 239: 2489 (June 9, 1978).

Nursing

Mosby's Current Practice and Perspectives in Nursing Series. St. Louis, MO: C. V. Mosby, 1976–.
The Mosby series includes *Current Concepts in Clinical Nursing; Current Perspectives in Nursing Education; Current Perspectives in Oncologic Nursing; Current Perspectives in Psychiatric Nursing; Current Practice in Family-Centered Community Nursing; Current Practice in Obstetric & Gynecologic Nursing; Current Practice in Oncologic Nursing; Current Practice in Pediatric Nursing;* etc.
R: *American Journal of Nursing* 79: 988 (May 1979).

Nutrition

Advances in Food Research. Vols. 1–. New York: Academic Press, 1948–.
Volume 25, 1979.
R: *Journal of Food Technology* 14: 332 (June 1979); Chen (p. 287); Wal (p. 485).

Advances in Modern Nutrition. Vols. 1–. Somerset, NJ: John Wiley, 1976–.
Volume 2, 1978.
R: *Nutrition Reviews* 36: 232 (July 1978).

Advances in Nutritional Research. Vols. 1–. New York: Plenum, 1977–.
Volume 2, 1979.
R: *American Journal of Clinical Nutrition* 31: 1292 (July 1978).

Bibliotheca Nutritio et Dieta. Nos. 1–. Basel: S. Karger, 1960–.
Number 28, 1979.

Recent Advances in Obesity Research. Vols. 1–. London: Newman Publishing, 1974–.
R: *BMJ* 1: 1081 (May 1, 1976); *Nutrition* 29: 316 (Sept.–Oct. 1975).

World Review of Nutrition and Dietetics. Vols. 1–. Basel: S. Karger, 1959–.

Volume 34, 1979.
R: *American Scientist* 62: 236 (Mar.–Apr. 1974); 64: 92 (Jan.–Feb. 1976); *BMJ* 2: 786 (June 30, 1973); 2: 619 (June 15, 1974).

ONCOLOGY AND NUCLEAR MEDICINE

Advances in Cancer Research. Vols. 1–. New York: Academic Press, 1953–.
Volume 30, 1980.
R: *American Scientist* 63: 355 (May–June 1975); 67: 111 (Jan.–Feb. 1979); *BMJ* 3: 351 (Aug. 3, 1974); *Quarterly Review of Biology* 49: 174 (June 1974); 50: 366 (1975); 51: 353 (1976); 51: 471 (1976); *ARBA* (1971, p. 529); Chen (p. 287). Also reviewed in *Science*.

Biosynthetic Products for Cancer Chemotherapy. Vols. 1–. New York: Plenum, 1977–.
Volume 3, 1978.

Breast Cancer: Advances in Research and Treatment. Vols. 1–. New York: Plenum, 1977–.
Volume 3, 1979.
R: *British Journal of Surgery* 66: 296 (Apr. 1979); *Lancet* 1: 1022 (May 13, 1978).

International Advances in Surgical Oncology. Vols. 1–. New York: Alan R. Liss, 1978–.
R: *Lancet* 2: 1130 (Nov. 25, 1978).

IARC Monographs on the Evaluation of Carcinogenic Risk of Chemicals to Humans. Vols. 1–. Lyon, France: International Agency for Research on Cancer, 1972–.
Volume 18 1978.
R: *Archives of Pathology & Laboratory Medicine* 101: 111 (Feb. 1977); *Journal of Clinical Pathology* 29: 367 (1976); 30: 295 (1977); 31: 209 (Feb. 1978); *Quarterly Review of Biology* 53: 86 (1978); 53: 357 (1978); *IBID* 7: 158 (Summer 1979).

Progress in Cancer Research and Therapy. Vols. 1–. New York: Raven Press, 1976–.
Volume 9, 1978.
R: *Archives of Pathology & Laboratory Medicine* 102: 390 (1978); 102: 942 (1978); 103: 208 (1979); *Nature* 275: iv (Sept. 14, 1978); *Science* 201: 248 (July 21, 1978).

Progress in Clinical Cancer. Vols. 1–. New York: Grune & Stratton, 1965–.
Volume 7, 1978.
R: *American Journal of Roentgenology* 133: 178 (July 1979); *Annals of Internal Medicine* 79: 617 (Oct. 1973); *Archives of Internal Medicine* 133: 875 (May 1974); *BMJ* 1: 1283 (May 22, 1976); *ARBA* (1971, p. 530).

Progress in Experimental Tumor Research. Vols. 1–. New York: S. Karger, 1960–.
Volume 15, 1979.

R: *Archives of Pathology & Laboratory Medicine* 95: 354 (May 1973); *BMJ* 2: 493 (May 26, 1973); *Journal of Neurosurgery* 39: 421 (Sept. 1973).

Progress in Nuclear Medicine. Vols. 1–. Baltimore, MD: University Park Press, 1972–.

Volume 4, 1978.
R: *Archives of Internal Medicine* 132: 141 (July 1973); 133: 157 (Jan. 1974); *Journal of Neurosurgery* 38: 395 (Mar. 1973).

Recent Advances in Clinical Nuclear Medicine. Nos. 1–. Edinburgh: Churchill Livingstone, 1975–.

R: *Physics in Medicine & Biology* 20: 1038 (Nov. 1975).

Recent Advances in Nuclear Medicine. Vols. 4–. New York: Grune & Stratton, 1974–.

Volumes 1–3, *Progress in Atomic Medicine*, 1965–1971; volume 5, 1978.
R: *American Scientist* 63: 472 (July–Aug. 1975); *Yale Journal of Biology and Medicine* 48: 460 (1975).

Recent Results in Cancer Research. Vols. 1–. New York: Springer-Verlag, 1965–.

Volume 69, 1979.
R: *British Journal of Haematology* 29: 367 (1975); 30: 373 (1975); 31: 415 (1975); *Quarterly Review of Biology* 49: 379 (1974).

OPHTHALMOLOGY

Abhandlungen Aus Der Augenheilkunde und Ihren Grenzgebieten. Vols. 1–. Basel: S. Karger, 1926–.

Continued by *Bibliotheca Ophthalmologica* with volume 28, 1939–.

Advances in Ophthalmology. Vols. 1–. Basel: S. Karger, 1949–.

Volume 40, 1979.
R: *American Journal of Ophthalmology* 75: 169 (Jan. 1973); 81: 113 (Jan. 1976); 81: 693 (May 1976); 84: 133 (July 1977); *Archives of Ophthalmology* 93: 92 (Jan. 1975); 94: 167 (Jan. 1976); 95: 902 (May 1977); 95: 1894 (Oct. 1977); 96: 919 (May 1978); 96: 1293 (July 1978).

Advances in Uveal Surgery, Vitreous Surgery, and the Treatment of Endophthalmitis. Vols. 1–. West Nyack, NJ: Prentice-Hall, 1975–.

R: *American Journal of Ophthalmology* 81: 540 (Apr. 1976); *Archives of Ophthalmology* 94: 1239 (July 1976).

Current Concepts in Ophthalmology. Vols. 1–. St. Louis, MO: C. V. Mosby, 1967–.

Volume 5, 1976; volume 6, 1979.
This series provides an up-to-date overview of the state of the art: recent advances, new diagnostic methods, current progress. The volumes are strongly oriented toward medical aspects of ophthalmology.

R: *American Journal of Ophthalmology* 75: 167 (Jan. 1973); *Archives of Ophthalmology* 89: 525 (June 1973); 93: 703 (Aug. 1975).

Current Topics in Eye Research. Vols. 1–. New York: Academic Press, 1979–.
Volume 2, 1980.

Major Problems in Ophthalmology. Vols. 1–. Philadelphia, PA: W. B. Saunders, 1975–.
Volume 2, 1976.
R: *American Journal of Ophthalmology* 84: 131 (1977).

Modern Problems in Ophthalmology. Vols. 1–. Basel: S. Karger, 1926–.
Volume 20, 1979.
R: *Annals of Otology, Rhinology and Laryngology* 85: 150 (1976).

Modern Trends in Ophthalmology. Vols. 1–. Glasgow, Scotland: Butterworths, 1940–.
Volume 5, 1973.
R: *American Journal of Ophthalmology* 76: 860 (Nov. 1977).

ORTHOPEDICS

Current Practice in Orthopaedic Surgery. Vols. 1–. St. Louis, MO: C. V. Mosby, 1963–.
Volume 6, 1975; volume 7, 1977.
American counterpart of British *Recent Advances in Orthopaedics*. State-of-the-art review of orthopedic surgery. Intended for orthopedic surgeons in practice or training.
R: *Canadian Medical Association Journal* 119: 1022 (Nov. 4, 1978); *Journal of Bone and Joint Surgery* 58B: 393 (Aug. 1976); *MRW* S1, p. 16.

Modern Trends in Orthopaedics. Vols. 1–. Washington, DC: Butterworths, 1950–.
Volume 6, 1972.
R: *MRW* S1, p. 16.

Progress in Orthopaedic Surgery. Vols. 1–. New York: Springer-Verlag, 1977–.
Volume 1, *Leg Length Discrepancy/The Injured Knee,* 1977; volume 2, *Acetabular Dysplasia-Skeletal Dysplasias in Childhood,* 1978; volume 3, *The Knee: Ligament and Articular Cartilage Injuries,* 1978.

Recent Advances in Orthopaedics. Nos. 1–. New York: Churchill Livingstone, 1969–.
Number 2, 1975.
R: *Journal of Bone and Joint Surgery* 58B: 148 (Feb. 1976).

OTORHINOLARYNGOLOGY

Advances in Oto-Rhino-Laryngology. Vols. 1–. Basel: S. Karger, 1953–.

Volume 25, 1979.
R: *Annals of Otology, Rhinology and Laryngology* 83: 265 (1974); 87: 883 (1978); *Archives of Neurology* 36: 389 (June 1979); *Electroencephalography & Clinical Neurophysiology* 37: 444 (Oct. 1974).

Recent Advances in Otolaryngology. Vols. 1–. Edinburgh: Churchill Livingstone, 1973–.
Volume 5, 1978.
R: *BMJ* 3: 703 (Sept. 29, 1973).

PATHOLOGY

Current Topics in Comparative Pathobiology. Vols. 1–. New York: Academic Press, 1971–.

International Review of Cytology. Vols. 1–. New York: Academic Press, 1952.
Volume 64, 1980.
R: *American Scientist* 66: 757 (Nov.–Dec. 1978). Also reviewed in *ASM News; Journal of Histochemistry and Cytochemistry; Quarterly Review of Biology.*

International Review of Experimental Pathology. Vols. 1–. **G. W. Richter and M. A. Epstein.** New York: Academic Press, 1962–.
Volume 20, 1979.
R: Chen (p. 288).

Major Problems in Pathology. Vols. 1–. Philadelphia, PA: W. B. Saunders, 1970–.
Volume 5, 1976.
R: *BMJ* 1: 241 (Jan. 22, 1977).

Methods and Achievements in Experimental Pathology. Vols. 1–. Basel: S. Karger, 1965–.
Volume 9, 1979.
R: *Journal of Clinical Pathology* 29: 368 (1976); *Canadian Medical Association Journal* 102: 767 (Apr. 11, 1970).

Monographs in Clinical Cytology. Vols. 1–. **G. L. Wied, ed.** Basel: S. Karger, 1965–. Irregular.
Volume 4, Part 1, *Aspiration Biopsy Cytology,* 1974; volume 7, Part 2, *Aspiration Biopsy Cytology,* 1979.
Text in English.

Progress in Clinical Pathology. Vols. 1–. New York: Grune & Stratton, 1967–.
Volume 7, 1978.
R: *Archives of Internal Medicine* 133: 324 (Feb. 1974); 135: 1273 (Sept. 1975); *Canadian Medical Association Journal* 103: 1017 (Nov. 7. 1970).

Progress in Histochemistry and Cytochemistry. Vols. 1–. Stuttgart: Gustav Fischer Verlag, 1970–.
Volume 9, 1976.
R: *Journal of Histochemistry and Cytochemistry* 23: 458 (June 1975).

Recent Advances in Clinical Pathology. Series 1–6. Edinburgh: Churchill Livingstone, 1973.
R: *Archives of Pathology & Laboratory Medicine* 99: 124 (1975); *British Journal of Haematology* 25: 553 (1973); *BMJ* 2: 721 (June 23, 1973).

Recent Advances in Neuropathology. Vols. 1–. London: Churchill Livingstone, 1979–.
R: *Lancet* 2: 15 (July 7, 1979).

Pediatrics

Advances in Pediatrics. Vols. 1–. Chicago, IL: Year Book Medical Publishers, 1942–.
Volume 24, 1978.
R: *American Family Physician* 16: 287 (Oct. 1977); *American Journal of Diseases of Children* 129: 1114 (Sept. 1975); 130: 219 (Feb. 1976); *BMJ* 2: 711 (Sept. 20, 1975); *Canadian Medical Association Journal* 115: 985 (Nov. 20, 1976); 117: 587 (Sept. 17, 1977); *Clinical Pediatrics* 17: 487 (June 1978).

Clinics in Developmental Medicine. Vols. 7–. Spastics International Medical Publications. Distributed by Philadelphia, PA: J. B. Lippincott, 1962–.
Continues *Little Club in Developmental Medicine,* vols. 1–6, 1960–61.
Volumes 69 and 70, 1979.
This is a series of books published four times a year on developmental medicine. Each volume is on a specific topic of the subject.

Pediatric and Adolescent Endocrinology. Vols. 1–. Basel: S. Karger, 1976–.
Volume 8, 1980.

Perspectives in Pediatric Pathology. Vols. 1–. Chicago, IL: Year Book Medical Publishers, 1973–.
Volume 2, 1975.
R: *American Journal of Diseases of Children* 127: 604 (Apr. 1974); *NEJM* 290: 413 (Feb. 15, 1974); *Pediatrics* 53: 96 (Jan. 1974); 59: 795 (May 1977).

Progress in Pediatric Radiology. Vols. 1–. Basel: S. Karger, 1967–.
Volume 7, 1979.
R: *American Journal of Human Genetics* 26: 418 (May 1974); *American Journal of Roentgenology* 131: 946 (Nov. 1978); *Archives of Neurology* 36: 325 (May 1979); *BMJ* 3: 180 (July 21, 1973); *Canadian Medical Association Journal* 119: 430 (Sept. 9, 1978); *Journal of Bone and Joint Surgery* 56B: 781 (Nov. 1974); *Journal of Neurosurgery* 46: 125 (Jan. 1977); *NEJM* 289: 1317 (Dec. 13, 1973).

Progress in Pediatric Surgery. Vols. 1–. Baltimore, MD: Urban & Schwar-

zenberg, 1971–.
Volume 10, 1977.
R: *British Journal of Surgery* 60: 418 (May 1973); 61: 926 (Nov. 1974); 62: 280 (Mar. 1975); 64: 74 (Jan. 1977); *Clinical Pediatrics* 16: 420 (May 1977); *JAMA* 238: 2642 (Dec. 12, 1977); *Pediatrics* 51: 1117 (June 1973).

Recent Advances in Paediatric Surgery. Nos. 1–. Edinburgh: Churchill Livingstone, 1963–.
Number 2, 1969; number 3, 1975.
R: *BMJ* 2: 344 (May 10, 1975).

Pharmacy and Pharmacology

Advances in Biochemical Psychopharmacology. Vols. 1–. New York: Raven Press, 1969–.
Volume 16, 1977.
R: *Brain* 96: 415 (June 1973); 101: 187 (Mar. 1978); *Neurology* 23: 387 (Apr. 1973).

Advances in Drug Research. Vols. 1–. New York: Academic Press, 1964–.
Volume 12, 1978.
R: *Journal of Pharmaceutical Sciences* 64: 899 (May 1975); *JAMA* 233: 186 (July 1975); *Pharmaceutical Journal* 215: 409 (1975); 217: 578 (1976); *ABL* 39: entry 215 (May 1974); 40: entry 115 (Apr. 1975); 43: entry 394 (Sept. 1978).

Advances in General and Cellular Pharmacology. Vols. 1–. New York: Plenum, 1977–.
Volume 2, 1977.
R: *Journal of Pharmaceutical Sciences* 67: 1195 (Aug. 1978); *Nature* 267: 292 (May 19, 1977).

Advances in Mass Spectrometry in Biochemistry & Medicine. Vols. 1–. Holliswood, NY: Spectrum Publications, 1976–.
Volume 2, 1977.
R: *Journal of Pharmaceutical Sciences* 66: 446 (Mar. 1977); 66: 1792 (Dec. 1977).

Advances in Pharmaceutical Sciences. Vols. 1–. New York: Academic Press, 1964–. Annual.
Volume 4, 1974.
R: *Journal of Pharmaceutical Sciences* 65: 1711 (Nov. 1976).

Advances in Pharmacology and Chemotherapy. Vols. 1–. New York: Academic Press, 1962–. Annual.
Volume 16, 1979.
R: *Quarterly Review of Biology* 51: 471 (1976).

Analytical Profiles of Drug Substances. Vols. 1–. New York: Academic Press, 1972–.
Volume 7, 1978.

R: *Journal of Pharmaceutical Sciences* 63: 1344 (Aug. 1974); 64: 1584 (Sept. 1975); 66: 1061 (July 1977); 68: 940 (July 1979).

Annual Reports in Medicinal Chemistry. Vols. 1–. **Division of Medicinal Chemistry, American Chemical Society.** New York: Academic Press, 1965–. Annual.

Volume 13, 1978.

R: *Journal of Pharmaceutical Sciences* 66: 1213 (Aug. 1977); *ARBA* (1971, p. 529).

Annual Review of Pharmacology. Palo Alto, CA: Annual Reviews, 1961–. Annual.

Volume 18, 1978.

A review of recent advances in pharmacology. Intended as an overview of progress for graduate students, researchers, and professors. Articles are written in advanced, scholarly manner. Lengthy bibliographies follow most articles.

R: *RSR* 2: 129 (Oct.–Dec. 1974); *ARBA* (1971, p. 539; 1976, p. 738); Chen (p. 288).

Current Developments in Psychopharmacology. Vols. 1–. New York: Spectrum Publications, 1975–.

Volume 5, 1978.

R: *American Journal of Psychiatry* 134: 1321 (Nov. 1977); 135: 880 (July 1978); *American Scientist* 65: 638 (Sept.–Oct. 1977).

Modern Problems in Pharmacopsychiatry. Vols. 1–. Basel: S. Karger, 1968–.

Volume 15, 1979.

Pharmacological and Biochemical Properties of Drug Substances. Vols. 1–. Washington, DC: American Pharmaceutical Association, 1977–.

Companion series to *Analytical Profiles of Drug Substances.*

Photochemical and Photobiological Reviews. Vols. 1–. New York: Plenum, 1976–.

Volume 4, 1979.

Progress in Drug Metabolism. Vols. 1–. New York: John Wiley, 1976–.

Volume 3, 1979.

R: *Journal of Pharmaceutical Sciences* 66: 1364 (Sept. 1977); 67: 1649 (Nov. 1978).

Progress in Drug Research/Fortschritte der Arzneimittelforschung/ Progres des Recherches Pharmaceutiques. Vols. 1–. Basel, Switzerland: Birkhaeuser Verlag, 1959–.

Volume 22, 1978.

R: *Journal of Pharmaceutical Sciences* 68: 806 (June 1979).

Progress in Medicinal Chemistry. Vols. 1–. New York: American Elsevier, 1961–.

Volume 15, 1978.

R: *Journal of Pharmaceutical Sciences* 63: 1344 (Aug. 1974); 65: 1562 (Oct. 1976).

Recent Advances in Clinical Pharmacology. Vols. 1–. New York/Edinburgh: Churchill Livingstone, 1978–.
R: *Lancet* 1: 901 (Apr. 28, 1979).

Side Effects of Drugs. Vols. 1–. Amsterdam: Excerpta Medica Foundation, 1957–.
Volume 7, 1971; volume 8, 1976; annual supplements to volume 8 (annual 1, 1977; annual 2, 1978; annual 3, 1979).
R: *Journal of Oral Surgery* 37: 366 (May 1979); *Pharmaceutical Journal* 223: 113 (1979).

Psychiatry and Psychology

Advances in Behavioral Biology. Vols. 1–. New York: Plenum, 1971–.
Volume 24, 1977.
R: *Archives of Neurology* 36: 182 (Mar. 1979); *Electroencephalography & Clinical Neurophysiology* 37: 111 (July 1974); *Neurology* 27: 1186 (Dec. 1977). Also reviewed in *Contemporary Psychology; Journal of Environmental Sciences; Medical Journal of Australia; Psychosomatics.*

Advances in Biological Psychiatry. Vols. 1–. Basel: S. Karger, 1978–.
Volume 3, 1979.

Advances in Clinical Child Psychology. Vols. 1–. New York: Plenum, 1977–.
Volume 2, 1978.

Advances in Human Psychopharmacology. Vols. 1–. Greenwich, CT: JAI Press, 1980–.

Advances in Mental Handicap Research. Vol. 1–. New York: John Wiley, 1979–.

Advances in Psychobiology. Vols. 1–. New York: John Wiley, 1972–.
Volume 3, 1976.
R: *Brain* 99: 394 (June 1976); *Journal of Nervous and Mental Disease* 163: 492 (1976).

Advances in Psychosomatic Medicine. Vols. 1–. Basel: S. Karger, 1960–.
Volume 10, 1979.
R: *American Journal of Psychiatry* 131: 613 (1974); 131: 729 (June 1974); *BMJ* 1: 120 (Jan. 13, 1973).

Advances in Sleep Research. Vols. 1–3. Flushing, NY: Spectrum Publications, 1974–1976.
R: *American Journal of Psychiatry* 134: 209 (June 1977); *Annals of Internal Medicine* 81: 426 (Sept. 1974); *Brain* 97: 613 (Sept. 1974); *BMJ* 1: 183 (July 17, 1975); *Pharmaceutical Journal* 212: 318 (1975); *Quarterly Review of Biology* 50: 124 (1975).

Advances in the Study of Behavior. Vols. 1–. New York: Academic Press. 1965–.

Volume 10, 1979.
R: *American Scientist* 58: 111 (Jan./Feb. 1970); Chen (p. 288).

Annual Progress in Child Psychiatry and Child Development. Vols. 1–. New York: Brunner/Mazel, 1968–. Annual.

Volume 11, 1979.
R: *American Journal of Psychiatry* 134: 1058 (Sept. 1977); 136: 1003 (July 1979); *Journal of Nervous and Mental Disease* 158: 82 (1974); *Pediatrics* 52: 761 (Nov. 1973).

Annual Review of Psychology. Vols. 1–. Palo Alto, CA: Annual Reviews, 1950–. Annual.

Volume 29, 1978.
Presents a broad overview of progress in selected areas of psychology. Topics vary annually. The review period spans two to three years. Articles are written by authors with recognized competency. A valuable tool for research psychologist.
R: *Archives of Physical Medicine and Rehabilitation* 54: 198 (Apr. 1973); 54: 447 (Sept. 1973); 56: 228 (May 1975); 57: 251 (May 1976); 58: 186 (Apr. 1977); 59: 397 (Aug. 1978).

Association for Research in Nervous and Mental Disease (ARNMD) Research Publications. Vols. 1–. Baltimore, MD: Williams & Wilkins, 1921–.

Volume 35, *The Neurologic and Psychiatric Aspects of the Disorders of Aging,* 1956; volume 57, *Congenital and Acquired Cognitive Disorders,* 1979.

Current Psychiatric Therapies. Vols. 1–. New York: Grune & Stratton, 1961–.

Volume 18, 1978.
R: *American Journal of Psychiatry* 135: 1256 (Oct. 1978).

Recent Advances in Clinical Psychiatry. Nos. 1–. New York: Churchill Livingstone, 1971–.

Number 2, 1976.

Reviews of Physiology, Biochemistry, and Pharmacology. Berlin and New York: Springer-Verlag.

Volume 71, 1974.
R: Chen (p. 292).

The Series in Clinical and Community Psychology. Vols. 1–. New York: John Wiley, 1976–.

Volume 5, *Stress and Anxiety,* 1978.
R: *Choice* 16: 292 (Apr. 1979).

PUBLIC HEALTH

Advances in Environmental Science and Technology. Vols. 1–. New York: Wiley-Interscience, 1969–.

Volume 2, 1972; volume 10, 1979.
R: *Science* 169: 463 (July 31, 1970); Chen (p. 297); Wal (p. 64, 367).

Advances in Forensic and Clinical Toxicology. Vols. 1–. Cleveland, OH: Chemical Rubber Company, 1972–.
R: *Annals of Internal Medicine* 80: 132 (Jan. 1974).

Advances in Modern Toxicology. Vols. 1–. New York: John Wiley, 1976–.
Volume 5, 1978.
R: *Archives of Dermatology* 114: 469 (Mar. 1978); *Journal of Pharmaceutical Sciences* 66: 1214 (Aug. 1977); *Lancet* 2: 1328 (Dec. 24, 1977); 2: 1328 (Dec. 31, 1977); 1: 587 (Mar. 17, 1979); *Nature* 265: vii (Feb. 10, 1977); *Pharmaceutical Journal* 217: 35 (1976).

Contributions to Epidemiology and Biostatistics. Vols. 1–. New York: S. Karger, 1979–.
Volume 2, 1980.

Currents in Alcoholism. Vols. 1–. New York: Grune & Stratton, 1977–.
Volume 3, 1978.

National Institute on Drug Abuse Research Monograph Series. Vols. 1–. Washington, DC: US Government Printing Office, 1975–.
Volume 13, *Cocaine*, R. C. Peterson and R. C. Stillman, eds., 1977.
R: *Journal of Pharmaceutical Sciences* 68: 1074 (Aug. 1979).

Occupational Safety and Health Series. Nos. 1–. Geneva: International Labour Office, 196?–.
Number 38, 1977.
R: *IBID* 6: 194 (June 1978).

Progress in Chemical Toxicology. Vols. 1–. New York: Academic Press, 1963–.
Volume 5, 1974.
R: *Yale Journal of Biology and Medicine* 48: 461 (1975).

Progress in Toxicology. Vols. 1–. New York: Springer-Verlag, 1973–.
Volume 2, 1976.
R: *American Scientist* 62: 608 (Sept.–Oct. 1974); *BMJ* 2: 338 (May 11, 1974); *Journal of Pharmaceutical Sciences* 66: 760 (May 1977); Chen (p. 289).

Recent Advances in Studies of Alcoholism. Vols. 1–. **Nancy K. Mello and Jack Mendelson, eds.** Washington, DC: US Government Printing Office, 1972–.

Research Advances in Alcohol and Drug Problems. Vols. 1–. New York: John Wiley, 1974–.
Volume 4, 1978.

R: *American Journal of Psychiatry* 132: 212 (1975); *BMJ* 3: 693 (Sept. 14, 1979); *Pharmaceutical Journal* 214: 117 (1975).

Radiology

Advances in Cerebral Angiography: Anatomy, Stereotaxy, Embolization, Computerized Axial Tomography. Vols. 1–. Berlin: Springer-Verlag, 1976–.
R: *Brain* 100: 207 (Mar. 1977).

Advances in Radiation Biology. Vols. 1–. New York: Academic Press,1964–.
Volume 8, 1979.
R: *Health Physics* 28: 637 (May 1975); 32: 123 (Feb. 1977); Chen (p. 288).

Advances in Radiation Chemistry. Vols. 1–. Chichester, Sussex, England: John Wiley, 1969–.
Volume 5, 1976.
R: *American Scientist* 58: 677 (Nov./Dec. 1970); *Chemistry in Britain* (Oct. 1971); *Physics in Medicine & Biology* 20: 853 (Sept. 1975); Chen (p. 282); Wal (p. 127).

Advances in Radiation Research. Vols. 1–. London: Gordon & Breach, 1973–.
Biology & Medicine, 3 vols., 1973; *Physics & Chemistry*, 2 vols., 1973.
R: *Physics in Medicine & Biology* 19: 392 (May 1974).

Bibliotheca Radiologica. Vols. 1–. Basel: S. Karger, 1959–.

Current Concepts in Radiology. Vols. 1–. St. Louis, MO: C. V. Mosby, 1972–.
Volume 3, 1977.
R: *JAMA* 238: 2198 (Nov. 14, 1977); *Radiology* 118: 558 (1976).

Current Problems in Diagnostic Radiology. Vols. 1–. Chicago, IL: Year Book Medical Publishers, 1971–.
Volume 2, *Radiation Exposure in Pregnancy*, 1972. Series title was *Current Problems in Radiology*.
R: *Health Physics* 25: 203 (Aug. 1973).

Current Topics in Radiation Research. Vols. 1–. Amsterdam: North-Holland, 1970–.
Volume 10, 1976.
R: *British Journal of Radiology* 48: 69 (1975); *International Journal of Radiation Biology* 27: 410 (1975); *Radiology* 115: 672 (1975); 118: 452 (1976).

Recent Advances in Radiology. Nos. 5–. Edinburgh: Churchill Livingstone, 1975–. (With revision).
Number 6, 1978.
R: *British Journal of Radiology* 48: 795 (1975).

Recent Advances in Ultrasound in Biomedicine. Vols. 1–. Forest Grove, OR:

Research Studies Press, 1977–.
R: *Physics in Medicine & Biology* 23: 1215 (Nov. 1978).

Respiratory System

Advances in Tuberculosis Research. Vols. 1–. Basel: S. Karger, 1948–.
Volume 20, 1980

Progress in Respiration Research. Vols. 1–. New York: S. Karger, 1963–.
Volume 13, 1979.

Rheumatology

Recent Advances in Myology. Vols. 1–. Amsterdam: Excerpta Medica, 1975–.
R: *Brain* 99: 613 (Sept. 1976).

Recent Advances in Rheumatology. Vols. 1–. Edinburgh: Churchill Livingstone, 1976–.
R: *Archives of Pathology & Laboratory Medicine* 101: 506 (Sept. 1977); *Archives of Physical Medicine and Rehabilitation* 58: 141 (Mar. 1977); *BMJ* 1: 1473 (June 12, 1976); *Lancet* 2: 347 (Aug. 14, 1976).

Urogenital System

Advances in Nephrology from the Necker Hospital. Vols. 1–. Chicago, IL: Year Book Medical Publishers, 1971–.
Volume 8, 1979.
R: *Annals of Internal Medicine* 82: 731 (May 1975); 84: 378 (Mar. 1976); 91: 148 (July 1979); *Archives of Internal Medicine* 133: 157 (Jan. 1974).

Advances in Prostaglandin Research. Vols. 1–. Baltimore, MD: University Park Press, 1976–.
Volume 2, 1976.
R: *Annals of Internal Medicine* 87: 260 (Aug. 1977).

Advances in Sex Hormone Research. Vols. 1–. Baltimore, MD: University Park Press, 1975–.
Volume 3, 1977.
R: *Archives of Internal Medicine* 138: 313 (Feb. 1978); *Lahey Clinic Foundation Bulletin* 25: 97 (Apr.–June 1976).

Contributions to Gynecology and Obstetrics. Vols. 1–. New York: S. Karger, 1976–.
Volume 7, 1979.

Contributions to Nephrology. Vols. 1–. New York: S. Karger, 1974–.
Volume 21, 1980.
R: *Radiology* 126: 110 (1978).

Progress in Gynecology. Vols. 1–. New York: Grune & Stratton, 1946–.
Volume 6, 1975.
R: *BMJ* 1: 101 (Jan. 10, 1976).

VETERINARY MEDICINE

Advances in Veterinary Science and Comparative Medicine. Vols. 1–. New York: Academic Press, 1953–.
Volume 23, 1980.
Volumes 1–12 under title *Advances in Veterinary Science.*
R: *American Scientist* 61: 361 (May–June 1973).

Comparative Animal Nutrition. Vols. 1–. Basel: S. Karger, 1976–. Irregular.
Volume 3, *Nitrogen, Electrolytes, Water and Energy Metabolism,* 1979.

OTHER REVIEWS OF PROGRESS

Besides the series selected for this chapter, there are numerous journal and nonjournal publications that provide authoritative reviews of progress in a subject field. For nonjournal review publications, readers are specifically referred to chapters 14 and 15, Treatises and Monographs, respectively. The following is a sample list of journal publications, a few of which have already been included in the chapter on periodicals, chapter 17.

TOOLS TO MEDICAL REVIEWS

Bibliography of Medical Reviews, DHEW Pub. no. (NIH) 77-1239, etc. Vols. 1–. **US National Library of Medicine.** Washington, DC: US Government Printing Office, 1955–. Annual.
Since 1968, also published monthly as *Monthly Bibliography of Medical Reviews.*
A multivolume bibliography of medical review articles. Appears in each monthly issue of *Index Medicus,* beginning in 1965. Abstracts from journals whose title appear in *Index Medicus,* cumulated annually.
R: Win (EJ26; EJ36; EK56; EK57; 1EJ5).

Index to Scientific Reviews. Vols. 1–. Philadelphia: Institute for Scientific Information, 1975–. Semiannual.
An eclectic index to scientific review articles. Contains author listings and permuted title-subject indexes. Indexes some 2,400 journals.
R: *ARBA* (1976, p. 639); Chen (p. 326); Mal (3-47).

Monthly Bibliography of Medical Reviews. Vols. 1–. **National Library of Medicine.** Washington, DC: US Government Printing Office, 1968–. Monthly.
Includes same material found in monthly issues of *Index Medicus.* Ready reference guide to biomedical journal literature. Topics should be of interest to biologists as well as physicians. Author and subject indexes.
R: Win (EJ36; 3EJ8).

REVIEWS

AAAS Reviews of Science. Washington, DC: American Association for the Advancement of Science, 1976–.
A series of compendium volumes that includes authoritative articles originally published in *Science.* Publications deal with today's critical issues. Although with heavy emphasis on science, many volumes are pertinent to those who are in the fields of health sciences. For example. *Food: Politics, Economics, Nutrition, and Research.*
R: Chen (p. 297).

Bacteriological Reviews. 1937–. Quarterly.

CRC Critical Reviews in Biochemistry. 1971–. Quarterly.

CRC Critical Reviews in Bioengineering. 1971–. Quarterly.

CRC Critical Reviews in Clinical Laboratory Sciences. 1970–. Quarterly.

CRC Critical Reviews in Clinical Radiology. Vols. 9–. 1977–. Quarterly.
Continues *CRC Critical Reviews in Radiological Sciences,* vols. 1–3, 1970–1972; and *CRC Critical Reviews in Radiological Sciences and Nuclear Medicine,* vols. 4–8, 1973–1976.

CRC Critical Reviews in Diagnostic Imaging. 1970–. Quarterly.

CRC Critical Reviews in Microbiology. 1971–. Quarterly.

CRC Critical Reviews in Toxicology. 1971–. Quarterly.

International Nursing Review. 1926–. Six issues/year.

Nutrition Reviews. 1942–. Monthly.

Physiological Reviews. 1921–. Quarterly.

Quarterly Review of Biology. Vols. 1–. Stony Brook, NY: Stony Brook Foundation, 1962–.
Volume 55, 1980.
Each volume provides critical review articles on topics of current interest in the biological sciences. Addressed to both researchers and students.
R: Chen (p. 298).

Viewpoints in Biology. London: Butterworths, 1962–. Irregular.
R: Chen (p. 298).

CHAPTER 14   TREATISES

This chapter includes mostly the multivolume treatises, which differ from those publications included in Important Series (chapter 13) and Monographs (chapter 15). Volumes in a treatise generally are published in irregular and indeterminate intervals, and the materials covered in each volume are generally comprehensive in nature. On the other hand, important series generally are published in established intervals, and each volume tends to report the current development of the field since the last volume; monographs are generally in one or two volume(s) which are less comprehensive in nature than those of the treatises.

GENERAL

Comprehensive Biochemistry. 34 vols. **Marcel Florkin and Elmer H. Stotz, eds.** New York: Elsevier, 1962–1979.

A comprehensive monographic series, projected to be 34 volumes, which covers all aspects of modern biochemistry. Should be useful to every biomedical scientist.
R: *BMJ* 2: 102 (Oct. 10, 1970); *Nature* 258: 27 (Nov. 6, 1975); *Science* 140: 1201 (1963); *Scientific American* 220: 126 (Feb. 1969); Chen (p. 300); Mal (9-57).

Computers in Biomedical Research. Vol. 4. **Ralph W. Stacy and Bruce D. Waxman, eds.** New York: Academic Press, 1974.

Volume 1, 1965; volume 2, 1965; volume 3, 1969.
A multivolume set covering computer applications to biomedical research; each volume with a different concentration. Geared more toward medical researchers than computer technologists, this book is clearly presented. Well recommended.
R: *Lancet* 1: 453 (Feb. 28, 1970); Allyn.

FASEB Monographs. Vols. 1–. **Karl F. Heumann, ed.** Federation of American Societies for Experimental Biology. New York: Plenum, 1975–.

Volume 1, *The Science of Life: Contributions of Biology to Human Welfare*, K. D. Fisher and A. U. Nixon, eds., 1975; volume 2, *Computers in Life Science Research*, William Siler and Donald A. B. Lindberg, eds., 1975; volume 3, *Biology of Aging and Development*, Geertruida J. Thorbecke, ed., 1976; volume 4, *Behavioral Pharmacology: The Current Status*, Bernard Weiss, ed., 1976; volume 5, *Membranes, Ions, and Impulses*, John W. Moore, ed., 1976; volume 6, *Primate Research*, William J. Goodman and James Augustine, eds., 1976.
An authoritative series of monographs on numerous topics of experimental biology.

Forensic Medicine: A Study in Trauma and Environmental Hazards. 3 vols. **C. G. Tedeschi, William G. Eckert, and Luke G. Tedeschi, eds.** Philadelphia, PA: W. B. Saunders, 1977.

Volume 1, *Mechanical Trauma*; volume 2, *Physical Trauma*; volume 3, *Environmental Hazards*.
Presentation of aspects of medicine that have actual or potential legal implications. Encyclopedic approach with 91 contributing authors offering readers an

overall approach to almost every medical, legal, and biological topic that falls into field of forensic medicine. Fine bibliography contains wealth of information.
R: *Archives of Pathology & Laboratory Medicine* 102: 607 (Nov. 1978); *Journal of Clinical Pathology* 31: 1006 (Oct. 1978).

Frontiers of Biology. Vols. 1–. Amsterdam: North-Holland, 1966–.
Volume 46, *Cytochalasins, Biochemical and Cell Biological Aspects,* 1978.
R: *Archives of Environmental Health* 29: 179 (1974).

Inter-University Electronics Series. Vol. 10. **Manfred Clynes and John H. Milsum.** New York: McGraw-Hill, 1970.
Volume 10, *Biomedical Engineering Systems.*
An important reference on biomedical engineering arranged in four parts: instrumentation, analysis, control of information and energy, and artificial devices. Coverage is thorough; well written. Contains excellent illustrations.
R: *ARBA* (1971, p. 530).

The Proteins. 3d ed. 8 vols. **Hans Neurath and Robert L. Hill, eds.** New York: Academic Press, 1975–.

Eight-volume series written by a group of outstanding contributors in the biochemical field. Volumes 1 through 3 devoted to general biochemical topics currently popular in the laboratory. The remaining five volumes concentrate on specific proteins. Attempts to relate the physicochemical properties of proteins to their biologic function. Aimed at biochemists and scientists in related fields.
R: *NEJM* 294: 1351 (June 10, 1976).

ALLERGY AND IMMUNOLOGY

The Antigens. Vols. 1–. **M. Sela, ed.** New York: Academic Press, 1973–.
Volume 5, 1979.
Excels in visual presentation with illustrations, diagrams, and charts. Includes good index. Noteworthy reference work for those interested in the molecular aspects of immunology.
R: *NEJM* 291: 684 (Sept. 26, 1974).

Clinical Immunobiology. Vols. 1–. **Fritz H. Bach and R. A. Good, eds,** New York: Academic Press, 1972–. Irregular.
Volume 3, 1976.
Clinically oriented essays on immunobiology. Valuable to clinicians and allergists.
R: *American Scientist* 61: 361 (May/June 1973); *Annals of Allergy* 38: 428 (1977).

Comprehensive Immunology. Vols. 1–. **Robert A. Good and Stacy B. Day, eds.** New York: Plenum, 1977–.

Volume 1, *Immunology and Aging,* 1977; volume 2, *Biological Amplification Systems in Immunology,* 1977; volume 3, *Immunopharmacology,* 1977; volume 4, *The Immunopathology of Lymphoreticular Neoplasms,* 1978; volume 5, *Immunoglobulins,* 1978; volume 6, *Cellular, Molecular, and Clinical Aspects of Allergic Disorders,* 1979.
R: *Annals of Internal Medicine* 91: 144 (July 1979); *Nature* 272: 194 (Mar. 9, 1978); 279: 172 (May 10, 1979).

Current Topics in Immunology. London: Edward Arnold, 1975–.
Number 1, *The Practice of Clinical Immunology*, 1975; number 2, *Cancer and the Immune Response*; number 3, *Blood Group Topics*; number 4, *Organ Grafts*; number 5, *Allergic Drug Reactions*; number 6, *Immunodeficiency*; number 7, *Immunology of the Rheumatic Diseases: Aspects of Autoimmunity*; number 8, *Immunology of Gastrointestinal and Liver Disease*; number 9, *HLA and H-L Basic Immunogenetics, Biology and Clinical Relevance*; number 10, *Immunology of the Lung*; number 11, *Immunopathology of the Kidney*, 1979.
R: *British Journal of Radiology* 48: 516 (1975); *British Medical Bulletin* 32: 291 (1976); *BMJ* 1: 427 (Aug. 14, 1976); 1: 499 (Feb. 25, 1978); 1: 334 (1979); 1: 1010 (Apr. 14, 1979); 1: 1418 (May 26, 1979); *Journal of Clinical Pathology* 32: 638 (June 1979); *Lancet* 1: 478 (Mar. 4, 1978); 1: 248 (Feb. 3, 1979).

Immunological Aspects of Allergy and Allergic Diseases. 8 vols. **E. Rajka and S. Korossy, eds.** New York: Plenum, 1974–1976.
Volume 1, *Basic Concepts in Experimental Immunology*, 1974; volume 2, *Methods in Experimental Immunology*, 1974; volume 3, *Clinical Aspects of Autoimmune Diseases*, 1976; volume 4, *Clinical Aspects of Immune Pathology*, 1976; volume 5, *Clinical Aspects of Allergic Diseases*, 1976; volume 6, *Antigen-Antibody Reactions in Different Organs*, 1976; volume 7, *Allergic Diseases of the Skin*, 1976; volume 8, *Allergic Responses to Infectious Agents*, 1976.

Immunological Diseases. 3d ed. 2 vols. **Max Samter, ed.** Boston, MA: Little, Brown, 1978.
Second edition, 1971.
Comprehensive and up-to-date reference on science of immunology and its clinical application. Completely revised edition reflects new knowledge of clinical aspects of disease and pathology and physiology of immunological response. Two volumes are well illustrated and referenced. Important for physicians and others interested in patients whose diseases are related to allergy or are in realm of clinical immunology.
R: *American Journal of Diseases of Children* 125: 298 (Feb. 1973); Allyn; Stearns & Ratcliff (*NEJM*, 1969; *NEJM*, 1970).

Immunological Reviews. Vols. 1–. Copenhagen: Munksgaard, 1969–. 4 issues/year.
Volume 46, 1979.
Formerly entitled *Transplantation Reviews.*

Monographs in Allergy. Vols. 1–. **P. Duker et al., eds.** Basel: S. Karger, 1966–.
Volume 16, 1979.

ANATOMY

Handbook of Physiology. Sections 1–. **American Physiological Society.** Baltimore, MD: Williams & Wilkins, 1962–. Second edition of some sections, 1977–.
Section 1, *The Nervous System* (Formerly *Neurophysiology*), 2 vols., 1977; section 2,

Circulation, 3 vols., 1979; section 3, *Respiration*, 2 vols., 1964–1965; section 4, *Adaptation to the Environment*, 1964; section 5, *Adipose Tissue*, 1965; section 6, *The Alimentary Canal*, 5 vols., 1967–1968; section 7, *Endocrinology*, 7 vols., 1972; section 8, *Renal Physiology*, 1973; section 9, *Reactions to Environmental Agents*, 1977. A multisection, multivolume treatise on the physiology of the nervous system, covering a broad range of topics comprehensively. Recommended especially for medical libraries.
R: *American Journal of Psychology* 135: 886 (July 1978); *American Scientist* 66: 628 (Sept.–Oct. 1978); *Annals of Internal Medicine* 81: 421 (1974); *Archives of Internal Medicine* 136: 375 (Mar. 1976); *Archives of Physical Medicine & Rehabilitation* 59: 348 (July 1978); *Brain* 102: 228 (Mar. 1979); *Journal of Neurosurgery* 48: 1050 (June 1978); *NEJM* 291: 1201 (Nov. 28, 1974); 293: 1375 (Dec. 25, 1975).

Physiology, Series One. 16 vols. **A. C. Guyton, ed.** Baltimore, MD: University Park Press, 1978.

Supersedes *International Review of Physiology.*
R: *Lancet* 1: 1134 (May 27, 1978).

ANESTHESIOLOGY AND GENERAL SURGERY

Operative Surgery: Fundamental International Techniques, Colon, Rectum and Anus. 3d ed. **Ian P. Todd.** Toronto: Butterworths, 1977.

Treatise on operative techniques of common problems in the colon, rectum, and anus. Lists contributions from eminent international surgeons; retains a British emphasis. Consists of nine broad sections from endoscopy to operations for diverticular diseases. Some techniques are controversial; others little used. Format of test is unusual. Material arranged in small blocks instead of whole pages. Side-by-side arrangement of text and illustrations (line drawings and black-and-white sketches) simplifies use. Contains short, pertinent references and a comprehensive index. Invaluable reference source for surgeons involved in colon, rectum, and anus operations.
R: *JAMA* 238: 1767 (Oct. 17, 1977).

Plastic and Reconstructive Surgery of the Breast. **Robert M. Goldwyn, ed.** Boston, MA: Little, Brown, 1976.

Definitive treatise on all aspects of plastic surgery of the breast. Outlines the anatomy, pathology, physiology, endocrinology, and radiology of the breast. Written by more than 50 contributing authors. Each chapter ends with a useful commentary. Illustrations present a slight weakness. Truly a classic, which belongs in the library of every plastic surgeon and medical institution.
R: *Archives of Surgery* 111: 1311 (Nov. 1976); *Plastic and Reconstructive Surgery* 59: 272 (1977).

Reconstruction Surgery and Traumatology. Vol. 16. **G. Luzern Chapchal, ed.** Basel: S. Karger, 1978.

This richly illustrated series offers a record of where international research in reconstruction surgery and traumatology is heading. Volumes creatively discuss vital problems so as to open new approaches to their solution. An emphasis on the practical value of material underlies the selection of articles in each volume.

BRAIN AND NERVOUS SYSTEM

The Central Nervous System of Vertebrates. 5 vols. **Hartwig Kuhlenbeck.** Basel: S. Karger, 1967-1978.

Volume 1, *Propaedeutics to Comparative Neurology,* 1967; volume 2, *Invertebrates and Origin of Vertebrates,* 1967; volume 3/Part I, *Structural Elements: Biology of Nervous Tissue,* 1970; volume 3/Part II, *Overall Morphologic Pattern,* 1973; volume 4, *Spinal Cord and Deuterencephalon,* 1975; volume 5/Part I, *Derivatives of the Prosencephalon: Diencephalon and Telencephalon,* 1977; volume 5/Part II, *Mammalian Telencephalon: Surface Morphology and Cerebral Cortex—The Vertebrate Neuroaxis as a Whole,* 1978. Subject and author indexes to volumes 1-5.

Clinical Neurology. 2d ed. 4 vols. **A. B. Baker, ed.** New York: Hoeber-Harper, 1962.

Encyclopedic, multi-authored volume of clinical neurology. Covers both rare and common syndromes, anatomy, physiology, pathology, biochemistry of the nervous system. Includes diagrams, references. A standard work, recommended to physicians, students, medical libraries.
R: Allyn.

Clinical Neurosurgery. Vol. 21. **Robert H. Wilkins et al.** Baltimore, MD: Williams & Wilkins, 1974.

Volume 20, 1973.
Deals with disorders of the spine. Provides a wide range of information. A good reference source for all physicians.
R: *JAMA* 227: 1308 (Mar. 18, 1974); 232: 75 (Apr. 7, 1975); *TBRI* 40: 288 (Sept. 1974).

Contemporary Neurology Series. Vols. 1–. Philadelphia, PA: F. A. Davis, 1971–.

Volume 1, *The Diagnosis of Stupor and Coma;* volume 2, *Epilepsy;* volume 3, *Special Techniques for Neurologic Diagnosis;* volumes 4 and 5, *Applied Neurochemistry;* volume 6, *Recent Advances in Neurology;* volume 7, *The Wernicke-Korsakoff Syndrome: A Clinical and Pathological Study of 245 Patients, 82 With Post Mortem Examinations;* volume 8, *Recent Advances in Parkinson's Disease;* volume 9, *Dementia;* volume 10, *The Diagnosis of Stupor and Coma;* volume 11, *Disorders of the Autonomic Nervous System;* volume 12, *Topics in Tropical Neurology;* volume 13, *Legal Aspects of Neurologic Practice;* volume 14, *Clinical Neuroendocrinology;* volume 15, *Dementia;* volume 16, *Pediatric Neurosurgery;* volume 17, *Mental Retardation and Related Disorders;* volume 18, *Clinical Neurophysiology of the Vestibular System;* volume 20, *Management of Head Injuries,* 1978.
R: *Archives of Internal Medicine* 131: 473 (Mar. 1973); *Journal of Neurosurgery* 41: 270 (Aug. 1974).

Functions of the Nervous System. 4 vols. **Marcel Monnier.** New York: American Elsevier, 1968-1975.

Volume 1, *General Physiology, Autonomic Functions,* 1968; volume 2, *Motor and Psychomotor Functions,* 1968; volume 3, *Sensory Functions and Perceptions,* 1975; volume 4, *Psychic Functions,* 1975.

Encyclopedic treatment of nervous system in four volumes with each covering a major category.

Major Problems in Neurology. Vols. 1–. Philadelphia, PA: W. B. Saunders, 1973–.

Volume 1, *Syringomyelia,* H. J. M. Barnett, ed., 1973; volume 2, *Muscle Biopsy: A Modern Approach,* 1973; volume 3, *The Neurology of Gastrointestinal Disease,* C. A. Pallis, 1974; volume 4, *Strokes: Natural History, Pathology and Surgical Treatment,* E. C. Hutchinson and E. J. Acheson, 1975; volume 5, *The Clumsy Child: A Study of Developmental Apraxic & Agnosic Ataxia,* G. Sasson, 1975; volume 6, *Pituitary & Parapituitary Tumors,* J. Hankinson, 1976; volume 7, *Neurology of Pregnancy,* J. O. Donaldson, 1978; volume 8, *Clinical Neuroimmunology,* P. O. Behan, 1978.
R: *Brain* 98: 528 (Sept. 1975); *BMJ* 4: 108 (Oct. 11, 1975).

Neurosciences Research. Vols. 1–5. New York: Academic Press, 1968–1973.
Volume 5, *Chemical Approaches to Brain Function.*

Pathology of the Nervous System. Vol. 3. **Jeff Minckler, ed.** New York: McGraw-Hill, 1972.

Encyclopedic coverage of neuropathology in English. Three volumes represent the efforts of 163 authorities from 23 countries. Emphasizes the structural aspects of nervous system disorders. Volume I deals with molecular pathobiological aspects; volume II emphasizes neuropathological disorders in accordance with standard classifications of disease entities; and volume III covers inflammatory diseases and special topics. Stresses comparative neuropathology in each volume. A comprehensive index and table of centents found in volume III. Geared toward researchers, students, and house officers in the field.
R: *American Scientist* 61: 594 (Sept.–Oct. 1973); *ARBA* (1973, p. 604).

Pathology of Tumours of the Nervous System. 4th ed. **Dorothy S. Russell and Lucien J. Rubinstein.** Baltimore, MD: Williams & Wilkins, 1977.
First edition, 1959; third edition, 1971.
Outstanding and authoritative treatise on tumors of the nervous system. Fourth edition features extensive revisions, considerable amounts of new data, and high-quality electron micrographs. Presents extensive new sections on the pathogenesis of brain tumors and experimental tumor production. Illustrations (electron micrographs) are numerous and excellent. References are thoroughly updated. Essential reference tool for neuropathologists, pathologists, neurosurgeons, and neurologists.
R: *Archives of Pathology & Laboratory Medicine* 102: 215 (Apr. 1978); *NEJM* 298: 1368 (June 15, 1978).

Slow Transmissible Diseases of the Nervous System. 2 vols. **Stanley B. Prusiner and William J. Hadlow, eds.** New York: Academic Press, 1979.
Proceedings of an International Symposium held at the Rocky Mountain Laboratory, Hamilton, Montana, in October 1978.

Studies of Brain Function. Vols. 1–. New York: Springer-Verlag, 1977–.

Volume 1, *Principles of Electrolocation and Jamming,* 1977; volume 2, *Neuronal Operations in the Vestibular System,* 1978.
A monograph series in neurobiology. The area covered extends from the sensory to the effector neuron, with methods ranging from those of basic science to those of clinical observation.

Topics on Tropical Neurology. Vol. 1. **R. W. Hornabrook, ed.** Philadelphia, PA: F. A. Davis, 1975.
A systematic summary of tropical neurology; papers discuss infections, metabolic disorders, degenerative diseases, dangers of tropical animals. Well illustrated and referenced. Recommended for all scientists.
R: *Brain* 99: 606 (Sept. 1976); *Neurology* 26: 701 (July 1976).

CARDIOVASCULAR SYSTEM

Cardiovascular Clinics Series. Vols. 1–. Philadelphia, PA: F. A Davis, 1968–.
Volumes 1–6, 1968–1975; volume 10, no. 1, *Congenital Heart Disease in Adults,* 1978.
A series on diagnosis and management of cardiac disorders; extensive coverage with contributions from authorities in their field.
R: Allyn.

Circulatory Physiology. 2d ed. 2 vols. **Arthur C. Guyton et al.** Philadelphia, PA: W. B. Saunders, 1973–1975.
Volume 1, *Cardiac Output and Its Regulation,* 1973; volume 2, *Dynamics and Control of the Body Fluids,* 1975.
Outlines research advances in cardiac physiology. Provides a basic understanding of cardiac problems; considered a principle reference on the subject for its in-depth coverage and concise presentation. Indexed, well referenced.
R: *Annals of Internal Medicine* 84: 627 (May 1976); Allyn.

Congenital Malformations of the Heart. 2d ed. 2 vols. **Helen B. Taussig.** Cambridge, MA: Harvard University Press, 1961.
Volume 1, *General Considerations,* 1960; volume 2, *Specific Malformations,* 1961.
Two volumes which deal with congenital heart malformations. Volume 1: a comprehensive introduction to diagnosis; volume 2: diagnostic materials. Complementary, informative volumes on cardiac malformations.

DENTISTRY

Enfermedades de la Boca: Semiologia, Patologia, Clinica y Terapeutica de la Mucosa Bucal. Vol. 3. **Julio Diaz et al.** Buenos Aires: Editorial Mundi, 1976.
Third volume of an encyclopedic treatise on diseases of the mouth. Eight chapters filled with charts and clinical photographs. Includes bibliographies. Valuable for dentists, oral pathologists, and dermatologists.
R: *Archives of Dermatology* 113: 860 (June 1977).

Frontiers of Oral Physiology. Vols. 1–. **Y. Kawamura, ed.** Basel: S. Karger, 1974–.

Volume 1, *Physiology of Mastication,* 1974; volume 2, *Physiology of Oral Tissues,* 1976.
Up-to-date reference tool for graduate students in any dental specialty.
R: *Journal of Oral Pathology*; *Journal of the American Dental Association.*

Monographs in Oral Science. Vols. 1–. Basel: S. Karger. 1972–.

Volume 1, *The Marmoset Periodontium in Health and Disease,* 1972; volume 2, *Saliva: Composition and Secretion,* 1974; volume 3, *The Crevicular Fluid,* 1974; volume 4, *The Tempo-romandibular Joint Syndrome,* out of print; volume 5, *Analysis of Human Mandibular Movement,* 1975; volume 6, *Phosphates and Dental Caries,* 1977; volume 7, *Fluorides and Dental Fluorosis,* 1978; volume 8, *The Biology of Pulp and Dentine,* 1979.
Classic monographic series covering dental medicine from oral physiology to the latest data on fluorides.
R: *British Dental Journal*; *Journal of Dentistry*; *Journal of Experimental Physiology*; *Journal of the American Dental Association*; *Laboratory Animal Science.*

DERMATOLOGY

Clinical Dermatology. 2d ed. 4 vols. **D. Joseph Demis et al.** New York: Harper & Row, 1974.

A comprehensive, systematic review of dermatology. Well referenced and indexed. Consists of five volumes which deal with classification, diagnosis, treatment of skin diseases. Well recommended for medical libraries.
R: *JAMA* 232: 404 (Apr. 28, 1975); *TBRI* 41: 266 (Sept. 1975).

Dermatology. 2d ed. 2 vols. **Samuel L. Moschella, Donald M. Pillsbury, and Harry J. Hurley, Jr.** Philadelphia, PA: W. B. Saunders, 1975.

First edition, 1956.
Considered a successor to the classic Pillsbury *Dermatology.* Extensively covers clinical matters in dermatology, such as metabolic disease, immunology, drug reactions. Contains over 1,000 black-and-white photographs, helpful tables, numerous references, and index. Well recommended for medical and dermatologic libraries.
R: *JAMA* 237: 277 (Jan. 17, 1977).

Major Problems in Dermatology. Vols. 1–. Philadelphia, PA: W. B. Saunders, 1974–.

Volume 1, *Urticaria,* by Robert P. Warin and R. H. Champion, 1974; volume 2, *Microbiology of Human Skin,* by W. C. Noble and Dorothy A. Somerville, 1974; volume 3, *Atopic Dermatitis,* by Georg Rajka, 1975; volume 4, *Dermatitis Herpetiformis,* by John O. Alexander, 1975; volume 5, *The Vulva,* by Constance M. Ridley, 1975; volume 6, *The Acnes: Clinical Features, Pathogenesis and Treatment,* by W. J. Cunliffe, 1975; volume 7, *Microvascular Injury: Vasculitis, Stasis & Ischaemia,* by T. J. Ryan, 1976; volume 8, *Psychophysiological Aspects of Skin Disease,* by Francis A. Whitlock, 1976.
R: *Annals of Internal Medicine* 83: 593 (Oct. 1975); *BMJ* 3: 634 (Sept. 7, 1974).

ENDOCRINOLOGY

Comprehensive Endocrinology. Vols. 1–. New York: Raven Press, 1979–.
Volume 1, *Endocrine Rhythms,* Dorothy T. Krieger, ed., 1979.
R: *Lancet* 2: 395 (Aug. 25, 1979).

The Enzymes. 3d ed. **Paul Boyer, ed.** New York: Academic Press, 1970–1976.
Volume 1, *Enzyme Structure-Control,* 1970; volume 2, *Kinetics-Mechanism,* 1970; volume 3, *Peptide Bond Hydrolysis,* 1971; volume 4, *Hydrolysis-Other C-N Bonds Phosphate Esters,* 1971; volume 5, *Hydrolysis-Sulfate Esters, Carboxyl Esters, Glycosides, Hydration,* 1971; volume 6, *Carboxylation and Decarboxylation (Nonoxidative) Isomerization,* 1972; volume 7, *Elimination and Addition, Aldol Cleavage and Condensation, Other C-C Cleavage, Phosphorolysis, Hydrolysis (Fats, Glycosides),* 1972; volume 8, *Group Transfer, Part A.,* 1973; volume 9, *Group Transfer, Part B.,* 1973; volume 10, *Protein Synthesis, DNA Synthesis and Repair, RNA Synthesis, Energy-Linked Atpases, Synthetases,* 1974; volume 11, *Oxidation-Reduction, Part A.,* 1975; volume 12, *Oxidation-Reduction, Part B.,* 1976; volume 13, *Oxidation-Reduction, Part C.,* 1976.

Hormones In Blood. 3d ed. 3 vols. **G. H. Gray and V. H. T. James.** New York: Academic Press, 1979–1980.
Considered the definitive work on endocrinology. Incorporates recent advances in the field written by international authorities.

Methods in Enzymology: a Multivolume Work. **Sidney P. Colowick and Nathan O. Kaplan, eds.** New York: Academic Press, 1955–.
Volume 68, 1980.
A multivolume, comprehensive treatise on the topic. Each volume has its own editor(s). It is intended for researchers in the field.

Monographs on Endocrinology. Vols. 1–. New York: Springer, 1967–.
Volume 12, 1979.

GASTROINTESTINAL SYSTEM

Colon, Rectum and Anus. 3d ed. **Ian P. Todd.** London: Butterworths, 1977.
An outstanding treatise with a practical approach to the operative treatment of proctological problems. Extensively indexed. A high-quality reference for surgeons.
R: *JAMA* 238: 1767 (Oct. 17, 1977).

GENETICS

Birth Defects: Original Article Series. Vols. 1–. **National Foundation-March of Dimes.** New York: Alan R. Liss, 1965–.

Volume 13, *Trends and Teaching in Clinical Genetics,* D. Bergsma et al., eds., 1977; volume 14, no. 3, *The Genetics of Hand Malformations,* by S. A. Temtamy and V. A. McKusick, 1978; volume 14, no. 6B, *Sex Differentiation and Chromosomal Ab-*

normalities, R. L. Summitt and D. Bergsma, eds., 1978.
R: *American Journal of Human Genetics* 31: 90 (Jan. 1979); 31: 391 (May 1979); *Yale Journal of Biology & Medicine* 52: 240 (Mar./Apr. 1979).

Chemical Mutagens. Vols. 1–. **A. Hollaender, ed.** New York: Plenum, 1973–.
Focuses on drug reactions from the special toxic mechanisms perspective. Written as a descriptive text.
R: *Clinical Pharmacology and Therapeutics* 15: 227 (1974).

Chromosome Techniques: Theory and Practice. 2d ed. **A. K. Sharma and A. Sharma.** Baltimore, MD: University Park Press, 1972.
First edition, 1965.
Comprehensive treatise on technological aspects of chromosome study. New edition incorporates recent advances in chromosome methodology. Numerous references and twenty full-page plates are included.
R: *American Journal of Human Genetics* 25: 460 (July 1973).

Human Cytogenetics. 2 vols. **John L. Hamerton.** New York: Academic Press, 1971.
Volume 1, *General Cytogenetics*; volume 2, *Clinical Cytogenetics*.
A two-volume treatise on general and clinical cytogenetics; deals with techniques in chromosomal research, aberrations, genetic counseling-related issues. A thorough reference source. Includes excellent bibliography, index, and illustrations.
R: *Annals of Human Genetics* 36: 363 (Jan. 1973); Allyn.

Monographs in Human Genetics. Vols. 1–. New York: S. Karger, 1966–.
Volume 7, *The HLA System*, 2d ed., 1979.
Up-to-date discussion of lymphocyte antigens of man. Over 200 references and an appendix enhance this concise monograph.
R: *BMJ* 1: 947 (Oct. 16, 1976).

GERONTOLOGY

Aging. Vols. 1–. New York: Raven Press, 1975–.
Volume 10, 1979.

HEMATOLOGY

Structure and Function of the Circulation. 3 vols. New York: Plenum, 1980–.
Comprehensive source book for cardiologists, hematologists, and physiologists.

INFECTIOUS DISEASES

Comprehensive Virology. Vols. 1–. **Heinz Fraenkel-Conrat and Robert R. Wagner, eds.** New York: Plenum, 1974–.
Volume 1, *Descriptive Catalogue of Viruses*, 1974; volume 2, *Reproduction: Small and Intermediate RNA Viruses*, 1974; volume 3, *Reproduction: DNA Animal Viruses*, 1974; volume 4, *Reproduction: Large RNA Viruses*, 1975; volume 5, *Structure and Assembly Virions, Pseudovirions, and Intraviral Nucleic Acids*, 1975; volume 6, *Reproduction:*

Small RNA Viruses, 1976; volume 7, *Reproduction: Bacterial DNA Viruses,* 1977; volume 8, *Regulation and Genetics: Bacterial DNA Viruses,* 1977; volume 9, *Regulation and Genetics: Genetics of Animal Viruses,* 1977; volume 10, *Regulation and Genetics: Viral Gene Expression and Integration,* 1977; volume 11, *Regulation and Genetics: Plant Viruses,* 1977; volume 12, *Newly Characterized Protist and Invertebrate Viruses,* 1978.
Interdisciplinary treatise. First encyclopedic analysis of current information in animal, plant, and bacterial virology. Intended to have about 25 volumes.
R: *Nature* 266: xvi (Apr. 28, 1977); *Science* 189: 989 (Sept. 19, 1975).

Flies and Disease. 2 vols. **Bernard Greenberg.** Princeton, NJ: Princeton University Press, 1971–1973.
Volume 1, *Ecology, Classification and Biotic Associations,* 1971; volume 2, *Biology and Disease Transmission,* 1973.
Two volumes present a comprehensive coverage of the literature on this insect. Well written and organized. Includes fine illustrations and useful references. Provides detailed technical information on the role of flies in disease. Valuable addition to the libraries of epidemiologists, medical entomologists, parasitologists, and microbiologists.
R: *Journal of Parasitology* 61: 94 (Feb. 1975); *Choice* 8: 532 (June 1971); *LJ* 96: 1961 (June 1, 1971); *ARBA* (1972, p. 633).

Principles and Practice of Infectious Diseases. 2 vols. **G. L. Mandell et al.** New York: John Wiley, 1979.
Covers clinical syndromes and their etiologic agents. Addresses new advances in hepatitis, viral gastroenteritis, Legionnaire's Disease, viruses and antiviral therapy and new antibiotics. The 261 state of the-art chapters reflect the work of some 170 specialists. Includes thousands of current literature references. Many color illustrations complement the text.

NURSING

Monitoring Quality of Nursing Care. **US Department of Health, Education, and Welfare. Bureau of Manpower. Division of Nursing.** Washington, DC: US Government Printing Office, 1976–.
Part 3, *Professional Review for Nursing: An Empirical Investigation,* 1978.
A series of publications which investigate the quality of nursing care in this country.

Nurse Planning Information Series. Hyattsville, MD: US Public Health Service, Health Resources Administration, Division of Nursing. 1977–.
The series is composed of selected monographs and bibliographies related to health planning. Sample titles are *Accountability: Its Meaning and Its Relevance to the Health Care Field,* 1977, and *Nursing Involvement in the Health Planning Process,* 1978.

Nursing Education Monographs. Vols. 1–. **Department for Nursing Education.** New York: Columbia University, Teachers College, 1962–.
Series includes the following: *Evaluation of Student Progress in Learning the Practice*

of Nursing, 1965; *Learning Needs of Registered Nurses,* 1967; *Asepsis: A Programmed Unit for Nurses,* 3d rev. ed. 1979.

Penguin Library of Nursing. 7 vols. Edinburgh: Churchill Livingstone, 1977.

Volume 1, *The Cardiovascular System,* by P. P. Turner; volume 2, *The Digestive System,* by R. J. Ryall; volume 3, *The Endocrine System,* by J. G. Lewis; volume 4, *The Neuromuscular System,* by R. S. Kocen; volume 5, *The Respiratory System,* by R. Grenville-Mathers; volume 6, *The Urological System,* by C. A. C. Charlton; volume 7, *The Special Senses,* by T. A. Casey and H. N. Waller.

Springer Series on the Teaching of Nursing. Vol. 1. New York: Springer Publishing, 1977–.
Volume 5, 1979.
Provides timely monographs of interest to nurse educators.

Study of Nursing Care: Research Project Series. Series 2. London: Royal College of Nursing and National Council of Nurses of the United Kingdom, 1973–.
Number 3, *Physiological Measures of Anxiety in Hospital Patients,* by Anne Munday, 1973.
R: *Nursing Research* 24: 65 (Jan.–Feb. 1975).

NUTRITION

Current Concepts in Nutrition. **Myron Winick, ed.** New York: John Wiley, 1972–.

Volume 4, *Nutrition and Aging,* 1976; volume 6, *Nutrition and Cancer,* 1977; volume 7, *Hunger Disease: Studies by the Jewish Physicians in the Warsaw Ghetto,* 1979; volume 8, *Nutritional Management of Genetic Disorders,* 1979.
Reviews current status of knowledge on nutrition and cancer. Covers experimental work, epidemiological evidence, and relation of food additives to cancer. For library collections in nutrition, medical science, and biology.
R: *Journal of the American Dietetic Association* 69: 348 (Sept. 1976); *Lancet* 1: 908 (Apr. 27, 1979); *Choice* 15: 576 (June 1978).

Food Science Series. Vols. 1–. New York: Marcel Dekker, 1971–.

Volume 1, *Flavor Research: Principles & Techniques,* R. Teranishi et al., eds., 1971; volume 2, *Principles of Enzymology for the Food Science,* by J. R. Whitaker, 4th printing, 1972; volume 3, *Low-Temperature Preservation of Foods and Living Matter,* Owen R. Fennema et al., eds., 1973; volume 4, *Principles of Food Science,* part I, *Food Chemistry,* Owen R. Fennema, ed., 3d printing, 1976; part II, *Physical Methods of Food Preservation,* 1975; part III, *Food Fermentations,* in preparation; volume 5, *Food Emulsions,* Stig Friberg, 1976.
A valuable multi-authored series. Designed for students of food science; presupposes a background in organic chemistry and biochemistry. Useful for all health workers and researchers in the field of nutrition and food metabolism.
R: *American Journal of Digestive Diseases* 22: 395 (Apr. 1977).

Human Nutrition: A Comprehensive Treatise. **Robert E. Hodges, ed.** New York: Plenum, 1979.

Volume 4, *Nutrition in Infectious and Metabolic Diseases,* 1979; volume 3A, *Nutrition and the Adult: Macronutrients,* 1980; volume 3B, *Nutrition and the Adult: Micronutrients,* 1980.

This series authoritatively examines the present state of knowledge concerning human nutrition and its relation to all aspects of health and disease, covering both basic research and field applications.

Nutrition: A Comprehensive Treatise. 3 vols. **George H. Beaton and Earle W. McHenry, eds.** New York: Academic Press, 1964–1966.

Volume 1, *Macronutrients and Nutrient Elements,* 1964; volume 2, *Vitamins, Nutrient Requirements and Food Selections,* 1964; volume 3, *Nutritional Status: Assessment and Application,* 1966.

Nutrition Intervention in Developing Countries. 8 vols. **Harvard Institute for International Development.** Boston, MA: G. K. Hall, 1980–.

Volume 1, *Overview,* James E. Austin and Marian Zeitlin, ed.; volume 2, *Supplementary Feeding,* Mary Ann Anderson et al., eds.; volume 3, *Nutrition Education,* Marian Zeitlin and Candelaria Formacion, eds.; volume 4, *Formulated Foods,* Jerianne Heimendinger, Marian Zeitlin, and James E. Austin, eds.; volume 5, *Fortification,* James E. Austin et al., eds.; volume 6, *Consumer Price Subsidies,* Beatrice Rogers et al., eds.; volume 7, *Agricultural Productivity,* Richard Goldman and Catherine Overholt, eds.; volume 8, *Integrated Nutrition and Primary Health Care Programs,* James E. Austin et al., eds.

A comprehensive view of the nature and potential of nutrition programs currently functioning in the Third World. Based on a review of published and unpublished studies, interviews with nutrition professionals, field analysis of individual projects, and a mail survey covering some 200 programs in 66 countries. Indispensable to nutrition planners, administrators, researchers, and scholars.

World Food and Nutrition Study. **Committee on International Relations, National Research Council.** Washington, DC: National Academy of Sciences.

Enhancement of Food Production for the United States, 1975.
Interim Report, 1975.
The Potential Contributions of Research, 1977.
Supporting Papers, 5 vols. 1977.

ONCOLOGY AND NUCLEAR MEDICINE

Cancer: A Comprehensive Treatise. 6 vols. **Frederick F. Becker, ed.** New York: Plenum, 1975–1977.

Volume 1, *Etiology: Chemical and Physical Carcinogenesis,* 1975; volume 2, *Etiology: Viral Carcinogenesis,* 1975; volume 3, *Biology of Tumors: Cellular Biology and Growth,* 1975; volume 4, *Biology of Tumors: Surfaces, Immunology, and Comparative Pathology,* 1975; volume 5, *Chemotherapy,* 1977; volume 6, *Radiotherapy, Surgery, and Immunotherapy,* 1977.

Multivolume set which is a systematic presentation of cancer, including etiology, biology, and therapeutics. Valuable to students, clinicians, and basic investigators.
R: *American Scientist* 64: 454 (July–Aug. 1976); *Lancet* 2: 1162 (Dec. 3, 1977); *NEJM* 295: 1485 (Dec. 23, 1976); 295: 1486 (Dec. 23, 1976); *ABL* 43: entry 105 (Feb. 1978); Allyn.

Frontiers of Radiation Therapy and Oncology. Vols. 1–. **J. M. Vaeth, ed.** Basel: S. Karger, 1965–. Irregular.

Volume 14, *Body Image, Self-Esteem, and Sexuality in Cancer Patients*, 1979 (14th Annual San Francisco Cancer Symposium, Mar. 1979).
R: *American Journal of Roentgenology* 133: 576 (Sept. 1979).

Methods in Cancer Research. Vols. 1–. **Harris Busch, ed.** New York: Academic Press, 1967–.

Volumes 1–3. 1977; volume 4, 1968; volume 5, 1970; volume 6, 1971; volumes 7–10, 1973; volume 11, 1975; volumes 12–13, 1976; volumes 14–15, 1978; volume 16A, *Cancer Drug Development*; volume 17B, *Cancer Drug Development*; volume 18, *Oncodevelopmental Antigens*, 1979.
R: *Archives of Pathology & Laboratory Medicine* 103: 547 (Sept. 1979); *Journal of Clinical Pathology* 32: 636 (June 1979).

National Cancer Institute Monograph. Vols. 1–. **National Cancer Institute.** Washington, DC: US Government Printing Office, 1959–.

Volume 48, *Cell, Tissue and Organ Culture*, Katherine K. Sanford, ed., 1978 (Third Decennial Review Conference, Lake Placid, Sept. 1978); volume 49, 1979. An important series on numerous topics related to cancer.
R: *British Journal of Haematology* 26: 511 (1975); *Journal of Neurosurgery* 51: 130 (July 1979).

OPHTHALMOLOGY

Clinical Ophthalmology. 5 vols. **Thomas Duane, ed.** Philadelphia, PA: Harper & Row, 1976.

A five-volume, loose-leaf format work which covers the field of ophthalmology. Multi-authored, with contributions by outstanding physicians. Contains thousands of illustrations, separately bound index. Subjects covered in volumes are ocular motility, neuro-ophthalmology, retina and glaucoma, external diseases, and systematic ophthalmology.
R: *American Journal of Ophthalmology* 84: 132 (July 1977).

The Eye. 2d ed. 6 vols. **Hugh Davson, ed.** New York: Academic Press, 1969–1977.

Volume 2A, *Visual Function in Man*, 1976; first edition, 1962.
Part of a multivolume treatise written by authorities in the field of visual function. In three parts: human vision, retina-neurophysiology, and color vision. Up-to-date, lucidly written text; includes extensive list of references. Highly recommended to students and researchers in ophthalmology.
R: *American Journal of Ophthalmology* 82: 946 (Dec. 1976); *BMJ* 1: 649 (Sept. 11, 1976).

System of Ophthalmology Series. Vols. 1–. **Sir Stewart Duke-Elder, ed.** St. Louis, MO: C. V. Mosby, 1958–.
Volume 2, *The Anatomy of the Visual System,* 1961; volume 3/1, *Normal and Abnormal Development: Embryology,* 1963; volume 3/2, *Congenital Deformities,* 1964; volume 4, *The Physiology of the Eye and of Vision,* 1968; volume 5, *Ophthalmic Optics and Refraction,* 1970; volume 6, *Ocular Motility and Strabismus,* 1973; volume 15, *Summary of Systemic Ophthalmology,* 1976.
R: *JAMA* 237: 1732 (Apr. 18, 1977).

ORTHOPEDICS

The Biochemistry and Physiology of Bone. 4 vols. 2d ed. **Geoffrey H. Bourne, ed.** New York: Academic Press, 1972–1976.
Volume 1, *Structure,* 1972; volume 2, *Physiology and Pathology,* 1972; volume 3, *Development and Growth,* 1972; volume 4, *Calcification and Physiology,* 1976.
First edition, 1956.
Multivolume text expands the one-volume first edition issued in 1956. Expert authors have contributed to this comprehensive treatise on bone. Clear photographs and diagrams and extensive bibliography enhance this work. Favorite with workers in the field.
R: *American Scientist* 61: 362 (May–June 1973); *JAMA* 237: 1873 (Apr. 28, 1977); *Journal of Oral Surgery* 31: 228 (Mar. 1973); *Yale Journal of Biology & Medicine* 46: 251 (1973).

OTORHINOLARYNGOLOGY

Scott-Brown's Diseases of the Ear, Nose and Throat. 3d ed. 4 vols. **John Ballantyne and John Groves, eds.** Philadelphia, PA: J. B. Lippincott, 1971.
Volume 1, *The Basic Sciences*; volume 2, *The Ear*; volume 3, *The Nose*; volume 4, *The Throat.*
Comprehensive coverage of ear, nose, and throat diseases. Reflects contributions of 39 distinguished physicians currently engaged in hospital and university research or practice. Consists of four volumes covering all aspects of otorhinolaryngology, from anatomy to diagnosis. Carefully highlights surgical procedures in a systematic manner. New topics include cancer of the larynx, diseases of middle ear cleft, speech therapy, and hearing disorders in children.

PATHOLOGY

Developmental and Cell Biology Series. Nos. 1–. New York: Cambridge University Press, 1973–.
Number 6, *Nuclear Cytology in Relation to Development,* by F. D'Amato, 1977.

International Academy of Pathology Monographs in Pathology Series. Baltimore, MD: Williams & Wilkins.
Number 13, *The Liver,* 1973; number 18, *The Gastrointestinal Tract,* 1977; number 19, *The Lung: Structure, Function and Disease,* 1978.
An important series of monographs which are based on series of lectures presented in course form by the International Academy of Pathology.
R: *Annals of Internal Medicine* 79: 148 (July 1973); *Lancet* 1: 1007 (May 5, 1979).

Major Problems in Pathology. Vols. 1–. Philadelphia, PA: W. B. Saunders, 1970–.
Volume 6, *Pathology of the Spinal Cord,* 2d ed., J. Trevor Hughes, ed., 1978; volume 7, *Pathology in the Placenta,* by Harold Fox, 1978; volume 9, *Pathology of Peripheral Nerve,* by A. K. Asbury and P. C. Johnson, 1978; volume 10, *The Pathogenesis of Colorectal Cancer,* by Basil C. Morson, 1978.
R: *Annals of Internal Medicine* 89: 1019 (Dec. 1978); *Archives of Neurology* 36: 525 (Aug. 1979); *Archives of Pathology & Laboratory Medicine* 103: 547 (Sept. 1979); *Journal of Clinical Pathology* 32: 309 (Mar. 1979); Journal of Neurosurgery 51: 421 (Sept. 1979); *Lancet* 1: 1008 (May 12, 1979).

Principles and Techniques of Electron Microscopy: Biological Applications. Vols. 1–. **M. A. Hayat, ed.** New York: Van Nostrand Reinhold, 1970–. Irregular.
Volume 2, 1972; volume 6, 1976.
A multivolume monograph series which extensively describes theoretical and practical techniques of electron microscopy. A valuable source for researchers of varied disciplines.
R: *Yale Journal of Biology and Medicine* 47: 140 (1974); 50: 432 (1977).

Scanning Electron Microscopy. 2 vols. **R. P. Becker and O. Johari, eds.** AMF O'Hare, IL: Scanning Electron Microscopy, Inc., 1978.
Volume 1, *Physical and Technical*; volume 2, *Biological.*
A state-of-the-art, two-volume publication which describes current techniques and theories in electron microscopy. Particularly helpful for biomedical applications. A good reference.
R: *Journal of Clinical Pathology* 32: 311 (Mar. 1979).

Systemic Pathology. 2d ed. 4 vols. **William St. C. Symmers, ed.** New York: Churchill Livingstone, 1976.
Volume 1, *Cardiovascular System Respiratory System.*
Consists of four volumes. Volume 1 devoted to diseases of cardiovascular and respiratory systems. Discusses disease entities in terms of pathogenesis and clinical aspects. Excellent black and white illustrations complement volume. Includes up-to-date and relevant references and comprehensive index.
R: *Archives of Pathology & Laboratory Medicine* 102: 111 (1978); *JAMA* 238: 519 (Aug. 8, 1977).

PEDIATRICS

Current Diagnostic Pediatrics. Vols. 1–. **A. Chrispin, ed.** New York: Springer-Verlag, 1977–.
Volume 1, *Current Concepts in Pediatric Radiology,* O. Eklöf, ed., 1977.
Written by international authorities, the self-contained volume reports diagnostic techniques and their applicability to individual problems. Reference source for practicing pediatricians. Future volumes will cover trauma, urology, and gastroenterology.

Major Problems in Clinical Pediatrics. Vols. 1–. Philadelphia, PA: W. B. Saunders, 1974–.

Volume 18, *Malignant Diseases of Infancy, Childhood and Adolescence,* 1978; volume 19, *Adolescent Dermatology,* 1978.
R: *American Journal of Digestive Diseases* 23: 380 (Apr. 1978); *Archives of Dermatology* 115: 115 (Jan. 1979); *British Journal of Surgery* 66: 445 (June 1979); *Journal of Neurosurgery* 44: 396 (Mar. 1976); *Lancet* 1: 1342 (June 24, 1978).

PHARMACY AND PHARMACOLOGY

Antibiotics. 3 vols. **John W. Corcoran and Fred E. Hahn, eds.** New York: Springer-Verlag, 1967–1975.
Volume 3, *Mechanism of Action of Antimicrobial and Antitumor Agents,* 1975.
Volume 3 of *Antibiotics* is an update of volume 1. Special features: new agents not previously covered; a wealth of information on structure, isolation and mechanisms of action. Experts in the field as well as the casual reader will find useful information.
R: *American Scientist* 64: 220 (Mar.–Apr. 1976); *Quarterly Review of Biology* 51: 199 (1976).

The Biological Basis of Medicine. 6 vols. **E. Edward Bittar and Neville Bittar, eds.** New York: Academic Press, 1968–1969.
Volumes 1–2, 1968; volumes 3–6, 1969.

Drugs and the Pharmaceutical Sciences Series. Vols. 1–. New York: Marcel Dekker, 1975–.
Volume 1, *Pharmacokinetics,* Milo Gibaldi and Donald Perrier, eds., 1975; volume 2, *Good Manufacturing Practices for Pharmaceuticals: A Plan for Total Quality Control,* Sidney H. Willig et al., eds., 1975; volume 3, *Microencapsulation,* J. R. Nixon, ed., 1976; volume 4, *Drug Metabolism: Chemical & Biochemical Aspects,* Bernard Testa and Peter Jenner, 1976; volume 5, *New Drugs: Discovery and Development,* Alan A. Rubin, ed., 1978.
R: *Journal of Pharmaceutical Sciences* 67: 1778 (Dec. 1978).

Medicinal Chemistry, A Series of Monographs. Vols. 1–. New York: Academic Press, 1963–.
Volume 15, *Anticonvulsants,* Julius A. Vida, ed., 1977.

Methods in Pharmacology. Vols. 1–. New York: Plenum, 1971–.
Volume 4B, *Renal Pharmacology,* 1978.
R: *Journal of Pharmaceutical Sciences* 68: 1074 (Aug. 1979).

Modern Pharmacology-Toxicology. Vols. 1–. New York: Marcel Dekker, 1973–.
Volume 14, *Developments in Opiate Research,* 1978.
Formerly *Modern Pharmacology.*
R: *Quarterly Review of Biology* 54: 210 (June 1979).

PSYCHIATRY AND PSYCHOLOGY

Attachment and Loss. 3 vols. **John Bowlby.** New York: Basic Books, 1973.
Volume 2, *Separation: Anxiety and Anger.*

The second volume in this series explores the processes of anxiety associated with separation and loss. Combines biological principles and related patterns in ethnology and psychology. Discusses various types of fear and corresponding behavior. Correlates childhood and adult behavior, influence of family structure. Provides explanation of mental and biological disorders due to conflict.
R: *American Jouranl of Psychiatry* 131: 6 (June 1974).

Current Topics in Mental Health. Vols. 1–. New York: Plenum, 1976–.

Some recent volumes include *The Principles and Techniques of Mental Health Consultation*; *Coping With Physical Illness*; and *State Mental Hospitals: What Happens When They Close.*

The Psychiatric Foundations of Medicine. 6 vols. **George U. Balis et al., eds.** Boston, MA: Butterworths, 1978.

Volume 1, *Dimensions of Behavior*; volume 2, *The Behavioral and Social Sciences and the Practice of Medicine*; volume 3, *Basic Psychopathology*; volume 4, *Clinical Psychopathology*; volume 5, *Psychiatric Clinical Skills in Medical Practice*; volume 6, *Problems in Medical Practice.*
A six-volume treatise which presents concepts of modern psychiatry. Adheres closely to the design of medical curriculum. Useful as a comprehensive reference, particularly for the nonspecialist.
R: *American Journal of Psychiatry* 136: 1239 (Sept. 1979); *Lancet* 1: 908 (Apr. 28, 1979).

Receptors and Recognition. Vols. 1–. New York: John Wiley, 1976–.

Volume 3, *Microbial Interactions*, J. L. Reissig, ed., 1978; volume 4, *Specificity of Embryological Interactions*, D. R. Garrod, ed., 1978.
R: *ASM News* (vol. 4, no. 7).

PUBLIC HEALTH

The Biology of Alcoholism. 5 vols. **Benjamin Kissin and Henri Begleiter, eds.** New York: Plenum, 1971–1976.

Volume 1, *Biochemistry,* 1971; volume 2, *Physiology and Behavior,* 1972; volume 3, *Clinical Pathology,* 1974; volume 4, *Social Aspects,* 1976; volume 5, *Treatment and Rehabilitation of the Chronic Alcoholic,* 1976.
Comprehensive study of the biological, psychological, and social aspects of alcoholism. Consists of contributions by authorities in the field.

Consumer Health and Produce Hazards. 2 vols. **Samuel S. Epstein and Richard D. Grundy, eds.** Cambridge, MA: MIT Press, 1974–1975.

Volume 1, *Chemicals, Electronic Products, Radiation,* 1974; volume 2, *Cosmetics, Drugs, Pesticides, Food Additives,* 1975.
Epstein is a pioneer in the field of consumer health. The books contain a wealth of information and citations useful to the specialists.
R: *Pharmaceutical Journal* 217: 438 (1976).

Geochemistry and the Environment. Vol. 1–. **US National Committee for Geochemistry, National Research Council.** Washington, DC: National Academy of Sciences, 1974–. Irregular.

Volume 1, *The Relation of Selected Trace Elements to Health and Disease*, 1974; volume 2, *The Relation of Other Selected Trace Elements to Health and Disease*, 1977; volume 3, *Distribution of Trace Elements Related to the Occurrence of Certain Cancers, Cardiovascular Diseases, and Urolithiasis*, 1979.

RADIOLOGY

Comprehensive Manuals in Radiology. Vols. 1–. **H. G. Jacobson, ed.** New York: Springer-Verlag, 1978–.

Volume 1, *Soft Tissues of the Extremities: A Radiologic Study of Rheumatic Disease*, by W. J. Weston and D. G. Palmer, 1978.

Multiple Imaging Procedures. Vols. 1–. New York: Grune & Stratton, 1979–.

Volume 1, Pulmonary System, 1979.

Radiology of the Skull and Brain. **Thomas H. Newton et al., eds.** St. Louis, MO: C. V. Mosby, 1971–.

Volume 1, *Skull*, 1971; volume 2, *Angiography*, 1974 (Book 1, *Technical Aspects*; Book 2, *Arteries*; Book 3, *Veins*; Book 4, *Specific Disease Processes*); volume 3, *Anatomy and Pathology*, 1977; volume 4, *Ventricles and Cisterns*, 1978.

A multivolume treatise which covers a vast amount of information in neuroradiology. Presents much detailed description of anatomy, radiological procedures, cerebral pathology. Highly recommended, considered an essential tool for neuroscientists. Excellent presentation, well indexed. An indispensable tool.

R: *American Journal of Roentgenology* 132: 514 (Mar. 1979); *Brain* 102: 231 (Mar. 1979); *British Journal of Radiology* 49: 576 (1976); *Journal of Neurosurgery* 47: 132 (Jan. 1976); 49: 322 (Aug. 1978); 51: 262 (Aug. 1979); *JAMA* 233: 1317 (Sept. 22, 1975); *Radiology* 118: 96 (1976); *RSR* 3: 32 (Apr.–June 1975).

RHEUMATOLOGY

The Structure and Function of Muscle. 2d ed. 4 vols. **Geoffrey H. Bourne, ed.** New York: Academic Press, 1972–1974.

Volume 1, part 1, *Structure*, 1972; volume 2, part 2, *Structure*, 1973; volume 3, *Physiology and Biochemistry*, 1973; volume 4, *Pharmacology and Disease*, 1974.

Four-volume set discusses structural features of muscle along with clinical and genetic aspects of muscle disease. Illustrations and bibliographies.

R: *JAMA* 228: 633 (Apr. 29, 1974); 229: 1509 (Sept. 9, 1974); *NEJM* 290: 580 (Mar. 7, 1974).

UROGENITAL SYSTEM

The Kidney. 2 vols. **Barry M. Brenner and Floyd C. Rector, eds.** Philadelphia, PA: W. B. Saunders, 1976.

Scholarly, comprehensive, and up-to-date study of renal disease. Eighty-eight experts contributed to this two-volume work. Helpful summaries in many chapters; clear illustrations and inclusive index. Over 13,000 references to original works. Valuable source of information for every practicing nephrologist.

R: *Annals of Internal Medicine* 86: 372 (1977); *Archives of Pathology & Laboratory*

Medicine 101: 395 (July 1977); *BMJ* 1: 452 (Feb. 12, 1977); *JAMA* 236: 1996 (Oct. 25, 1976); *Kidney International* 10: 481 (1976); *NEJM* 295: 1268 (1976); Brandon.

Major Problems in Obstetrics and Gynecology. 11 vols. **Erich Burghardt.** Philadelphia, PA: W. B. Saunders, 1970–1977.
Volume 1, *Laparoscopy, Colposcopy and Gynecography,* 1970; volume 2, *Lymphatic System of the Female Genitalia,* 1971; volume 3, *Thyroid Gland in Pregnancy,* 1972; volume 4, *Ovarian Tumors,* 1973; volume 5, *Response to Contraception,* 1973; volume 6, *Early Historical Diagnosis of Cervical Cancer,* 1973; volume 7, *Menstrual Cycle,* 1977; volume 8, *Hysteroscopy,* 1975; volume 9, *Vulvar Disease,* 1976; volume 10, *Colposcopy,* 1976; volume 11, *Septic Shock in Obstetrics and Gynecology,* 1977.
R: *NEJM* 290: 581 (Mar. 7, 1974); *Obstetrics and Gynecology* 44: 628 (Oct. 1974).

Pathophysiology of Gestation. 3 vols. **Nicholas S. Assali and Charles R. Brinkman, eds.** New York: Academic Press, 1972.
Volume 3, *Fetal and Neonatal Disorders.*
Comprehensive treatise on maternal and fetal disorders in pregnancy. Three volumes concentrate on basic scientific and clinical data. Volume I deals specifically with maternal disorders, volume 2 with the normal and abnormal functioning of the fetoplacental unit, and volume 3 with the fetal condition at term and the early neonatal period. A standard reference source on human gestation worthy of inclusion in university and departmental libraries specializing in reproductive biology.
R: *BMJ* 2: 313 (May 5, 1973); *Obstetrics and Gynecology* 44: 784 (Nov. 1974).

Scientific Foundations of Urology. 2 vols. **David I. Williams and Geoffrey D. Chisholm, eds.** London: Heinemann, 1976.
Volume 2, *Congenital Tract, Oncology and the Urological Armamentarium.*
Two-volume set reflecting the development of urology. Volume 1 focuses on renal diseases; volume 2 concentrates on urodynamics, tumors of the urogenital system and the development of endoscopic equipment. Recommended reference source for every urologist and nephrologist.
R: *British Journal of Surgery* 64: 226 (Mar. 1977); *BMJ* 1: 849 (Mar. 26, 1977).

VETERINARY MEDICINE

Design and Analysis of Experiments in the Animal and Medical Sciences. 3 vols. **John L. Gill.** Ames, IA: Iowa State University Press, 1978.

CHAPTER 15 MONOGRAPHS

Medical monographs exist for various purposes, such as textbooks for students at different levels of sophistication, research monographs on specific subject matter, etc. It is impossible to present an adequate listing of titles under each subject in this chapter since the volume of medical books is enormous. The titles listed indicate the types of useful monographs that one can easily locate through the use of subject-review journals and available "core lists" and/or regular bibliographical tools. For collection development purposes, it is important to keep in mind the information consumer's need since each book is written with specific groups of readers in mind.

The monographs included here are mostly single-volume works. They are frequently included in numerous core lists prepared and recommended for various health sciences libraries, for example, Allyn, Brandon, Stearns & Ratcliff, etc., as indicated in the "R" section at the end of each entry. For these core lists, readers are referred to "Core Lists" in the Reference List at the end of the book for complete listings and bibliographical information.

For monographic volumes in a series or a set of publications, see chapter 13, Important Series, and chapter 14, Treatises.

GENERAL

The ABC of Acid-Base Chemistry. 6th ed. **H. W. Davenport.** Chicago, IL: University of Chicago Press, 1974

Lucid description of chemistry and extensive use of diagrams result in excellent book for students.
R: *Annals of Internal Medicine* 81: 865 (Dec. 1974); *Clinical Chemistry* 21: 790 (May 1975); *TBRI* 41: 54 (Feb. 1975).

Acid-Base Balance. **A. Gorman Hills.** Baltimore, MD: Williams & Wilkins, 1973.

Thoroughly reviews historic tenets of acid-base physiology, and pertinent developments in field are presented in clear, readable form. Material is presented logically and has been written for physicians interested in renal contribution to acid-base balance as well as those responsible for diagnosis and treatment of respiratory insufficiency.
R: *Anesthesiology* 41: 530 (Nov. 1974); Allyn.

An Analysis of Health Care Delivery. **James M. Rosser and Howard E. Mossberg.** New York: John Wiley, 1977.

Focuses on the health care delivery system in the United States. Complete with comprehensive tables and graphs. Includes useful references. Points out information presently available for the general public. Cites many inadequacies and discrepancies in the literature.
R: *Choice* 14: 1096 (Oct. 1977).

Assessing Quality in Health Care. **Institute of Medicine.** Washington, DC: National Academy of Sciences, 1977.

Basic Medical Statistics. **Anita K. Bahn.** New York: Grune & Stratton, 1972.

A programmed guide to medical statistics which includes many exercises and problem sets. Concepts and definitions are clearly explained; contains helpful diagrams and glossary. Considered an excellent introductory book, recommended to students, teachers, and practitioners as a reference source on statistical methodology.

R: *Annals of Internal Medicine* 78: 466 (Mar. 1, 1973); *Archives of Internal Medicine* 133: 874 (May 1974).

Biochemistry: The Molecular Basis of All Structure and Function. 2d ed. **Albert L. Lehninger.** New York: Worth, 1975.

First edition, 1970.
Considered a basic and valuable reference text in biochemistry. Includes summaries, references, extensive index. Classic, comprehensive work.

Biomedical Instrumentation and Measurements. **Leslie Cromwell et al.** Englewood Cliffs, NJ: Prentice-Hall, 1973.

An introduction to biomedical instrumentation, written for those with a technical background in electronics, engineering, or physiology. Deals with instrumental measurements of cardiovascular, respiratory, nervous functions. Covers basic principles of physiology, laboratory medicine, radioisotopes, but is technically oriented in regard to electronic setup of instruments. Recommended as a useful reference.

R: *Biomedical Engineering* 10: 315 (1975); *NTB* 58: 252 (July 1973); Allyn.

Biomedical Physics and Biomaterials Science. **H. Eugene Stanley, ed.** Cambridge, MA: MIT Press, 1975.

An interdisciplinary, multi-authored work on biomedical physics, covering the application of materials science to medical problems.

R: *Biomedical Engineering* 10: 231 (1975).

Continuing Medical Education: Perspectives, Problems, Prognosis. **Robert K. Richards.** New Haven, CT: Yale University Press, 1978.

Presents an overview of continuing medical education in the United States in three major parts: the development of medical education since the 1930s; current forces in continuing education; recommendations for change. Uniformly informatic, comprehensive. Well referenced.

R: *Journal of Medical Education* 54: 600 (July 1979).

Ethical Constraints and Imperatives in Medical Research. **M. B. Visscher.** Springfield, IL: Charles C. Thomas, 1975.

Deals with the ethics of medical research, covering such topics as syphillis experiments on Alabama prisoners, research practice of the Third Reich. Recommended for those interested in ethical practice in research medicine.

R: *Physical Therapy* 56: 1315 (Nov. 1976).

Evolution. **T. Dobzhansky et al.** San Francisco, CA: W. H. Freeman, 1977.

Up-to-date discussion of evolution divided into two parts. The first covers cytogenetic basis of response of individuals and populations to evolution, while the second covers evolutionary record from origin of life to evolution of mankind. Highly readable volume, recommended to students of biology.
R: *Heredity* 40: 469 (June 1978).

Experimentation with Human Beings: The Authority of the Investigator, Subject, Professions, and State in the Human Experimentations Process. **Jay Katz, Alexander M. Capron, and Eleanor S. Glass.** New York: Russell Sage Foundation, 1972.

A major work in medicolegal field which treats such questions as, "What constitutes harm?" Written in casebook text methods format. Includes newspaper and magazine articles as well as appeal court decisions. Can easily be used as keystone for research, interdisciplinary seminars and lectures.
R: *American Journal of Psychiatry* 130: 228 (Feb. 1973).

The Future of Medical Education. **William G. Anlyan et al.** Durham, NC: Duke University Press, 1973.

Deals with a wide range of problems that confront medical educators. Includes critical analysis of current trends and problems. Helpful in setting up curriculum. Considered a well-organized volume.
R: *Medical Care* 12: 626 (July 1974).

Goodale's Clinical Interpretation of Laboratory Tests. 8th ed. **Frances K. Widmann.** Philadelphia, PA: F. A. Davis, 1979.
Seventh edition, 1973.
Extensively updated and revised. Describes a full range of laboratory tests. Useful for clinicians. Provides numerous up-to-date references.

Human Experimentation and the Law. **Nathan Hershey and Robert D. Miller.** Germantown, MD: Aspen Systems Corp., 1976.

Written by lawyers, book discusses legal implications of medical experiments involving human subjects. Describes institutional process by which proposals for research with human subjects are evaluated. Informative treatments of topics such as fetal research, psychosurgery, drug study protocols, and informed consent. Recommended for those who participate in research with human subjects as a reference for clarification and guidance.
R: *American Journal of Psychiatry* 134: 106 (Jan. 1977); *Nursing Research* 26: 94 (Mar.–Apr. 1977).

Issues in the Design and Evaluation of Medical Trials. **John M. Weiner.** Boston, MA: G. K. Hall, 1979.

Step-by-step guide to the methodology necessary for the collection, translation, and communication of patient information. Reliable source for physicians involved in research projects and graduate and undergraduate students studying health sciences and research methodology.

Laboratory Safety Monograph: A Supplement to the NIH Guidelines for Recombinant DNA Research. **US National Institutes of Health.** Washington, DC: US Government Printing Office, 1978.

The Law Relating to the Misuse of Drugs. **P. W. H. Lydiate.** London: Butterworth Law Publishers, 1977.

Highlights legislation and legal aspects concerning abused drugs in the United Kingdom. Comprehensive treatment of decided court cases enhances its reference value. Immensely valuable to lawyers involved in drug abuse cases.
R: *Pharmaceutical Journal* 219: 87 (1977).

Medical Engineering. **Charles D. Ray, ed.** Chicago, IL: Year Book Medical Publishers, 1974.

Covers the following subjects: medical engineering, research, diagnosis and treatment, safety hazards of machinery, electronics and instrumentation, materials handling methods, application of medical engineering principles. A large reference volume with bibliographies at the end of each chapter. Considered an excellent work; recommended to medical libraries, teaching hospitals, and medical engineers.
R: *Archives of Physical Medicine and Rehabilitation* 57: 251 (1976); *Biomedical Engineering* 10: 32 (Jan. 1975); *Lancet* 2: 1182 (Nov. 16, 1974); *NEJM* 291: 1203 (Nov. 28, 1974); *Physical Therapy* 56: 1191 (Oct. 1976); Allyn.

Medical Jurisprudence. **Jon R. Waltz and Fred E. Inbau.** Riverside, NJ/New York: Macmillan, 1971.

A comprehensive, dry-as-dust guide to philosophical and ethical problems of medical jurisprudence. Written mainly for practitioners and medical students. This work covers judicial opinions, statutes, rules and regulations, liability, etc. Bibliography after each chapter.

Medical Malpractice Law. 2d ed. **Angela R. Holder.** New York: John Wiley, 1978.

First edition, 1975.
Revised edition presents full range of malpractice issues concerning physician-patient relationships. Description of biomedical and constitutional issues is illustrated by over 2,000 actual cases, which are alphabetically indexed. Alerts the physician to areas prone to malpractice suits. Primarily a reference source for legal aspects of medical practice; recommended to doctors, medical students, lawyers, as a basic information source.
R: *Radiology* 129: 248 (1978); *RSR* 3: 31 (Apr.–June 1975); *TBRI* 41: 388 (Dec. 1975).

Medical, Moral and Legal Issues in Mental Health Care. **Frank J. Ayd, Jr., ed.** Baltimore, MD: Williams & Wilkins, 1974.

Explores role of doctor and patient in mental health treatment. Contributions from twelve essayists with some overlap and repetition. For use by psychiatrists, lawyers, and behavioral scientists.
R: *American Journal of Psychiatry* 132: 8 (Aug. 1975).

Medical Nemesis: The Expropriation of Health. **Ivan Illich.** London: Calder & Boyars, 1975.
R: *American Journal of Public Health* 66: 299 (1976).

Nonparametric Methods for Quantitative Analysis. **J. D. Gibbons.** New York: Holt, Rinehart and Winston, 1976.
Reference in nonparametric statistics for average researcher. Written at low mathematical level and includes student exercises drawn from actual research. Emphasizes hypothesis-testing situations. Procedures are presented under headings that reflect questions they are designed to answer.
R: *Physical Therapy* 57: 756 (1977).

Principles of Biochemistry. 6th ed. **Abraham White et al.** New York: McGraw-Hill, 1978.
An extensive text; details human biochemistry.
R: Allyn; Stearns & Ratcliff (*AJN*; *NEJM*, 1969; *NEJM*, 1970).

Principles of Medical Statistics. 9th rev. ed. **Austin B. Hill.** New York: Oxford University Press, 1971.
R: Stearns & Ratcliff (*NEJM*, 1970).

Review of Physiological Chemistry. 17th ed. **Harold A. Harper et al.** Los Altos, CA: Lange Medical Publications, 1979.
Twelfth edition, 1969; fifteenth edition, 1975; sixteenth edition, 1977.
R: Allyn.

Statistics: A Biomedical Introduction. **B. W. Brown and M. Hollander.** New York: John Wiley, 1977.
An introductory text based on lecture notes; serves to illustrate the application of statistical techniques to medicine. Concise format provides introductions, sample problems, discussions, and appropriate references. Contains three appendixes: glossary of terms, answers to problems, and mathematical and statistical tables. Employs all standard notation; helpful to those who wish to apply statistics to biomedical problems.
R: *Physical Therapy* 59: 78 (1979).

ALLERGY AND IMMUNOLOGY

The Antibody Molecule. **Alfred Nisonoff, John E. Hopper, and Susan B. Spring.** New York: Academic Press, 1975.
Introduces the reader to the basic mechanisms of protein chemistry and molecular immunology. Includes summaries by outstanding immunologists. A comprehensive monograph which will prove useful to both the clinician and the researcher. Lucidly written text and accompanying illustrations are of high quality.
R: *Annals of Internal Medicine* 84: 111 (Jan. 1976); *Immunological Communications* 5: 114 (1976).

Basic and Clinical Immunology. 2d ed. **H. H. Fudenberg et al.** Los Altos, CA: Lange Medical Publications, 1978.

First edition, 1976.
Acknowledges immunology as an independent discipline in its own right. Highlights clinical immunology. Includes laboratory procedures and comprehensive references.
R: *Immunogenetics* 5: 191 (1977); Brandon.

Clinical Aspects of Immunology. 4th ed. **P. G. H. Gell, R. R. Coombs, and P. J. Lachmann.** Oxford, England: Blackwell Scientific Publications, 1979.

Second edition, 1968; third edition, 1975.
A comprehensive, encyclopedic volume of immunology, revised and updated. Highly recommended as a reference for allergists, immunology researchers.
R: *Annals of Allergy* 35: 393 (Dec. 1975); *Archives of Pathology & Laboratory Medicine* 100: 564 (Oct. 1976); *Immunology* 30: 779 (1976); *International Archives of Allergy & Applied Immunology* 53: 195 (1977); *JAMA* 235: 1060 (Mar. 8, 1976); *TBRI* 42: 98 (Mar. 1976); 42: 184 (May 1976); 42: 384 (Dec. 1976); Allyn; Brandon; Inke.

Essential Immunology. 3d ed. **Ivan M. Roitt.** Philadelphia, PA: J. B. Lippincott, 1977.

First edition, 1971; second edition, 1974.
Text which covers subject of immunology from basic principles through clinical application. Chapter summaries, index, references, charts, tables, drawings and photographs are included. Valuable for both students and researchers.
R: *Immunological Communications* 4: 296 (1975); *Immunology* 29: 221 (1975); *JAMA* 239: 1442 (Apr. 3, 1978); Allyn.

The Immune System: A Course on the Molecular and Cellular Basis of Immunity. **I. McConnell and M. J. Hobart, eds.** Oxford, England: Blackwell Scientific Publications, 1976.

Collection of lectures delivered in Department of Immunology, Royal Postgraduate Medical School, London. Contains four sections which treat chemistry, biology, genetics, and pathology as they relate to immunology. Excellent, informative book for the advanced reader.
R: *Immunology* 32: 605 (Apr. 1977); *JAMA* 236: 1893 (Oct. 18, 1976).

Immunochemistry of Proteins. **M. Z. Atassi, ed.** New York: Plenum, 1977.
Gathers research which is relevant to immunochemical studies of proteins.
R: *Nature* 267: 652 (June 16, 1977).

Immunology: An Introduction to Molecular and Cellular Principles of the Immune Responses. **Herman N. Eisen.** Hagerstown, MD: Harper & Row, 1974.

Immunology section of Bernard Davis's *Microbiology* which stands by itself as an excellent monograph. Homogeneity of style and organization. Highly recommended to all physicians, medical students, and researchers in immunology, microbiology, pathology, and related fields.

R: *British Journal of Haematology* 27: 679 (Aug. 1974); *Health Laboratory Science* 11: 313 (Oct. 1974); *Immunological Communications* 3: 197 (1974); *Military Medicine* 141: 472 (June 1974); *New Zealand Medical Journal* 80: 525 (Dec. 11, 1974); *TBRI* 40: 362 (Nov. 1974); 41: 13 (Jan. 1975); 41: 172 (May 1975).

Immunology, Immunopathology and Immunity. 2d ed. **Stewart Sell.** Hagerstown, MD: Harper & Row, 1975.

Covers essentials of immunology; divided into instructive, well-illustrated and documented sections. Especially noteworthy is discussion of immunology of cancer which is complete and current. Useful for audience ranging from biology and medical students to physicians.
R: *Annals of Allergy* 37: 142 (Aug. 1976); *Annals of Internal Medicine* 83: 922 (Dec. 1975); *Immunology* 30: 780 (1976); *TBRI* 42: 67 (Feb. 1976).

Medical Mycology. 3d ed. **Chester W. Emmons et al.** Philadelphia, PA: Lea & Febiger, 1977.

Third edition adds to knowledge of medical mycology. Complete, current work has cross-referenced index, substantial bibliography for each chapter, and beautiful color plates. Reference for dermatologists, internists, surgeons, and researchers.
R: *Archives of Dermatology* 113: 860 (June 1977).

Principles of Immunology. 2d ed. **Noel R. Rose, Felix Milgrom, and Carel J. van Oss, eds.** New York: Macmillan, 1979.

A multi-authored volume which extensively covers the scope of immunology. The volume is divided into three units: basic immunology, clinical immunology, and applied immunology. Useful as both a reference and textbook.

Principles of Modern Immunobiology: Basic and Clinical. **Byung H. Park and Robert A. Good.** Philadelphia, PA: Lea & Febiger, 1974.

Section 1 covers basic immunobiologic principles. Section 2 is intended as a guide to clinical specialties. Includes useful appendix, covering identification of T & B lymphocytes by their properties and a guide for active and passive immunizations. A broad overview for the student and teacher of immunobiology.
R: *Immunological Communications* 4: 96 (1975).

ANATOMY

Essentials of Human Anatomy. 6th ed. **Russell T. Woodburne.** New York: Oxford University Press, 1978.

Maintains a regional approach rather than a systematic one. Concise coverage of basic concepts and anatomical functions. Up-to-date, discusses such topics as EMG. Contains illustrations. Highly recommended as a companion volume in dissection anatomy courses.
R: *Physical Therapy* 59: 804 (June 1979).

Hamilton, Boyd and Mossman's Human Embryology. 4th ed. **W. J. Hamilton, J. D. Boyd, and H. W. Mossman.** Baltimore, MD: Williams & Wilkins, 1972.

Extensive revision and enlargement make this new fourth edition even more valuable than previous editions.
R: *Journal of Anatomy* 113: 264 (Nov. 1972); *Obstetrics and Gynecology* 44: 628 (Oct. 1974); *TBRI* 39: 160 (Apr. 1973).

Human Embryology. 5th ed. **W. J. Hamilton, J. B. Boyd, and H. W. Mossman.** Baltimore, MD: Williams & Wilkins, 1980.
R: *Obstetrics and Gynecology* 44: 628 (Oct. 1974).

Medical Physiology. 13th ed. 2 vols. **Vernon B. Mountcastle, ed.** St. Louis, MO: C. V. Mosby, 1974.
Substantial revision of a classic textbook. Includes new sections on endocrinology, renal physiology, gastrointestinal physiology, and autonomic nervous system.
R: *Annals of Internal Medicine* 80: 440 (Mar. 1974); Allyn.

Primary Anatomy. 7th ed. **John V. Basmajian.** Baltimore, MD: Williams & Wilkins, 1976.
An introduction to gross and functional anatomy. Briefly outlines the microscopic structure of important tissues and basic developmental anatomy. New seventh edition features sixteen chapters with a new chapter on regional anatomy. There are 691 outstanding illustrations and 30 colored plates to complement the text. Book available in French, Spanish, and Italian. Designed primarily for the nonmedical student. Useful reference for medical and paramedical students.
R: *Archives of Physical Medicine and Rehabilitation* 58: 45 (Jan. 1977).

Structure of the Human Body. 2d ed. **W. D. Gardner and W. A. Osburn.** Philadelphia, PA: W. B. Saunders, 1973.
Introductory text on systemic gross anatomy for college students. Anatomical descriptions are clear. It discusses embryology, reviews connective tissue, respiratory system, digestive system, and integumentary systems, and includes illustrations.
R: *Physical Therapy* 54: 209 (1974).

Textbook of Medical Physiology. 5th ed. **Arthur C. Guyton.** Philadelphia, PA: W. B. Saunders, 1976.
Fourth edition, 1971.
A classic text, covers all aspects of physiology. Excellent format and bibliography. Includes tables, illustrations, indexes. A fundamental source.
R: Allyn; Stearns & Ratcliff (*AJN*; *NEJM*, 1969; *NEJM*, 1970).

ANESTHESIOLOGY AND GENERAL SURGERY

Acupuncture Anesthesia in the People's Republic of China: A Trip Report of the American Acupuncture Anesthesia Study Group. Washington, DC: US National Academy of Sciences, 1976.

Alexander's Care of the Patient in Surgery. 6th ed. **Marie Rhodes, Barbara J. Gruendemann, and Walter F. Ballinger.** St. Louis, MO: C. V. Mosby, 1978.

Fifth edition, 1972.
Revised edition contains over 2,000 illustrations, many of which are new. Also includes new information on operating room procedures for nurses. Contributors from many different fields and regions account for representative sampling of different nursing procedures.
R: Brandon (NO).

Analgesic Drugs. **J. Parkhouse, B. J. Pleuvry, and J. M. H. Rees.** Oxford, England: Blackwell Scientific Publications, 1979.
Attempts to outline the current state of analgesic drugs. First section deals with introductory material (anatomy and physiology of pain) and progresses to the general pharmacology of analgesics. Analgesic trials and statistics comprise the remainder of the volume. Lists some 300 references. Lacks a sought after cohesive, comprehensive summary. Intended audience: medical students and residents.
R: *BMJ* 1: 1619 (June 16, 1979).

Hamilton Bailey's Demonstrations of Physical Signs in Clinical Surgery. 15th ed. **Allan Clain, ed.** Baltimore, MD: Williams & Wilkins, 1973.
Considered the standard reference in clinical surgery. Well written; contains good photographs and index and is encyclopedic in scope. There are many helpful references, biographical footnotes. Text is succinct. Well recommended.
R: *Archives of Surgery* 108: 750 (May 1974); *JAMA* 227: 666 (Feb. 11, 1974).

Hamilton Bailey's Emergency Surgery. 10th ed. **H. A. F. Dudley, ed.** Bristol, England: John Wright, 1977.
First edition, 1930.
A classic book on emergency surgery. Provides clear guidance on all aspects of emergency treatment. Well indexed. Recommended.
R: *ABL* 43: entry 109 (Feb. 1978).

Implants in Surgery. **D. F. Williams and Robert Roaf.** Philadelphia, PA: W. B. Saunders, 1973.
Recent and comprehensive book about alloplastic materials used in surgery. Basic discussion of materials; clinical and medical considerations in surgery are covered. Terms are defined and chapters are well referenced. Pictures, diagrams, and tables enhance value as reference for those interested in generalities or specific details.
R: *Plastic and Reconstructive Surgery* 54: 480 (1974).

Kazanjian and Converse's Surgical Treatment of Facial Injuries. 3d ed. 2 vols. **John M. Converse.** Baltimore, MD: Williams & Wilkins, 1974.
Complete coverage of field of facial traumas. For collections in medical libraries.
R: *JAMA* 231: 523 (Feb. 3, 1975).

Monitoring in Anesthesia. **Lawrence J. Saidman and N. Ty Smith, eds.** Chichester, Sussex, England: John Wiley, 1978.
A guide to monitoring.
R: *Nature* 274: 96 (July 6, 1978).

Organ Preservation for Transplantation. **Armand M. Karow, Jr., George J. M. Abouna, and Arthur L. Humphries, Jr.** Boston, MA: Little, Brown, 1974.

Seriously analyzes experimental and clinical activity associated with preserving the functional integrity of tissues and organs. Provides essential background material and pertinent references.
R: *Archives of Surgery* 110: 852 (July 1975).

Plastic Surgery. **Tord Skoog.** Philadelphia, PA: W. B. Saunders, 1975.

Emphasizes the author's preference for particular surgical procedures. Format of volume is magnificent. Features 701 colored plates and black-and-white drawings. Destined to be a classic due to the extraordinary union of surgical procedures and art. Informative text for plastic surgeons in training and senior members of the specialty.
R: *Archives of Surgery* 110: 1520 (Dec. 1975); *NEJM* 294: 231 (Jan. 22, 1976).

Recent Advances in Anaesthesia and Analgesia. 13th ed. **C. L. Hewer and R. S. Atkinson, eds.** Edinburgh: Churchill Livingstone, 1979.

First edition, 1932; twelfth edition, 1976.
R: *Anaesthesia* 28: 215 (Mar. 1973); 31: 806 (July 1976); *BMJ* 1: 1408 (June 5, 1976); 1: 1282 (June 30, 1979); *Lancet* 1: 1326 (June 23, 1979).

A Synopsis of Anaesthesia. 7th ed. **J. Alfred Lee and R. S. Atkinson.** Baltimore, MD: Williams & Wilkins, 1973.

Summarizes current practice and teaching of anesthesia and includes significant developments of the last decade. Many footnote references and 66-page index with approximately 6,000 entries. Source of reference for student, resident anesthetist, and practitioner.
R: *Anesthesiology* 41: 420 (Oct. 1974).

Treatment of Hand Injuries: Preservation and Restoration of Function. **Elden C. Weckesser.** Chicago, IL: Year Book Medical Publishers, 1974.

Primer for treatment of hand injuries which is an excellent introduction for surgical students.
R: *NEJM* 292: 487 (1975).

Vascular Surgery. **Robert B. Rutherford, ed.** Philadelphia, PA: W. B. Saunders, 1977.

Reviews material on surgical treatment of peripheral vascular conditions within the last 25 years. Discusses arterial occlusion, aneurysms, renovascular hypertension, and cerebrovascular insufficiency. Recommended to vascular surgeons, residents, and students.
R: *JAMA* 239: 865 (Feb. 27, 1978).

BRAIN AND NERVOUS SYSTEM

Bing's Local Diagnosis in Neurological Diseases. 15th ed. **Webb D. Haymaker.** St. Louis, MO: C. V. Mosby, 1969.

First edition titled *Bing's Kompendium,* 1909.

Brain's Clinical Neurology. 5th ed. **Rev. by Roger Bannister.** London: Oxford University Press, 1978.
Third edition, 1969; fourth edition, 1973.
Textbook explains diagnosis and treatment of neurological disorders. References, glossary, and colored plates are included.
R: *Archives of Neurology* 29: 286 (Oct. 1973).

Brain's Diseases of the Nervous System. 8th ed. **Rev. by John N. Walton.** Oxford, England: Oxford University Press, 1977.
First edition, 1933; seventh edition, 1969.
Revised eighth edition covers entire field of clinical neurology. Chapter on psychological aspects of neurology has been revamped. One of the best chapters is devoted to disorders of spinal cord and cauda equina. Illustrations are new, and bibliography has been expanded. Contains excellent index. Essential single-volume reference for neurologists and those in training.
R: *American Journal of Psychiatry* 135: 259 (Feb. 1978); *Brain* 100: 795 (Dec. 1977); *BMJ* 1: 497 (Feb. 25, 1978); *Journal of Neurosurgery* 48: 1047 (June 1978).

Brock's Injuries of the Brain and Spinal Cord and Their Coverings. 5th ed. **Emanuel H. Feiring, ed.** New York: Springer Publishing, 1974.
Information about traumatic diseases affecting the central nervous system. Appropriate for neurologists, psychiatrists, and those in the legal profession.
R: *Archives of Neurology* 31: 143 (Aug. 1974); *Journal of Neurosurgery* 41: 646 (Nov. 1974); *JAMA* 229: 1926 (Sept. 20, 1974); *TBRI* 40: 277 (Sept. 1974); 40: 405 (Dec. 1974).

The Concept of a Blood-Brain Barrier. **M. Bradbury.** New York: John Wiley, 1979.
Deals with physiological and biochemical aspects of the subject in detail; includes helpful illustrations and diagrams. Contains a wealth of information, extensive bibliography, and end-of-chapter summaries.
R: *Lancet* 2: 335 (Aug. 18, 1979).

Current Controversies in Neurosurgery. **T. P. Morley, ed.** Philadelphia, PA: W. B. Saunders, 1976.
A standard work for neurosurgeons; of interest to both practitioners and residents. Has an excellent text and is recommended for reference collections.
R: *JAMA* 238: 897 (Aug. 22, 1977); *TBRI* 43: 305 (Oct. 1977).

Developmental Neuropathology. **Reinhard L. Friede.** New York: Springer-Verlag, 1975.
Considered a thorough reference on neuropathology in infancy and childhood. Highly recommended to pediatric neurosurgeons and others who deal with children.
R: *Journal of Clinical Pathology* 29: 763 (Aug. 1976); *JAMA* 236: 1893 (Oct. 18, 1976); *Physical Therapy* 57: 972 (Aug. 1977); *TBRI* 42: 346 (Nov. 1976); 42: 384 (Dec. 1976).

Diseases of the Nervous System, Described for Practitioners and Students. 11th repr. ed. **Francis M. R. Walshe.** Baltimore, MD: Williams & Wilkins, 1973.

Eleventh edition, 1970.
Classic text with two parts. The first discusses foundation of neurological diagnosis and the second gives an account of common nervous diseases.

Electrical Activity of the Nervous System. 4th ed. **Mary A. B. Brazier.** Baltimore, MD: Williams & Wilkins, 1977.

First edition, 1951; third edition, 1967.
Well-organized, concise presentation of select neuroelectric fundamentals. Introductory book which is recommended for students in the neurosciences and practicing clinicians in neurological areas.
R: *Journal of Neurosurgery* 48: 842 (May 1978).

EEG of Human Sleep. **R. M. Williams, I. Karacan, and C. Hursch.** Chichester, Sussex, England: John Wiley, 1974.

Compendium of information based on thirteen years of study of electroencephalography of night sleep. Basic reference work with excellent documentation, 33 tables, and 59 figures. For all those interested in study of sleep.
R: *Electroencephalography & Clinical Neurophysiology* 40: 445 (Apr. 1976).

EEG Technology. **R. Cooper, J. W. Osselton, and J. C. Shaw.** London: Butterworths, 1974.

Extensive and critical analysis of EEG signal techniques. Discusses theoretical problems as well as logistics of the mechanics. Contains many illustrations, making the book instructive and descriptive. Includes references and index. A book of wide scope, useful to those working with EEG.
R: *Electroencephalography & Clinical Neurophysiology* 40: 554 (May 1976).

Epilepsy: A Study of the Idiopathic Disease. **William A. Turner.** New York: Raven Press, 1973. Originally published in London: Macmillan, 1907.

Facsimile reproduction of treatise on etiology of epilepsy with emphasis on genetic and precipitating causes of seizures. Milestone in history of epilepsy which provides modern neurologists with account of epilepsies at a transitional period. Merits reading by epileptologists, clinicians, social scientists, rehabilitation and vocational counselors.
R: *Journal of Neurosurgery* 41: 401 (Sept. 1974).

Essentials of Clinical Neuroanatomy and Neurophysiology. 5th ed. **Ronald G. Clark.** Philadelphia, PA: F. A. Davis, 1975.

Revised text contains recent advances in knowledge of the nervous system. Current terminology and accurate illustrations.

Essentials of Neuropathology. **Sydney S. Schochet, Jr., and William F. McCormick.** New York: Appleton-Century-Crofts, 1979.

Concise text surveys neuropathologic disorders. Over 100 photographs and diagrams and extensive lists of references augment this aid for medical students.

Functional Neuroanatomy of Man. **Peter L. Williams and Roger Warwick.** Philadelphia, PA: W. B. Saunders, 1975.
Represents neurological section of 35th edition of *Gray's Anatomy*. Up-to-date account of modern neuroanatomy begins with principles of neurobiology and continues with topographic anatomy. Short accounts of functional and practical clinical aspects follow each section. Complete in itself with its own index. Clearly organized text has high-quality illustrations. Excellent reference for both students and practitioners.
R: *Archives of Neurology* 33: 521 (July 1976); *Brain* 99: 388 (June 1976).

Fundamentals of Electroencephalography. 2d ed. **Kenneth A. Kooi, Richard P. Tucker, and Robert E. Marshall.** New York: Harper & Row, 1978.
Clinically oriented text should be useful to students of electroencephalography as well as neurologists, psychiatrists, and allied health personnel.

Greenfield's Neuropathology. 3d ed. **W. Blackwood and J. A. N. Coresellis, eds.** London: Edward Arnold, 1976.
First edition, 1958.
Standard British contribution on histopathology of the nervous system. Has a complete index, excellent illustrations, and reference to both English and foreign literature. For students and neurosurgeons.
R: *Brain* 99: 795 (Dec. 1976); *Journal of Neurosurgery* 46: 557 (Apr. 1977).

Grinker's Neurology. 7th ed. **Nicholas A. Vick, ed.** Springfield, IL: Charles C. Thomas, 1976.
First edition, 1934.
Extensively revised seventh edition incorporates advances in the field of neurobiology. Over 1,000 references have been added. Includes nearly 400 illustrations and has extensive index. Reference work for neurosurgeons and neurologists.
R: *Journal of Neurosurgery* 46: 695 (May 1977); *JAMA* 237: 68 (Jan. 3, 1977); Brandon.

Human Neuropsychology. **Henri Hécaen and Martin L. Albert.** New York: John Wiley, 1978.
Encyclopedic volume which makes a major contribution to fields of neuropsychology, neurology, neurosurgery, and linguistics. Indexed by author and subject. Bibliography covers 66 pages. Useful for those with knowledge of basic terminology as reference text and bibliographic source.
R: *Journal of Neurosurgery* 50: 266 (Feb. 1979).

Multiple Sclerosis Research. **A. N. Davison et al., eds.** London: Her Majesty's Stationery Office, 1975.
Written as a result of joint conference of Medical Research Council and Multiple Sclerosis Society of Great Britain and Northern Ireland. Covers research up to 1975 and discusses such subjects as modern concepts of diagnostic criteria, epidemiological studies, histocompatibility testing, and role of linoleic acid. Comprehensive bibliography and adequate index. Important reading for clinical

neurologists and research workers in multiple sclerosis.
R: *British Medical Bulletin* 33: 86 (1977).

Neurosurgical Management of the Epilepsies. **D. P. Purpura et al., eds.** New York: Raven Press, 1975.

Authoritative review of status of surgical treatment of all epilepsies. In-depth and useful reference source for those working in this area.
R: *JAMA* 235: 210 (Jan. 12, 1976).

Neurotoxicology. Vol. 1. **Leon Roizin, Hirotsugu Shiraki, and Nenad Grĉevic, eds.** New York: Raven Press, 1978.

Multidisciplinary volume on neurotoxicology. Includes discussions on toxic effects of tranquilizers, stimulants, antidepressants, etc. Beautifully illustrated with electron microscopic evidence. Reference source for pathologists, neuropathologists, and neurologists.
R: *Journal of Neurosurgery* 49: 937 (Dec. 1978).

Normal and Abnormal Development of the Human Nervous System. **Ronald J. Lemire et al.** Hagerstown, MD: Harper & Row, 1975.

Covers the neuroanatomy and neuropathology of the developing CNS. Divided into six sections: embryonic and fetal development, neural tube development, segmental structures, suprasegmental structures, CNS anatomy, related anatomy. Contains tables and diagrams as well as numerous references. A definitive work, highly recommended to neurologists, pathologists, pediatricians, embryologists.
R: *Archives of Neurology* 33: 666 (Sept. 1976); *Archives of Pathology & Laboratory Medicine* 101: 162 (Mar. 1977); *Electroencephalography & Clinical Neurophysiology* 41: 444 (Oct. 1976); *Journal of Neurosurgery* 45: 235 (Aug. 1976).

Recent Advances on Pain: Pathophysiology and Clinical Aspects. **John J. Bonica et al., eds.** Springfield, IL: Charles C. Thomas, 1974.

R: *American Family Physician* 11: 186 (June 1975); *Brain* 98: 186 (Mar. 1975); *Journal of Neurosurgery* 42: 485 (Apr. 1975); *Neurology* 25: 1097 (Nov. 1975).

A Review of Anatomical Neurology. **Walter R. Ingram.** Baltimore, MD: University Park Press, 1976.

A timely reference to neuroanatomical concepts. Emphasizes neurophysiological functions. Contains numerous references. A basic and valuable reference source for neuroscientists.
R: *Journal of Neurosurgery* 47: 639 (Oct. 1977).

The Spinal Cord: Basic Aspects and Surgical Considerations. 2d ed. **George Austin, ed.** Springfield, IL: Charles C. Thomas, 1972.

Revised second edition has increased information on effects and actions of spinal cord neurotransmitter substances. Well-referenced with good radiographic illustrations. Recommended to practicing neurosurgeons and residents.
R: *Journal of Neurosurgery* 42: 738 (June 1975).

Spinal Cord Injuries: Comprehensive Management and Research. 2d ed. **Ludwig Guttman.** Oxford, England: Blackwell Scientific Publications, 1976.

First edition, 1973.
Reflects the personal experience of Dr. Guttman, gained in 30 years of care for patients with neurological injury. Comprehensive treatment of basic principles, complications, neurophysiologic and clinical features of spinal cord damage, rehabilitation, and legal aspects. Includes a detailed bibliography. Classical text for neurologists, neurosurgeons, and all hospital and university libraries.
R: *Archives of Neurology* 30: 424 (May 1974); *Journal of Bone and Joint Surgery* 56B: 596 (Aug. 1974); *Journal of Neurosurgery* 47: 137 (July 1977); *JAMA* 228: 1434 (June 10, 1974); *Lancet* 2: 1129 (Nov. 17, 1973).

The Spine. 2 vols. **Richard H. Rothman and Frederick A. Simeone, eds.** Philadelphia, PA: W. B. Saunders, 1975.

Compendium of articles by 27 authors which discusses diagnosis and treatment of spinal disease. Contributions are from a variety of medical disciplines. Descriptions are well annotated, and most sections are provided with extensive bibliographies. Excellent half-tone and line drawing illustrations. Recommended for use by residents, practitioners of orthopedic surgery and neurosurgery, and physical therapists.
R: *Journal of Neurosurgery* 44: 395 (Mar. 1976); *JAMA* 233: 1006 (Sept. 1, 1975); *Physical Therapy* 56: 369 (Mar. 1976).

A Textbook of Neurology. 6th ed. **Houston Merritt.** Philadelphia, PA: Lea & Febiger, 1979.

Discusses the pathology, diagnosis, and treatment of specific neurological diseases. Includes references.
R: *Annals of Internal Medicine* 79: 931 (Dec. 1973); *TBRI* 40: 76 (Feb. 1974); Allyn; Stearns & Ratcliff (*NEJM,* 1969; *NEJM,* 1970).

Therapeutics in Neurology. **Donald B. Calne.** Oxford, England: Blackwell Scientific Publications, 1975.

Neurological text on drug therapy offers answers to clinical problems and guidance to further reading. Valuable reference book.
R: *Brain* 98: 724 (Dec. 1975).

CARDIOVASCULAR SYSTEM

Advances in Cardiovascular Surgery. **John W. Kirklin, ed.** New York: Grune & Stratton, 1973.

Considered a valuable reference on cardiovascular surgery. Detailed discussion of congenital heart disease as well as valvular disease. Authoritative, important work for cardiac surgeons.
R: *British Journal of Surgery* 62: 587 (July 1975); *JAMA* 228: 909 (May 13, 1974); Allyn.

Angina Pectoris. **Desmond G. Julian, ed.** New York: Churchill Livingstone, 1977.

An up-to-date review of the disease. Concise discussions of pathology, history, diagnosis, and treatment of angina pectoris written by sixteen contributors. Pro-

vides full references, detailed account of coronary artery disease. A beneficial reference for all physicians.
R: *American Heart Journal* 96: 841 (1978); *Lancet* 2: 226 (July 30, 1977).

Cardiac and Vascular Diseases. 2 vols. **Hadley L. Conn, Jr., and Orville Horwitz.** Philadelphia, PA: Lea & Febiger, 1971.

Cardiac Catheterization and Angiography. **William Grossman, ed.** Philadelphia, PA: Lea & Febiger, 1974.
A multi-authored compendium on cardiac catheterization; constitutes a practical guide to evaluating cardiac functions. Extensive coverage; highly recommended.
R: *Archives of Internal Medicine* 135: 1407 (Oct. 1975); Allyn.

Cardiac Diagnosis and Treatment. 2d ed. **Noble O. Fowler.** Hagerstown, MD: Harper & Row, 1976.
A clinically oriented book; contains good illustrations, references. Highly recommended to physicians, medical students.
R: *American Heart Journal* 93: 135 (1977); *Chest* 71: A20 (Jan. 1977); *JAMA* 236: 1511 (Sept. 27, 1976); *TBRI* 42: 345 (Nov. 1976); 43: 101 (Mar. 1977); Allyn; Brandon.

Cardiac Mechanics: Physiological, Clinical, and Mathematic Considerations. **Israel Mirsky et al., eds.** New York: John Wiley, 1974.
Assessment of cardiac function in clinical situation. Primarily for academic institutions, the book is of interest to physiologists, cardiologists, biophysicists, and medical engineers.
R: *NTB* 59: 217 (June 1974).

Cardiovascular Physiology. **A. C. Guyton and C. E. Jones, eds.** Baltimore, MD: University Park Press, 1974.
Succinct review of cardiovascular physiology with emphasis on circulation. Carefully outlines significant developments in the field. Problems discussed include pulmonary circulation, control of arterial blood pressure, and myocardial excitation and contraction. Includes extensive bibliographies.
R: *American Heart Journal* 90: 129 (1975).

Cerebral Arterial Disease. **R. W. Ross Russell, ed.** New York: Churchill Livingstone, 1976.
Series of chapters on all aspects of cerebral arterial disease written by notable authorities in the field. Reviews recent advances such as methods of measuring cerebral blood flow and metabolism and improved diagnostic techniques. Provides a useful guide for clinicians.
R: *Brain* 100: 613 (Sept. 1977).

Chest, Heart, and Vascular Disorders for Physiotherapists. **Joan E. Cash, ed.** Philadelphia, PA: J. B. Lippincott, 1975.
Summary of physical management of patients with chest, cardiac, and peripheral vascular problems. Written on level appropriate for students. Also reference for physical therapists.

R: *Physical Therapy* 56: 622 (May 1976).

Clinical Cardiovascular Physiology. **Herbert J. Levine, ed.** New York: Grune & Stratton, 1976.

Reviews common problems in cardiac pathophysiology. A multi-authored book; informative; recommended to clinicians dealing with cardiac disease and to medical libraries.

R: *American Heart Journal* 94: 418 (1977); *JAMA* 236: 2110 (Nov. 1, 1976).

Clinical Disorders of the Heart Beat. 3d ed. **Samuel Bellet.** Philadelphia, PA: Lea & Febiger, 1971.

This is a standard reference which deals with heart beat irregularities. Covers diagnosis and therapy. Includes diagrams, glossary, and bibliographies.

R: Allyn.

Clinical Phonocardiography and External Pulse Recording. 3d ed. **Morton E. Travel.** Chicago, IL: Year Book Medical Publishers, 1978.

New edition includes materials which correlates echocardiogram to other body sounds. Covers all fundamental information. Serves as a text and reference book. One of the standard such books in the field.

R: *Annals of Internal Medicine* 91: 146 (July 1979).

Clinical Scalar Electrocardiography. 6th ed. **B. S. Lipman et al.** Chicago, IL: Year Book Medical Publishers, 1972.

Considered a classic book in scalar interpretation. Well recommended.

R: Allyn; Stearns & Ratcliff (*NEJM,* 1969; *NEJM,* 1970).

Clinical Vectorcardiography. 2d ed. **Te-Chuan Chou et al.** New York: Grune & Stratton, 1974.

Intended for those who interpret vectorcardiograms. Includes clear illustrations. Highly recommended for clinicians.

R: *American Heart Journal* 89: 407 (1975); *Circulation* 51: 574 (Mar. 1975); *TBRI* 41: 181 (May 1975); Allyn; Brandon.

d'Abreu's Practice of Cardiothoracic Surgery. 4th ed. **J. Leigh Collis, D. B. Clarke, and R. Abbey Smith.** Baltimore, MD: Williams & Wilkins, 1976.

Provides a broad perspective of cardiothoracic surgical techniques with step-by-step explanations to therapy approach. Illustrations are an excellent accompaniment to the systematic presentation. Contains many helpful references. A beneficial reference for students and surgeons.

R: *JAMA* 237: 276 (Jan. 17, 1977).

Development of Angiography and Cardiovascular Catheterization. **T. Doby.** Littleton, MA: Publishing Sciences Group, 1976.

Classic book which traces history of angiography as diagnostic and therapeutic tool. Closing chapter followed by biographies of 62 scientists who contributed to its development. Contains interesting anecdotes and illustrations.

R: *Chest* 72: 32 (1978).

Diagnosis of Diseases of the Chest. 2d ed. 2 vols. **Robert G. Fraser and J. A. Peter Pare.** Philadelphia, PA: W. B. Saunders, 1978.
First edition, 1970.
Comprehensive work in chest radiology has been expanded from two volumes to four. Serves as a diagnostic review of chest disease. Over 6,000 citations, detailed table of contents, and quality reproductions. For radiologists and physicians involved with chest disease.
R: *American Journal of Roentgenology* 131: 1128 (Dec. 1978); *Radiology* 128: 300 (1978).

Diagnostic Methods in Cardiology. **Noble O. Fowler, ed.** Philadelphia, PA: F. A. Davis, 1975.
A highly recommended book on cardiac diagnosis. Update includes recent methods. A fine book; well organized. For physicians interested in cardiovascular technique.
R: Allyn.

Diseases of the Heart. **Noble O. Fowler.** New York: Harper & Row, 1968.
Contributions from authorities in the field. Well referenced; recommended.
R: Allyn; Stearns & Ratcliff (*AJN*; *NEJM,* 1969; *NEJM,* 1970).

Diseases of the Heart. 3d. ed. **Charles K. Friedberg.** Philadelphia, PA: W. B. Saunders, 1966.
A classic book on cardiac examination and treatment of cardiac disease.
R: Allyn; Stearns & Ratcliff (*AJN*; *NEJM,* 1969; *NEJM,* 1970).

Echocardiography. 2d ed. **Harvery Feigenbaum.** Philadelphia, PA: Lea & Febiger, 1976.
First edition, 1972.
A revised edition of this comprehensive book on echocardiography. Discusses the most recent techniques in the field with an extensive amount of references. Recommended as a good source on ultrasonic imaging of the heart.
R: *Radiology* 124: 470 (1977); Allyn.

Exercise Testing and Exercise Training in Coronary Heart Disease. **John P. Naughton and Herman K. Hellerstein, eds.** New York: Academic Press, 1973.
A monograph on stress testing; contains a large amount of data and references. For cardiologists.
R: *American Heart Journal* 88: 131 (July 1974); *NEJM* 291: 109 (July 11, 1974); *TBRI* 40: 323 (Oct. 1974); Allyn.

Gibbon's Surgery of the Chest. 3d ed. **David C. Sabiston and Frank C. Spencer, eds.** Philadelphia, PA: W. B. Saunders, 1976.
Third edition has expanded section on coronary disease, including authoritative chapters on arteriography, resuscitation, and therapy of arteriosclerosis. Excellent section on cardiovasuclar surgery.
R: *British Journal of Surgery* 64: 453 (June 1977); *JAMA* 236: 1751 (Oct. 11, 1976); Allyn; Brandon; Inke; Stearns & Ratcliff (*NEJM,* 1970).

Grant's Clinical Electrocardiography. 2d ed. **J. Beckwith.** New York: Mc-Graw-Hill, 1970.

Purpose of text is to present basics of electrocardiography.
R: Allyn.

The Heart. 4th ed. 2 vols. **J. Willis Hurst, ed.** New York: McGraw-Hill, 1978.

Second edition, 1970; third edition, 1974.
An extensive reference text, considered a valuable addition to medical library. Clear format. Highly recommended.
R: *American Journal of Cardiology* 35: 593 (1973); *Canadian Family Physician* 21: 157 (1974); Allyn; Stearns & Ratcliff (*NEJM,* 1969; *NEJM,* 1970).

Heart Disease. **Earl N. Silber and Louis N. Katz.** New York: Macmillan, 1975.

Written for practicing physicians, text presents physiological, pathological, and electrocardiographic aspects of cardiology. References, illustrations, and tables, cross-references, and detailed index are included.
R: *American Heart Journal* 91: 542 (1976); *RSR* 3: 37 (July–Dec. 1975); Allyn.

The Lymphatics: Diseases, Lymphography and Surgery. **John B. Kinmonth, ed.** Baltimore, MD: Williams & Wilkins, 1972.

Summarizes author's efforts in delineating more closely the problem of lymphatic disease. Text is well written, photographs are clear, and bibliographies include basic, pertinent references. For all physicians interested in vascular diseases.
R: *Annals of Internal Medicine* 81: 130 (July 1974); *BMJ* 1: 181 (Jan. 20, 1973).

The Mammalian Myocardium. **Glenn A. Langer and Allen J. Brady, eds.** New York: John Wiley, 1974.

Comprehensive text on subcellular function of myocardium. Expert editors have created an organized, readable monograph which is excellent beginning reference for students and practicing specialists who wish to improve understanding of recent advances in mechanisms governing cardiac performance.
R: *American Journal of Cardiology* 36: 414 (1975).

Mechanisms of Contraction in the Normal and Failing Heart. 2d ed. **Eugene Braunwald et al.** Boston, MA: Little, Brown, 1976.

A review of hemodynamics in relation to heart problems. Contributions from research authorities; an up-to-date presentation of interest to all cardiologists.
R: *American Heart Journal* 92: 545 (1976); *Annals of Internal Medicine* 85: 413 (Sept. 1976); *Connecticut Medicine* 40: 573 (Aug. 1976); *Lahey Clinic Foundation Bulletin* 25: 198 (Oct.–Dec. 1976); *Medical Journal of Australia* 2: 653 (Oct. 23, 1976); *TBRI* 42: 343 (Nov. 1976); 43: 18 (Jan. 1977); 43: 99 (Mar. 1977); Allyn.

Myocardial Diseases. **Noble O. Fowler.** New York: Grune & Stratton, 1973.

Compendium of present knowledge of myocardial diseases covers pathological findings, familial aspects, immunologic studies, role of viruses, etc. Sections on

clinical findings provide information on evaluation of patients with myocardial disorders. Enumerates advances in the field in the last decade.
R: *American Journal of Cardiology* 34: 749 (1974); Allyn.

Myocardial Infarction. **Eliot Corday and H. J. C. Swan.** Baltimore, MD: Williams & Wilkins, 1973.

Gathers together concepts, physiological findings, diagnosis, and treatment techniques of myocardial infarctions. Also discusses pathophysiology and echocardiography. Well written and illustrated; analysis of the literature on myocardial infarction. Includes information on patient care. Recommended to cardiologists, internists, and pathologists as a standard reference.
R: *American Journal of Cardiology* 33: 322 (1974); Allyn.

Noninvasive Evaluation of Human Circulation: Clinical, Clinicopharmacological and Data Processing Aspects. **J. Simonyi.** New York: International Publications Service, 1977.

Contribution to theory and practice of noninvasive cardiology. Acquaints American physicians with foreign work in this area.
R: *JAMA* 237: 692 (Feb. 14, 1977).

Non-Invasive Methods in Cardiology. **Samuel Zoneraich.** Springfield, IL: Charles C. Thomas, 1975.

Fundamental discussion of recordings of heart sounds, venous and arterial pulses, and electrical activity of the heart. Clearly written text.
R: *American Heart Journal* 90: 813 (1976).

Peripheral Arterial Disease. 2d ed. Vol. 4. **W. F. Barker.** Philadelphia, PA: W. B. Saunders, 1975.

Features excellent illustrations. Outstanding reference source for students, house officers, and workers in the field of vascular disorders.
R: *Annals of Surgery* 184: 59A (Sept. 1976); Allyn.

Practical Echocardiology. **J. Roelandt.** Forest Grove, OR: Research Studies Press, 1977.

Part of the *Ultrasound in Medicine* series, orients those who read echocardiograms. Covers basics of ultrasound, instrumentation, etc., various structures of the heart as seen by echo, and specific disease processes. Well-organized volume includes real-time illustrations that provide cross-sectional illustrations in comparison with M-mode strips.
R: *American Journal of Roentgenology* 129: 960 (Nov. 1977).

Pulmonary Emboli: A Progress in Cardiovascular Diseases Reprint. **Arthur A. Sasahara, Edmund H. Sonnenblick, and Michael Lesch, eds.** New York: Grune & Stratton, 1975.

A collection of papers originally published as a symposium in *Circulation* in 1974. Presents experimental data as well as practical information on diagnosis and therapy of pulmonary embolic disease. The 1973 urokinase pulmonary embolism trial provides most of the material for discussion. Highly recommended to internists and chest physicians.

R: *Annals of Internal Medicine* 84: 377 (Mar. 1976); Allyn.

Recent Advances in Cardiology. 7th ed. Edinburgh: Churchill Livingstone, 1977.

First edition, 1929.
R: *American Heart Journal* 87: 266 (1974); *American Journal of Cardiology* 33: 322 (1974); *BMJ* 1: 1470 (Mar. 12, 1977).

Recent Trends in Cardiovascular and Thoracic Surgery. **Joseph B. Borman, ed.** New York: Grune & Stratton, 1975.

Essays from international centers about heart disease, lung and esophageal surgery. Valuable information on selection of patients for operations and evaluation of long-term care.
R: *Annals of Thoracic Surgery* 22: 403 (Oct. 1976); *JAMA* 235: 211 (Jan. 12, 1976).

Surgical Diseases of the Chest. 3d ed. **Brian Blades, ed.** St. Louis, MO: C. V. Mosby, 1974.

Twenty-two chapters written by different surgeons on surgical treatment of diseases of the chest, with over half on heart surgery. Subject index; 788 photographs and drawings. Intended for surgeons, medical practitioners, and students.
R: *RSR* 2: 130 (Oct.–Dec. 1974); Allyn.

Surgical Treatment of Congenital Heart Disease. 2d ed. **Grady L. Hallman and Denton A. Cooley.** Philadelphia, PA: Lea & Febiger, 1975.

Well-illustrated surgical book on techniques of performing majority of cardiovascular operations. Sections on cardiopulmonary bypass and operations within the heart. Reference for medical students and residents.
R: *Annals of Surgery* 184: 534 (Oct. 1976); *Archives of Surgery* 111: 726 (June 1976).

DENTISTRY

Burket's Oral Medicine: Diagnosis and Treatment. 7th ed. **Malcolm A. Lynch, ed.** Philadelphia, PA: J. B. Lippincott, 1977.

Thorough revision reflects latest developments and current literature in field of oral medicine. Authoritative standard work for dentists and dental students.

Cleft Lip and Palate: Surgical, Dental, and Speech Aspects. **William C. Grabb et al.** Boston, MA: Little, Brown, 1971.

A comprehensive monograph; covers all aspects of cleft lip including surgical and dental procedures, speech and hearing problems. Useful as both a reference work and a manual. A classic source, highly recommended.
R: *Archives of Otolaryngology* 95: 285 (Mar. 1972).

Cost and Benefit of Fluoride in the Prevention of Dental Caries, WHO Offset Pub. no. 9. **G. N. Davies.** Geneva: World Health Organization, 1974.

Reviews different methods of fluoride application. Includes numerous tables and

references. Discusses side effects, cost-benefit ratios.
R: *RSR* 4: 43 (Jan.–Mar. 1976).

The Dental Assistant. 5th ed. **Richard E. Richardson and Roger E. Barton.** New York: McGraw-Hill, 1978.

Fourth edition, 1970.
A basic reference source for dental assistants, detailing fundamental, clinical procedures, management of instruments, and other subjects relevant to the dental assistant. Expanded edition now contains a chapter on oral diagnosis. Profusely illustrated; thoroughly revised. Gathers together core information for dental assistants.
R: *Journal of Allied Health* 2: 196 (Fall 1973).

Dental X-ray Protection. US National Council of Radiation Protection and Measurements Report no. 35. **US National Council of Radiation Protection and Measurements.** Washington, DC: US Government Printing Office, 1972.

Discusses the design of dental equipment, including structural shielding of X-rays. Offers guidelines to radiation protection; answers questions most frequently asked by patients concerned with radiation exposure.
R: *Journal of Oral Surgery* 31: 948 (Dec. 1973).

Oral Pathology. 6th ed. 2 vols. **Robert Gorlin and Henry Goldman.** St. Louis, MO: C. V. Mosby, 1970.

A classic in the field of tooth, jaw, and oral mucosa pathology. Copiously illustrated with many color plates. Includes numerous bibliographies. Well indexed.
R: Stearns & Ratcliff (*NEJM,* 1969; *NEJM,* 1970).

Oral Surgery. 5th ed. 2 vols. **Kurt H. Thoma.** St. Louis, MO: C. V. Mosby, 1969.

Comprehensive coverage of oral surgery. Emphasizes surgical procedures and proper patient handling. Includes illustrations, bibliographies, and index. Aimed at the general practitioner.

Orthodontics: Principles and Practice. 3d ed. **Touro M. Graber.** Philadelphia, PA: W. B. Saunders, 1972.

Integration of theory and practical management. Systematic approach to the art of orthodontics. Emphasizes biomechanical methods of tooth removal. Copiously illustrated; complete with references and index.

An Outline of Dental Materials and Their Selection. **William J. O'Brien and Gunnar Ryge.** Philadelphia, PA: W. B. Saunders, 1978.

Concise summary of major topics in dental materials also provides programmed reviews in the following areas: viscoelasticity, ceramics, clinical research programming, polymer systems for composites, etc.

Principles of Dental Public Health. 3d ed. **James M. Dunning.** Cambridge, MA: Harvard University Press, 1979.

First edition, 1962; second edition, 1970.

Totally revised introduction to the field of public health. Recognized as the most authoritative and comprehensive publication in this field. Lists the specifics of planning, operating, and evaluating dental public health programs. Includes current references.
R: *NEJM* 301: 448 (Aug. 23, 1979).

DERMATOLOGY

Acne: Morphogenesis and Treatment. **Gerd Plewig and Albert M. Kligman.** New York: Springer-Verlag, 1975.

Photographic and conceptual treatise on morphology, pathogenesis, and treatment of acne. Magnificent color close-ups are valuable additions. Recommended for dermatologists.
R: *Archives of Dermatology* 112: 901 (June 1976).

Cancer of the Skin: Biology, Diagnosis, Management. 2 vols. **Rafael Andrade et al., eds.** Philadelphia, PA: W. B. Saunders, 1976.

Well-organized text stresses multidisciplinary approach to skin cancer. Reflects over 25 years of experience at New York University Skin and Cancer Unit. Prolific references; excellent black-and-white photographs and complete index. Comprehensive work highly recommended for medical libraries.
R: *BMJ* 1: 1653 (June 25, 1977); *JAMA* 238: 428 (Aug. 1, 1977).

Consultations in Dermatology II. **Walter B. Shelley.** Philadelphia, PA: W. B. Saunders, 1974.

Consists of 50 essays presenting clinical and physiological viewpoints in dermatology. Includes illustrations, annotated bibliography, index. A well written reference of interest not only to dermatologists but to general physicians as well.
R: *Archives of Dermatology* 110: 648 (Oct. 1974); *TBRI* 41: 31 (Jan. 1975).

Dermatoglyphics in Medical Disorders. **B. Schaumann and M. Alter.** New York: Springer-Verlag, 1976.

An excellent, detailed book on dermatoglyphics. Presents interpretative techniques in a systematic manner. Highly recommended to dermatologists and clinical geneticists.

Differential Diagnosis in Dermatology. **G. W. Korting and R. Denk.** Philadelphia, PA: W. B. Saunders, 1976.

Discusses little- and well-known subjects in dermatologic diagnosis. Well organized; includes excellent photographs. A classic reference for dermatologists.
R: *Dermatologica* 154: 128 (1977); *JAMA* 237: 2336 (May 23, 1977).

Histopathology of the Skin. 5th ed. **Walter F. Lever and Gundula Schaumburg-Lever.** Philadelphia, PA: J. B. Lippincott, 1975.

Latest edition of classic textbook has been extensively revised to reflect latest advances. Contains expanded sections on cutaneous biology and electron microscopy. Clinical descriptions are concise and informative; updated histopathological descriptions remain lucid and precise. Well-selected photomicrographs. Bibliographies include important literature and are up-to-date. Detailed index refers to

principal discussions and illustrative material as well as regular text items. Should be handy to every pathologist and dermatologist who reads skin biopsies; required reading for residents.
R: *Journal of Investigative Dermatology* 67: 288 (Aug. 1976); *JAMA* 235: 543 (Feb. 2, 1976); *RSR* 4: 46 (Jan.–Mar. 1976).

Microbiology of Human Skin. **W. C. Noble and Dorothy A. Somerville.** Philadelphia, PA: W. B. Saunders, 1974.

Major compendium on human cutaneous microbiology. Reflects vast personal experience of authors. Recommended reading for residents, dermatologists, general practitioners, and research workers.
R: *Archives of Dermatology* 111: 404 (Mar. 1975).

New Concepts in Surgical Pathology of the Skin. **Richard J. Reed.** New York: John Wiley, 1976.

An excellent reference text for all pathologists and medical libraries.
R: *Archives of Pathology & Laboratory Medicine* 101: 335 (June 1977); 101: 455 (Aug. 1977).

Recent Advances in Dermatology. 4th ed. **Arthur Rook, ed.** New York: Churchill Livingstone, 1977.

Third edition, 1974.
Contributions of well-known dermatologists are contained in this volume which reviews numerous topics on dermatology in detail. Subjects such as viral infections, contact dermatitis, and acne were chosen because of their frequent occurrence or their reflection of notable recent developments. Comprehensive lists of references and well-reproduced figures. Recommended to practitioner, student, and research worker in dermatology.
R: *Archives of Dermatology* 110: 649 (Oct. 1974); 114: 140 (Jan. 1978); *BMJ* 2: 126 (Apr. 13, 1974); 2: 629 (Sept. 3, 1977); *JAMA* 230: 906 (Nov. 11, 1974).

Recent Advances in Dermato-Pharmacology. **Philip Frost, Edward C. Gomez, and Nardo Zaias, eds.** New York: Spectrum Publications, 1978.
R: *Archives of Dermatology* 114: 1863 (Dec. 1978); *Lancet* 1: 970 (May 6, 1978).

Skin Signs of Systemic Disease. **Irwin M. Braverman.** Philadelphia, PA: W. B. Saunders, 1975.

Not intended as a comprehensive treatment of skin disorders. Emphasizes common skin diseases and processes. Also focuses on manifestations of rare and unusual metastases, from carcinoma to endocrine disorders. Beautifully illustrated with 192 high-quality color plates. Includes extensive bibliographies and complete index. Ready reference tool of the common and unusual for dermatologists, general practitioners, internists, and plastic surgeons.
R: *Plastic and Reconstructive Surgery* 57: 657 (1976).

Skin Surgery. 4th ed. **E. Epstein and E. Epstein, Jr.** Springfield, IL: Charles C. Thomas, 1977.

Reference text for dermatologists who perform skin surgery. Chapters cover traditional aspects such as electrosurgery and dermabrasion as well as new ones

such as chemosurgery, cryosurgery, and investigative surgical therapy. Volume is very well organized and illustrated.
R: *Archives of Dermatology* 113: 1146 (Aug. 1977); *Plastic and Reconstructive Surgery* 60: 442 (1977).

ENDOCRINOLOGY

Complications of Diabetes. **Harry Keen and John Jarrett, eds.** London: Edward Arnold, 1975.

Reviews the state of the art of research related to the complications of diabetes. Each chapter is a separate essay with thorough bibliographic references. Subjects covered include: biochemical changes, pregnancy and diabetes, pathology, etiology, metabolic disorders, retinopathy. A good ready reference source; provides much basic information.
R: *Diabetes* 25: 533 (June 1976).

The Diabetic Foot. **Marvin E. Levin and Lawrence W. O'Neal.** St. Louis, MO: C. V. Mosby, 1977.

Information on practical management of diabetes which is valuable for all those who treat this disease and its complications.
R: *Annals of Internal Medicine* 80: 435 (1974).

Duncan's Diseases of Metabolism. 8th ed. 2 vols. **Philip K. Bondy and Leon E. Rosenberg, eds.** Philadelphia, PA: W. B. Saunders, 1979.

Volume 1, *Genetics and Metabolism*; volume 2, *Endocrinology.*
Provides basis for understanding, diagnosis, and treatment of various metabolic disorders. Reference text for students, house officers, and endocrinologists.
R: *Annals of Internal Medicine* 81: 573 (1974).

Endocrinology, Metabolism & Gastroenterology. 3 vols. **Leslie J. DeGroot, ed.** New York: Grune & Stratton, 1979.

Volume 1, *Neuroendocrinology*; volume 2, *Disorders of Bone and Bone Mineral Metabolism: Parathyroid Hormone, Calcitonin, and Vitamin D*; volume 3, *Sexual Differentiation.*
Three-volume text presents functional and anatomical knowledge of endocrinology. Detailed, concise, and complete in scope. Pertinent for those concerned with research and patient care.

Endocrinology of Pregnancy. 2d ed. **Fritz Fuchs and A. Klopper, eds.** Hagerstown, MD: Harper & Row, 1977.

Timely material, clinically oriented. Provides basic understanding of the subject.
R: *JAMA* 237: 2651 (June 13, 1977).

Epidemiology of Diabetes and Its Vascular Lesions. **Kelly M. West.** New York: Elsevier North-Holland, 1978.

Author provides in-depth coverage of all aspects of diabetes except treatment. Ten chapters cover range from epidemiological and laboratory methods to comprehensive review of courses of types of diabetes. Up-to-date and comprehen-

sive; includes about 2,500 references up to 1977. Recommended to those who study diabetes.
R: *BMJ* 1: 539 (1979).

Gynecologic Endocrinology. 2d ed. **Jay J. Gold, ed.** Hagerstown, MD: Harper & Row, 1975.
Lucid review of subject; will serve as reference for students and clinicians.
R: *Annals of Internal Medicine* 83: 922 (Dec. 1975); *JAMA* 235: 1273 (1976); *TBRI* 42: 61 (Feb. 1976).

Hormone Chemistry. 2d ed. **W. R. Butt.** New York: John Wiley, 1977.
Provides basic facts about structure, metabolism, and functions of vertebrate hormones. Each section also includes data about synthetic analogues of the natural hormones. Well produced and illustrated with many clear diagrams. Carefully selected bibiographies include references to over 1,400 original papers and reviews.
R: *Heredity* 40: 321 (Apr. 1978).

Human Endocrinology: A Developmental Approach. **Dorothy B. Villee.** Philadelphia, PA: W. B. Saunders, 1975.
Investigates the biochemistry of fetal development; proceeds systematically, explaining prenatal hormone activity from fertilization to placenta development. Well referenced and indexed. An authoritative book on endocrinology and reproductive physiology.
R: *American Journal of Diseases of Children* 130: 788 (July 1976); Allyn.

Joslin's Diabetes Mellitus. 12th ed. **Alexander Marble et al., eds.** Philadelphia, PA: Lea & Febiger, 1979.
First edition, 1916: 11th edition, 1971.
Solid survey of current and past knowledge of diabetes balanced as to clinical application and scientific information. Twenty-six authors cooperated on 32 chapters. Well organized; generous use of figures; extensively referenced. Source book for all physicians and students of diabetes.
R: *Archives of Internal Medicine* 131: 308 (Feb. 1973); *Diabetes* 22: 68 (Jan. 1973); Allyn.

The Prostaglandins. 3 vols. **Peter W. Ramwell, ed.** New York: Plenum, 1973–1977.
Reports on the chemistry and physiology of the prostaglandins; discusses developments in related male and female reproductive functions, cardiovascular implications, and asthma.
R: *Journal of Pharmaceutical Science* 62: 1908 (Nov. 1973).

Stress in Health and Disease. **Hans Selye.** London: Butterworths, 1976.
Deals mainly with the adrenal secretions which can act as stressors. History of ideas of stress-disease mechanisms and medicolegal implications. Discusses nervous and hormonal mediators and related diseases. Summarizes developments in neuropharmacology and neuroendocrinology in the past twenty years. Consid-

ered a state-of-the-art volume, most useful to those seeking an outline of general concepts in stress and disease. Extensive bibliographies.
R: *Archives of Neurology* 34: 202 (Mar. 1977).

Textbook of Endocrinology. 5th ed. **Robert H. Williams, ed.** Philadelphia, PA: W. B. Saunders, 1974.
Fourth edition, 1968.
Extensive coverage of common principles of endocrinology. Describes normal and abnormal functions. Signed chapters. Standard reference text for beginning student and experienced physician.
R: *Annals of Internal Medicine* 82: 292 (Feb. 1975); *Journal of the American Osteopathic Association* 74: 255 (Nov. 1974); *TBRI* 41: 33 (Jan. 1975); 41: 150 (Apr. 1975); Allyn; Stearns & Ratcliff (*NEJM,* 1969; *NEJM,* 1970).

GASTROINTESTINAL SYSTEM

Clinical Gastroenterology. 2d ed. **Howard M. Spiro.** New York: Macmillan, 1977.
This is an authoritative, comprehensive monograph on clinical aspects of gastroenterology. It includes useful photographs from gross specimens, and X-rays. Format is organized generally by anatomic section (i.e. pancreas, esophagus, small intestine). Includes an up-to-date bibliography. Recommended to clinicians, medical students, and departmental libraries in gastroenterology.
R: *American Journal of Clinical Nutrition* 30: 1568 (Sept. 1977); *Annals of Internal Medicine* 87: 254 (Aug. 1977); Stearns & Ratcliff (*NEJM.* 1970).

Cope's Early Diagnosis of the Acute Abdomen. 15th ed. **William Silen, rev.** London: Oxford University Press, 1979.
First edition, 1921.
Provides detailed descriptions and diagrams of acute conditions of the abdomen. A classic monograph of diagnostic descriptions.
R: *BMJ* 2: 485 (Aug. 25, 1979).

Diseases of the Esophagus. **G. Vantrappen and J. Hellemans.** New York: Springer-Verlag, 1974.
A classic volume on the details of normal and abnormal esophageal behavior. Well-documented analysis of normal anatomic and physiological data and methods of investigation of pathologies. Clear roentgenographic reproductions, current references, and readable text. Valuable addition to hospital libraries.
R: *British Journal of Radiology* 48: 884 (1975); *Chest* 72: 27 (1978).

Diseases of the Gallbladder and Biliary System. **Leslie J. Schoenfield.** New York: John Wiley, 1977.
Provides current information on pathophysiology and treatment of major diseases of the liver and gastrointestinal tract. Some subjects covered are congenital abnormalities, parasitic disorders of gallbladder, and detailed attention to gallstones. Illustrations and radiographs of high quality; extensively referenced. Recommended to surgical or medical gastroenterologists, general internists, and students and for inclusion in medical libraries.

R: *Digestive Diseases & Science* 24: 89 (Jan. 1979); *Lancet* 1: 588 (Mar. 18, 1978); *NEJM* 298: 1097 (May 11, 1978).

Diseases of the Liver. 4th ed. **Leon Schiff, ed.** Philadelphia, PA: J. B. Lippincott, 1975.

Third edition, 1969.
Revised and expanded. Deals with epidemiology prevention, and management of liver disease. New material includes information on laproscopy, treatment of gall stones, immunologic disorders. A volume of wide scope; indexed. Well recommended as a standard reference source.
R: *Gastroenterology* 71: 708 (Oct. 1976); *RSR* 4: 91 (Apr.–June 1976); Allyn.

Diseases of the Liver and Biliary System. 5th ed. **Sheila Sherlock.** Oxford, England: Blackwell Scientific Publications, 1975.

First edition, 1945; fourth edition, 1968.
Rewritten text shows advances pertaining to hepatitis B virus, immunology of liver disease, therapy of acute hepatic failure, and evaluation of new radiological techniques. Thirty-eight percent of illustrations are new, references are current, and 21-page index is comprehensive. Recommended for medical libraries.
R: *Gastroenterology* 70: 630 (Apr. 1976); *RSR* 4: 91 (Apr.–June 1976); Allyn; Stearns & Ratcliff (*NEJM*, 1969; *NEJM*, 1970).

The Double Contrast Examination of the Colon: Experiences With the Welin Modification. **Solve Welin and Grethe Welin.** Littleton, MA: Publishing Sciences Group, 1976.

Provides valuable information for radiologists performing air contrast examinations in addition to being an excellent introduction to those just starting to perform the procedures. For medical school libraries and radiology departments.
R: *Radiology* 121: 306 (Nov. 1976).

The Early Diagnosis of the Acute Abdomen. 14th ed. **Zachary Cope.** New York: Oxford University Press, 1972.

First edition, 1921.
Emphasizes the relationship between anatomy, neuroanatomy, and physiology of the abdomen. Attempts to correlate these factors to diagnosis of disease. Chapters arranged by symptoms of abdominal disease. Considered a valuable guide and reference for students and physicians.
R: *Gastroenterology* 64: 1062 (May 1973).

Endoscopy. **George Berci, ed.** New York: Appleton-Century-Crofts, 1976.

Complete reference book includes work from 58 contributing authors. Well illustrated.
R: *Clinical Pediatrics* 17: 589 (July 1978).

The Esophagus. **W. Spencer Payne and Arthur M. Olsen.** Philadelphia, PA: Lea & Febiger, 1974.

Valuable text about the diagnosis and management of diseases of the esophagus. Illustrations are numerous and excellent. Designed for surgeons, gastroenterologists, and medical students.

R: *Archives of Otolaryngology* 100: 481 (Dec. 1974).

Gastrointestinal Angiography. 2d ed. **S. R. Reuter and H. C. Redman.** Eastbourne, England: Holt-Saunders, 1977.

First edition, 1972.
Second edition reflects changes in application of angiography. Detailed description of catheterization techniques has been added while those on tumors, trauma, and vascular diseases remain excellent. Illustrations are of high quality; bibliographies follow each chapter.
R: *Digestion* 18: 295 (1978).

Gastrointestinal Disease: Pathophysiology, Diagnosis, Management. 2d ed. **Marvin H. Sleisenger and John S. Fordtran.** Philadelphia, PA: W. B. Saunders, 1978.

First edition, 1973.
Major contribution to gastroenterological literature from leading authorities. Begins with discussions of nutritional factors and immunological disturbances which are related to intestinal tract. Second half of book treats subjects of diagnosis and management. Consistent in style and content; written for students as well as gastroenterologists.
R: *BMJ* 1: 463 (Feb. 22, 1975); Allyn.

Ileostomy: Surgery, Physiology and Management. **Graham L. Hill.** New York: Grune & Stratton, 1976.

Comprehensive monograph covers all aspects of ileostomy surgery. Operation is described and well illustrated in one chapter which, along with others, combines to give a total picture of ileostomy, its function and problems. Excellent source book for those who treat ileostomy patients. Authoritative text, clear presentation, and references cover significant literature.
R: *American Journal of Proctology* 28: 12 (Apr. 1977); *Archives of Surgery* 111: 1412 (Dec. 1976).

Inflammatory Bowel Disease. **Joseph B. Kirsner and Ray G. Shorter, eds.** Philadelphia, PA: Lea & Febiger, 1975.

Thorough and balanced coverage of ulcerative and granulomatous colitis. Makes a valuable contribution to knowledge of inflammatory bowel disease. Includes useful references and is well edited. Recommended highly to surgeons, gastroenterologists, and their residents.
R: *Gastroenterology* 69: 1028 (Oct. 1975); *JAMA* 234: 541 (Nov. 3, 1975); *Journal of the American Osteopathic Association* 74: 1191 (Aug. 1975); *Mayo Clinic Proceedings* 50: 675 (Nov. 1975); *NEJM* 294: 617 (Mar. 11, 1976); *Surgery, Gynecology and Obstetrics* 142: 95 (Jan. 1976); *TBRI* 41: 346 (Nov. 1975); 41: 388 (Dec. 1975); 42: 24 (Jan. 1976); 42: 100 (Mar. 1976); 42: 224 (June 1976); Brandon.

The Liver: Normal and Abnormal Functions. **Frederick F. Becker, ed.** New York: Marcel Dekker, 1975.

Emphasis is placed on pathogenesis and relation of liver tests to clinical abnormalities. Recommended for those who function in hepatology, pathology, and gastroenterology.

R: *American Journal of Digestive Diseases* 20: 898 (Sept. 1975); *Johns Hopkins Medical Journal* 137: 249 (Nov. 1975); *Medical Journal of Australia* 1: 170 (Feb. 7, 1976); *TBRI* 41: 342 (Nov. 1975); 42: 20 (Jan. 1976); 42: 219 (June 1976).

Radiology of the Gallbladder and Bile Ducts. **Robert N. Berk and Arthur R. Clemett.** Philadelphia, PA: W. B. Saunders, 1977.

A basic reference text; excellent format covers biliary tract radiology. Emphasizes techniques and procedures. Recommended for radiologists and gastroenterologists.
R: *Annals of Internal Medicine* 89: 294 (Aug. 1978).

Recent Advances in Gastroenterology. 3d ed. **Ian A. Bouchier, ed.** Baltimore, MD: Williams & Wilkins, 1977.

Second edition, 1972.
R: *Annals of Internal Medicine* 80: 128 (Jan. 1974); *BMJ* 2: 251 (Apr. 28, 1973); *Gastroenterology* 66: 632 (Apr. 1974); *JAMA* 238: 2544 (Dec. 5, 1977).

Strauss and Welt's Diseases of the Kidney. 3d ed. **Lawrence E. Early and Carl W. Gottschalk, eds.** Boston, MA: Little, Brown, 1979.

Second edition, *Diseases of the Kidney,* 1971.
Extensively covers the diagnosis and treatment of kidney diseases. A multi-authored compendium which includes extensive bibliographies.

GENETICS

Chromosome Techniques: Theory and Practice. 2d ed. **A. K. Sharma and A. Sharma.** Baltimore, MD: University Park Press, 1972.

First edition, 1965.
Comprehensive treatise on technological aspects of chromosome study. New edition incorporates recent advances in chromosome methodology and examination techniques. Numerous references and twenty full-page plates are included. Considered a worthy reference source.
R: *American Journal of Human Genetics* 25: 460 (July 1973).

Congenital Deformities of the Hand and Forearm. **H. Kelikian.** Philadelphia, PA: W. B. Saunders, 1974.

A compendious work on the subject of congenital deformities of the limbs. Chapters organized by general type of deformity. Illustrations include radiographs, photographs, drawings. Clear presentation, selective bibliography. A classic treatise, recommended to all hospitals, orthopedic surgeons.
R: *Archives of Pathology & Laboratory Medicine* 100: 452 (Aug. 1976); *Journal of Bone and Joint Surgery* 57A: 589 (June 1975); *JAMA* 231: 1291 (Mar. 24, 1975).

Davidson's Biochemistry of the Nucleic Acids. 8th ed. **Revised by R. L. P. Adams et al.** London: Chapman & Hall, 1976.

First edition, 1950.
An essential reference for researchers who work with nucleic acids. Contains a comprehensive bibliography, information on research techniques. A handy reference; highly recommended.

R: *Heredity* 41: 116 (Aug. 1978).

Elements of Medical Genetics. 4th ed. **Alan E. H. Emery.** Edinburgh: Churchill Livingstone, 1975.

Fourth edition provides a thorough overview of field of genetics. Covers historical development, biochemical genetics, radiation, and other topics. Includes a good glossary. Adds valuable information to nature-nurture controversy.
R: *Pharmaceutical Journal* 215: 562 (1975).

Genetic Screening Programs: Principles and Research. **Committee for the Study of Inborn Errors of Metabolism, US National Research Council.** Washington, DC: US National Academy of Sciences, 1975.

Comprehensive discussions of genetic screening of such diseases as Tay-Sachs, PKU, Down's Syndrome. Covers ethical and legislative aspects of genetic testing. Contains appendixes of supporting material. Includes a great deal of information; especially recommended to those interested in preventive medicine.
R: *American Journal of Human Genetics* 29: 109 (Jan. 1977); *Annals of Internal Medicine* 86: 514 (Apr. 1977).

The Genetics of Human Populations. **L. L. Cavalli-Sforza and W. F. Bodmer.** San Francisco, CA: W. H. Freeman, 1971.

Outstanding book which presents theory of genetics in light of the origins and maintenance of differences among men. New figures and tables; terminates with a series of problems. A major reference for human geneticists.
R: *American Journal of Human Genetics* 25: 112 (Jan. 1973); *Science* 176: 659 (May 12, 1972).

Human Chromosomes. **S. Makino.** Oxford, England: North-Holland, 1975.

Comprehensive account of current state of knowledge in human chromosome research. Greater part of volume describes chromosome features of normal and affected states derived from studies on Japanese populations. Highly informative section on irradiation gives detailed account of findings from survivors of Hiroshima and Nagasaki bombings. Useful for comparisons with data obtained in studies on other racial groups. New methods of chromosome staining described but not used in illustrations. Contains wealth of information.
R: *Heredity* 37: 135 (Aug. 1976).

Lysosomes and Storage Diseases. **H. G. Hers and F. Van Hoof, eds.** New York: Academic Press, 1973.

Devoted to storage diseases associated with a disruption of lysosomal function. Remarkable in depth of coverage and ability to integrate clinical and biochemical material. Comprehensive coverage; adequately referenced; subject and author index.
R: *American Journal of Human Genetics* 26: 664 (Sept. 1974).

The Metabolic Basis of Inherited Disease. 4th ed. **John B. Stanbury, James B. Wyngaarden, and Donald S. Fredrickson, eds.** New York: McGraw-Hill, 1978.

First edition, 1960; third edition, 1972.

Authoritative work discusses disorders of inherited diseases, described in biochemical terms. Encyclopedic coverage of contributions from laboratory to clinical medicine. Extensive references and well-constructed diagrams and illustrations are included. Valuable for biomedical and health science libraries.
R: *Archives of Environmental Health* 26: 286 (1973); *Archives of Internal Medicine* 132: 458 (Sept. 1973); *ARBA* (1973, p. 604); Allyn.

Oral-Facial Genetics. **R. E. Stewart and G. H. Prescott.** St. Louis, MO: C. V. Mosby, 1976.

Provides a comprehensive review of genetic disorders affecting oral and facial structures. First half of text devoted to detailed descriptions of heritable diseases. Diseases discussed in terms of embryology, histology, and biochemistry of defective oral tissue. Remainder of text predominantly an atlas of oral-facial disorders. Some repetition and fragmentation results from the two diverse sections. Graduate students and clinicians form the intended audience.
R: *American Journal of Human Genetics* 29: 645 (Nov. 1977).

Principles of Genetics. 4th ed. **E. J. Gardner.** New York: John Wiley, 1972.
R: Chen (p. 313).

The Principles of Human Biochemical Genetics. 2d ed. **Harry Harris.** New York: North-Holland/American Elsevier, 1975.

First edition, 1969.
Thoroughly revised state-of-the-art summary of human biochemical genetics. Initial chapters deal with various aspects of gene action. Further chapters concentrate on enzyme variability, mutation rates in man, inborn errors of metabolism, etc. Desptie the weighty material, the text is extremely readable. Richly illustrated. Recommended to advanced undergraduates, graduate and medical students, hematologists, general practitioners, and researchers in the field of biochemical genetics.
R: *American Journal of Human Genetics* 28: 532 (Sept. 1976); *British Journal of Haematology* 31: 264 (1975); *Science* 170: 1071 (Dec. 4, 1970); Chen (p. 313); Allyn.

Sickle Cell Disease: Diagnosis, Management, Education and Research. **Harole Abramson, John F. Bertles, and Doris L. Weathers, eds.** St. Louis, MO: C. V. Mosby, 1973.

Based on the symposium proceedings of a program sponsored by the National Foundation-March of Dimes and the Foundation for Research and Education in Sickle Cell Disease. Exhaustive presentation of sickle-cell disease. Represents contributions from 36 distinguished scholars. Bulk of book devoted to individual scientific developments. Despite the format, little repetition. Exhaustive bibliographies conclude sections. Valuable reference aid for physicians, health workers, and scientists.
R: *American Journal of Diseases of Children* 128: 261 (Aug. 1974).

The Thalassaemia Syndromes. 2d ed. **D. J. Weatherall and J. B. Clegg.** Oxford, England: Blackwell Scientific Publications, 1972.
First edition, 1964.

Second edition comprehensively details the clinical aspects of thalassaemia syndromes. In a broad, general framework. Provides historical discussion, details of laboratory diagnosis, genetic information. Comprises an excellent guide for both the genetic researcher and the clinician.
R: *Annals of Human Genetics* 37: 235 (Oct. 1973); Allyn.

Understanding Inherited Disorders. **Lucille F. Whaley.** St. Louis, MO: C. V. Mosby, 1974.

Presentation of basic concepts of human genetics with emphasis on inherited disorders in humans and effects of genetics on total population. New terms are explained in text and listed in glossary. Of value to students, nurses, health professionals concerned with rehabilitation, and the lay reader.
R: *Archives of Physical Medicine and Rehabilitation* 56: 48 (Jan. 1975); *RSR* 3: 33 (Apr.–June 1975).

GERONTOLOGY

Aging: The Process and the People. **Gene Usdin, ed.** New York: Brunner/Mazel, 1978.

The Biology of Aging. **J. A. Behnke, C. E. Finch, and G. B. Moment, eds.** New York: Plenum, 1978.

A multi-authored study of theories of aging. Contains illustrations and diagrams, discusses the topic on many different levels (i.e. molecular, state of the art in research, etc.). Primarily for physicians and biologists.
R: *Lancet* 1: 475 (Mar. 3, 1979); *Nature* 279: 87 (May 3, 1979).

Clinical Aspects of Aging. **W. Reichel, ed.** Baltimore, MD: Williams & Wilkins, 1978.

Emphasizes caring for the geriatric patient as a whole, with an awareness of problems created by aging. A multi-authored book which covers important topics. Well written; recommended to physicians, nurses, health professionals.
R: *Physical Therapy* 58: 1552 (1978).

Clinical Geriatrics. 2d ed. **Isadore Rossman, ed.** Philadelphia, PA: J. B. Lippincott, 1979.

First edition, 1971.
Considered an important contribution to the geriatric literature. Contains illustrations, tables of drug names, both British and American. A highly technical approach; well edited. Recommended to practitioners and students who work with the elderly.
R: *Geriatrics* 27: 164 (Nov. 1972); Allyn; Brandon.

Cowdry's Care of the Geriatric Patient. 5th rev. ed. **Franz U. Steinberg, ed.** St. Louis, MO: C. V. Mosby, 1976.

Third edition, 1968.
This classic handbook details problems in the field of geriatrics, with attention to sociological as well as physiological aspects. Deals with doctor-patient relation-

ship, home care of the patient. Contains an excellent index. Recommended for both the professional and lay person.
R: *Annals of Internal Medicine* 87: 133 (July 1977); Allyn; Brandon; Stearns & Ratcliff (*AJN*).

Developmental Physiology and Aging. **P. S. Timiras.** New York: Macmillan, 1972.
R: *Science* 180: 1048 (June 8, 1973); Chen (p. 310).

Normal Aging I: Reports from the Duke Longitudinal Study 1955–1969. **Erdman Palmore, ed.** Durham, NC: Duke University Press, 1970.
Comprehensive report of the Duke University Longitudinal Study of Aging. Destined to be the definitive research compendium in the field of gerontology and geriatrics.
R: *Choice* 9: 1661 (Feb. 1973).

Normal Aging II: Reports from the Duke Longitudinal Study, 1970–1973. **Erdman Palmore, ed.** Durham, NC: Duke University Press, 1974.

Practical Management of the Elderly. 3d ed. **Ferguson Anderson.** Philadelphia, PA: J. B. Lippincott, 1976.
Focuses on the preventive approach. Comprehensive study of the aging process. Features useful appendixes on methods of training physicians in the field of geriatrics, drugs and their interactions, and special equipment. Aimed at a British audience. Good introduction for any student, resident, nurse, or practitioner.
R: *Annals of Internal Medicine* 87: 133 (July 1977); *JAMA* 237: 903 (Feb. 28, 1977).

Textbook of Geriatric Medicine and Gerontology. 2d ed. **John C. Brocklehurst, ed.** Edinburgh & London: Churchill Livingstone, 1978.
First edition, 1973.
Monumental work in the field of geriatrics. Exhibits definite British slant. Volume of references attests to its completeness and high scholarship. Its price could be a disadvantage. Noteworthy addition to all geriatric libraries.
R: *Annals of Internal Medicine* 87: 133 (July 1977); *British Medical Bulletin* 30: 287 (Sept. 1974); *Experimental Gerontology* 9: 95 (Apr. 1974); *Journal of Gerontology* 29: 589 (Sept. 1974); *NEJM* 291: 369 (Aug. 15, 1974); *The Practitioner* 212: 171 (Feb. 1974); *TBRI* 40: 229 (June 1974); 40: 312 (Oct. 1974); 40: 401 (Dec. 1974); Allyn; Brandon.

HEALTH SERVICES ADMINISTRATION

Comparative National Policies on Health Care. **Milton I. Roemer.** New York: Marcel Dekker, 1977.
Details the health care delivery systems in over 45 nations. Major topics covered are economic support of health care, facilities, patterns of delivery. Discussed with the context of economic status of nation: free enterprise, underdeveloped, transitional, socialist. Indispensable reference for medical schools, health care administrators, planners.
R: *Canadian Medical Association Journal* 118: 781 (Apr. 8, 1977).

Ethics and Health Policy. **Robert M. Veatch and Roy Branson, eds.** Cambridge, MA: Ballinger, 1976.

The outgrowth of an institute on ethics and science. This book discusses links between ethics and medicine in three sections: health care delivery, ethics and allocating medical resources, and ethics and health care planning. Maintains an interdisciplinary approach. Considered a valuable reference in the field of medical ethics.
R: *American Journal of Psychiatry* 134: 1055 (Sept. 1977).

Governing Hospitals: Trustees and the New Accountabilities. **Robert M. Cunningham, Jr.** Chicago, IL: American Hospital Association, 1976.

Discusses the structure of hospital administration, including such topics as financial management, planning, public relations, staffing of hospitals.

Health Care Administration: A Managerial Perspective. **Samuel Levey and Narendra P. Loomba.** Philadelphia, PA: J. B. Lippincott, 1973.

Relates new management concepts to health field. Of greatest value for students in programs of health care and hospital administration responsible for managing health service organizations.
R: *Hospitals* 48: 26 (June 1, 1974); *JAMA* 224: 1651 (June 18, 1973); Brandon.

Health Service Research. Washington, DC: US National Academy of Sciences, 1979.

Hospital Computer Systems. **M. F. Collen, ed.** New York: John Wiley, 1974.

Description of use of computerized systems in hospitals. Focuses on administrative aspects
R: *Journal of Nursing Administration* 1: 46 (June 1976); Allyn.

Hospital Management Systems: Multi-unit Organization and Delivery of Health Care. **Montague Brown and Howard L. Lewis.** Germantown, MD: Aspen Systems Corp., 1976.

Illustrates the development of hospital systems. Discusses various systems and factors associated with changes. For hospital administrators.
R: *Hospital and Health Services Administrations* 22: 92 (1977); Brandon.

A Manpower Policy For Primary Health Care. **Institute of Medicine.** Washington, DC: US National Academy of Sciences, 1978.

New Directions in Public Health Care: An Evaluation of Proposals for National Health Insurance. **Cotton M. Lindsay, ed.** San Francisco, CA: Institute for Contemporary Studies, 1980.

First edition, 1976.
Assesses the impact of various proposals for national health insurance on the nation's medical care delivery system. Highly recommended by legislators and educators.

Organization and Administration of Health Care: Theory, Practice, Environ-

ment. 2d ed. **Richard L. Durbin and W. Herbert Springall.** St. Louis, MO: C. V. Mosby, 1974.

Confronts the problem of administration and management. Sets up a concrete and viable system applicable to hospital administration.
R: *Hospital Administration* 20: 106 (Winter 1975); Brandon.

Principles of Hospital Administration. 2d ed. **John R. McGibony.** New York: G. P. Putnam's, 1969.

R: Brandon; Stearns & Ratcliff (*NEJM,* 1970).

Quality Control in Blood Banking: Quality Controls in the Clinical Laboratory. **Byron A. Myhre.** New York: John Wiley, 1974.

Standard reference in the area of quality control. Valuable addition to large hospital and community blood bank libraries.
R: *Transfusion* 15: 387 (July.–Aug. 1975); *TBRI* 41: 313 (Oct. 1975).

HEMATOLOGY

The Acid-Base Status of the Blood. 4th ed. **Ole Siggaard-Andersen.** Copenhagen: Munksgaard, 1974.

Comprehensive treatment of all known factors concerned in acid-base blood chemistry. Excellent bibliography. Suitable for clinical chemists.
R: *Journal of Clinical Pathology* 28: 599 (1975).

Blood Groups in Man. 6th ed. **R. R. Race and Ruth Sanger.** Oxford, England: Blackwell Scientific Publications, 1975.

First edition, 1950: fifth edition, 1968.
Major reference work on blood group systems. Expanded and updated text provides broad framework and detailed documentation assessing the vast body of literature accumulated in last 50 years on ABO system. For immunologists, human geneticists, and all those involved in blood transfusion and serology.
R: *American Journal of Human Genetics* 28: 306 (May 1976); *British Journal of Haematology* 31: 413 (1975); *JAMA* 235: 950 (Mar. 1, 1976); Allyn.

Clinical Hematology. 7th ed. **Maxwell M. Wintrobe.** Philadelphia, PA: Lea & Febiger, 1973.

The classic text on hematology; recommended for inclusion in medical reference collections.
R: Allyn.

Comprehensive Management of Hemophilia. **Donna C. Boone, ed.** Philadelphia, PA: F. A. Davis, 1976.

A concise multidisciplinary "how-to" reference which covers the management of hemophilia. Discusses medical, dental, nursing, surgical problems. Clearly presented information, emphasizes care of patient in different stages of hemophilia. Recommended to all practitioners.
R: *Archives of Physical Medicine and Rehabilitation* 58: 502 (Nov. 1977); *JAMA* 237: 691 (Feb. 14, 1977); *Physical Therapy* 57: 601 (1977).

Current Topics in Haematology, Immunology and Blood Transfusion. **I. Bernat, ed.** Budapest, Hungary: Akademiae Kiado, 1975.

A multi-authored reference source on hematology, immunohematology, and blood tranfusions. Authors are authorities in their fields, who presented these papers in honor of Prof. Susan Hollan for her significant contributions to the field.
R: *British Journal of Haematology* 32: 463 (1976).

The Distribution of the Human Blood Groups and Other Polymorphisms. 2d ed. **A. E. Mourant, Ada C. Kopec, and Kazimiera Domaniewska-Sobczak.** London: Oxford University Press, 1976.

First edition, 1954.
Informative volume provides data on human blood groups as well as thirty other polymorphisms. Initial chapters contain descriptions of biochemistry of inherited characteristics, which are followed by chapters containing gene frequency calculations and distributions of significant polymorphisms. Provides data bank of tabulated facts, figures, and maps for quick reference. Extensive bibliography, subject and author indexes. For use by geneticists, anthropologists, and transfusionists.
R: *British Medical Bulletin* 32: 292 (1976); *BMJ* 1: 1472 (June 12, 1976); *Journal of Clinical Pathology* 30: 3923 (1977).

Fundamentals of Clinical Hematology. 4th ed. **Byrd S. Leavell and Oscar A. Thorup.** Philadelphia, PA: W. B. Saunders, 1976.

Third edition, 1971.
A technical reference source, well recommended to specialists in hematology.
R: Allyn.

Haematological Aspects of Systemic Disease. **M. C. G. Israels and I. W. Delamore, eds.** Philadelphia, PA: W. B. Saunders, 1976.

Comprehensive discussion of problems for hematologists and clinicians. Chapters on hematological aspects of liver disease, geriatric medicine, neurobiology, and adverse drug reactions have been added. Extensive bibliographies and illustrations. For general physicians, hematologists, and pathologists.
R: *Archives of Pathology & Laboratory Medicine* 102: 112 (1978); *British Journal of Haematology* 35: 687 (1977).

Hematology. 2d ed. **William S. Beck, ed.** Cambridge, MA: MIT Press, 1977.

First edition, 1973.
This manual contains hematology lecture notes from the Harvard Medical School. Second edition maintains high quality of scholarship; deals with clinical and diagnostic procedures. Contains bibliography and index.
R: *NEJM* 289: 1316 (Dec. 13, 1973).

Hematology. 2d ed. **W. J. Williams et al.** New York: McGraw-Hill, 1977.

First edition, 1972.
A standard reference in the field. Extensive coverage; well organized. Can be used as a ready source of information in medical libraries.

R: *Annals of Internal Medicine* 77: 822 (1972).

Hematology: Physiologic, Pathophysiologic, and Clinical Principles. **James W. Linman.** New York: Macmillan, 1975.

Comprehensive treatise on all aspects of hematology. Well-organized volume is cross-indexed and contains a rich bibliography and illustrations, a large number of which are electron micrographs. Of practical value to general clinicians, hematologists, pediatricians, and students. A tool for all medical and hospital libraries.

R: *American Journal of Diseases of Children* 130: 1379 (Dec. 1976); *RSR* 4: 89 (Apr.–June 1976).

Laboratory Medicine: Hematology. 5th ed. **John B. Miale.** St. Louis, MO: C. V. Mosby, 1977.

Fourth edition, 1972.
A classic text on laboratory medicine.
R: Allyn.

Lupus Erythematosus: A Review of the Current Status of Discoid and Systemic Lupus Erythematosus and Their Variants. 2d ed. **Edmund L. Dubois, ed.** Los Angeles, CA: University of Southern California Press, 1974.

First edition, 1965.
Updates experimental and clinical knowledge of systemic and discoid lupus erythematosus through supplements to chapters. Comprehensive, well-illustrated, standard reference for lupus erythematosus. Over 3,000 sources. For pathologists in addition to medical libraries.

R: *Archives of Internal Medicine* 135: 1276 (Sept. 1975); *Archives of Pathology & Laboratory Medicine* 102: 215 (1978); *Arthritis and Rheumatism* 18: 94 (Jan.–Feb. 1975); *BMJ* 3: 418 (Aug. 10, 1974).

Man's Haemoglobins, Including the Haemoglobinopathies and Their Investigation. 2d ed. **H. Lehmann and R. G. Huntsman.** Philadelphia, PA: J. B. Lippincott, 1974.

An extensive account of the biology of hemoglobins. Includes historical and current references, diagrams, and a comprehensive index. Highly recommended to clinicians and researchers and for all medical library collections.

R: *RSR* 3: 31 (Apr.–June 1975); Allyn.

The Morphology of Human Blood Cells. 3d ed. **L. W. Diggs, Dorothy Sturm, and Ann Bell.** North Chicago, IL: Abbott Laboratories, 1975.

The third edition of this popular bench atlas contains clear illustrations. It emphasizes cellular features, cytochemical stains. Considered a useful working atlas for hematologists.

R: *Archives of Pathology & Laboratory Medicine* 100: 509 (Sept. 1976).

Platelets: Physiology and Pathology. **J. P. Caen, S. Cronberg, and P. Kubisz.** New York: Stratton Intercontinental Medical Book Corporation, 1977.

Presents an overview of current knowledge concerning platelets. Features over 1,140 references, including some published in 1977. Style is brusque and stac-

cato. Certainly a worthwhile addition to all medical libraries.
R: *British Journal of Haematology* 37: 164 (1977).

The Red Blood Cell. 2d ed. 2 vols. **Douglas M. Surgenor, ed.** New York: Academic Press, 1975.

First edition, 1964.
Volume 1 of expanded second edition presents analysis of composition of red cells while volume 2 is a more detailed approach to function of the cell. Valuable reference for advanced hematologists as well as students.
R: *Blood* 45: 596 (1975); 46: 995 (1975); *British Journal of Haematology* 30: 255 (1975).

INFECTIOUS DISEASES

Anaerobic Bacteria: Role in Disease. **A. Balows et al., eds.** Springfield, IL: Charles C. Thomas, 1974.

A compendium of microbial diseases. An excellent reference for microbiologists as well as clinicians.
R: *Annals of Internal Medicine* 82: 862 (1975); *Gastroenterology* 68: 420 (Feb. 1975); *TBRI* 41: 178 (May 1975).

Anaerobic Bacteria in Human Disease. **Sidney M. Finegold.** New York: Academic Press, 1977.

This treatise clearly presents clinical and technical aspects of bacteria and disease. Among subjects covered are infections of respiratory tract, female genital tract, abdomen, skin, and muscle. Contains index, valuable list of references. Recommended; considered an encyclopedic work.
R: *Annals of Internal Medicine* 87: 501 (Oct. 1977).

Bacterial and Mycotic Infections of Man. 4th ed. **Rene J. Dubos and James G. Hirsch, eds.** Philadelphia, PA: J. B. Lippincott, 1965.

A classic text; covers all aspects of bacteriology including morphology, physiology, disease vectors, therapy, and treatment of disease. Maintains a clinical approach; well referenced.
R: Stearns & Ratcliff (*AJN*).

Bacteriology, Virology and Immunity for Students of Medicine. 10th ed. **F. S. Stewart and T. S. L. Beswick.** New York: Macmillan, 1978.

Encompasses recent advances in immunology, with completely revised sections on immunity and virology. In four parts: general microbiology, immunity, systematic bacteriology, and virology.

Bailey and Scott's Diagnostic Microbiology: A Textbook for the Isolation and Identification of Pathogenic Microorganisms. 5th ed. **Sydney M. Finegold, William J. Martin, and Elvyn G. Scott.** St. Louis, MO: C. V. Mosby, 1978.

A classic text of microbiology; updated and revised edition contains current information, including new chapters on anaerobic cocci, diagnostic parasitology.

Contains photographs, line drawings, full-color plates, summary tables, glossary, and appendix.

Clinical Concepts in Infectious Disease. 2d ed. **Leighton E. Cluff and Joseph E. Johnson, III.** Baltimore, MD: Williams & Wilkins, 1978.
First edition, 1972.
Emphasizes concepts and principles of infectious diseases for those interested in clinical management of disease. Well recommended.
R: *Annals of Internal Medicine* 81: 721 (1974); *JAMA* 226: 1063 (Nov. 20, 1972); *TBRI* 39: 38 (Jan. 1973); Allyn.

Clinical Microbiology. **Hugh L. Moffet, ed.** Philadelphia, PA: J. B. Lippincott, 1975.
Reviews all disciplines in clinical microbiology. Informative; includes an extensive bibliography. Recommended to those working with infectious disease.
R: *American Journal of Diseases of Children* 129: 1462 (Dec. 1975); *American Journal of Medical Technology* 42: 57 (July 1976); *Annals of Internal Medicine* 83: 592 (1975); *TBRI* 42: 55 (Feb. 1976); 42: 298 (Oct. 1976).

Craig & Faust's Clinical Parasitology. 8th ed. **Ernest C. Faust, Paul F. Russell, and Rodney C. Jung.** Philadelphia, PA: Lea & Febiger, 1970.
Deals with protozoa, helminthes, and arthropods. A comprehensive international classic that deals with etiology, pathology, and diagnosis of pathological diseases.

Diseases Transmitted From Animals to Man. 6th ed. **William T. Hubbert, William F. McCulloch, and Paul R. Schnurrenberger, eds.** Springfield, IL: Charles C. Thomas, 1975.
First edition, 1930; fifth edition, 1963.
Sixth edition is a new book, related to earlier editions by tradition. Emphasizes epidemiologic characteristics of each disease as affected by distribution, reactions of specific human or animal populations, and use of these factors in disease prevention. Useful parasitology-microbiology textbook for human or veterinary medicine as well as standard reference for zoonotic infections.
R: *Quarterly Review of Biology* 51: 197 (1976).

The Epidemiology of Human Mycotic Diseases. **Yousef Al-Doory, ed.** Springfield, IL: Charles C. Thomas, 1975.
Covers major factors in the epidemiology of mycotic diseases, compiling data according to geographic and clinical distribution. Also discusses predisposing factors in mycotic infections. A useful ready reference source for libraries of medical schools and for mycologists, epidemiologists.
R: *Journal of Parasitology* 63: 205 (Apr. 1977).

Essentials of Immunology and Microbiology. 2d ed. **Robert G. White and Morag C. Timbury.** Philadelphia, PA: J. B. Lippincott, 1973.
Authoritative overview of bacteria, fungi, and viruses and their relationship to man. Insert of 38 illustrations consisting of photo and electron micrographs is important feature.

Fundamentals of Microbiology. 9th ed. **Martin Frobischer et al.** Philadelphia, PA: W. B. Saunders, 1974.
R: Chen (p. 313).

General Parasitology. 2d ed. **Thomas C. Cheng.** New York: Academic Press, 1973.
Second edition extensively organizes large amount of information on parasites and their hosts. Well-written text includes excellent illustrations and tables. Good indexes as well as numerous lists of references to original literature are included in this monumental treatise.
R: *Journal of Parasitology* 60: 988 (Dec. 1974).

Human Viral Hepatitis. 2d ed. **A. J. Zuckerman.** New York: American Elsevier, 1976.
First edition, 1972.
Complete review of recent developments in human viral hepatitis. Set in a historical perspective. Problems in clinical management, diagnosis, and prospects for prevention are discussed. Required reading for all those interested in hepatitis.
R: *Lancet* 2: 664 (Sept. 25, 1976).

Infectious Diseases of Children. 6th ed. **Saul Krugman et al.** St. Louis, MO: C. V. Mosby, 1977.
Fifth edition, 1973.
Thorough discussion of 31 infectious diseases. Covers pathology, diagnosis, treatment. Includes color illustrations, suggestions for immunization and prevention. A highly technical text for medical students and physicians.
R: Allyn.

Influenza: The Viruses and the Disease. **Charles H. Stuart-Harris and Geoffrey C. Schild.** London: Edward Arnold, 1976.
Detailed commentary on modern research of influenza viruses and prospects for control and treatment. Illustrated with good photographs, charts, and tables. Much recent work is mentioned; good selection of references for further exploration. Useful for novice interested in basic understanding of influenza virus infections as well as those who wish to know the present state of the subject.
R: *American Journal of Public Health* 67: 629 (1977); 67: 690 (July 1977); *BMJ* 1: 718 (Mar. 12, 1977); *Pharmaceutical Journal* 219: 87 (1977).

Insects and Other Arthropods of Medical Importance. 2d ed. **Kenneth G. V. Smith, ed.** New York: John Wiley, 1978.
First edition, 1975.
Reference which identifies arthropods and discusses general structure of insects, classification, nomenclature, and methods of collection and preservation. Chapters by different contributors vary in content. Text is lucid and includes some obscure information. Index to authors cited and subject index included. Over 200 beautiful line drawings. Intended for teachers and advanced students. Recommended for libraries where tropical medicine is studied.
R: *BMJ* 1: 677 (June 22, 1974).

Manson's Tropical Diseases. 17th ed. **C. Wilcocks and P. E. C. Manson-Bahr.** New York: Macmillan, 1972.
First edition, 1898; sixteenth edition, 1966.
Standard source on tropical diseases. Contains photos, plates, and maps along with a table of drugs for treatment, with their origins and dosages.
R: Allyn.

Parasitology: The Biology of Animal Parasites. 4th ed. **Elmer R. Noble and Glenn A. Noble.** Philadelphia, PA: Lea & Febiger, 1976.
Explains parasite-host reactions in humans and domestic animals. Includes information on physiology, biochemistry, immunology, and pathology. Contains illustrations. Updated edition, recommended for undergraduate students.

Scabies and Pediculosis. **Milton Orkin et al., eds.** Philadelphia, PA: J. B. Lippincott, 1977.
Covers the biology, immunology, and epidemiology of scabies. Concise, easy-to-read. Contains color photographs.
R: *American Family Physician* 18: 255 (Sept. 1978); *American Journal of Public Health* 68: 508 (May 1978).

Textbook of Microbiology. 21st ed. **William Burrows.** Philadelphia, PA: W. B. Saunders, 1979.
Widely used textbook, revised frequently to reflect new concepts. Primary concern is with microorganisms and the effects of chemical agents.

Topley and Wilson's Principles of Bacteriology, Virology and Immunity. 6th ed. 2 vols. **Graham S. Wilson and Ashley Miles.** Baltimore, MD: Williams & Wilkins, 1975.
Fifth edition, 1964.
The classic text in bacteriology and infectious disease encompasses much information which is presented in a clear format. New edition includes up-to-date information. Considered a trustworthy and indispensable reference.
R: *JAMA* 235: 95 (Jan. 5, 1976); Allyn.

The Treatment and Control of Infectious Diseases in Man. **P. J. Imperato.** Springfield, IL: Charles C. Thomas, 1974.
Focuses on effect of infectious diseases on the patient and community. Intended for nurses, physicians' assistants, and paramedical personnel.
R: *Annals of Internal Medicine* 81: 722 (1974).

Tropical Medicine. 5th ed. **George W. Hunter, J. Clyde Swartzwelder, and David F. Clyde.** Philadelphia, PA: W. B. Saunders, 1976.
First edition, 1945.
Clinically oriented text covers virus infections; rickettsial, spirochetal, and bacterial diseases; nutritional diseases; infections caused by fungi; etc. Reference tool for practicing physicians.
R: *American Journal of Tropical Medicine and Hygiene* 26: 193 (1977); *Journal of Parasitology* 63: 140 (Feb. 1977); Stearns & Ratcliff (*NEJM*, 1970).

Viral Infections of Humans. **Alfred S. Evans, ed.** New York: Plenum, 1976.

Covers all major viral infections in humans, emphasizing epidemiology. Includes illustrations and tables, which enhance comprehension. Also discusses viral aspects of cancer and neurological diseases. Highly recommended for both specialists and family physicians.
R: *American Family Physician* 16: 291 (Oct. 1977).

Zinsser Microbiology. 16th ed. **Wolfgang K. Joklik and Hilda P. Willett, eds.** New York: Appleton-Century-Crofts, 1976.

Fifteenth edition under the title *Microbiology,* 1972.
A classic in the field of microbiology.
R: Chen (p. 313).

INTERNAL MEDICINE

Artificial Organs. **W. J. Kloff.** New York: Halsted Press, 1976.

Discusses artificial kidney, heart, and heart-assist devices. Includes detailed bibliography; written by an authority in the field.
R: *Biomaterials, Medical Devices and Artificial Organs* 5: 119 (1977).

Best and Taylor's Physiological Basis of Medical Practice. 10th ed. **John R. Brobeck, ed.** Baltimore, MD: Williams & Wilkins, 1979.

A classic text on physiology; covers all basic physiological processes: digestion, respiration, sensory control, etc. A comprehensive and well-written work.
R: *Annals of Internal Medicine* 80: 429 (Mar. 1974); *NEJM* 290: 60 (Jan. 1974); Allyn.

Cecil-Loeb Textbook of Medicine. 15th ed. **Paul B. Beeson and Walsh McDermott, eds.** Philadelphia, PA: W. B. Saunders, 1979.

Multi-authored text. Describes major diseases and their treatment. Arranged by disease type. A basic reference for practicing physicians.
R: Stearns & Ratcliff (*AJN*; *NEJM,* 1969).

Current Medical Diagnosis & Treatment. 17th ed. **Marcus A. Krupp and Milton J. Chatton, eds.** Los Altos, CA: Lange Medical Publications, 1978.

Considered a standard reference in medical diagnosis; covers an extensive list of subjects and for each syndrome lists diagnosis, treatment, prognosis, and references. Contains charts and tables, including a section on computerized tomography. An encyclopedic desk reference, indispensable in reference collections.
R: *American Family Physician* 18: 253 (Sept. 1979); *Gastroenterology* 75: 550 (Sept. 1978); *NEJM* 298: 1B71 (June 15, 1978); *ARBA* (1975, p. 731).

Early Care of the Injured Patient. **Committee on Trauma, American College of Surgeons.** Philadelphia, PA: W. B. Saunders, 1972.

This is a revised and combined publication by the American College of Surgeons which deals with emergency trauma situations. The book is highly recommended for its concise and coherent presentation.
R: *Lancet* 1: 702 (Mar. 31, 1973); Allyn.

Family Medicine: Principles and Practice. **Robert B. Taylor, ed.** New York: Springer, 1978.

For general practitioners. Includes information on a wide range of topics in family medicine. Useful as both a reference manual and a monograph.
R: *Lancet* 1: 136 (Jan. 20, 1979).

Harrison's Principles of Internal Medicine. 8th ed. **George W. Thorn et al.** New York: McGraw-Hill, 1977.

Seventh edition, 1974.
Basic reference textbook for internist. Well-organized, problem-oriented book. Selective bibliographies; well indexed.
R: Allyn; Stearns & Ratcliff (*NEJM,* 1970).

The Healing Hand: Man and Wound in the Ancient World. **Guido Majno.** Cambridge, MA: Harvard University Press, 1975.

A scholarly work which covers the history of wound healing from prehistoric to ancient times. Contains many illustrations. Recommended for public, college, and medical libraries.
R: *Journal of Bone and Joint Surgery* 58A: 582 (June 1976); *RSR* 3: 36 (July–Dec. 1975).

Interferon 1 1979. **Ion Gressler et al., eds.** New York: Academic Press, 1980.

First volume in the series *Essays in Biochemistry.* Contains readings by international experts on interferon research.

An Introduction to Clinical Research. **W. P. Small and Urban Krause.** Baltimore, MD: Williams & Wilkins, 1972.

Introduction to problems of clinical research, collection and evaluation of data, and presentation of results. Brief, well-written monograph is designed to show how interested clinicians can contribute to professionals' knowledge of disease.
R: *Journal of Oral Surgery* 31: 566 (July 1973).

An Introduction to the Study of Disease. 7th ed. **William Boyd and Huntington Sheldon.** Philadelphia, PA: Lea & Febiger, 1977.

Completely updated, includes new material on the heart, liver, and central nervous system. Each chapter contains a summary and glossary. For students in the allied health sciences.

MGH Textbook of Emergency Medicine: Emergency Care as Practiced at the Massachusetts General Hospital. **E. W. Wilkins, Jr., J. J. Bineen, and A. C. Moncure, eds.** Baltimore, MD: Williams & Wilkins, 1978.

Combines a practical and theoretical approach to emergency medicine. Considers basic systems of life support in cardiology, pulmonary disease, etc. Covers a full range of emergency situations, including a chapter on angiography. An outstanding reference source.
R: *Plastic and Reconstructive Surgery* 64: 399 (Sept. 1979).

Modern Medical Treatment. 2d ed. **Henry Miller and Reginald Hall, eds.** Oxford, England: Blackwell Scientific Publications, 1975.

Emphasizes the therapy of diseases, including infectious disease, tropical, gynecological, and psychiatric diseases. Also deals with alcoholism, drug reactions, preventive medicine. Well-organized, concise format with contributions from authorities in their field. A short, clear guide to medical therapy.
R: *Annals of Internal Medicine* 83: 745 (Nov. 1975); *RSR* 4: 46 (Jan.–Mar. 1976); Allyn.

Mountain Medicine: A Clinical Study of Cold and High Altitudes. **Michael Ward.** London: Granada Publishing, 1975.

Summarizes current knowledge about clinical effects of the mountain environment and the impact of these effects on populations inhabiting these areas. Author has summarized aspects of mountain medicine such as effects of cold, accidents, etc. Of interest to physiologists and clinicians.
R: *Archives of Environmental Health* 30: 563 (1975).

Principles and Practice of Medicine. 19th ed. **A. McGehee Harvey et al., eds.** New York: Appleton-Century-Crofts, 1976.

The classic introduction to patient diagnosis and treatment. Scope is extensive, covering the full range of physical and mental disorders.

Progress in Clinical Medicine. 7th ed. **A. R. Horler and J. B. Foster, eds.** New York: Churchill Livingstone, 1978.

Seventh revised edition includes wide range of topics: body systems, genetics, pharmacology, geriatrics. Excellent format, numerous references. Well recommended.
R: *Lancet* 2: 242 (July 29, 1978).

Recent Advances in Medicine. 17th ed. **D. N. Barron, N. Compston, and A. M. Dawson, eds.** Edinburgh: Churchill Livingstone, 1977.
R: *Lancet* 1: 310 (Feb. 11, 1978).

Scientific American Medicine. **E. Rubenstein and D. D. Federman, eds.** New York: Scientific American, 1978.

Two volumes in loose-leaf format. Monthly supplements keep text and index completely up to date. Text covers, in detail, all areas of internal medicine and can be used as a base for continuing education. Provides clear, well-presented discussions. Recommended for physicians needing to be kept up to date; an important tool in professional education.
R: *NEJM* 301: 220 (July 26, 1979).

Sports Medicine. 2d ed. **J. G. P. Williams and P. N. Sperryn.** Baltimore, MD: Williams & Wilkins, 1977.

First edition, 1974.
Comprehensive coverage of sports medicine. Emphasizes four main sections: medical supervision and care of athlete, physical education programs, prevention of chronic degenerative disease, and exercise relating to physical disorders and diseases. Special sections devoted to nutrition, injury management, problems of

female athletes, exercise prescription, and specific disease entities. Reflects contributions from 29 prominent specialists. Illustrations consist mainly of photographs. Standard text for physicians in sports medicine, general practitioners, physical and occupational therapists and athletic training and physical education departments.
R: *Archives of Physical Medicine and Rehabilitation* 59: 50 (Jan. 1978); *Physical Therapy* 56: 126 (1976); 57: 1433 (Dec. 1977).

Trauma Management. **E. F. Cave, J. F. Burke, and R. J. Boyd.** Chicago, IL: Year Book Medical Publishers, 1974.
Practical volume explores daily problems of surgeons and methods of solution. Organization and illustrations are excellent.
R: *Plastic and Reconstructive Surgery* 59: 566 (1977).

Urinalysis in Clinical Laboratory Practice. **Alfred H. Free and Helen M. Free.** Cleveland, OH: Chemical Rubber Company, 1975.
Fifty chapters contain information on a wide range of urinary studies. Useful in training of laboratory technicians.
R: *Clinical Chemistry* 22: 697 (1976); *Medical Laboratory Sciences* 33: 240 (July 1976); *TBRI* 42: 265 (Sept. 1976).

NURSING

Acute Coronary Care. **Gerald H. Whipple, et al.** Boston, MA: Little, Brown, 1979.
R: Brandon (*NO*).

Administration in Nursing. 2d ed. **Mary D. Shanks and Dorothy A. Kennedy.** New York: McGraw-Hill, 1970.

Advanced Concepts in Clinical Nursing. 2d ed. **Kay C. Kintzel.** Philadelphia, PA: J. B. Lippincott, 1977.
Extensively revised, multi-authored text which aims to develop concepts in clinical nursing. Among topics covered are the allergic patient, mechanisms of shock, burns, psychological aspects of health and disease. Valuable for students and practitioners.
R: Brandon (*NO*).

Basic Nursing Techniques: A Programmed Introduction to Nursing Fundamentals. **Maja C. Anderson.** Philadelphia, PA: W. B. Saunders, 1968.
Emphasizes nursing fundamentals. Follows patient through a hospital day. Concentrates on practical aspects but includes some theoretical sections. Volume concludes with question-and-answer quiz. Complements basic nursing textbooks.

Basic Statistics for Nurses. **Rebecca G. Knapp.** New York: John Wiley, 1978.
Introductory text in statistics, emphasizing nursing applications. Includes examples, exercises, and tables. Necessary for all students and professionals.
R: *Journal of Nursing Administration* 9: 9 (May 1979); Brandon (*NO*).

Cardiovascular Nursing: Prevention, Intervention, Rehabilitation. **Jennie M. Holland.** Boston, MA: Little, Brown, 1977.
R: Brandon (*NO*).

Care of the Adult Patient. 3d ed. **Dorothy W. Smith and Carol P. Germain.** Philadelphia, PA: J. B. Lippincott, 1975.
Second edition, 1966.
Concentrates on the treatment of the adult patient as a total individual. Stresses mental and physical needs of the patient. Covers nurse-patient relationships, therapy, pain, and various diseases and accidents. Well referenced with bibliography, tables, and index. Contains illustrations. Written for nurses in the area of medical-surgical practice and paramedical personnel.
R: Stearns & Ratcliff (*AJN*); Brandon (*NO*).

Carini and Owens' Neurological and Neurosurgical Nursing. 7th ed. **Barbara L. Conway.** St. Louis, MO: C. V. Mosby, 1978.
Fifth edition, 1970.
Major revisions of text reflect the expanded role of the nurse. In three sections: anatomy and physiology of the nervous system, disorders of the neurologic structure, and care of disorders. Includes much updated information. A standard reference.
R: Brandon (*NO*).

The Case for Consultation in Nursing: Designs for Professional Practice. **Mary F. Kohnke.** New York: John Wiley, 1978.
R: Brandon (*NO*).

Childbearing: A Nursing Perspective. 2d ed. **Ann Clark and Dyanne D. Affonso.** Philadelphia, PA: F. A. Davis, 1979.
R: Brandon (*NO*).

Child Health Maintenance: A Guide to Clinical Assessment. 2d ed. **Peggy I. Chinn.** St. Louis, MO: C. V. Mosby, 1979.
R: Brandon (*NO*).

Child Health Maintenance: Concepts in Family Centered Care. 2d ed. **Peggy I. Chinn.** St. Louis, MO: C. V. Mosby, 1979.

Clinical Nursing. 3d ed. **Irene L. Beland and Joyce Y. Passos.** New York: Macmillan, 1975.
Second edition, 1970.
Encompasses all aspects of clinical nursing: psychological, pathological, neurological, rehabilitative, etc. Includes illustrations and bibliography. Geared toward the nursing student.
R: Brandon (*NO*); Stearns & Ratcliff (*AJN*; *NEJM*, 1970).

Clinical Perspectives in Nursing Research. **M. J. Nelson, ed.** New York: Columbia University, Teachers College Press, 1978.
Proceedings from the fourteenth annual Stewart Conference on Research in

Nursing; presents papers analyzing the role of the nurse in medicine. Clear organization presents many relevant topics. Provides much research data and supplementary information for students. Contains many new insights into the field of nursing.
R: *American Journal of Nursing* 79: 992 (May 1979).

Communicating Nursing Research. **Marjorie V. Batey, ed.** Boulder, CO: Western Interstate Commission for Higher Education (WICHE), 1968–. Annual.
Papers presented at the annual WICHE Conferences on nursing research.

Community Health Nursing Practice. **Ruth B. Freeman.** Philadelphia, PA: W. B. Saunders, 1970.
Provides a good overview of public health nursing. Standard text for beginning nurses in this field.
R: Brandon (*NO*); Stearns & Ratcliff (*NEJM*, 1970).

Comprehensive Pediatric Nursing. 2d ed. **Gladys M. Scipien et al.** New York: McGraw-Hill, 1979.
R: Brandon (*NO*).

Concepts and Practices of Intensive Care for Nurse Specialists. 2d ed. **Lawrence E. Meltzer et al., eds.** Bowie, MD: Charles Press, 1976.
Consists of contributions from authorities in all medical specialties as they relate to intensive care situations. Concise descriptions of the role of nursing personnel. Comprehensive coverage of most biological crises for nurse specialists.
R: *Choice* 13: 854 (Sept. 1976); Stearns & Ratcliff (*AJN*; *NEJM*, 1970).

Creative Teaching in Clinical Nursing. **Jean E. Schweer and Kristine M. Gebbie.** St. Louis, MO: C. V. Mosby, 1976.
R: Brandon (*NO*).

Critical Care Nursing. 2d ed. **Carolyn M. Hudak, Barbara M. Gallo, and Thelma Lohr.** Philadelphia, PA: J. B. Lippincott, 1977.
First edition, 1973.
Includes *Work Manual for Critical Care Nursing*, 2d ed, 1977.
Second edition incorporates new and revised data. Still emphasizes the "core body systems" of the previous edition.
R: Brandon (*NO*).

Curriculum Building in Nursing: A Process. 2d ed. **Olivia E. Bevis.** St. Louis, MO: C. V. Mosby, 1978.
R: Brandon (*NO*).

Dynamics of Law in Nursing and Health Care. **Mary D. Hemelt and Mary E. Mackert.** Reston, VA: Reston, 1978.
R: Brandon (*NO*).

Dynamics of Oncology Nursing. **Pamela Burkhalter.** New York: McGraw-Hill, 1978.
R: Brandon (*NO*).

Elements of Research in Nursing. 2d ed. **Eleanor W. Treece and James W. Treece.** St. Louis, MO: C. V. Mosby, 1977.
R: Brandon (*NO*).

Essentials of Nursing: A Medical-Surgical Text for Practical Nurses. 4th ed. **Claire B. Keane.** Philadelphia, PA: W. B. Saunders, 1979.
A beginning text for nursing students. Contains vocabulary lists, study outlines, learning highlights.

Essentials of Nursing Research. 2d ed. **Lucille E. Notter.** New York: Springer, 1978.
R: Brandon (*NO*).

Essentials of Psychiatric Nursing. 10th ed. **Dorothy A. Mereness and Cecelia M. Taylor.** St. Louis, MO: C. V. Mosby, 1978.
Standard text. Extensively revised edition contains information on community health crisis intervention. Provides chapter outlines and summaries.
R: *American Journal of Nursing* 79: 765 (Apr. 1979); Stearns & Ratcliff (*AJN*).

Ethical Dilemmas and Nursing Practice. **Anne J. Davis and Mila A. Aroskar.** New York: Appleton-Century-Crofts, 1978.
R: Brandon (*NO*).

Fundamentals of Nursing. 15th ed. **Elinor V. Fuerst et al.** Philadelphia, PA: J. B. Lippincott, 1979.
Emphasizes a holistic approach to nursing.
R: Brandon (*NO*).

Fundamentals of Nursing Practice: Concepts, Roles and Functions. **Fay L. Bower and E. Olivia Bower.** St. Louis, MO: C. V. Mosby, 1979.

Fundamentals of Operating Room Nursing. 2d ed. **Shirley M. Brooks.** St. Louis, MO: C. V. Mosby, 1979.
R: Brandon (*NO*).

Gastroenterology in Clinical Nursing. 3d ed. **Barbara A. Given and Sandra A. Simmons.** St. Louis: C. V. Mosby, 1979.
R: Brandon (*NO*).

Health Care of Women. **Leonide L. Martin.** Philadelphia, PA: J. B. Lippincott, 1978.
An obstetrics and gynecology text aimed specifically at nurses. Includes good illustrations.
R: Brandon (*NO*).

Intensive Nursing Care. 2d ed. **Lenette O. Burrell and Zeb L. Burrell, Jr.** St. Louis, MO: C. V. Mosby, 1973.
First edition, 1969.
R: Stearns & Ratcliff (*AJN*; *NEJM*, 1970).

Introduction to Patient Care: A Comprehensive Approach to Nursing. 3d ed. **Beverly W. Du Gas.** Philadelphia, PA: W. B. Saunders, 1971.
R: Brandon (*NO*).

Issues in Nursing Research. **Florence S. Downs and Juanita W. Fleming.** New York: Appleton-Century-Crofts, 1979.
Outlines historical, theoretical, clinical, educational, and conceptual perspectives of research in nursing. All topics written by a nurse authority with valuable research experience. All chapters are well documented with concise summaries, up-to-date references, and comprehensive bibliographies. Designed primarily for graduate students anticipating a research program. Useful reference tool for educators, administrators, and consumers of nursing research.
R: *Choice* 16: 1056 (Oct. 1979); Brandon (*NO*).

Key Concepts for the Study and Practice of Nursing. 2d ed. **Marjorie Byrne and Lida F. Thompson.** St. Louis, MO: C. V. Mosby, 1978.
R: Brandon (*NO*).

Legal Accountability in the Nursing Process. **Irene Murchison et al.** St. Louis, MO: C. V. Mosby, 1978.
R: Brandon (*NO*).

Levels of Health Intervention. **Ann Wobert Burgess.** Englewood Cliffs, NJ: Prentice-Hall, 1978.

Maternal and Infant Drugs and Nursing Intervention. **Elizabeth J. Dickason, Martha O. Schult, and Elaine M. Morris, eds.** New York: McGraw-Hill, 1978.
Comprehensive review of the pharmacological literature for nurses specializing in maternal and infant care. Provides results from current drug studies and research on teratogens. Tabular format increases its reference value. Each chapter concludes with generous bibliography. Appendixes outline information on simple measurement calculations and injection procedures. Lacks any description of nurse communication skills. Written for nurse-teachers specializing in drug administration during childbirth and infancy.
R: *American Journal of Nursing* 79: 1473 (Aug. 1979); Brandon (*NO*).

Medical-Surgical Nursing. 6th ed. **Kathleen N. Shafer et al.** St. Louis, MO: C. V. Mosby, 1975.
Fifth edition, 1971.
Updates classic book on medical-surgical nursing. Includes new section on ecology and health. Features modifications, additions, and deletions in areas of neurology and musculoskeletal injuries. Standard text for hospital staff.

R: *The Canadian Nurse* 72: 51 (May 1976); Brandon (*NO*); Stearns & Ratcliff (*AJN*; *NEJM*, 1970).

Medical-Surgical Nursing: A Conceptual Approach. **Dorothy A. Jones, Claire F. Dunbar, and Mary M. Jirovac.** New York: McGraw-Hill, 1978.

Textbook approach to modern medical-surgical nursing. Features strong points in nursing intervention. Carefully integrates basic nursing assessment skills. Relays unifying theme of human-environmental interaction. Geared toward the professional nurse.
R: *American Journal of Nursing* 79: 988 (May 1979); Brandon (*NO*).

Medical-Surgical Nursing: A Psychophysiologic Approach. 2d ed. **Karen Sorensen and Joan Luckmann.** Philadelphia, PA: Saunders, 1979.

R: Brandon (*NO*).

Mosby's Comprehensive Review of Critical Care. **Donna A. Zschoche, ed.** St. Louis, MO: C. V. Mosby, 1976.

Comprehensive overview of critical care. Contains contributions from experts in the field. Handy reference tool for all critical care units. Recommended to practitioners and nurses with a critical care specialty.
R: *American Journal of Nursing* 77: 329 (Feb. 1977); Brandon (*NO*).

Mosby's Comprehensive Review of Nursing. 9th ed. **Dolores F. Saxton, ed.** St. Louis, MO: C. V. Mosby, 1977.

Eighth edition, 1973.
Extensively revised text, covers fundamentals of nursing. Uses a patient-centered approach. Helpful for students; includes blank answer sheets, bibliographies, and cross-references.
R: Brandon (*NO*).

Mosby's Review of Practical Nursing. 7th ed. **Eva W. Caldwell et al.** St. Louis, MO: C. V. Mosby, 1978.

Sixth edition, 1974.
An outline review for students. Updated edition reflects current trends in the profession.
R: Brandon (*NO*).

Newton's Geriatric Nursing. 5th ed. **Helen C. Anderson.** St. Louis, MO: C. V. Mosby, 1971.

Standard text on aging and nursing care. Concentrates on prevention of illness. Outlines common disease afflicting the aged. Fine illustrations.

Normal and Therapeutic Nutrition. 15th ed. **Corinne H. Robinson and Marilyn R. Lawler.** New York: Macmillan, 1977.

Covers all aspects of nutrition: economic, psychologic, and cultural factors. Intended for students of nursing and dietetics.
R: Brandon (*NO*).

Nursing and the Law. 3d ed. **Mary W. Cazalas, ed.** Germantown, MD: Aspen Systems Corp., 1978.
R: Brandon (*NO*).

Nursing Audit. **Dorothy B. Doughty and Norma J. Mash.** Philadelphia, PA: F. A. Davis, 1977.
R: Brandon (*NO*).

The Nursing Audit: Self Regulation in Nursing Practice. **Maria C. Phaneuf.** New York: Appleton-Century-Crofts, 1976.

Nursing Care in Eye, Ear, Nose and Throat Disorders. **William Saunders et al.** St. Louis, MO: C. V. Mosby, 1979.
R: Brandon (*NO*).

Nursing Care of Patients With Urologic Diseases. 4th ed. **C. C. Winter and Alice Morel.** St. Louis, MO: C. V. Mosby, 1977.
Third edition, 1972.
Highlights basic principles of urology. Covers procedures and materials in urologic nursing. Question-and-answer section completes each chapter. Contains fine illustrations.
R: Stearns & Ratcliff (*AJN*); Brandon (*NO*).

Nursing Care of the Alcoholic and Drug Abuser. **Pamela K. Burkhalter.** New York: McGraw-Hill, 1975.
A valuable reference on nursing care of alcoholism and drug abuse. Deals with the effects on mind and body, emphasizing skills and caring attitude of nurses. Well referenced, an excellent source of reference in the field.
R: *ARBA* (1976, p. 730); Brandon (*NO*).

Nursing Care of the Growing Family: A Maternal-Newborn Text. **Adele Pillitteri.** Boston, MA: Little, Brown, 1976.
R: Brandon (*NO*).

Nursing Care of the Labor Patient. **Janet S. Malinowski.** Philadelphia, PA: F. A. Davis, 1978.
R: Brandon (*NO*).

Nursing Care of the Patient With Burns. 2d ed. **Florence G. Jacoby.** St. Louis, MO: C. V. Mosby, 1976.
First edition, 1972.
Emphasizes pathological, physiological, and psychological aspects of treating burn patients. Outlines specific techniques and materials commonly employed by nurses in this specialized area.
R: Brandon (*NO*).

Nursing in the Intensive Respiratory Care Unit. 2d ed. **Hannelore Sweetwood, ed.** New York: Springer Publishing, 1979.

First edition, 1971.
Concentrates on the care of patients suffering from respiratory problems. Introduction outlines physiology, basic principles, and common procedures. Valuable section on administration of medication and the function of mechanical equipment. Final sections devoted to common respiratory ailments (emphysema, asthma, bronchitis, chest injuries, etc.). Aimed at the nurse in intensive respiratory care units.
R: *ARBA* (1972, p. 630).

Nursing Management of Diabetes Mellitus. **D. W. Guthrie and R. Guthrie.** St. Louis, MO: C. V. Mosby, 1977.
Emphasizes nursing management of diabetic patients. Discusses chronic care, Special problems, patient education, and psychological aspects. An up-to-date text.

The Nursing Profession: Views Through the Mist. **Norma L. Chaskar.** New York: McGraw-Hill, 1978.
R: Brandon (*NO*).

Nursing Research: Development, Collaboration and Utilization. **Janelle Kreuger et al.** Germantown, MD: Aspen Systems Corp., 1978.
R: Brandon (*NO*).

Nursing Research: Principles and Practice. **Denise Polit and Bernadette Hungler.** Philadelphia, PA: J. B. Lippincott, 1978.
R: Brandon (*NO*).

Nursing Standards and Nursing Process. **Marion E. Nicholls & Virginia G. Wessells.** Wakefield, MA: Contemporary Publishing, 1977.
A multi-authored compendium of articles on various important topics in nursing. Examples of articles are: problem-oriented medical records, Patients' Bill of Rights, nursing processes, and quality care. Each chapter contains bibliography. Easily understood articles. A valuable reference, particularly for nursing management courses.
R: *The Canadian Nurse* 74: 37 (Dec. 1978); *Nurse Educator* 3: 21 (Nov.–Dec. 1978); *Supervisor Nurse* 9: 12 (July 1978); Brandon (*NO*).

Nursing Theory: Analysis, Application, Evaluation. **Barbara J. Stevens.** Boston, MA: Little, Brown, 1979.
R: Brandon (*NO*).

Obstetric Nursing. 7th ed. **Erna E. Ziegal and Mecca S. Cranley.** New York: Macmillan, 1978.
Discusses both psychological and physiological aspects of nursing care in obstetrics. Emphasizes the role of the nurse in professional practice and presents coverage of antepartum, intrapartum, postpartum, and newborn nursing. A standard reference.
R: Brandon (*NO*).

Orthopedic Nursing. 9th ed. **Carroll B. Larson and Marjorie Gould.** St. Louis, MO: C. V. Mosby, 1978.
Seventh edition, 1970.
R: Stearns & Ratcliff (*AJN*); Brandon (*NO*).

Parent-Child Nursing: Psychosocial Aspects. 2d ed. **Gladys B. Lipkin.** St. Louis, MO: C. V. Mosby, 1978.
R: Brandon (*NO*).

Patient-Nurse Interaction: A Study of Interaction Patterns in Acute Psychiatric Wards. **Annie T. Altschul.** Edinburgh: Churchill Livingstone, 1972.
R: *Nursing Research* 24: 146 (Mar.–Apr. 1975).

Pediatric Neurologic Nursing. **Barbara L. Conway.** St. Louis, MO: C. V. Mosby, 1977.
R: Brandon (*NO*).

Perinatal Nursing: Care of Newborns and Their Families. **Florence B. Roberts.** New York: McGraw-Hill, 1977.
R: Brandon (*NO*).

The Pharmacologic Basis of Patient Care. 3d ed. **Mary K. Asperheim and Laurel A. Eisenhower.** Philadelphia, PA: W. B. Saunders, 1977.
Teacher's manual accompanies text.
R: Brandon (*NO*).

Pharmacology in Nursing. 14th ed. **Betty S. Bergersen.** St. Louis, MO: C. V. Mosby, 1979.
Outlines current concepts of pharmacology for nurses.
R: Brandon (*NO*).

Practical Nursing Review. **Sister Mary Redempta Grawunder.** New York: Arco Publishing, 1976.

Prenatal Intensive Care. **Silvio Aladjem and Audrey Brown.** St. Louis, MO: C. V. Mosby, 1977.
R: Brandon (*NO*).

Principles and Practice of Nursing. 6th ed. **Virginia Henderson and Gladys Nite.** New York: Macmillan, 1978.
R: Brandon (*NO*).

Principles of Obstetrics and Gynecology For Nurses. 2d ed. **Josephine Iorio.** St. Louis, MO: C. V. Mosby, 1971.

The Process of Patient Teaching in Nursing. 3d ed. **Barbara K. Redman.** St. Louis, MO: C. V. Mosby, 1976.
R: Brandon (*NO*).

Providing Safe Nursing Care for Ethnic People of Color. **Marie F. Branch and Phyllis P. Paxton, eds.** New York: Appleton-Century-Crofts, 1976.
R: Brandon (*NO*).

Psychiatric Nursing. 10th ed. **Marguerite L. Manfreda and Sydney D. Krampitz.** Philadelphia, PA: F. A. Davis, 1977.
Updated, contains much new information, including discussions of human sexuality, psychiatric disorders, and drug and alcohol abuse. Provides illustrations and bibliographies. A comprehensive text.
R: Brandon (*NO*).

Psychiatric Nursing. 7th ed. **Mary Topalis and Donna Aguilera.** St. Louis, MO: C. V. Mosby, 1978.
Fifth edition, 1970.
Emphasizes community nursing and mental health. New material includes psychotherapeutic techniques, crisis intervention, and aging information. Describes psychotropic drugs.
R: Stearns & Ratcliff (*AJN*).

Readings in Gerontology. 2d ed. **Mollie Brown, ed.** St. Louis, MO: C. V. Mosby, 1978.
R: Brandon (*NO*).

Research in Nursing Practice. **Donna Diers.** Philadelphia, PA: J. B. Lippincott, 1979.

Saunders Review for Practical Nurses. **Claire Brackman Keane.** Philadelphia, PA: W. B. Saunders, 1977.

Scientific Principles in Nursing. 8th ed. **Dorothy Elhart et al.** St. Louis, MO: C. V. Mosby, 1978.
Revised edition features concepts of nursing care, including definitions, charts, references. Outlines nursing responsibilities and problems. Provides performance checklists.
R: *American Journal of Nursing* 79: 535 (March 1979); Brandon (*NO*).

Sociology: Nurse and Their Patients in a Modern Society. 9th ed. **Lida F. Thompson, Michael H. Miller, and Helen F. Bigler.** St. Louis, MO: C. V. Mosby, 1975.
Illustrates sociological principles as they relate to nursing. Discusses population, culture, and hospital administration.

A Textbook for Nursing Assistants. 3d ed. **Gertrude D. Chereseavich.** St. Louis, MO: C. V. Mosby, 1973.
Good introduction to nursing procedures for the assistant. Includes illustrations of basic techniques.
R: Brandon (*NO*).

Textbook of Medical-Surgical Nursing. 3d ed. **Lillian Brunner et al., eds.** Philadelphia, PA: J. B. Lippincott, 1975.

Second edition, 1970.
Focuses on the care of the medical and surgical patient. Special emphasis on emergency and disaster nursing and the control of communicable diseases. Lists sources of patient education. Contains individualized glossaries of various clinical specialties.
R: Stearns & Ratcliff (*AJN*).

Textbook of Pediatric Nursing. 5th ed. **Dorothy R. Marlow.** Philadelphia, PA: W. B. Saunders, 1977.

Fourth edition, 1973.
R: Stearns & Ratcliff (*AJN*; *NEJM*, 1970).

Travelbee's Intervention in Psychiatric Nursing. 2d ed. **Mary E. Doona.** Philadelphia, PA: F. A. Davis, 1979.

Women in Stress: A Nursing Perspective. **Diane Kjervik and Ida Martinson, eds.** New York: Appleton-Century-Crofts, 1978.
R: Brandon (*NO*).

NUTRITION

Clinical Nutrition. **Meredith Overton and Barbara Lukert.** Chicago, IL: Year Book Medical Publishers, 1977.

Succinct discussion of diet and nutrition, including chapters on hyperlipidemias, infant and child nutrition, and malnourishment.
R: *American Journal of Diseases of Children* 133: 562 (May 1979).

A Diet of Living. **Jean Mayer.** New York: McKay, 1975.

Eating Disorders: Obesity, Anorexia Nervosa, and the Person Within. **Hilde Bruch.** New York: Basic Books, 1973.

Contains a wealth of clinical descriptions, superb vignettes, and the reflections of a talented clinician. Spans author's research work from mid-1930s to the present in area of eating disorders. Particularly important is her discussion of anorexia nervosa. Little emphasis on promise of treatments now becoming available.
R: *American Journal of Psychiatry* 131: 334 (Mar. 1974); *Journal of Nervous and Mental Disease* 160: 380 (1975).

Food, Nutrition and Diet Therapy. 6th ed. **Marie V. Krause and L. Kathleen Mahan.** Philadelphia, W. B. Saunders, 1979.

Useful as a comprehensive text and reference tool. Incorporates new material on diet nutrition and cancer, nutritional diseases of infancy and childhood, interaction between drugs, nutrition and nutritional status.

Fundamentals of Quantity Food Preparation: Desserts and Beverages. **Geraline B. Hardwick and Robert L. Kennedy.** Boston: Cahners Books, 1975.

Presents the standardization of food formulas. Includes 250 quantity desserts

and beverages, as well as many basic preparations and variations. Reference book for all libraries that need basic food information.
R: *ARBA* (1976, p. 748); Chen (p. 317).

Infant Nutrition. 2d ed. **Samuel J. Fomon.** Philadelphia, PA: W. B. Saunders, 1974.
First edition, 1967.
Current, extensive review of infant nutrition, covering period from birth to three years. Objective source reference. Contains many excellent citations and is valuable for those interested in a concentrated study of infant nutrition.
R: *American Journal of Diseases of Children* 129: 266 (Feb. 1975).

Introduction to Food Science and Technology. **G. F. Stewart and M. A. Amerine.** New York: Academic Press, 1973.
A reference to the vast field of food science. An introductory text.
R: *Journal of Nutrition Education* p. 216 (July/Sept. 1973); Chen (p. 317).

Modern Nutrition in Health and Disease: Dietotherapy. 6th ed. **Robert S. Goodhart and Maurice E. Shils.** Philadelphia, PA: Lea & Febiger, 1979.
First edition, 1955; fourth edition, 1968; fifth edition, 1973.
Extensively revised standard text on nutrition. Contains monographs on topics such as basic nutritional science, diagnosis of nutritional deficiencies, and the role of nutrition in disease. Includes an appendix, bibliographies, and an index. Reference for students and practitioners in nutrition, medicine, and public health.
R: *American Journal of Digestive Diseases* 19: 1169 (Dec. 1974); Win (EK180); Allyn; Stearns & Ratcliff (*AJN; NEJM,* 1969; *NEJM,* 1970).

Nutrition and Cardiovascular Disease. **Elaine B. Feldman, ed.** New York: Appleton-Century-Crofts, 1976.
Maintains an epidemiologic approach to cardiovascular disease. Discusses fats, cholesterol, and other nutrients as they relate to heart disease. Also details related factors such as obesity, kidney disease, metabolic factors, atherosclerosis. Information is accompanied by figures and tables. A good source for those interested in the dietary prevention of heart disease.
R: *Journal of the American Dietetic Association* 71: 90 (July 1977).

Nutrition, Immunity, and Infection: Mechanisms of Interactions. **R. K. Chandra and P. M. Newberne.** New York: Plenum, 1977.
Concise summary of research findings on relationships between diet, morbidity, and mortality. Assesses the significance and limitations of data. Work deals with such topics as mechanism of host defense and nutritional, metabolic, and immunological effects of infection.
R: *American Journal of Public Health* 68: 912 (Sept. 1978).

Nutrition Reviews' Present Knowledge in Nutrition. 4th ed. Washington, DC: Nutrition Foundation, 1976.
Fourth edition updates other volumes; includes such topics as carbohydrates and sucrose, vitamins which are fat soluble, fiber, nutrition, and immunology. Con-

tains bibliographies. Helpful as a ready source of current knowledge in the field.
R: *Journal of the American Dietetic Association* 71: 91 (July 1977).

Principles of Food Science. 2 vols. **George Borgstrom.** New York: Macmillan, 1968.
Volume 1 treats food technology and volume 2 deals with food microbiology and biochemistry.
R: *Choice* 6: 243 (1969); *LJ* 94: 529 (1969); Jenkins (J115).

Trace Elements and Iron in Human Metabolism. **Ananda S. Prasad.** New York: Plenum, 1978.
Familiarizes the physician with recent research concerning the role of trace elements in human nutrition. Analyzes each element, summarizing biochemistry, toxicity, and role in metabolic processes.

U. S. Nutrition Policies in the Seventies. **Jean Mayer, ed.** San Francisco, CA: W. H. Freeman, 1973.
Examines policies concerning groups such as infants and pregnant women, food manufacturing, education of the public, as well as those affected by government at all levels.

The World Food Situation: Problems and Prospects to 1985. 2 vols. **Joseph W. Willet, comp.** Dobbs Ferry, NY: Oceana, 1976.
Includes reproductions of three United Nations reports on the world food problem resulting from World Food Conference held in November 1974.
R: *IBID* 4: 226 (Sept. 1976).

ONCOLOGY AND NUCLEAR MEDICINE

Biology of Cancer. 2d ed. **E. J. Ambrose and F. J. C. Roe.** Chichester, Sussex, England: Ellis Horwood, 1975.
Details the biochemistry of cancer in two sections: characteristics of malignancy and treatment of cancer. Copious references. A valuable source for researchers and clinicians.
R: *Pharmaceutical Journal* 219: 199 (1977).

Bone Tumors. 5th ed. **Louis Lichtenstein.** St. Louis, MO: C. V. Mosby, 1977.
Fourth edition, 1972.
In-depth survey of tumor and tumorlike lesion pathology; emphasizes accurate diagnosis and treatment. Contains bibliographies.
R: *Human Pathology* 4: 451 (Sept. 1973); *Journal of Bone and Joint Surgery* 54B: 1811 (Dec. 1972); *JAMA* 226: 1313 (Dec. 4, 1972); *TBRI* 39: 82 (Feb. 1973); 39: 359 (Nov. 1973); Brandon.

Brain Metastasis. **Leonard Weiss, Harvey A. Gilbert, and Jerome Posner, eds.** Boston, MA: G. K. Hall, 1979.
In three sections: brain metastasis; diagnosis; indications for radiotherapy, chemotherapy, and surgery. Includes drawings, tables, graphs, photographs, bibliog-

raphy. Comprehensive multidisciplinary book, essential to a wide range of medical specialists.

Cancer: Diagnosis, Treatment, and Prognosis. 5th ed. **J. A. del Regato and H. J. Spjut.** St. Louis, MO: C. V. Mosby, 1977.

Fourth edition, 1970, by Lauren V. Ackerman and J. A. del Regato.
Definitive work which covers malignant neoplasm except central nervous system tumors. Reference tool for oncologists as well as other specialists.
R: *Plastic and Reconstructive Surgery* 63: 722 (1979); Allyn; Stearns & Ratcliff (*AJN*; *NEJM,* 1969; *NEJM,* 1970).

Cancer Chemotherapy. 2d ed. **Martin J. Cline and Charles M. Haskell.** Philadelphia, PA: W. B. Saunders, 1975.

A concise monograph; includes timely information, extensive bibliography. A useful introductory text for students, general internists.
R: *Annals of Internal Medicine* 84: 513 (Apr. 1976); *Mayo Clinic Proceedings* 51: 317 (May 1976); *New Zealand Medical Journal* 84: 214 (Sept. 8, 1976); Allyn.

Cancer Chemotherapy. 2d ed. **Edward S. Greenwald.** Flushing, NY: Medical Examination Publishing, 1973.

Discusses chemotherapeutic agents, mode of action, and clinical applications. New edition includes information on management of leukemia. A concise format of chapters, each accompanied by a bibliography. An extensive compendium; recommended for internists and residents.
R: *Gastroenterology* 65: 181 (July 1973); Allyn; Stearns & Ratcliff (*NEJM,* 1969; *NEJM,* 1970).

Cancer Chemotherapy III. **Isadore Brodsky and S. B. Kahn, eds.** New York: Grune & Stratton, 1978.

Details the clinical aspects of chemotherapy. Covers hematologic malignancies, including bone marrow physiology, immunotherapy of leukemia.
R: Stearns & Ratcliff (*NEJM,* 1969).

Cancer, Epidemiology and Prevention: Current Concepts. **David Schottenfeld, ed.** Springfield, IL: Charles C. Thomas, 1975.

Focuses on aspects of cancer problems, ranging from economics to immunology. Thirty-seven contributors have presented information of value to those involved in cancer research.
R: *Archives of Dermatology* 113: 1146 (Aug. 1977).

Cancer Medicine. **James F. Holland and Emil Frei III et al., eds.** Philadelphia, PA: Lea & Febiger, 1973.

Valuable as both a reference source and textbook; covers a wide spectrum of information with subsection breakdowns. Discusses both diagnosis and management. For medical students and oncologists.
R: *NEJM* 290: 524 (Feb. 28, 1974).

Chemical Carcinogens. **Charles E. Searle.** Washington, DC: American Chemical Society, 1976.

Presents facts and theories concerning chemical carcinogens.
R: *Nature* 265: 666 (Feb. 17, 1977); *TBRI* 43: 147 (Apr. 1977).

Chemotherapy of Cancer. **Warren H. Cole, ed.** Philadelphia, PA: Lea & Febiger, 1970.
R: Brandon.

Clinical Cancer Medicine: Treatment Tactics. **Jacob J. Lokich.** Boston, MA: G. K. Hall, 1979.
Surveys treatment tactics and strategies in the management of cancer and its complications. Liberally illustrated with drawings, graphs, charts, tables, and photographs. Provides chapter summaries for easy reference. Geared toward primary care physicians without special training in oncology.

Clinical Scintillation Imaging. 2d ed. **Leonard M. Freeman and Philip M. Johnson, eds.** New York: Grune & Stratton, 1975.
First edition, 1969.
In two parts: nuclear medicine instrumentation and clinical aspects of nuclear medicine. The book is well organized; includes glossary, appendix. Recommended as a reference source for radiologists.
R: *Radiology* 119: 166 (1976); Allyn.

Disease of the Breast. 2d rev. ed. **C. D. Haagensen.** Philadelphia, PA: W. B. Saunders, 1974.
First edition, 1951; second edition, 1971.
A classic monograph on breast cancer and breast diseases. Includes discussions of surgical methods, physiology, aspects of disease based on case studies. Updated edition includes developments in radiology.
R: *Plastic and Reconstructive Surgery* 58: 218 (1976); Allyn; Brandon.

Early Breast Cancer: Its History and Results of Treatment. **Carl M. Mansfield.** A. Wolsky, ed. New York: S. Karger, 1976.
Considered an objective reference source; clear presentation. Recommended to physicians who deal with breast cancer.
R: *JAMA* 238: 1559 (Oct. 3, 1977).

Gynaecological Oncology. **Felix Rutledge et al.** New York: John Wiley, 1976.
Recommended for those with interest in gynecological cancer.
R: *British Journal of Cancer* 34: 576 (Nov. 1976).

Hodgkin's Disease. **Henry S. Kaplan.** Cambridge, MA: Harvard University Press, 1973.
Detailed consideration of entire range of knowledge in area of Hodgkin's Disease. Spans epidemiology, management, clinical evaluation, treatment. Photomicrographs are informative and well reproduced. Quality volume recommended for all those whose work is associated with disease.
R: *British Journal of Radiology* 47: 345 (1974); *Lancet* 2: 241 (Aug. 4, 1973); Allyn.

Investigation of Oncogenic Viruses: I. Recent Articles and Research in Progress. New York: MSS Information, 1974.

Collection of primarily technical reprints of five papers on RNA tumor viruses as causative factors in malignancy and twelve reprints related to the analysis of tumor viruses.

R: *Quarterly Review of Biology* 51: 353 (1976).

Leukemia. 3d ed. **Frederick Gunz and Albert G. Baikie.** New York: Grune & Stratton, 1974.

First edition, 1958; second edition, 1964.
Reviews developments in problems of leukemia. Brings together information on which modern management and research is based. Some repetition of earlier editions. Numerous references in each section. Addition to medical library of physicians dealing with leukemic patients.

R: *Annals of Internal Medicine* 83: 439 (Sept. 1975); *Blood* 46: 993 (Dec. 1975); *British Journal of Haematology* 31: 126 (1975).

The Management of Malignant Disease Series. No. 1. **Cicely M. Saunders, ed.** London: Edward Arnold, 1978.

Number 1, *The Management of Terminal Disease.*
Volume provides information to those concerned with the care of patients in the terminal stages of malignant disease. Contributors include physicians, nurses, psychiatrists, lawyers, and others. Practical advice on how to relieve pain and problems of communication with families are just two of the areas which are discussed.

R: *BMJ* 1: 110 (1979).

Medical Oncology: Medical Aspects of Malignant Disease. **K. D. Bagshawe, ed.** Oxford, England: Blackwell Scientific Publications, 1975.

Presents an overview of cancer; covers such topics as genetics, immunology, metabolic processes. Authors are specialists in their fields. A well-edited survey of selected topics in oncology. A useful book for medical libraries.

R: *Annals of Internal Medicine* 83: 591 (Oct. 1975); *British Journal of Radiology* 48: 941 (1975); *RSR* 3: 33 (July–Dec. 1975); Allyn.

Nuclear Medicine: Clinical and Technological Bases. **J. T. Andrews and M. Jean Milne.** New York: John Wiley, 1977.

Half the text is devoted to clinical bases of nuclear medicine procedures and the rest to conventional coverage of instrumentation and technology. For students in training as nuclear medicine technologists.

R: *NEJM* 298: 1371 (June 15, 1978).

Oncogenic Viruses. 2d ed. **Ludwik Gross.** New York: Pergamon, 1970.

Gold mine of information on oncogenic viruses in animals. Extremely valuable because of historical content. Similarity between human and animal tumors allows for comparison. Monograph not fully up to date or complete. Regarded as a useful source book.

R: *Lancet* 2: 82 (July 11, 1970).

The Physiopathology of Cancer. 3d ed. **F. Homburger, ed.** Basel: S. Karger, 1974–1976.

First edition, 1953; second edition, 1959.
A helpful work for oncologists in the clinic and research laboratory. Emphasizes those areas of clinical application.

A Primer of Cancer Management. **Jacob J. Lokich.** Boston, MA: G. K. Hall, 1979.

Provides basic facts about the management of the cancer patient and the expanding role of support services in cancer care. Concept of total care is emphasized throughout the book. Provides pertinent information to a wide range of personnel in the medical field.

Radiation Oncology: Rationale, Technique, Results. 5th ed. **William T. Moss, William N. Brand, and Hector Battifora.** St. Louis, MO: C. V. Mosby, 1979.

Third edition entitled *Therapeutic Radiation: Rationale, Technique, Results,* 1969; fourth edition, 1973.
Volume explores not only administration of radiation but also patient care from diagnosis to clinical management, treatment, and follow-up care. More than 300 illustrations.
R: *NEJM* 291: 858 (Oct. 17, 1974); *Radiology* 111: 420 (May 1974); Allyn; Brandon; Inke; Stearns & Ratcliff (*NEJM,* 1969; *NEJM,* 1970).

Recent Advances in Cancer and Radiotherapeutics: Clinical Oncology. **K. E. Halnan, ed.** Edinburgh: Churchill Livingstone, 1972.

R: *British Medical Bulletin* 29: 87 (1973); *Physics in Medicine & Biology* 18: 296 (Mar. 1973).

Tumors of the Head and Neck. **John G. Batsakis.** Baltimore, MD: Williams & Wilkins, 1974.

Complete and up-to-date reference which represents clinicopathological presentation of material. Devoid of therapeutic recommendations. Classification of tumors conforms to modern nomenclature.
R: *Plastic and Reconstructive Surgery* 54: 479 (1975).

OPHTHALMOLOGY

Adler's Physiology of the Eye. 6th ed. **Robert A. Moses, ed.** St. Louis, MO: C. V. Mosby, 1975.

Fifth edition, 1970.
A comprehensive text; covers all subjects relevant to ocular physiology. Deals with basic fields of science and ophthalmology. Sixth edition includes a chapter on mechanism of sensation. Good format; recommended for core reference collections in medical libraries.
R: *American Journal of Ophthalmology* 80: 962 (Nov. 1975); *Journal of the American Optometric Association* 47: 1091 (Aug. 1976); 48: 253 (Feb. 1977).

Becker-Shaffer's Diagnosis and Therapy of the Glaucomas. 4th ed. **Allan E. Kolker and John Hetherington.** St. Louis, MO: C. V. Mosby, 1976.
First edition, 1961.
An essential reference for physicians managing glaucomas. Updated edition contains many illustrations, stereoscopic goniophotographs, descriptions of surgical techniques. Highly recommended.
R: *American Journal of Ophthalmology* 83: 426 (1977).

Cataract Surgery and Its Complications. 2d ed. **Norman S. Jaffe.** St. Louis, MO: C. V. Mosby, 1976.
Volume on cataract surgery discusses subjects such as progress in surgical procedures as well as improved materials and instruments. Includes chapter on intraocular lenses written largely as a result of author's experiences. Contains abundant illustrations, and text reflects attention to detail.
R: *American Journal of Ophthalmology* 83: 139 (1977).

Contact Lens Practice. **Montague Ruben, ed.** Baltimore, MD: Williams & Wilkins, 1975.
For all optometrists who fit contact lenses. Discusses nature of contact lens material, manufacturing. Contains excellent illustrations. Also includes information on prosthetic appliances. Well written, highly recommended.
R: *American Journal of Ophthalmology* 81: 697 (May 1976).

The Eye: Comparative Physiology. Vol. 5. **Hugh Davson and L. T. Graham, Jr., eds.** New York, Academic Press, 1974.
Part of a series which reviews ophthalmological research. This issue focuses on physiology of lower vertebrate, particularly the lens. The volume is recommended as a useful reference for workers in the field.
R: *Yale Journal of Biology and Medicine* 49: 102 (1976).

Eye Surgery. 5th ed. **H. B. Stallard.** Baltimore, MD: Williams & Wilkins, 1973.
Survey of the field of ophthalmic surgery. Contains 287 new illustrations of procedure in step-by-step fashion. Recommended for ophthalmic surgery.
R: *American Journal of Ophthalmology* 78: 351 (1974).

General Ophthalmology. 8th ed. **D. Vaughn et al.** Los Altos, CA: Lange Medical Publications, 1977.
Considered a standard text book for medical students, residents, and ophthalmologists.
R: *Journal of the Medical Society of New Jersey* 72: 90 (1975); *West Virginia Medical Association* 71: xix (1975); Brandon.

Immunopathology of the Eye. **A. H. S. Rahi and A. Garner.** Philadelphia, PA: J. B. Lippincott, 1976.
First English-language text that deals comprehensively with immunology of the eye. Contains documented immunological properties of eye diseases. First section is concise view of immunological mechanisms, while remaining section evaluates

published works on immunopathology of various ocular conditions. For those interested in immunology and ocular disease.
R: *American Journal of Ophthalmology* 83: 139 (1977); *Annals of Allergy* 37: 372 (Nov. 1976).

The Ocular Adnexa. **Stewart Duke-Elder and Peter A. MacFaul.** St. Louis, MO: C. V. Mosby, 1974.
Authoritative account of diseases of ocular adnexa. First part covers territory shared by ophthalmology and dermatology while the second treats such topics as diseases of lacrimal secretory apparatus and the orbit. Wealth of information for ophthalmologists.
R: *JAMA* 235: 1379 (Mar. 29, 1976).

Ocular Syndromes. 3d ed. **Walter J. Geeraets.** Philadelphia, PA: Lea & Febiger, 1976.
Lists 436 syndromes, which should be an aid in identification of ocular disorders. Valuable section on synonyms and eponyms of syndromes. Each syndrome includes a bibliography. Includes references up to 1975. Fills the literature gap in descriptions of syndromes of pediatric ophthalmology.
R: *American Journal of Ophthalmology* 81: 859 (June 1976).

Ocular Therapeutics and Pharmacology. 5th ed. **Philip P. Ellis.** St. Louis, MO: C. V. Mosby, 1977.
Emphasis on proper administration of medication for treatment of ocular diseases. New edition features updated and condensed pharmacology section. Volume highlights the use of ocuserts and pilocarpine in glaucoma treatment and expanded pediatric dosage tables.

Ophthalmic Plastic Surgery. 5th ed. **Sidney A. Fox.** New York: Grune & Stratton, 1976.
Encyclopedic approach to ophthalmic plastic surgery. Detailed descriptions of techniques and procedures clearly reflect the author's opinion and choice. Most of the procedures represent classic surgical procedures. History and scope of problems in ophthalmic plastic surgery receive full treatment. Well-illustrated text recommended to all residents and eye physicians.
R: *American Journal of Ophthalmology* 83: 764 (May 1977); Brandon.

Ophthalmology: Principles and Concepts. 4th ed. **Frank W. Newell and J. T. Ernest.** St. Louis, MO: C. V. Mosby, 1978.
Second edition, 1969; third edition, 1974.
A treatise on ophthalmology. Serves as a guide to minor and serious diseases with ocular symptoms. Bridges the gap between the anatomy, pharmacology, physiology, and clinical examinations and diseases of the eye. References conclude each chapter. Recommended to undergraduate and graduate students.
R: *British Journal of Ophthalmology* 58: 111 (Mar. 1974); 58: 832 (Sept. 1974); *JAMA* 229: 339 (July 15, 1974); *TBRI* 40: 367 (Nov. 1974); 41: 108 (Mar. 1975); Allyn; Brandon; Inke; Stearns & Ratcliff (*NEJM*, 1969; *NEJM*, 1970).

Practical Ophthalmic Plastic and Reconstructive Surgery. **Merrill J. Reeh,**

Charles K. Beyer, and Gerard M. Shannon. Philadelphia, PA: Lea & Febiger, 1976.

Comprehensive coverage of major areas of ophthalmic plastic and reconstructive surgery. A compendium of up-to-date surgical procedures and techniques. Attempts to evaluate the patient in terms of proper procedure. Features useful references and clear illustrations. Recommended to residents and general ophthalmologists interested in plastic and reconstructive surgery.
R: *American Journal of Ophthalmology* 82: 807 (Nov. 1976).

Surgery of the Eyelids and Lacrimal System. **Lester T. Jones and John L. Wobig.** Birmingham, AL: Aesculapius, 1976.
R: *Archives of Ophthalmology* 94: 1817 (1976).

Textbook of Ophthalmology. 9th ed. **Harold G. Scheie and Daniel M. Albert.** Philadelphia, PA: W. B. Saunders, 1977.
Eighth edition entitled *Adler's Textbook of Ophthalmology,* 1969.
R: Brandon.

Toxicology of the Eye. 2d ed. **W. Morton Grant.** Springfield, IL: Charles C. Thomas, 1974.

Comprehensive index of chemicals, drugs, venoms, and plants and their related toxic effects on the eye. Lists common and exotic compounds. Outlines standard types of toxic effects in introductory section. Includes numerous, up-to-date references. Extensive cross-referencing within index facilitates ease in identifying generic, trade, common, industrial, and scientific names, signs, symptoms, toxic processes, and visual disturbances. A must for every ophthalmologist.
R. *American Journal of Ophthalmology* 77. 775 (1974); *Archives of Ophthalmology* 91: 428 (May 1974); *Canadian Journal of Ophthalmology* 9: 488 (1974).

Tumors of the Eye. 3d ed. **Algernon B. Reese.** Hagerstown, MD: Harper & Row, 1976.

Subchapters contributed by specialists supplement author's discourse on diagnosis and therapy. Highly recommended to ophthalmic residents and practicing ophthalmologists.
R: *American Journal of Ophthalmology* 83: 426 (Mar. 1977).

Ultrasonography of the Eye and Orbit. **D. Jackson Coleman, Frederic L. Lizzi and Robert L. Jack.** Philadelphia, PA: Lea & Febiger, 1977.

Comprehensive text on diagnostic and therapeutic ultrasound as applied to ophthalmology. Four sections cover basic physics, biometry and ocular and retrobulbar diagnoses. Excellent line drawings accompany ultrasonogram. Compilation of cited bibliography and additional references listed by subject.
R: *American Journal of Ophthalmology* 85: 578 (Apr. 1978).

Vitroretinal Disorders: Diagnosis and Management. **Felipe I. Tolentino. Charles L. Schepens, and H. Mackenzie Freeman.** Philadelphia, PA: W. B. Saunders, 1976.

Encyclopedic text presents material on anatomy, physiology, and biochemistry of vitreous as well as physiological and pathological appearances of vitreoretinal

diseases. Clinical significance, methods of treatment, and complications in diseases are also discussed. References are current and integrated in the text. For vitreoretinal surgeons and ophthalmologists.
R: *American Journal of Ophthalmology* 83: 140 (Jan. 1977).

ORTHOPEDICS

Backache. **Ian McNab.** Baltimore, MD: Williams & Wilkins, 1977.
Classic monograph on backache. Author's fine reputation and credentials speak for themselves. Analysis of backache utilizes simple, uncluttered line illustrations. Relates concrete facts on low back pain. Recommended to general practitioner, industrial physician, and surgeon.
R: *American Family Physician* 17: 299 (Jan. 1978); *British Journal of Surgery* 65: 67 (Jan. 1978).

Classics of Orthopaedics. **Edgar M. Bick, ed.** Philadelphia, PA: J. B. Lippincott, 1976.
A one-volume compendium of important orthopedic literature. Recommended for medical libraries as a tool which illustrates the development of orthopedics.
R: *NEJM* 295: 680 (1976).

Disease of Bone and Joints. 2d ed. **Louis Lichtenstein.** St. Louis, MO: C. V. Mosby, 1975.
First edition, 1970.
Second edition of book on disorders of bones and joints has been enlarged and rewritten. Expanded chapters on osteoporosis, infections, and chemical and radiation effects on bone. Inlcudes over 700 references and 50 new roentgenograms and photomicrographs. Contains much useful information and is a guide to further reading for all those in field of orthopedics.
R: *Archives of Otolaryngology* 102: 63 (Jan. 1976); *British Journal of Surgery* 63: 165 (Feb. 1976); *Journal of Bone and Joint Surgery* 57A: 733 (1975); *RSR* 3: 36 (July–Dec. 1975).

DuVries' Surgery of the Foot. **Verne T. Inman, ed.** St. Louis, MO: C. V. Mosby, 1973.
A much revised edition, containing a wealth of information. Recommended for medical libraries.
R: *Journal of Bone and Joint Surgery* 57B: 126 (1975).

Foot Disorders: Medical and Surgical Management. 2d ed. **Nicholas J. Giannestras, ed.** Philadelphia, PA: Lea & Febiger, 1973.
Revised and expanded edition guides the physician to care of foot problems. Explains procedures. Considered a useful book on the subject. Recommended for the library of the physician.
R: *Journal of Bone and Joint Surgery* 57A: 220 (1975).

Fractures. 2 vols. **Charles A. Rockwood, Jr., and David P. Green, eds.** Philadelphia, PA: J. B. Lippincott, 1975.
Two-volume text provides current material on fractures in a well-organized

manner. Written primarily for practicing orthopedic surgeons.
R: *Archives of Physical Medicine and Rehabilitation* 57: 303 (June 1976); *Archives of Surgery* 111: 306 (1976); *Journal of Bone and Joint Surgery* 57A: 1177 (1975); 58B: 269 (May 1976); *JAMA* 234: 977 (1975).

Heritable Disorders in Orthopaedic Practice. **Ruth Wynne-Davies.** Oxford, England: Blackwell Scientific Publications, 1973.

Concise reference on heritable orthopedic problems, described both clinically and genetically. One appendix catalogues 200 phenotypes according to patterns of inheritance, while a second appendix lists genetic advisory centers in Great Britain. Directed primarily toward orthopedic surgeons.
R: *Teratology* 10: 209 (Oct. 1974).

Mercer's Orthopaedic Surgery. 7th ed. **Robert B. Duthie and Albert B. Ferguson, Jr.** Baltimore, MD: Williams & Wilkins, 1973.

Sixth edition, 1964.
Seventh edition of classic in field of orthopedic surgery. Reflects current concerns by devoting space to amputations, prosthetics, physical therapy, and rehabilitation. Written with continued attention to scientific basis of orthopedics. Contains clear radiographs. For inclusion in medical libraries and collections of practicing orthopedists.
R: *Journal of Bone and Joint Surgery* 56B: 395 (May 1974); 57A: 437 (1975).

Metabolic, Degenerative, and Inflammatory Diseases of Bones and Joints. **Henry L. Jaffe.** Philadelphia, PA: Lea & Febiger, 1972.

A monograph on bone diseases; includes over 1,000 illustrations which relate radiograms to histological findings. Depicts many different syndromes, discusses bone growth rates. A comprehensive work for radiologists, orthopedists, and pathologists.
R: *Archives of Internal Medicine* 133: 154 (Jan. 1974); Allyn.

Orthopedic Diseases: Physiology, Pathology, Radiology. 4th ed. **Ernest E. Aegerter and John A. Kirkpatrick, Jr.** Philadelphia, PA: W. B. Saunders, 1975.

Approaches orthopedic diseases from a basic science viewpoint. Profusely illustrated; written in relatively simple language. Highly recommended to physiatrists, physical therapists, and occupational therapists.
R: *Annals of Internal Medicine* 84: 114 (1976); *Archives of Physical Medicine and Rehabilitation* 57: 46 (1976); *Journal of Bone and Joint Surgery* 57A: 1177 (1975).

Outline of Orthopaedics. 8th ed. **J. Crawford Adams.** New York: Churchill Livingstone, 1977.

First edition, 1956.
Text discusses clinical methods of approach to orthopedic disorders; provides general survey and overview of regional approaches. Omits diagnosis and treatment of fractures. Illustrations such as line drawings, X-rays, and photographs are clear. Designed for medical students and practitioners with occasional contact with orthopedic problems.
R: *Archives of Physical Medicine and Rehabilitation* 59: 51 (Jan. 1978).

Textbook of Orthopaedic Medicine. 9th ed. **J. Cyriax and Gillean Russell.** London: Macmillan, 1979.

Volume 2, *Treatment by Manipulation, Massage, and Injection.*
Seventh edition, 1978; volume 1, *Diagnosis of Soft Tissue Lesions.*
Well-known textbook. Describes diagnosis of orthopedic symptoms. Covers all major topics.

OTORHINOLARYNGOLOGY

Diseases of the Ear. 3d ed. **Stuart Mawson.** Baltimore, MD: Williams & Wilkins, 1975.

First edition, 1973.
Newest concepts are included in this third edition of classic text on otology. Covers basic anatomy and diagnostic procedures as well as pathological abnormalities and diseases. Describes surgical procedures illustrated with drawings. Important for surgeons, residents, and students in field of otology.
R: *Archives of Otolaryngology* 102: 518 (Oct. 1976).

Diseases of the Nose, Throat and Ear. 12th ed. **John J. Ballenger, ed.** Philadelphia, PA: Lea & Febiger, 1977.

In five parts: the nose and sinuses, the pharynx, the larynx, the ear, and bronchoesophagology. Comprises a thorough review. A standard reference in the field.
R: *Plastic and Reconstructive Surgery* 62: 607 (1978).

Pathology of the Ear. **I. Friedmann.** Philadelphia, PA: F. A. Davis, 1974.

A synthesis of recent advances in the field of otorhinolaryngologic pathology, the author's clinical work, and ear research with tissue culture and electron microscopy. Divided into three sections: pathology of the external and middle ears, pathology of the inner ear and deafness, and laboratory procedures and techniques. Profusely illustrated. Includes very comprehensive bibliography and reliable index. Written mainly for the teacher and advanced student in otorhinolaryngology or pathology.
R: *Archives of Otology, Rhinology and Laryngology* 84: 133 (1975); *Lancet* 2: 199 (July 27, 1974).

Pathology of the Ear. **Harold F. Schuknecht.** Cambridge, MA: Harvard University Press, 1974.

A complete compendium of otopathology. Treats the histology, anatomy, and pathophysiology of otologic diseases. Illustrations are mainly black-and-white photographs, sections, and diagrams. Includes a complete reference list and index. A selected slide set of relevant illustrations accompany this volume. Described as a must for practicing otologists and an essential reference source for otolaryngology training programs.
R: *Annals of Otology, Rhinology and Laryngology* 84: 404 (1975); *Archives of Otolaryngology* 101: 588 (Sept. 1975); *RSR* 3: 45 (Jan.–Mar. 1975).

PATHOLOGY

Applied Surgical Pathology. **Angus E. Stuart, A. N. Smith, and Eric Samuel, eds.** Philadelphia, PA: J. B. Lippincott, 1975.

Attempts to integrate the fields of pathology, radiology, and surgery, providing systematic accounts of disease. Profusely illustrated; contains X-rays, photomicrographs, and diagrams. An excellent reference combining the viewpoints of three different fields. Recommended.
R: *Journal of Clinical Pathology* 29: 763 (Aug. 1976); *South African Medical Journal* 50: 1418 (Aug. 21, 1976); *Surgery, Gynecology and Obstetrics* 143: 287 (Aug. 1976); *TBRI* 42: 310 (Oct. 1976); 42: 350 (Nov. 1976); 42: 387 (Dec. 1976).

Bailey's Textbook of Histology. 17th ed. **W. M. Copenhaver, D. E. Kelly, and R. L. Wood.** Baltimore, MD: Williams & Wilkins, 1978.

A well-written and referenced text which assists the student in integrating human embryology and histology. Includes photomicrograph and electron micrograph methods of studying cells. For medical students and laboratory workers.
R: *Journal of Anatomy* 129: 189 (Aug. 1979).

Basic Pathology. 2d ed. **Stanley L. Robbins and Marcia Angell.** Philadelphia, PA: W. B. Saunders, 1976.

Second edition of the standard pathology text. Contains new information. Lucid text which describes the basis of disease at a cellular level. Divided into two sections: basic and systematic. A useful reference for the medical library and as a text for core curriculum in pathology.
R: *Annals of Internal Medicine* 86: 681 (May 1977); *Archives of Pathology & Laboratory Medicine* 101: 392 (July 1977).

The Essentials of Forensic Medicine. 3d ed. **Cyril J. Polson and D. J. Gee.** New York: Pergamon, 1973.

Second edition, 1965.
Third edition of authoritative textbook of forensic medicine. Book is in two sections: forensic pathology comprises the larger and law relating to medical practice the smaller. Standard of research has been high, resulting in extensive bibliography. Directed to postgraduate students and specialists and practitioners in forensic medicine.
R: *BMJ* 2: 1178 (May 1, 1965); 2: 395 (Apr. 18, 1974); *Journal of Clinical Pathology* 27: 434 (May 1974); *Journal of Pathology* 117: 63 (Sept. 1975).

Fine Structure of Cells and Tissues. 4th ed. **Keith R. Porter and Mary A. Bonneville.** Philadelphia, PA: Lea & Febiger, 1973.

A concise text of histology and cell biology. Contains many high-resolution micrographs. Instructive for students; a supplement in lectures and labs.

General Pathology. 4th ed. **Lord Florey.** Philadelphia, PA: W. B. Saunders, 1970.

Revised edition of Florey's classic lectures. Includes newer information. Combines fact with hypothesis; covers all major topics. Recommended for students of pathology.

R: *Canadian Medical Association Journal* 102: 1114 (May 1970).

Histopathologic Technic and Practical Histochemistry. 4th ed. **R. D. Lillie and Harold M. Fullmer.** New York: McGraw-Hill, 1976.

Encyclopedic histopathology-histochemistry text has been expanded to include enzyme and fluorescent histochemistry and electron microscopic techniques. In-depth approach to topics exemplified in well-documented chapter on endogenous pigments. Characterized by extensive detailed coverage of histologic techniques. Highly recommended to both beginner and expert.

R: *Journal of Histochemistry and Cytochemistry* 25: 473 (June 1977).

Histopathology of the Bone Marrow. **Arkadi M. Rywlin.** Boston, MA: Little, Brown, 1976.

A systematic account of bone marrow histopathology in various diseases. Provides meticulous, scholarly descriptions. A comprehensive ready reference. Includes helpful photographs and illustrations. Most useful for histopathologists and hematologists.

R: *Annals of Internal Medicine* 86: 677 (May 1977); *British Journal of Haematology* 35: 168 (1977).

Microbiology and Pathology. 11th ed. **Alice L. Smith.** St. Louis, MO: C. V. Mosby, 1976.

R: Brandon (*NO*).

Molecular Pathology. **Robert A. Good et al.** Springfield, IL: Charles C. Thomas, 1975.

A basic reference source for pathologists on both a clinical and research level.

R: *Delaware Medical Journal* 48: 115 (Feb. 1976); *JAMA* 235: 656 (Feb. 9, 1976); *TBRI* 42: 139 (Apr. 1976); 42: 184 (May 1976).

Pathologic Basis of Disease. 2d ed. **Stanley L. Robbins and Ramzi S. Cotran.** Philadelphia, PA: W. B. Saunders, 1979.

The best-known book in the field. Complete, reliable reference for medical students.

R: *JAMA* 229: 1808 (Sept. 23, 1974); *TBRI* 40: 368 (Nov. 1974); Allyn.

Pathologic Physiology: Mechanism of Disease. 6th ed. **W. A. Sodeman, Jr., and W. A. Sodeman, eds.** Philadelphia, PA: W. B. Saunders, 1979.

Fifth edition, 1974.

Discusses the biochemical and natural history of disease, covering a wide range of topics. This is an extensive collection of information, valuable to the clinician.

R: *Physical Therapy* 55: 199 (Feb. 1975); Allyn.

Pathology. 7th ed. 2 vols. **William A. D. Anderson and John M. Kissane.** St. Louis, MO: C. V. Mosby, 1977.

Sixth edition, 1971.

Expanded and updated, this new, multi-authored edition details general and then systematic pathology. Emphasizes clinical and pathologic correlation. Encyclopedic in scope. Includes good quality black-and-white plates and extensive

bibliographies. Useful for pathologists of all levels.
R: *JAMA* 238: 2730 (Dec. 19, 1977); Allyn; Stearns & Ratcliff (*NEJM*, 1969).

Pathology of Pulmonary Hypertension. **C. A. Wagenvoort and Noeke Wagenvoort.** New York: John Wiley, 1977.

Billed as an authoritative review of current information regarding pulmonary hypertension pathology. Covers etiology, pathogenesis, pathology, pathophysiology, and even therapy. Each chapter ends with a diagrammatic summary. Important reference source for the practicing pathologist and research worker.
R: *Archives of Pathology & Laboratory Medicine* 102: 331 (1978).

The Pathology of the Heart. **E. G. J. Olsen.** New York: Stratton Intercontinental Medical Book Corporation, 1973.

Bridges the literature gap between voluminous texts and standard textbooks. Summarizes the pathology of cardiovascular disease in a pocket-size text. Classic, terse descriptions of almost every condition are mentioned. The twenty chapters are divided into four parts: normal heart and structural and functional changes, acquired conditions, congenital anomalies, and cardiomyopathies. Black-and-white gross and microscopic photographs are excellent. Most references quoted from American sources. Perfect companion for every student of pathology, general medicine, or cardiology.
R: *American Journal of Cardiology* 34: 880 (1974); *BMJ* 1: 81 (Jan. 12, 1974); *Journal of Gerontology* 31: 487 (July 1976).

Pathology of the Kidney. 2d ed. 2 vols. **Robert H. Heptinstall.** Boston, MA: Little, Brown, 1974.

First edition, 1966.
Comprehensive two-volume text on the pathology of the kidney. Deserves the same attention and praise as Dr. Heptinstall's first edition in 1966. Second edition contains updated and expanded sections on embryological developments, congenital malformations, and transplantation of the kidney. Incorporates additional high-quality electron micrographs and immunofluorescent photomicrographs. Billed as a combination reference source and atlas on all phases of renal pathology. Highly recommended to nephrologists and pathologists in training, physicians and medical and graduate students.
R: *Annals of Internal Medicine* 83: 295 (Aug. 1975); *Archives of Pathology & Laboratory Medicine* 99: 510 (Sept. 1975); *Archives of Surgery* 111: 96 (Jan. 1976); Allyn.

Pathology of the Lung (Excluding Pulmonary Tuberculosis). 3d ed. 2 vols. **H. Spencer.** Philadelphia, PA: W. B. Saunders, 1977.

Second edition, 1968.
Standard reference work covering both common and rare conditions of the lung. Incorporates data on pulmonary diseases accumulated within the last decade. Special and complete emphasis given to the areas of embryology, anatomy, and congenital anomalies. Includes in-depth discussion of occupational diseases.
Third edition appears in two-column format. No references supplied to numerous studies conducted since 1968. Useful as general reading and for specific reference cases.
R: *JAMA* 239: 651 (Feb. 13, 1978); *Nature* 266: x (Apr. 28, 1977); Allyn.

Pathophysiology: Altered Regulatory Mechanisms in Disease. 2d ed. **Edward D. Frohlich, ed.** Philadelphia, PA: J. B. Lippincott, 1976.

A timely updated edition. Correlates pathophysiology to clinical practice, as in first edition.
R: *JAMA* 237: 809 (Feb. 21, 1977); Allyn.

Principles and Techniques of Scanning Electron Microscopy: Biological Applications. 2 vols. **M. A. Hayat, ed.** New York/Princeton, NJ: Van Nostrand Reinhold, 1974–1975.

Details the techniques of scanning electron microscopy. A useful tool for biologists. Accompanied by extensive bibliographies.
R: *Quarterly Review of Biology* 50: 528 (1975).

Recent Advances in Forensic Pathology. **F. E. Camps.** London: Churchill Livingstone, 1969.

Short, concise, readable, illustrated work.

Scanning Electron Microscopy. 2 vols. Chicago, IL: Illinois Institute of Technology Research Institute, 1976.

A two-volume monograph which discusses applications and trends in scanning electron microscopy research. Format is concise, yet comprehensive. Accompanying illustrations are of high quality. Useful for biologists and pathologists.
R: *Archives of Pathology & Laboratory Medicine* 101: 333 (June 1977).

Surgical Pathology. 5th ed. **Lauren V. Ackerman and Juan Rosai.** St. Louis, MO: C. V. Mosby, 1974.

Fourth edition, 1968.
The fifth edition of this basic text on surgical pathology has been expanded and updated. Organ systems provide outline of book, and format includes descriptions, incidences, behavior, und prognosis. Excellent illustrations and extensive bibliography. Recommended as a reference for surgeons.
R: *Chest* 66: 738B (1974); *Gastroenterology* 67: 563 (Sept. 1974); Allyn.

PEDIATRICS

Adolescents in Health and Disease. **William A. Daniel, Jr.** St. Louis, MO: C. V. Mosby, 1977.

In two parts: gives an overview of the health care needs of the adolescent with reference to emotional needs of young adults and details health care concerns and practice as well as diseases inherent to adolescents. A practical and valuable reference.
R: *Canadian Medical Association Journal* 118: 1042 (May 6, 1978).

Assessment of Medical Care for Children. **Institute of Medicine.** Washington, DC: US National Academy of Sciences, 1974. (*Contrasts in Health Status* series, vol. 3).

Babies: Human Development During the First Year. **B. Zachau-Christiansen and E. M. Ross.** New York: John Wiley, 1975.

Based on a study conducted on some 9,000 mothers in the Copenhagen University Hospital between 1959 and 1961. Emphasis on factors in pregnancy and prenatal period affecting the infant (particularly its development after one year of life). Data processed in tabular form for quick and easy understanding. Highlights the influences of maternal health, birth weight, and social background. Fine addition to most medical libraries.
R: *British Journal of Obstetrics and Gynecology* 83: 591 (July 1976).

Basic Pediatrics for the Primary Health Care Provider. **Catherine DeAngelis.** Boston, MA: Little, Brown, 1975.
Introduction to the field of pediatrics. Aimed at pediatricians in practice and in classroom instructor positions.

Beck's Obstetrical Practice and Fetal Medicine. 10th ed. **Stewart Taylor.** Baltimore, MD: Williams & Wilkins, 1976.
Authoritative volume on obstetrics. Includes information on neonatal and intensive care practice. Especially useful for residents.

Behavior Disorders of Childhood and Adolescence. **Richard J. Jenkins.** Springfield, IL: Charles C. Thomas, 1973.
Classifies personality disorders of children and adolescents. Employs psychoanalytic and more general analysis of commonly encountered problems. A valuable treatise for physicians, paramedics, community mental health workers.
R: *Pediatrics* 53: 595 (Apr. 1974).

Cancer in Children: Clinical Management. **H. J. G. Bloom et al., eds.** New York: Springer-Verlag, 1975.
Comprehensive treatment of subject of childhood cancer. Concise text for medical students and physicians interested in care of children with cancer.
R: *Annals of Internal Medicine* 86: 678 (May 1977).

Clinical Paediatric Surgery. **Peter G. Jones.** Philadelphia, PA: J. B. Lippincott, 1977.
A ready reference to surgical conditions in infancy and childhood. Systematic presentation. Inlcudes information on such topics as genetic counseling, tonsillectomy. Appendix includes normal values of blood and its components. Recommended to any physician who cares for infants and children.
R: *American Family Physician* 17: 299 (Jan. 1978).

Clinical Pediatric Oncology. 2d ed. **Wataru W. Sutow, Teresa J. Vietti, and Donald J. Fernbach, eds.** St. Louis, MO: C. V. Mosby, 1977.
First edition, 1973.
Expanded, authoritative edition. Details etiology, genetic, and environmental factors in pediatric oncology. New edition includes information on nuclear medicine, radiation therapy, and comprehensive coverage of leukemia. Well referenced; extensive bibliography. A classic reference source.
R: *Clinical Pediatrics* 14: 802 (Sept. 1975); *JAMA* 239: 1911 (May 5, 1978).

Clinical Perinatology. **Silvio Aladjem and Audrey K. Brown, eds.** St. Louis, MO: C. V. Mosby, 1974.

A well-organized and presented book on perinatology. Multi-authored, with contributions from European and American authorities. Among topics discussed are placental function, neonatal pneumonia, genetic counseling, protection of fetus and newborn. Valuable index and list of references. Recommended to obstetricians, pediatricians.
R: *Journal of the Medical Society of New Jersey* 72: 268 (Mar. 1975); *Lancet* 2: 212 (Aug. 2, 1975); *Mayo Clinic Proceedings* 50: 157 (Mar. 1975); *Rhode Island Medical Journal* 58: 134 (Mar. 1975); *TBRI* 41: 177 (May 1975); 41: 222 (June 1975).

Current Pediatric Diagnosis & Treatment. 5th ed. **C. Henry Kempe, Henry K. Silver, and Donough O'Brien.** Los Altos, CA.: Lange Medical Publications, 1978.

Describes current methods of diagnosis and treatment in pediatrics. Includes line drawings, charts. Discusses common disorders. A usual ready reference.
R: *American Family Physician* 18: 259 (Nov. 1978).

Current Pediatric Therapy. 8th ed. **Sydney S. Gellis and Benjamin M. Kagan.** Philadelphia, PA: W. B. Saunders, 1978.

Recent edition of this multi-authored compendium discusses treatment of disease in children and parents of diseased children. Includes tables of drug dosage and information on sudden infant death. A valuable guide for the practicing pediatrician.
R: *American Family Physician* 18: 257 (Nov. 1978).

Davison's Compleat Pediatrician. 9th ed. **Jay M. Arena, ed.** Philadelphia, PA: Lea & Febiger, 1969.

Diseases of the Nervous System in Infancy, Childhood, and Adolescence. 6th ed. **Frank R. Ford.** Springfield, IL: Charles C. Thomas, 1973.

Major reference text for pediatricians and neurologists. Clear presentation of clinical picture of pathology of symptoms affecting the nervous systems of children and adolescents. Surgical information is not extensive or current. For inclusion in neurological and neurosurgical libraries.
R: *Journal of Neurosurgery* 44: 267 (Feb. 1976).

Disorders of the Respiratory Tract in Children. 3d ed. **Edwin L. Kendig, Jr., and Victor Chernick, eds.** Philadelphia, PA: W. B. Saunders, 1977.

Third edition reflects revision and the addition of seven new chapters. Discusses pathophysiology of pediatric chest disease, diagnosis, and therapy. High-quality reproduction of roentgenograms. Essential resource for physicians who cope with children's chest disease.
R: *JAMA* 239: 1800 (Apr. 28, 1978).

The Fetus and Newly Born Infant: Influences of the Perinatal Environment. 2d ed. **Roger E. Stevenson.** St. Louis, MO: C. V. Mosby, 1977.

Discusses prenatal influences that govern development of the product of conception. Bibliography is extensive; graphic and tabular material excellent; text writ-

ten with clarity. Should appeal to obstetricians, pediatricians, and residents.
R: *Clinical Pediatrics* 14: 802 (Sept. 1975).

The First Three Years of Life. **Burton L. White.** Englewood Cliffs, NJ: Prentice-Hall, 1975.
Chronological reference of child development in the first three years. Emphasizes practical advice for recognition of behavioral phases, educational needs, and child rearing practices. Includes index and annotated reading list. Helpful for parents, public and school libraries.
R: *RSR* 4: 92 (Apr.–June 1976).

Hematology of Infancy and Childhood. **David G. Nathan and Frank A. Oski.** Philadelphia, PA: W. B. Saunders, 1974.
Covers all hematologic diseases of children, with contributions from authorities that emphasize biochemistry, immunology, enzymology, and physiology. Contains a comprehensive list of references as well as electron and photomicrographs. A superb text for medical students, hematologists, researchers.
R: *Blood* 46: 470 (1975); *Journal of Pediatrics* 88: 349 (Feb. 1976); *Pediatrics* 58: 469 (Sept. 1976); Allyn.

Infectious Diseases of the Fetus and Newborn Infant. **Jack S. Remington and Jerome O. Klein, eds.** Philadelphia, PA: W. B. Saunders, 1976.
Comprehensive collection of data published on major infectious diseases which afflict fetus and newborn. Twenty chapters written by experts span epidemiology, diagnosis, and treatment of infection. Critical review of current state of the art with excellent tables and graphs. Exhaustive bibliographies, some containing over 600 citations. Recommended as a standard reference work and definitive volume for use by pediatricians, family practitioners, obstetricians, and medical students.
R: *American Family Physician* 16: 161 (Aug. 1977); *American Journal of Diseases of Children* 132: 825 (Aug. 1978); *Annals of Internal Medicine* 87: 139 (July 1977); *British Journal of Obstetrics & Gynaecology* 84: 638 (Aug. 1977); *JAMA* 237: 2126 (May 9, 1977); *Mayo Clinic Proceedings* 54: 260 (1977).

Leukemia in Childhood. **Andre D. Lascari.** Springfield, IL: Charles C. Thomas, 1973.
Summarizes information about treatment of childhood acute leukemia. At once a practical primer and reference source. Concise, logical format and simply written. Contains over 1,750 references. Illustrations are of poor quality. For use in hospital libraries.
R: *Archives of Internal Medicine* 134: 1142 (Dec. 1974); *Clinical Pediatrics* 14: 323 (Apr. 1975); *NEJM* 291: 110 (July 11, 1974); *Pediatrics* 57: 290 (Feb. 1976).

Medical Complications During Pregnancy. **Gerard N. Burrow and Thomas F. Ferris.** Philadelphia, PA: W. B. Saunders, 1975.
Composed of 22 reviews written by authorities about the effect of pregnancy on medical disease. Includes glossary. Text for both beginning students and practicing internists and obstetricians.
R: *JAMA* 237: 159 (Jan. 10, 1977); *Mayo Clinic Proceedings* 51: 396 (June 1976).

Metabolic, Endocrine and Genetic Disorders of Children. 3 vols. **Vincent C. Kelley, ed.** New York: Harper & Row, 1974.

Recommended as a reference text for practicing physicians.
R: *JAMA* 231: 768 (Feb. 17, 1975); *TBRI* 41: 145 (Apr. 1975).

Neonatal Medicine. **Forrester Cockburn and Cecil M. Drillien, eds.** London: Blackwell Scientific Publications, 1974.

Textbook of neonatal physiology and disorders. Excellent reference in neonatal ward.
R: *BMJ* 1: 1408 (June 5, 1976).

Neonatology: Pathophysiology and Management of the Newborn. **Gordon B. Avery, ed.** Philadelphia, PA: J. B. Lippincott, 1975.

A complex and thorough presentation of the pathophysiology of the newborn; covers an encyclopedic amount of information, including a section on surgery of the neonate. Contains useful references, appendixes. Extensive and well organized; an excellent reference source for those who manage the care of high-risk infants.
R: *American Family Physician* 13: 225 (Mar. 1976); *American Journal of Diseases of Children* 130: 788 (July 1976).

Neuroradiology in Infants and Children. 3 vols. **Derek C. Harwood-Nash and Charles R. Fitz.** St. Louis, MO: C. V. Mosby, 1976.

Definitive work covers such topics as computed tomography, normal and abnormal skulls, neoplasms, abnormalities of cerebral arteries, and congenital malformations. Well-organized book which includes outstanding photographs. Very useful to neurosurgeons, pediatric neurologists, and radiologists concerned with childhood neurological problems and to students and residents.
R: *Radiology* 125: 164 (1977).

Orthopaedic Surgery in Infancy and Childhood. 4th ed. **Albert B. Ferguson, Jr.** Baltimore, MD: Williams & Wilkins, 1975.

A compendium of pediatric orthopedics. Outlines facts and procedures in surgery. Incorporates the experience of twelve additional contributors. Suited to the needs of advanced residents and clinicians. Valuable addition to libraries serving teaching facilities.
R: *Journal of Bone and Joint Surgery* 58A: 292 (1976); *NEJM* 294: 677 (1976).

Paediatric Gastroenterology. **Charlotte M. Anderson and Valerie Burke, eds.** Philadelphia, PA: J. B. Lippincott, 1975.

A reference source for pediatricians and physicians interested in the gastrointestinal tract in children.
R: *American Journal of Diseases of Children* 130: 903 (Aug. 1976).

Paediatric Kidney Disease. 2 vols. **C. M. Edelmann, Jr., ed.** Boston, MA: Little, Brown, 1978.

A multi-authored, two-volume work which covers all aspects of kidney anatomy and physiology of children. Text is clear, comprehensive; includes illustrations,

index, and bibliography. Written by authorities in the field, recommended as a standard reference.
R: *BMJ* 2: 381 (Aug. 11, 1979); *Lancet* 2: 15 (July 7, 1979).

Pathology of Infancy and Childhood. 2d ed. **John M. Kissane and Margaret G. Smith.** St. Louis, MO: C. V. Mosby, 1975.
Includes recent data and new ideas. Highly recommended to general and pediatric pathologists and residents in pathology.
R: *JAMA* 235: 542 (Feb. 2, 1976).

Pediatric Cardiology. 3d ed. **Alexander S. Nadas and Donald C. Fyler.** Philadelphia, PA: W. B. Saunders, 1972.
Considered a basic text on the subject.
R: Allyn.

Pediatric Clinical Gastroenterology. 2d ed. **Claude C. Roy, Arnold Silverman, and Frank J. Cozzetto.** St. Louis, MO: C. V. Mosby, 1975.
First edition, 1971.
A state-of-the-art publication. Places great emphasis on clinical information. Organized in three major sections: common symptoms and signs, 25 common disease entities, and laboratory procedures and tests. Particularly strong in methods of management. Richly illustrated with line drawings, X-rays, and tables. Key references conclude each section; some classic papers are omitted. Aimed at pediatricians, primary care physicians dealing with children, and gastroenterologists.
R: *American Journal of Digestive Diseases* 21: 839 (Sept. 1976); *Gastroenterology* 71: 176 (July 1976); *Pediatrics* 51: 962 (May 1973).

Pediatric Nephrology. **Mitchell I. Rubin and T. Martin Barratt, eds.** Baltimore, MD: Williams & Wilkins, 1975.
A compendium of information on renal disease in children. Written by leading authorities in the field. A reference text directed to both nephrologists and practitioners.
R: *JAMA* 234: 1185 (Dec. 15, 1975); *TBRI* 42: 26 (Jan. 1976).

Pediatric Nuclear Medicine. **A. Everette James, Jr., Henry N. Wagner, Jr., and Robert E. Cooke, eds.** Philadelphia, PA: W. B. Saunders, 1974.
Fourteen sections devoted to pediatric nuclear medicine rather than to isotope scanning in pediatrics. Written by 85 contributing authors in the field. Bulk of text emphasizes the biological implications of the use of radioactive materials. Some repetition in chapters of choice of agent, sedation, etc. Bone scanning section is excellent. Suggested reference source for pediatricians, radiologists, and surgeons.
R: *American Journal of Roentgenology* 123: 857 (Apr. 1975).

Pediatric Orthopedics. 2 vols. **Mihran O. Tachdjian.** Philadelphia, PA: W. B. Saunders, 1972.
Devoted to common and rare conditions. Valuable reference source.
R: *NEJM* 289: 51 (1973).

Pediatric Surgery. Repr. 2d ed. 2 vols. **W. T. Mustard et al., eds.** Chicago, IL: Year Book Medical Publishers, 1972.
First edition, 1962; second edition, 1969.
Two-volume monumental reference work. Consists of contributions from 80 authorities in the field. Specialty sections offer only brief overviews rather than thorough presentations. General chapters (anesthesia, antibiotics, genetic principles, etc.) tend to be somewhat dated. Contains excellent illustrations of patients. Aimed at surgeons with an interest in pediatrics.
R: *Plastic and Reconstructive Surgery* 58: 496 (1976).

Pediatrics. 16th ed. **Abraham M. Rudolph, ed.** New York: Appleton-Century-Crofts, 1977.
First edition, 1896; fourteenth edition, 1968; fifteenth edition, 1972.
A practical one-volume reference source. Emphasizes diagnosis, management, and treatment of pediatric conditions. Provides in-depth discussion on genetic disorders, hematology, psychological disorders, prenatal care and diagnosis, etc. Delineates recent developments and current approaches to growth and development. Includes detailed index.
R: *American Family Physician* 17: 265 (Feb. 1978); *American Journal of Diseases of Children* 124: 790 (1972); Allyn.

Perinatal Medicine. **James W. Goodwin, John O. Godden, and Graham W. Chance, eds.** Baltimore, MD: Williams & Wilkins, 1976.
Praised as a comprehensive and well-written text on perinatal medicine.
R: *British Journal of Obstetrics & Gynaecology* 84: 636 (Aug. 1977); *Canadian Medical Association Journal* 117: 444 (Sept. 3, 1977); *Lancet* 2: 70 (July 9, 1977).

Practical Neonatal Pediatrics. 3d ed. **R. J. K. Brown and H. B. Valman.** Philadelphia, PA: J. B. Lippincott, 1976.
Second edition, 1973.
Emphasis on the management of the newborn infant in the average hospital setting. Sound, practical advice on differential diagnosis from symptoms and signs. Various common conditions and treatments briefly outlined. Appendixes list tables and nomograms for gestation age and developmental assessments. Fills the literature gap for the obstetric house surgeon, pediatrician, midwife, nursery nurse, and medical students.
R: *Clinical Pediatrics* 13: 611 (July 1974); 17: 342 (Apr. 1978).

The Practice of Pediatric Neurology. 2 vols. **Kenneth F. Swaiman and Francis S. Wright.** St. Louis, MO: C. V. Mosby, 1975.
A comprehensive review of child neurology. Encyclopedic in scope, it covers diagnostic procedures and treatments of various neurologic disorders. Both volumes abundantly referenced with classic and up-to-date citations. Includes high-quality illustrations and helpful summary tables. Volume 1 contains a comprehensive index. Designed as a reference source in physical medicine for residents and physiatrists.
R: *Archives of Physical Medicine and Rehabilitation* 58: 45 (Jan. 1977).

The Prenatal Diagnosis of Hereditary Disorders. **Aubrey Milunsky.** Springfield, IL: Charles C. Thomas, 1973.

An excellent review of the field of genetic counseling and basic principles of genetics until 1972. Composed of nine chapters mainly concerned with the techniques, interpretations, limitations, and pitfalls of amniocentesis. Additional techniques and procedures involved in prenatal diagnosis are discussed. Features clear illustrations, extensive bibliography (891 references), and complete index. Monograph aimed at obstetricians, pediatricians, general practitioners, genetic counselors, and pediatric neurologists.

R: *American Journal of Human Genetics* 26: 276 (Mar. 1974); *Neurology* 24: 799 (Aug. 1974); *Teratology* 11: 331 (June 1975).

Progress in Paediatric Neurosurgery. **K. A. Bushe, O. Spoerri, and J. Shaw, eds.** Stuttgart: Hippokrates Verlag, 1974.

R: *Brain* 97: 613 (Sept. 1974); *Journal of Neurosurgery* 42: 242 (Feb. 1975).

Pulmonary Physiology of the Fetus, Newborn and Child. **Emile M. Scarpelli.** London: Henry Kimpton, 1976.

Surveys the pulmonary function during the prenatal period. This multi-authored volume features numerous well-chosen references for advanced study. Aimed at research workers in this progressive new field.

R: *BMJ* 1: 1217 (May 15, 1976).

Radiology of the Newborn and Young Infant. **Leonard E. Swischuh.** Baltimore, MD: Williams & Wilkins, 1973.

Radiology text which contains excellent reproductions and up-to-date literature references.

R: *Clinical Pediatrics* 13: 612 (July 1974).

Recent Advances in Pediatrics. 5th ed. **D. Hull, ed.** Baltimore, MD: Williams & Wilkins, 1976.

Fourth edition, 1971.

R: *American Journal of Diseases of Children* 123: 267 (1972); *BMJ* 1: 1567 (Dec. 12, 1976).

Review of Urology in Childhood. **Innes Williams, ed.** New York: Springer-Verlag, 1974.

Text incorporates large volume of information from many disciplines in its modern approach to pediatric urological problems. Forty-five pages of pertinent references are included.

R: *Pediatrics* 59: 488 (Mar. 1977).

Smith's Blood Diseases of Infancy and Childhood. 4th ed. **Carl H. Smith, Denis R. Miller, and Howard A. Pearson, eds.** St. Louis, MO: C. V. Mosby, 1978.

Third edition, 1972.

Textbook of Pediatrics. 11th ed. **Waldo E. Nelson et al.** Philadelphia, PA: W. B. Saunders, 1979.

Ninth edition, 1969.
A well-organized and basic reference text which extensively covers the field of pediatrics.
R: Stearns & Ratcliff (*AJN*; *NEJM*, 1969; *NEJM*, 1970).

Tumours of Childhood: A Clinical Treatise. **I. G. Williams.** London: Heinemann Medical, 1972.
Includes chapters on surgical problems of treatment, radiotherapy, and chemotherapy of tumors. Sections on acute leukemia, intracranial tumors, nursing aspects, and parent counseling. Illustrated with case histories. Important reference for pediatricians and surgeons.
R: *Lancet* 2: 26 (July 7, 1973).

PHARMACY AND PHARMACOLOGY

Antibiotics: A Critical Review. **W. Kurylowicz, ed.** Warsaw, Poland: Polish Medical Publishers, 1976.
A valuable introduction to the subject of antibiotics in a very small book. The book is divided into two principal parts: antibiotics in microbial metabolism and antibiotics as therapeutic agents. Its condensed form prevents its use as a sole source of information about these compounds.
R: *Journal of Pharmaceutical Sciences* 66: 911 (June 1977).

Benzodiazepines in Clinical Practice. **David J. Greenblatt and Richard I. Shader.** New York: Raven Press, 1974.
Synthesizes the literature of benzodiazepines into a concise volume. Cites some 2,000 references, reviews biochemical, neurophysiological, neuropharmacological, and behavioral manifestations of these commonly taken tranquilizers. A reference for medical libraries.
R: *American Journal of Psychiatry* 132: 206 (Feb. 1975); *Lancet* 2: 500 (Aug. 31, 1974).

Burger's Medicinal Chemistry. 4th ed. 3 parts. **M. E. Wolff, ed.** New York: John Wiley, 1979–.
Three-part classic in medicinal chemistry. Concentrates on advances in the field within the past ten years. Part I examines general principles of medicinal chemistry. Part II focuses on individual drug classes. Part III offers additional individual drug classes.

Cannabis and Health. **J. D. P. Graham, ed.** London: Academic Press, 1976.
Comprehensive account of current status on cannabis: its nature, pharmacological action, and social issues which surround it. Valuable contribution to the literature; recommended for medical libraries.
R: *American Journal of Psychiatry* 134: 705 (June 1977); *BMJ* 1: 1139 (Nov. 6, 1976).

Cocaine. **Lester Grinspoon and James B. Bakalar.** New York: Basic Books, 1976.

A monograph on cocaine. Covers all aspects of the drug.
R: *Journal of Nervous and Mental Disease* 166: 452 (1978).

Cooper and Gun's Dispensing for Pharmaceutical Students. 12th ed. **S. J. Carter, ed.** Turnbridge Wells, Kent, England: Pitman Medical, 1975.

Written as a companion to *Tutorial Pharmacy.* Describes the whole process of pharmaceutical dispensing, complete with theoretical background. Ideal reference tool for students and pharmacists.
R: *ABL* 41: entry 16 (Jan. 1976).

Drug Disposition and Pharmacokinetics With a Consideration of Pharmacological and Clinical Relationships. **Stephen H. Curry.** Oxford, England: Blackwell Scientific Publications, 1977.

Drug-Induced Ocular Side Effects and Drug Interactions. **F. T. Fraunfelder.** Philadelphia, PA: Lea & Febiger, 1976.

Quick reference source to adverse reactions affecting the ocular system caused by medication and/or the interactions of several drugs. Tabular format lists generic and proprietary names with corresponding ocular effects in order of importance. A gold mine of information for ophthalmologists, physicians, and pharmacists.
R: *American Journal of Ophthalmology* 84: 130 (July 1977); *Archives of Ophthalmology* 95: 530 (Mar. 1977); *ARBA* (1977, p. 723).

Drug Metabolism in Man. **J. W. Gorrod and A. H. Beckett, eds.** London: Taylor & Francis, 1978.

Drugs and the Elderly: Social and Pharmacological Issues. **David M. Petersen, Frank J. Whittington, and Barbara P. Payne, eds.** Springfield, IL: Charles C. Thomas, 1979.

Based on results from a series of conferences conducted by the Duke University Center for the Study of Aging and Human Development in North Carolina. Concentrates on the plight of the elderly at home and in nursing homes faced with drug misuse and abuse.
R: *BMJ* 2: 267 (July 28, 1979).

Gaddum's Pharmacology. 8th ed. **A. S. V. Burgen and J. F. Mitchell.** New York: Oxford University Press, 1978.

Seventh edition, 1972.
Eighth edition describes advances in pharmacology over past few years. Covers drug action and its relevance to modern pharmacology. Concentrates on centrally acting drugs, analgesics, and catecholamines. Drug action is carefully reviewed for each physiological system and includes a discussion of pertinent individual drugs.

An Introduction to Human Pharmacology. **J. D. P. Graham.** London: Oxford University Press, 1979.

Basic introduction to the clinical manifestations of drugs on the human body. Outlines mechanisms of drug action. Discusses principles from pharmacokinetics

through significant groups of medicine. Concentrates on the nervous system drugs. Features various illustrations of disease processes. Geared toward beginning medical students and students of pharmacology.
R: *BMJ* 1: 1555 (June 9, 1979).

LSD: A Total Study. **D. Siva Sankar et al.** Westbury, NY: PJD Publications, 1975.
Emphasizes various aspects of LSD: molecular, genetic, biochemical, psychological, pharmacological, and physiological. Includes illustrations of plants which produce drugs. A drug abuse bibliography and drug slang glossary comprise the appendixes. Subject and author indexes included.
R: *RSR* 3: 71 (July–Dec. 1975).

The Pharmacological Basis of Therapeutics. 5th ed. **Louis S. Goodman and Alfred Gilman, eds.** New York: Macmillan, 1975.
First edition, 1940; third edition, 1965; fourth edition, 1970.
Comprehensive treatment of all phases of therapeutic drugs. A classic in the field, known as the "blue bible." Extensive bibliographies, well indexed. Should be on the shelf of every practicing physician.
R: *Journal of Parasitology* 62: 208 (Apr. 1976); *Journal of Pharmaceutical Sciences* 65: 781 (May 1976); *RSR* 4: 44 (Jan.–Mar. 1976); Allyn; Stearns & Ratcliff (*AJN*; *NEJM,* 1969; *NEJM,* 1970).

Pharmacology and Therapeutics. 7th ed. **Arthur Grollman and Evelyn Grollman.** Philadelphia, PA: Lea & Febiger, 1970.
First edition, 1951.
Relates the science of pharmacy to basic biological sciences. Attempts to interpret the actions and uses of drugs from a medical viewpoint.

Pharmacology of Steroid Contraceptive Drugs. **S. Garattini and H. W. Berendes, eds.** New York: Raven Press, 1977.
Provides full-scale reports on the metabolic effects of steroid contraceptive drugs. A detailed reference source which outlines risks associated with oral contraceptives.
R: *Quarterly Review of Biology* 53: 504 (1978).

Remington's Pharmaceutical Sciences. 15th ed. Easton, PA: Mack Publishing, 1975.
Fourteenth edition, 1970.
A reference work which provides overview of pharmaceutical industry as well as pharmaceutical and medicinal agents. Important for pharmacists, physicians, and other medical scientists.
R: Stearns & Ratcliff (*NEJM,* 1970).

Review of Medical Pharmacology. 6th ed. **Frederick H. Meyers, Ernest Jawetz, and Alan Goldfien.** Los Altos, CA: Lange Medical Publications, 1978.
First edition, 1968; fourth edition, 1974; fifth edition, 1976.
Succinctly reviews major drug categories and properties. Arranged alphabeti-

cally. Major subject headings include system drugs, nutritional and metabolic drugs, endocrine drugs. Appendix and table of drug interactions, laboratory procedures, and toxicity levels are included. For medical students.
R: *American Family Physician* 19: 226 (Apr. 1979); *Nurse Educator* 3: 6 (Mar.–Apr. 1978); *ARBA* (1975, p. 751).

Sprowl's American Pharmacy: An Introduction to Pharmaceutical Techniques and Dosage Forms. 7th ed. **Lewis W. Dittert, ed.** Philadelphia, PA: J. B. Lippincott, 1974.
Special emphasis on standard preparation and stability of large-scale manufactured pharmaceuticals. New edition covers particle size and volume, emulsions, powders, and tablets. Despite its title, has universal applications. Characterized by comprehensive bibliography. A must for science libraries and educational and manufacturing pharmacy departments.
R: *Pharmaceutical Journal* 214: 508 (1975).

The Theory and Practice of Industrial Pharmacy. 2d ed. **Leon Lachman, Herbert A. Lieberman, and Joseph L. Kanig, eds.** Philadelphia, PA: Lea & Febiger, 1976.
First edition, 1970.

Theory of Pharmaceutical Systems. 3 vols. **J. Thuro Carstensen, ed.** New York: Academic Press, 1973.
A text on the compounds of drugs.

Toxicology: The Basic Science of Poisons. **Louis J. Casarett and John Doull, eds.** London: Bailliere Tindall, 1975.
Text covers general principles of toxicology, systemic toxicology, specific toxic agents, and application of the subject in various disciplines. Provides current account of major hazards. Many references and good index are found in this text for students of toxicology and related disciplines.
R: *Pharmaceutical Journal* 217: 156 (1976).

The Use of Antibiotics: A Comprehensive Review With Clinical Emphasis. 2d ed. **A. Kucers.** Philadelphia, PA: J. B. Lippincott, 1975.
Reviews antibiotics as they relate to infection. Information is up to date and well organized. An excellent reference for oncologists, microbiologists, clinicians.
R: *Annals of Internal Medicine* 84: 762 (1976).

PHYSICAL MEDICINE AND REHABILITATION

The Child with Disabling Illness: Principles of Rehabilitation. **John A. Downey and Neils L. Low, eds.** Philadelphia, PA: W. B. Saunders, 1974.
Discusses selected chronic disorders with emphasis on management and the team approach. Excellent text for pediatric rehabilitation which is of special interest to practicing pediatricians and residents in neurology, orthopedics, and physical medicine and rehabilitation.
R: *American Journal of Diseases of Children* 129: 1113 (Sept. 1975); *Archives of Physical Medicine and Rehabilitation* 58: 47 (Jan. 1977); *TBRI* 41: 344 (Nov. 1975).

Contemporary Vocational Rehabilitation. 2d ed. **Herbert Rusalem and David Malikin.** New York: New York Press, 1976.

First edition, 1968.
A revised and expanded edition of a definitive work on vocational rehabilitation. Comprehensive; recommended to all rehabilitation professionals.
R: *Archives of Physical Medicine and Rehabilitation* 58: 186 (1977); 58: 465 (Oct. 1977).

Physical Activities for the Handicapped. **Maryhelen Vannier.** Englewood Cliffs, NJ: Prentice-Hall, 1976.

Covers a wide spectrum of handicaps, from mental retardation to visual and/or auditory impairment. Emphasizes the need for physical activity, organizational and administrative problems, methods and techniques, and required equipment and facilities. Diagrams and illustrations complement the text. Useful appendix lists names of equipment suppliers, associations, and societies related to the handicapped. Directed toward persons concerned with physical, educational, and recreational programs for the handicapped.
R: *Archives of Physical Medicine and Rehabilitation* 58: 279 (June 1977).

Prostheses and Rehabilitation After Arm Amputation. **Leonard F. Bender.** Springfield, IL: Charles C. Thomas, 1974.

Fills the literature gap on prosthetics. Authoritative and complete reference source for all those concerned with amputee rehabilitation.
R: *Physical Therapy* 55: 687 (June 1975).

Rehabilitation Medicine: A Textbook on Physical Medicine and Rehabilitation. 4th ed. **Howard A. Rusk, ed.** St. Louis, MO: C. V. Mosby, 1977.

Third edition, 1971.
Basic textbook on principles and application of rehabilitation medicine. References follow each chapter. Helpful to physicians learning specialized skills and techniques of rehabilitation.
R: *Archives of Physical Medicine and Rehabilitation* 60: 189 (Apr. 1979); Allyn; Stearns & Ratcliff (*AJN*).

Speech Pathology and Audiology in Medical Settings. **Raphael M. Haller and Neil Sheldon, eds.** New York: Stratton Intercontinental Medical Book Corporation, 1976.

Describes how audiology and speech pathology services should function in various medical settings. Specialists in disciplines such as pediatrics and dentistry define how they work with those in audiology and speech pathology. Those in the field discuss their roles as well as issues such as credentials, new technology, and future directions. Recommended for professionals in speech and hearing.
R: *Archives of Otolaryngology* 103: 180 (Mar. 1977).

Spinal Injury. **David Yashon.** New York: Appleton-Century-Crofts, 1978.

Encyclopedic volume contains information about spinal cord and vertebral injury. Includes extensive bibliographies. Recommended for residents as well as specialists who desire a review of the subject.
R: *Archives of Physical Medicine and Rehabilitation* 60: 91 (Feb. 1979).

Stroke and Its Rehabilitation. **S. H. Licht, ed.** Baltimore, MD: Waverly Press, 1975.

Presents material relevant to stroke rehabilitation. Excellent source for residents, students, and practitioners.
R: *Archives of Physical Medicine and Rehabilitation* 56: 461 (1975); *Physical Therapy* 55: 1161 (Oct. 1975).

Treatment of Injuries to Athletes. 3d ed. **Don H. O'Donoghue.** Philadelphia, PA: W. B. Saunders, 1976.

First edition, 1962.
A gold mine of information on the prevention, diagnosis, and treatment of sports-related injuries. Concentrates entirely on acute injuries. Edition plagued by small and hard-to-interpret photographs. Lacks a bibliography. Not geared toward the junior surgeon. Highly recommended to therapists and physicians involved with rehabilitation and athletic medicine.
R: *Journal of Bone and Joint Surgery* 59A: 286 (Mar. 1977); *JAMA* 237: 1988 (May 2, 1977); *Physical Therapy* 57: 1219 (1977).

Willard and Spackman's Occupational Therapy. 5th ed. **Helen L. Hopkins and Helen D. Smith, eds.** Philadelphia, PA: J. B. Lippincott, 1978.

Fourth edition, 1970.
A comprehensive text on occupational therapy; covers topics from administration to physical and psychological development of patient. Arranged by chapters, which include bibliographies.
R: Brandon; Stearns & Ratcliff (*NEJM*, 1970).

PSYCHIATRY AND PSYCHOLOGY

Aging and Mental Health: Positive Psychosocial Approaches. **Robert N. Butler and Myrna I. Lewis.** St. Louis, MO: C. V. Mosby, 1973.

Evaluates the treatment and prevention of mental illness in the aged and focuses on the nature of the problems of the elderly. Thorough and comprehensive. Clearly written; recommended to lay people, mental health specialists, and students in a wide variety of disciplines.
R: *Journal of Gerontology* 29: 588 (1974); Brandon (*NO*).

The Battered Child. 2d ed. **Ray E. Helfer and C. Henry Kempe.** Chicago, IL: University of Chicago Press, 1974.

First edition, 1968.
Second edition of a classic work on child abuse; includes useful information on radiological aspects of syndromes of battered children, pathological findings, legal matters. Emphasizes the role of the physician in recognizing and treating cases of child abuse. An excellent reference source.
R: *Journal of Nervous and Mental Disease* 162: 437 (1975).

Behavior and Adaptation in Late Life. **Ewald W. Busse and Eric Pfeiffer, eds.** Boston, MA: Little, Brown, 1969.

Useful compendium of papers on the problems of adaptation among the aged. Based on material gathered from longitudinal studies of the Duke Center for the

Study of Aging and Human development. Relates basic information on adaptation or maladaptation of the aged. Chapter on functional disorders particularly noteworthy. Draws little attention to the aged.
R: *Journal of Nervous and Mental Disease* 156: 444 (1973).

Beyond the Best Interests of the Child. **Joseph Goldstein, Anna Freud, and Albert J. Solnit.** New York: The Free Press, 1973.
Emphasis on lawful rights of children, specifically in placement situations. New and familiar terminology defined equally well. Based on outstanding legal reference material. The definitive monograph of this topic.
R: *American Journal of Psychiatry* 132: 75 (Jan. 1975).

Comprehensive Textbook of Psychiatry. 2d ed. 2 vols. **Alfred M. Freedman, Harold I. Kaplan, and Benjamin J. Sadock.** Baltimore, MD: Williams & Wilkins, 1975.
First edition, 1967.
A two-volume compendium on psychiatry and mental health; covers a wide range of topics, with over 200 contributions from authorities in the field. Among areas covered are abnormal psychology, human sexuality, circadian rhythm. Includes copious references. An authoritative book for special school and public libraries.
R: *JAMA* 233: 1399 (Sept. 29, 1975); *RSR* 3: 35 (July–Dec. 1975); Stearns & Ratcliff (*NEJM*, 1970).

Depression: Clinical, Biological and Psychological Perspectives. **Gene Usdin, ed.** New York: Brunner/Mazel, 1977.
A series of monographs based on the annual meetings of the American College of Psychiatrists.
R: *American Journal of Psychiatry* 134: 943 (Aug. 1977).

Depression: Theory and Research. **Joseph Becker.** New York: Halsted Press, 1974.
Systematic review of recent research on all aspects of depression except treatment modes. Thorough and critical discussion of nosology, epidemiological and psychosocial data, and biological factors. Discusses many aspects of depression. A clearly combined presentation of theory and research.
R: *Journal of Nervous and Mental Disease* 161: 63 (1975).

Male and Female Homosexuality: A Comprehensive Investigation. **M. T. Saghir and E. Robins.** Baltimore, MD: Williams & Wilkins, 1973.
Reference work for students and practitioners concerned with human sexuality. A compendium of data.
R: *NEJM* 290: 114 (Jan. 10, 1974).

Medical Sociology. 2d ed. **David Mechanic.** New York: The Free Press, 1978.
First edition, 1968.
Wide ranging coverage of the subject; discusses health care organizations, services, medical economics, psychosocial problems in medicine. Includes behavioral

science perspectives as well as social and cultural perspectives. Considered an excellent account of the field of medical sociology.
R: *Journal of Nervous and Mental Disease* 167: 513 (Aug. 1979).

Mental Health in the Metropolis: The Midtown Manhattan Study. 2 books. **Leo Srole et al.** Leo Srole and Anita K. Fischer, eds. New York: Harper & Row, 1977.
A classic of its genre, the Midtown Manhattan Study is a model for collaboration of sociology and psychiatry. Book 2 carries mental health study into the community. Important for psychiatrists. Recommended for inclusion in residents training programs.
R: *American Journal of Psychiatry* 135: 1448 (Nov. 1978).

Mental Illness in Later Life. **Ewald W. Busse and Eric Pfeiffer.** Washington, DC: American Psychiatric Association, 1973.
Provides foundation for better understanding of psychological and physical problems of the old. Good index and current citations. Geared for practicing physicians.
R: *Journal of Gerontology* 30: 712 (Nov. 1975).

Modern Clinical Psychiatry. 9th ed. **Lawrence C. Kolb.** Philadelphia, PA: W. B. Saunders, 1977.
Seventh edition, 1968; eighth edition, 1973. Both entitled *Noyes' Modern Clinical Psychiatry,* Arthur P. Noyes and Lawrence C. Kolb, eds.
Maintains a practical and clinical approach.
R: Allyn.

Nature of Schizophrenia: New Approaches to Research and Treatment. **Lyman C. Wynne, R. Cromwell, and S. Matthysse, eds.** New York: John Wiley, 1978.
Describes etiology, treatment, and prognosis of schizophrenia.
R: *Nature* 274: 724v (Aug. 17, 1978).

The Opium Problem. **Charles E. Terry and Mildred Pellens.** Montclair, NJ: Bureau of Social Hygiene, 1928. Repr. Montclair, NJ: Patterson Smith, 1970.
Reprint of this classic treatment of the opium problem provides valuable information for those involved in the study of drug addiction.
R: *ARBA* (1973, p. 622).

The Origin and Treatment of Schizophrenic Disorders. **Theodore Lidz.** New York: Basic Books, 1973.
Concentrates on theories and research of Theodore Lidz and his team. Composed of three chapters based on the Salmon lectures given in December 1967.
R: *Journal of Nervous and Mental Disease* 162: 295 (1976).

Problems of Drug Dependence 1975. **Division of Medical Sciences, US National Research Council.** Washington, DC: US National Academy of Sciences, 1975.

Proceedings of the 37th Annual Scientific Meeting of the Committee on Problems of Drug Dependence.

Psychiatric Medicine. **Gene Usdin, ed.** New York: Brunner/Mazel, 1977.

Psychopharmacology: From Theory to Practice. **Jack D. Barchas et al., eds.** New York: Oxford University Press, 1977.

Deals with the theoretical and biological aspects of psychiatry and pharmacology. Describes most recent developments; psychotic disorders, such as schizophrenia. Devotes space to use of drugs in relation to sleep disorders, geriatric care, drug dosages, and interactions. Up to date, authoritative book for physicians.
R: *American Journal of Psychiatry* 135: 1005 (Aug. 1978).

Psychopharmacology of Affective Disorders: A British Association for Psychopharmacology Monograph. **E. S. Paykel and A. Coppen, eds.** London: Oxford University Press, 1979.

Up-to-date summary of pharmacodynamics, particularly in relation to antidepressive drugs. Includes authoritative accounts on lithium, ECT, tricyclic and tetracyclic drugs. Considered a valuable source for psychiatrists.
R: *BMJ* 1: 946 (Apr. 7, 1979).

Psychosomatic Medicine: Current Trends and Clinical Applications. **Z. J. Lipowski, Don R. Lipsitt, and Peter C. Whybrow, eds.** New York: Oxford University Press, 1977.

A current state-of-the-art review of psychosomatic medicine. Consists of five major sections: psychosomatic theory, intermediate mechanisms, current trends in psychosomatic research, psychosomatic approach in the practice of medicine, and teaching psychosomatic medicine. Includes many tidbits and facts not found elsewhere. In-depth discussion of new diagnostic procedures and treatments is a definite strength. A must for those involved with psychosomatic medicine.
R: *American Family Physician* 17: 327 (Mar. 1979); *American Journal of Psychiatry* 134: 1460 (Dec. 1977); *Journal of Nervous and Mental Disease* 166: 455 (1978).

Rape Victimology. **Leroy G. Schultz, ed.** Springfield, IL: Charles C. Thomas, 1975.

Important articles previously published on rape victims are divided into six sections which focus on such topics as sociology of rape, legal aspects, policy, etc. Written for curricula in social work, nursing, and medicine.
R: *American Journal of Psychiatry* 132: 1341 (Dec. 1975).

Realities in Childbearing. **Mary Lou Moore.** Philadelphia, PA: W. B. Saunders, 1978.

A comprehensive approach to the social, ethical, and psychological realities of childbearing. Discusses ethnic groups, rural and urban populations, and raises controversial questions. Contains much information, including charts and bibliographies.
R: *American Journal of Nursing* 79: 1151 (June 1979).

The Technique of Psychoanalytic Psychotherapy. Vol. 2. **Robert J. Langs.** New York. Jason Aronson, 1974.

Comprehensive coverage of psychoanalytic psychotherapy. Divided into three main sections: responses to interventions, the patient-therapist relationship, and the phases of psychotherapy. Includes clinical vignettes, describing steps of progression, regression, or impasse drawn extensively from author's practice. Despite extensive repetition, this volume is an outstanding ready reference source for every therapist.
R: *American Journal of Psychiatry* 132: 93 (1975).

Tredgold's Mental Retardation. 11th ed. **Roger Tredgold and Kenneth Soddy.** London: Bailliere Tindall & Cassell, 1970.

First edition, 1908.
An authoritative reference text, greatly revised. Provides current ideas. Considered a comprehensive and classic volume in the field of mental retardation and psychiatry.
R: *Lancet* 2: 346 (Aug. 15, 1970).

The Use of Drugs in Psychiatry. **John Crammer, Brian Barraclough, and Bernard Heine.** Ashford, Kent, England: Headley Brothers, 1978.

Pocket-size text contains much clinical information along with the pharmacology. Discusses commonly used drugs, daily problems, and important side effects. Index and appendix.
R: *BMJ* 1: 257 (1979).

PUBLIC HEALTH

Asbestos and Disease. **Irving J. Selikoff et al.** New York: Academic Press, 1978.

A comprehensive monograph that covers all aspects of asbestos as it relates to changes in the lung and respiratory system. Discusses statistical incidence in relation to disease, historical events and findings, clinical descriptions. Contains photographs, X-rays, charts and tables, identification of asbestos fibers in the environment. A high-quality work for public health workers, epidemiologists, physicians, and industrial hygienists.
R: *BMJ* 1: 112 (1979).

Coal Workers' Pneumoconiosis: A Critical Review. **Withold W. Zahorski, ed.** Hanover, NH: University Press of New England, 1974.

A thorough summary of pneumoconiosis research efforts in Britain and the United States. Covers pathogenic properties of dust and silica, frequency of respiratory impairment in coal miners. A ready reference for libraries, physicians interested in occupational diseases.
R: *Annals of Internal Medicine* 83: 752 (1975).

Control of Communicable Disease in Man. 12th ed. **Abram S. Beneson, ed.** Washington, DC: American Public Health Association, 1975.

R: *Annals of Internal Medicine* 91: 145 (July 1979).

Dangerous Plants, Snakes, Arthropods & Marine Life. Toxicity & Treatment. **Michael D. Ellis, ed.** Hamilton, IL/Washington, DC: Drug Intelligence Publications, 1978.

Ready access to important information in toxicology in four parts: toxic agents and taxonomic and common names, toxic elements, symptoms of toxicity, and current methods of treatment. Contains close to 400 color photographs of agents defined. Valuable for poison control centers, emergency rooms.
R: *Annals of Internal of Medicine* 91: 342 (Aug. 1979).

Drinking Water and Health. **Committee on Drinking Water, US National Research Council.** Washington, DC: US National Academy of Sciences, 1978.

The Effects of Irradiation on the Skeleton. **Janet M. Vaughn.** New York: Oxford University Press, 1973.

Discusses the adverse effects of radiation, including radium, strontium, and plutonium. Clinically oriented, includes numerous tables and graphs. Well organized, recommended to physicians concerned with biological effects of radiation.
R: *Archives of Internal Medicine* 134: 790 (Oct. 1974).

Epidemiology and Community Medicine. **Sidney L. Kark.** New York: Appleton-Century-Crofts, 1974.

For community health workers; discusses epidemiology and health care on a community level. Recommended to public health libraries.
R: *American Journal of Diseases of Children* 129: 1464 (Dec. 1975).

Health Hazards of the Human Environment. **World Health Organization.** Geneva: World Health Oranization, 1972.

A hundred specialists provide summaries of areas of concern to those medical and scientific workers involved with public health, pollution, and the environment. Wide survey of environmental hazards as well as nutritional and mental diseases, accidents, and infectious diseases. Comprehensive and extensive bibliography. Good review of state of the art of many other environmental sciences in addition to being a useful reference document.
R: *Health Physics* 28: 89 (Jan. 1975); *Lancet* 2: 1364 (Dec. 15, 1973).

Industrial Environmental Health: The Worker and the Community. **Lester V. Cralley, ed.** New York: Academic Press, 1972.

Maxcy-Rosenau's Preventive Medicine and Public Health. 10th ed. **Philip E. Sartwell, ed.** New York: Appleton-Century-Crofts, 1973.

Ninth edition, 1965.
A comprehensive text of preventive medicine. Organized by subject, some of which are infectious disease, chronic illness, public health methods. Includes references. Well-written technical account, useful in medical libraries.
R: Allyn.

The Nuclear Fuel Cycle: A Survey of the Public Health, Environmental, and

National Security Effects of Nuclear Power. Rev. ed. **Union of Concerned Scientists.** Cambridge, MA: MIT Press, 1975.
R: *American Scientist* 64: 686 (Nov./Dec. 1976).

Occupational and Environmental Cancers of the Urinary System. **Wilhelm C. Hueper.** New Haven, CT: Yale University Press, 1969.
An extensive study of the occupational and environmental causes of cancer of the urinary tract. Combines epidemiological and experimental results. Includes an extensive bibliography. Two inherent weaknesses: inaccurate references and unsubstantiated statements. Despite these faults, the book contains essential material for the experimentalist, epidemiologist, industrial medical officer, and clinician.
R: *Lancet* 1: 338 (Feb. 14, 1970).

Occupational Lung Diseases. **William K. C. Morgan and Anthony Seaton.** Philadelphia, PA: W. B. Saunders, 1975.
Designed as a medical reference work on industrial lung diseases. Volume begins with a useful glossary. Initial chapters are most informative and cover historical and legal aspects of industrial disease. Bulk of book presents a detailed description of pneumoconiosis and other occupational lung diseases. Final chapter focuses on pulmonary neoplasms. Despite small volume size, subject coverage is comprehensive. Between 50 and 100 selective references conclude each section. Highly recommended to internists, pathologists, radiologists, and specialists in respiratory disease.
R: *American Journal of Public Health* 66: 98 (Jan. 1976); *Chest* 69: 25 (Jan. 1976); *Physical Therapy* 56: 873 (1976); *TBRI* 42: 102 (Mar. 1976).

Patty's Industrial Hygiene and Toxicology. 3rd rev. ed. 3 vols. **George D. Clayton and Florence E. Clayton, eds.** New York: John Wiley, 1978–1979.
Second revised edition, volume 1, *General Principles*, 1958; volume 2, *Toxicology*, 1963.
Practical reference for persons responsible for safeguarding health of others in industry. Comprehensive survey of basic knowledge and techniques.
R: Allyn.

School Health Practice. 6th ed. **C. L. Anderson and William H. Creswell.** St. Louis, MO: C. V. Mosby, 1976.

Supervision in Social Work. **Alfred Kadushin.** New York: Columbia University Press, 1976.
Contains sections on administrative, educational, and supportive supervision, with chapters covering evaluation, group supervision, and supervision of paraprofessionals.
R: *Social Service Review* 51: 366 (June 1977).

Venom Diseases. **Sherman A. Minton, Jr.** Springfield, IL: Charles C. Thomas, 1974.
Information on many types of venomous bites and stings. Bibliography of over

600 references concentrates mainly on current research.
R: *Lancet* 2: 500 (Aug. 31, 1974).

A World Geography of Human Diseases. **G. Melvyn Howe, ed.** New York: Academic Press, 1977.

A multi-authored volume which discusses geographic variation of diseases such as smallpox, tuberculosis, cancer. Details complex relationships between mortality and rainfall, latitude, temperature, water supply. An excellent reference, recommended to medical libraries.
R: *BMJ* 1: 707 (Mar. 18, 1977); *Nature* 270: 126 (Nov. 10, 1977).

RADIOLOGY

Advances in Radiation Research: Biology and Medicine. **J. F. Duplan and A. Chapiro, eds.** New York: Gordon & Breach, 1973.

Alimentary Tract Roentgenology. 2d ed. 2 vols. **Alexander R. Margulis and H. Joachim Burhenne, eds.** St. Louis, MO: C. V. Mosby, 1973.

Emphasizes the role of the radiologist in the diagnosis of gastrointestinal diseases. Updated edition contains numerous illustrations, new information on mechanisms of digestion and on the liver and biliary tract. A valuable, basic reference for all radiologists and physicians.
R: *Gastroenterology* 66: 633 (Apr. 1974); *Radiology* 111: 432 (1974); Allyn.

Analysis of Roentgen Signs in General Radiology. **Isadore Meschan.** Philadelphia, PA: W. B. Saunders, 1973.
R: *Radiology* 111: 288 (May 1974); Allyn.

Biomedical Ultrasonics. **P. N. T. Wells.** New York: Academic Press, 1977.

This work concerns itself with the biophysical and biological aspects of ultrasound. A comprehensive discussion is provided, making this a standard reference for all departments of ultrasound and all medical and technical researchers.
R: *Lancet* 2: 690 (1977).

Clinical Cardiac Radiology. **Keith Jefferson and Simon Rees.** London: Butterworths, 1973.

Guides the user to techniques in cardiac radiology. A standard book for medical libraries, X-ray and cardiology departments.
R: *Lancet* 1: 662 (Apr. 13, 1974); Allyn.

Diagnostic Ultrasound. **Donald L. King, ed.** St. Louis, MO: C. V. Mosby, 1974.

Authoritative survey of diagnostic ultrasound from a series of lectures at Columbia University presented by pioneers in this discipline. Chapters are readable and clear. Includes high-quality illustrations, index, and bibliographies. Useful addition to medical school and hospital libraries.
R: *Radiology* 115: 678 (1975); *RSR* 3: 42 (Jan.–Mar. 1975).

Diagnostic Ultrasound: Text and Cases. **Dennis A. Sarti and W. Frederick Sample, eds.** Boston, MA: G. K. Hall, 1979.

Surveys the latest developments in the field. Each chapter deals with a particular organ system and is divided into two major sections: text and case studies. Some 1,200 high-quality scan images accompany over 350 case studies. Essential text for primary care physicians, medical students, radiology residents, and practicing ultrasonographers and radiologists.

The Essentials of Roentgen Interpretation. 3d ed. **Lester W. Paul and John H. Juhl.** Hagerstown, MD: Harper & Row, 1972. (New edition in preparation).

Emphasizes radiologic diagnosis. Includes short description of disease process and anatomy. Over 1,200 illustrations, good bibliographies, index. Recommended for radiology department libraries.
R: Allyn; Stearns & Ratcliff (*NEJM,* 1969; *NEJM,* 1970).

Fundamentals of Radiation Therapy and Cancer Chemotherapy. **Sidney Lowry.** New York: Arco Publishing, 1975.

A how and why presentation of radiation therapy. Chapters arranged by organ systems; basic summary of clinical and laboratory details. Features good index and helpful end-of-chapter references. Despite a choppy style, good subject coverage. Manual essentially for nonradiotherapist physicians involved with cancer patients.
R: *Annals of Internal Medicine* 83: 441 (Sept. 1975).

Fundamentals of Radiology. 2d ed. **Lucy F. Squire.** Cambridge, MA: Harvard University Press, 1975.

Excellent introduction to radiology and its fundamentals. Clear explanations, high-quality illustrations, and index characterize this second edition. Suitable not only for medical students but also for medical professionals at every level.
R: *JAMA* 236: 1065 (Aug. 30, 1976); *Radiology* 121: 18 (Oct. 1976); *BMLA* 59: 597 (Oct. 1971).

Paleopathological Diagnosis and Interpretation. Bone Diseases in Ancient Human Populations. **R. T. Steinbock.** Springfield, IL: Charles C. Thomas, 1976.

Combined discussion of anthropology and bone pathology in ancient human populations. Author describes skeletal material from Egyptian mummies, Eskimos, New Mexican Indians, and correlates the incidence of metabolic bone disease, hematologic disorders, and infections. Considered a scholarly work, providing a clear picture of bone pathology. Contains much illustrative material. Considered a worthy reference source for radiologists, osteologists, and pathologists.
R: *Radiology* 124: 674 (1977).

Principles of Diagnostic Radiology. **E. James Potchen, P. Ruben Koehler, and David O. Lewis, eds.** New York: McGraw-Hill, 1971.

Systematically presents manifestations and diagnosis of disease. Presentation emphasizes use of radiology as a diagnostic tool; also outlines the hazards of radiation and appropriate precautions.
R: *ARBA* (1972, p. 620).

Principles of Successful Radiation Therapy: Introduction to Treatment Planning. **Stanley E. Order, Joyce Kopicky, and Steve Liebel.** Boston, MA: G. K. Hall, 1979.

Emphasizes treatment planning in therapeutic radiology. Concentrates on Hodgkin's, prostate, pituitary and head and neck cancer. Compact introduction to the field of radiation oncology for beginning residents, technology students, and surgical, gynecological, and medical oncologists.

Radiology of Bone Diseases. 2d ed. **George B. Greenfield.** Philadelphia, PA: J. B. Lippincott, 1975.

Covers metabolic aspects of bone disease, grouping each disease according to radiologic symptoms. Text is concise, informative, and thorough. Contains numerous references, over 1,000 illustrations, and a comprehensive bibliography. Recommended as a valuable and practical reference book. Useful in radiology libraries and to those working with musculoskeletal disease.
R: *British Journal of Radiology* 49: 787 (1976); *NEJM* 293: 615 (Sept. 18, 1975); *Radiology* 117: 418 (Nov. 1975).

Radiology of the Gallbladder and Bile Ducts. **Philip M. Hatfield and Robert E. Wise.** Baltimore, MD: Williams & Wilkins, 1976.

This monograph, which is section 22 of *Golden's Diagnostic Radiology,* concisely presents information on all aspects of biliary radiology. Among topics included are embryology, radiology, cholecystography. Excellent format includes high-quality illustrations. Considered an essential reference.
R: *Radiology* 126: 618 (1978).

Radiology of the Pancreas and Duodenum. **S. Boyd Eaton, Jr., and Joseph T. Ferrucci.** Philadelphia, PA: W. B. Saunders, 1973.

Volume 3 of *Monographs in Clinical Radiology.*
A fine combination of clinical and pathophysiologic data. Comprehensive coverage of literature relating to radiologic diagnosis of pancreatic and duodenal diseases. Includes outstanding illustrations, line drawings, and tables useful for radiological examinations. Features an accurate, up-to-date bibliography. Only brief mention of the techniques of endoscopic retrograde cholangiography and pancreatography reflects a serious omission. Valuable reference work and general text for internists.
R: *Annals of Internal Medicine* 80: 786 (June 1974); *British Journal of Radiology* 47: 789 (Nov. 1974).

Radiology of the Small Intestine. 2d ed. **Richard H. Marshak and Arthur E. Lindner.** Philadelphia, PA: W. B. Saunders, 1976.

Updated second edition includes three new chapters on metastatic cancer, angiography of small bowel, and lesions of small bowel. Excellent illustrations. Recommended to radiologists, gastroenterologists, and residents.
R: *Radiology* 124: 306 (1977); Allyn.

Roentgen Diagnosis of Diseases of Bone. 2d ed. 2 vols. **Jack Edeiken and Philip J. Hodes.** Baltimore, MD: Williams & Wilkins, 1973.

Extensively revised and expanded, a two-volume reference work for radiologists,

orthopedists, and others who work with skeletal diseases. Considered an excellent source.
R: *JAMA* 228: 765 (May 6, 1974).

Roentgen Examinations in Acute Abdominal Diseases. 3d ed. **J. Frimann-Dahl.** Springfield, IL: Charles C. Thomas, 1974.
Classic text on radiological diagnosis of abdominal diseases. Bibliography is complete, and reproductions are of good quality.
R: *JAMA* 232: 306 (Apr. 21, 1975).

Textbook of Radiotherapy. 2d ed. **Gilbert H. Fletcher.** Philadelphia, PA: Lea & Febiger, 1973.
Discusses practical aspects of radiotherapy. Highly recommended to all specialists.
R: *JAMA* 228: 1434 (June 10, 1974); *Radiology* 111: 410 (May 1974); Allyn; Brandon; Inke.

RESPIRATORY SYSTEM

Bronchial Carcinoma. **Thomas W. Shields and Roy E. Ritts, Jr.** Springfield, IL: Charles C. Thomas, 1974.
Clear and concise summary of present knowledge of lung cancer. Published for physician or surgeon who needs brief review of subject. Contains over 200 references; recommended to medical students, physicians, and surgeons.
R: *Annals of Internal Medicine* 83: 295 (Aug. 1975); *Surgery, Gynecology and Obstetrics* 141: 105 (July 1975).

Cancer of the Lung. **H. Gunter Seydel, Arnold Chait, and John T. Cmclich.** New York: John Wiley, 1975.
Documents the natural history, pathology, and management of lung cancer. Contains historical references, discussions of the prognosis of lung cancer. Recommended to libraries, physicians. Useful as a guide to the understanding of the phases of lung cancer.
R: *Chest* 70: 26 (1976).

Chest Roentgenology. **Benjamin Felson.** Philadelphia, PA: W. B. Saunders, 1973.
Basic primer in chest roentgenology. Contains analytic evaluation of normal and abnormal chest radiographs. Includes helpful bibliography and index. Recommended to all radiologists.
R: *JAMA* 227: 566 (Feb. 4, 1974); *NEJM* 289: 1317 (Dec. 13, 1973); *New Zealand Medical Journal* 79: 937 (May 8, 1974); *Radiology* 112: 68 (July 1974); *TBRI* 40: 71 (Feb. 1974); 40: 110 (Mar. 1974); 40: 278 (Sept. 1974); Allyn; Brandon.

Immunologic and Infectious Reactions in the Lung. **Charles H. Kirkpatrick and Herbert Y. Reynolds, eds.** New York: Marcel Dekker, 1976.
Collation of 24 chapters written on immunologic components of host-defense operating in lungs. Three sections cover basic molecular biology, diseases, and treatment. Authors appropriately critical of data about various therapeutic mo-

dalities. Presentations have orderly sequence and are well cross-referenced. All chapters referenced, with many having more than 100 citations. Exceptional reference for clinical immunologists, chest physicians, general internists, and allergists.
R: *Annals of Allergy* 37: 370 (Nov. 1976); *Annals of Internal Medicine* 87: 139 (July 1977); *Clinical Immunology and Immunopathology* 7: 151 (1977).

Lung Biology in Health and Disease: Bioengineering Aspects of the Lung. Vol. 3. **John B. West, ed.** New York: Marcel Dekker, 1977.
A bioengineering approach to lung problems, covering the following topics: mechanical properties of lung, gas exchange, structure function relationships. Provides excellent descriptions, photomicrographs. Excellently edited, contains a wealth of information for all those interested in the lung.
R: *Chest* 75: 24 (1978).

Lung Cancer: Natural History, Prognosis and Therapy. **Lucien Israel and A. Philippe Chahinian.** New York: Academic Press, 1976.
Presents multidisciplinary approach to management of patients with carcinoma of the lung. Chapters deal with etiological and risk factors, current status of immunotherapy, and proposals for combined therapeutic approaches. Valuable to physicians caring for those with lung cancer.
R: *Chest* 72: 30 (1978).

Lung Function: Assessment and Application in Medicine. 3d ed. **J. E. Cotes.** Oxford, England: Blackwell Scientific Publications, 1975.
A theoretical text on pulmonary function, reviews basic terminology and equipment involved in the measurement of lung function. Assesses function of both normal and diseased lung. Third edition contains minor revisions. Considered a good text for those concerned with pulmonary function.
R: *Annals of Internal Medicine* 83: 920 (1975); Allyn.

Lung Sounds. **Paul Forgacs.** London: Bailliere Tindall, 1978.
Outlines mechanisms by which noises detected by careful listening in normal subjects and those with lung disease may be produced. First chapter on terminology of lung sounds defines the noises, and following chapters deal with physiology of generation of lung sounds. Precise book on sounds heard daily in clinical practice; useful for chest physicians, clinical tutors, and general practitioners.
R: *Lancet* 1: 640 (Mar. 25, 1978).

Pulmonary Diagnostic Techniques. **Thomas L. Petty.** Philadelphia, PA: Lea & Febiger, 1975.
An introductory survey of pulmonary diagnostic techniques. Twelve chapters attempt to integrate procedures with various disease entities. Designed as a ready reference source with a multitude of references for further detail. Extremely simple and readable text. A gem of a book for primary physicians, house officers, advanced medical students, and researchers in the field of pulmonary service.
R: *Annals of Internal Medicine* 84: 235 (1976).

Pulmonary Metastasis. **Leonard Weiss and Harvey A. Gilbert, eds.** Boston, MA: G. K. Hall, 1979.
In three sections: basic mechanisms and pathways in pulmonary metastasis; patterns of pulmonary metastasis; treatment information essential to all those involved in pulmonary care and research.

Regional Differences in the Lung. **John B. West, ed.** New York: Academic Press, 1977.
Complete account of regional lung function. Contains comprehensive list of references from 1855 to 1976. Illustrated with clear diagrams.
R: *BMJ* 1: 1404 (May 28, 1977).

Respiratory Diseases. 2d ed. **John Crofton and Andrew Douglas.** Philadelphia, PA: J. B. Lippincott, 1975.
First edition, 1969.
An updated edition of this comprehensive reference work; deals with basic principles of pulmonary disease, including epidemiology, immunology, and structure and function. Includes copious references, illustrations, X-rays. Well recommended to researchers and practitioners who specialize in pulmonary medicine.
R: *Chest* 70: 30 (1975); *JAMA* 236: 308 (July 19, 1976); Allyn.

Respiratory Failure. 2d ed. **M. K. Sykes, M. W. McNicol, and E. J. M. Campbell.** Philadelphia, PA: J. B. Lippincott, 1976.
Second edition details advances in laboratory and patient monitoring of respiratory failure. Contains much practical information. Recommended to personnel in respiratory and intensive care units.
R: *JAMA* 237: 808 (1977).

Respiratory Research in the People's Republic of China, DHEW Pub. no. (NIH) 75-770. **Frederick S. Kao.** Washington, DC: US Government Printing Office, 1975.
Discusses the history of Chinese medicine and health systems, particularly in relation to respiratory disease. Contains photographs, bibliography. A well-researched volume concerning Chinese medical practice.
R: *Annals of Internal Medicine* 84: 376 (1976).

Textbook of Pulmonary Diseases. 2d ed. **Gerald L. Baum, ed.** Boston, MA: Little, Brown, 1974.
Emphasizes the clinical aspects of pulmonary disease, dealing with diagnosis and treatment. Includes X-ray reproductions and color plates. Excellent format; contains much information for those working in the field of chest diseases. Considered a basic reference source.
R: *Annals of Internal Medicine* 83: 442 (1975); Allyn; Stearns & Ratcliff (*NEJM*, 1970).

Tuberculosis. **Guy P. Youmans.** Philadelphia, PA: W. B. Saunders, 1979.
Standard reference work on tuberculosis. Emphasis on microbiology. Written by an international specialist.

Viral and Mycoplasmal Infections of the Respiratory Tract. **Vernon Knight, ed.** Philadelphia, PA: Lea & Febiger, 1973.
Compendium of clinical knowledge, epidemiology, and diagnostic laboratory procedures for viral and *Mycoplasma pneumoniae* respiratory infections. Illustrated with excellent electron micrographs. Recommended reading for students, physicians, microbiologists, and inhalation therapists.
R: *NEJM* 289: 594 (1973).

RHEUMATOLOGY

Age Changes in the Neuromuscular System. **E. Gutman and V. Hanzlikova.** Baltimore, MD: Williams & Wilkins, 1972.
Describes biochemical, structural, and functional changes in motor behavior, emphasizing changes at the intracellular level. Includes diagrams, photomicrographs, and approximately 400 references. Fairly technical. An excellent reference for physical therapists and physiologists.
R: *Physical Therapy* 54: 322 (1974).

The Aging of Connective Tissue. **David A. Hall.** New York: Academic Press, 1976.
A treatise that will serve as a standard reference, summing up the major changes in aging connective tissue. Sequentially presents macrostructural and microstructural, chemical, and biochemical changes associated with age changes. Copious references, highly recommended.
R: *Quarterly Review of Biology* 53: 359 (1978).

Arthritis and Allied Conditions: A Textbook of Rheumatology. 9th ed. **Daniel J. McCarthy, ed.** Philadelphia, PA: Lea & Febiger, 1979.
Most recent edition combines clinical and basic science information. Includes a new section on pharmacology of anti-arthritic drugs. A standard reference for rheumatologists.

Copeman's Textbook of the Rheumatic Diseases. 5th ed. **J. T. Scott.** New York: Churchill Livingstone, 1978.
A comprehensive reference on rheumatology. Covers natural history, etiology, immunology of rheumatic diseases, as well as diagnostic and therapeutic techniques. Authoritative and well written; considered one of the best reference sources in rheumatology.
R: *American Family Physician* 19: 257 (Nov. 1978); *Arthritis and Rheumatism* 21: 870 (Sept.–Oct. 1978).

Diseases of Muscle: A Study in Pathology. 3d ed. **Raymond D. Adams.** Hagerstown, MD: Harper & Row, 1975.
First edition, 1953; second edition, 1962.
Third edition of this standard reference on muscle pathology contains much new information concerning both clinical and basic research in muscle pathology. Provides excellent descriptions and illustrations of muscle tumors, inflammatory diseases, neuromuscular atrophy. Also details new techniques in experimental

pathology. Considered an essential and permanent reference for both clinicians and pathologists.
R: *Archives of Pathology & Laboratory Medicine* 100: 227 (Apr. 1976); *JAMA* 235: 210 (Jan. 12, 1976); *Neurology* 27: 102 (Jan. 1977).

Disorders of Voluntary Muscle. **John N. Walton, ed.** New York: Churchill Livingstone, 1974.

A standard reference on muscle disorders; contributions from experts in their field. A classic, recommended to all libraries.
R: *Archives of Neurology* 31: 281 (Oct. 1974).

Rheumatism in Populations. **J. S. Lawrence.** London: Heinemann Medical, 1977.

An epidemiological account of rheumatic disease. Discusses such topics as occupational aspects of diseases, incidence of lupus, congenital deformities. Extensively reviews literature, contains numerous references and quality radiographs. Considered a standard reference source on the epidemiology of rheumatic diseases.
R: *Arthritis and Rheumatism* 21: 398 (Apr. 1978).

The Striated Muscle. **C. M. Pearson and F. K. Mostofi.** Baltimore, MD: Williams & Wilkins, 1973.

Summarizes recent advances in myopathology on topics from normal muscle structure to concepts in pathogenesis of certain diseases. Well illustrated with excellent photographs. Concise reference concerning muscle and related diseases.
R: *Archives of Pathology & Laboratory Medicine* 97: 259 (Apr. 1974).

Total Management of the Arthritic Patient. **George E. Ehrlich, ed.** Philadelphia, PA: J. B. Lippincott, 1973.

Focuses on the management of patients plagued by arthritis and similar problems. Special section devoted to rehabilitation aspects of chronic arthritis sufferers. Reflects treatments and therapy considered current in 1973. Numerous charts, graphs, and illustrations complement text. Serves as an excellent review for orthopedic surgeons and physiatrists. A must for all internists and practitioners involved in the management of patients with arthritic problems.
R: *Archives of Physical Medicine and Rehabilitation* 55: 47 (Jan. 1974).

UROGENITAL SYSTEM

Advances in Obstetrics and Gynecology. **Ronald M. Caplan and William J. Sweeney.** Baltimore, MD: Williams & Wilkins, 1978.

Reviews a wide range of topics in obstetrics and gynecology. Some areas covered are complications of pregnancy, amenorrhea, thyroid problems, ovulation induction, androgen metabolism. Recommended for specialists in the field.
R: *Canadian Medical Association Journal* 119: 1394 (Dec. 23, 1978).

Artificial Insemination. 2d ed. **Wilfred J. Finegold.** Springfield, IL: Charles C. Thomas, 1976.

An extensive monograph which covers all topics pertinent to artificial insemination. An excellent format provides for a clear introduction and good reference.
R: *Australian & New Zealand Journal of Obstetrics & Gynecology* 17: 120 (May 1977); *Fertility and Sterility* 28: 214 (Feb. 1977); *TBRI* 43: 183 (May 1977); 43: 302 (Oct. 1977).

Bonney's Gynaecological Surgery. 8th ed. **John Howkings and John Stallworthy, eds.** London: Bailliere Tindall, 1974.
Seventh edition, 1964.
Reflects changes in thought and practice in gynecological surgery. Revision has been extensive. Important for general as well as gynecological surgeons.
R: *British Journal of Surgery* 62: 415 (May 1975).

Corscaden's Gynecologic Cancer. 5th ed. **S. B. Gusberg and H. C. Frick.** Baltimore, MD: Williams & Wilkins, 1978.
Fourth edition, 1970; fourth reprinted edition, 1977.
Considered a basic reference in gynecological cancer; emphasizes surgical and radiological therapy. Also includes information on pathology and cytology.
R: Brandon.

Female Sex Anomalies. **Cary M. Dougherty and Rowena Spencer.** New York: Harper & Row, 1972.
Well-organized reference for physician who examines and identifies sex anomalies in females. Well diagrammed.
R: *Clinical Pediatrics* 13: 285 (Mar. 1974).

General Urology. 9th ed. **Donald R. Smith.** Los Altos, CA: Lange Medical Publications, 1978.
Eighth edition, 1975.
Comprehensive textbook for medical students, interns, and residents. Deals with basic topics in urology; recommended for medical libraries and practitioners.
R: *British Journal of Surgery* 63: 503 (June 1976); *International Surgery* 61: 119 (Feb. 1976); *Journal of the Medical Society of New Jersey* 73: 87 (Jan. 1976); *TBRI* 42: 106 (Mar. 1976); 42: 189 (May 1976); Allyn; Brandon.

Gynecology: Essentials of Clinical Practice. 3d ed. **Thomas H. Green, Jr.** Boston, MA: Little, Brown, 1977.

Hermaphroditism, Genital Anomalies and Related Endocrine Disorders. 2d ed. **Howard W. Jones, Jr., and William W. Scott.** Baltimore, MD: Williams & Wilkins, 1971.
Most comprehensive work on this subject written in this country.
R: *Obstetrics and Gynecology* 41: 321 (Feb. 1973).

Human Multiple Reproduction. **Ian MacGillivray, P. S. S. Nylander, and Gerald Corney.** Philadelphia, PA: W. B. Saunders, 1975.
Comprehensive work on all aspects of twin pregnancies and development. Extensive bibliography of about 550 entries.
R: *Lancet* 2: 70 (July 9, 1977).

Human Reproductive Physiology. **E. S. E. Hafez.** Ann Arbor, MI: Ann Arbor Science, 1978.

Human Sexuality: A Health Practitioner's Text. **Richard Green, ed.** Baltimore, MD: Williams & Wilkins, 1975.
Human sexuality is discussed by contributors involved in disciplines ranging from research in reproductive biology through psychiatry to divinity. Topics include instructions on taking a sex history; sexual anatomy and physiology; heterosexual and homosexual relationships; and treatment of sexual dysfunction. Excellent chapter on pelvic examination of women. References and index included. Should be in all medical, hospital, and public libraries.
R: *RSR* 4: 88 (Apr.–June 1976).

Infectious Diseases in Obstetrics and Gynecology. **Giles R. G. Monif.** Hagerstown, MD: Harper & Row, 1974.
Comprehensive, current, and readily available text.
R: *JAMA* 233: 372 (July 28, 1975); *TBRI* 41: 271 (Sept. 1975); Brandon.

The Kidney. **Jan Brod.** London: Butterworths, 1973.
Lucid interpretation of the functional kidney in health and disease. Covers an enormous amount of material on a wide variety of renal topics. Only an occasional unfamiliar term detracts from this excellent monograph. Informative source for all medical libraries.
R: *BMJ* 2: 429 (May 19, 1973); *Kidney International* 4: 175 (1973).

The Kidney: A Clinico-Pathological Study. **Priscilla Kincaid-Smith.** Oxford, England: Blackwell Scientific Publications, 1975.
Organized, illustrated review of clinicopathological correlation of renal disease. Useful to nephrologists, renal pathologists, and physicians caring for patients with kidney disease.
R: *Annals of Internal Medicine* 86: 515 (1977); *JAMA* 236: 1064 (1976).

Normal and Abnormal Development of the Kidney. **Edith L. Potter.** Chicago, IL: Year Book Medical Publishers, 1972.
A detailed examination of kidney disease, including illustrations of histology and microdissection. Thorough discussion of disease classifications, diagnosis, and history. An expert reference; highly recommended to medical libraries.
R: *American Journal of Diseases of Children* 129: 1244 (Oct. 1975); *Lancet* 2: 26 (July 7, 1973).

Novak's Gynecological and Obstetric Pathology With Clinical and Endocrine Relations. 8th ed. **Edmund R. Novak and J. Donald Woodruff.** Philadelphia, PA: W. B. Saunders, 1979.
Classic text. Includes numerous new illustrations.

Novak's Textbook of Gynecology. 9th ed. **E. R. Novak et al.** Baltimore, MD: Williams & Wilkins, 1975.
Eighth edition, 1970.
A systematic discussion of diseases in gynecology, covering anatomy, physiology,

and embryology. Ninth edition includes chapters on sex education, abortion, family planning. Well referenced.
R: Allyn.

Obstetric and Perinatal Infections. **David Charles and Maxwell Finland, eds.** Philadelphia, PA: Lea & Febiger, 1973.
Focuses on obstetric and perinatal infections. First section of the monograph deals with fetal infections, second with maternal diseases, and final section with diseases involving both mother and fetus. All contributors are acknowledged authorities in their field. Bibliographies are comprehensive. Geared toward obstetricians and pediatricians.
R: *Archives of Internal Medicine* 136: 624 (May 1976).

Obstetrics: Essentials of Clinical Practice. **Kenneth R. Niswander, ed.** Boston, MA: Little, Brown, 1976.
Initiates a new approach to a wider concept of the physiology and well-being of mother and baby. Recommended to students and postgraduates in the field of clinical obstetrics.
R: *Australian & New Zealand Journal of Obstetrics & Gynecology* 17: 120 (May 1977); *TBRI* 43: 305 (Oct. 1977).

Operative Urology: The Kidneys, Adrenal Glands and Retroperitoneum. **Bruce H. Stewart.** Baltimore, MD: Williams & Wilkins, 1975.
Focuses on operations for kidney conditions. Magnificent illustrations complement the detailed text. Geared toward medical students and residents; too introductory for experienced surgeons.
R: *British Journal of Surgery* 64: 75 (Jan. 1977).

Progress in Infertility. 2d ed. **S. J. Behrman and Robert W. Kistner, eds.** Boston, MA: Little, Brown, 1975.
First edition, 1968.
Contributions from 62 international experts comprise this volume for those with an interest in managing patient with reproductive problems. Aspects treated are structural and functional aspects of female reproductive system, endometriosis, reproductive endocrinology, immunologic factors in infertility, etc. Authors provide editorial comments. Many illustrations; 1,000 references. For physicians interested in problems concerning human reproduction.
R: *BMJ* 1: 530 (Feb. 28, 1976); *JAMA* 235: 1619 (Apr. 12, 1976).

Recent Advances in Urology. 2d ed. **W. F. Hendry, ed.** New York: Churchill Livingstone, 1976.
R: *BMJ* 1: 534 (Aug. 28, 1976).

Renal Disease. 3d ed. **Douglas Black.** Philadelphia, PA: F. A. Davis, 1973.
R: Allyn; Stearns & Ratcliff (*NEJM,* 1969; *NEJM,* 1970).

Surgery of the Anus, Rectum and Colon. 3d ed. **J. C. Goligher.** Springfield, IL: Charles C. Thomas, 1976.
First edition, 1961.

Survey of current knowledge of diseases of large bowel and guide to surgical treatment. Sources listed at close of chapters. Valuable reference for proctologists.
R: *American Journal of Proctology* 24: 78 (Feb. 1973); *British Journal of Urology* 47: 581 (Oct. 1975); *Postgraduate Medical Journal* 52: 59 (Jan. 1976); *TBRI* 42: 184 (May 1976); Brandon; Stearns & Ratcliff (*NEJM,* 1969; *NEJM,* 1970).

Synopsis of Gynecology. 9th ed. **Daniel W. Beacham and Woodard D. Beacham, eds.** St. Louis, MO: C. V. Mosby, 1977.

Eighth edition, 1972.
General reference work intended for family physicians and general practitioners.
R: Brandon.

Synopsis of Obstetrics. 10th ed. **Eugene Sandberg.** St. Louis, MO: C. V. Mosby, 1978.

Concise new edition of text on obstetric principles. Includes much timely information.

Trauma in Pregnancy. **Herbert J. Buchsbaum, ed.** Philadelphia, PA: W. B. Saunders, 1979.

Comprehensive overview of obstetric trauma. Relates research material to clinical situations. Covers physiological alternations of pregnancy, psychological trauma, legal issues, etc. Practical guide for the attending physician.

Tumors of the Kidney, Renal Pelvis, and Ureter. **James L. Bennington and J. Bruce Beckwith.** Washington, DC: Armed Forces Institute of Pathology, 1975.

Explores, in depth, all aspects of renal tumor pathology. Correlates radiologic diagnosis to pathological findings. Devotes space to both major and minor tumors. Includes electron micrographs of ultrastructure. An invaluable source for radiologists, oncologists, and urologists.
R: *Archives of Pathology & Laboratory Medicine* 100: 562 (Oct. 1976); *British Journal of Surgery* 64: 304 (Apr. 1977).

Tumors of the Ovary. **H. Fox and F. A. Langley.** Chicago, IL: Year Book Medical Publishers, 1976.

Discusses clinical features and treatment of ovarian tumors. Recommended to pathologists and gynecologists.
R: *British Journal of Obstetrics & Gynaecology* 83: 990 (Dec. 1976); *South African Medical Journal* 51: 52 (Jan. 8, 1977).

The Uterus. **Henry J. Norris and Arthur T. Hertig, eds.** Baltimore, MD: Williams & Wilkins, 1973.

Comprehensive monograph discusses aspects of uterus functioning in state of health and disease. Written by 23 authorities; volume is well illustrated with diagrams, tables, and photographs; bibliography contains extensive references. For students of female genital tract as well as pathologists.
R: *Archives of Pathology & Laboratory Medicine* 98: 288 (Oct. 1974); *Obstetrics and Gynecology* 44: 785 (Nov. 1974).

The Vulva. **Constance M. Ridley.** Philadelphia, PA: W. B. Saunders, 1975.
Inclusive monograph covering anatomy, infections, dermatitis, and tumors of the vulva. Many photographs and excellent references enhance this book, which is recommended to gynecologists and dermatologists.
R: *Archives of Dermatology* 112: 1484 (Oct. 1976).

Williams Obstetrics. 15th ed. **Jack A. Pritchard and Paul C. MacDonald.** New York: Appleton-Century-Crofts, 1976.
Fourteenth edition, 1971.
Standard text on study of reproduction, pregnancy, and birth. Presents current consensus in obstetric diagnosis and therapy. Newest edition contains updated chapters on fetal health, abortion, and contraception. Well illustrated.
R: Allyn; Brandon; Stearns & Ratcliff (*AJN; NEJM,* 1969).

VETERINARY MEDICINE

Animal Agents and Vectors of Human Disease. 4th ed. **Ernest C. Faust, Paul C. Beaver, and Rodney C. Jung.** Philadelphia, PA: Lea & Febiger, 1975.
First edition, 1955; second edition, 1962; third edition, 1968.
Fourth revised edition details the transmission of parasites; provides fundamental information on protozoa, helminths, arthropods, and their role in human disease. Discusses diagnostic technique. Contains useful black-and-white photographs. Recommended for medical school and public health libraries.
R: *Journal of Parasitology* 61: 949 (Oct. 1975); 23: 164 (Feb. 1976); *RSR* 3: 35 (July–Dec. 1975).

Animal Science. 7th ed. **M. Eugene Ensminger.** Danville, IL: Interstate Printers and Publishers, 1977.
Useful for veterinary students.
R: *Food Technology* 31: 82 (Dec. 1977).

Avian Physiology. 3d ed. **P. D. Sturkie, ed.** New York: Springer-Verlag, 1976.

Canine Neurology; Diagnosis and Treatment. 3d ed. **B. F. Hoerlein.** Philadelphia, PA: W. B. Saunders, 1978.
State-of-the-art text in veterinary neurology. Incorporates up-to-date information on all aspects of canine neurology and some major contributions to feline neurology. Highly recommended to veterinarians.

General Veterinary Pathology. **R. G. Thomson.** Philadelphia, PA: W. B. Saunders, 1978.
Covers recent developments in veterinary technology, animal health technology, animal science and husbandry. Geared toward practitioners and students of veterinary medicine.

Veterinary Applied Pharmacology and Therapeutics. 3d ed. **G. C. Brander and D. M. Pugh.** Philadelphia, PA: Lea & Febiger, 1977.

Veterinary Gastroenterology. **Neil V. Anderson, ed.** Philadelphia, PA: Lea & Febiger, 1980.

Veterinary Pathology. 4th ed. **Hilton A. Smith, Thomas C. Jones, and Ronald D. Hunt.** Philadelphia, PA: Lea & Febiger, 1972.

Veterinary Pharmacology and Therapeutics. 4th ed. **L. Meyer Jones et al.** Ames, IO: Iowa State University, 1977.

Veterinary Reproduction and Obstetrics. 4th ed. **Geoffrey H. Arthur.** Philadelphia, PA: Lea & Febiger, 1975.

Numerous illustrations, some in color, complement text.

CHAPTER 16   ABSTRACTS AND INDEXES, AND CURRENT-AWARENESS SERVICES

ABSTRACTS AND INDEXES

For abstracts and indexes in machine-readable form, see chapter 24, Data Bases. For those in microforms, see chapter 22, Nonprint Materials.

GUIDES TO ABSTRACTS AND INDEXES

The following are examples of sources that provide both a guide to available abstracts and indexes in science and technology and an insight into the role that such publications play throughout the disciplines:

Abstracting Scientific and Technical Literature. **Robert E. Maizell, Julian F. Smith, and T. E. R. Singer.** New York: Wiley-Interscience, 1971.

An introductory guide and text for scientists, abstractors, and indexers.
R: Chen (p. 325).

Abstracting Services, FID Pub. no. 445-456. 2d ed. 2 vols. **International Federation for Documentation.** The Hague, The Netherlands: International Federation for Documentation, 1969.

First edition, 1965.
This multilingual text lists 1,500 abstracting services in science, technology, agriculture, social sciences, humanities. Text in English, Russian, Spanish, French. Arranged alphabetically by abstract name. Title, subject, and country indexes.
R: *MRW* S2, p. 2.

Abstracts and Indexes in Science and Technology: A Descriptive Guide. **Dolores B. Owen and Marguerite M. Hanchey.** Metuchen, NJ: Scarecrow Press, 1974.

Provides a comprehensive listing of indexing tools in scientific and technical subjects. Entries, described in outline form, are arranged under general headings.
R: *Choice* 11: 1459 (Dec. 1974); *ARBA* (1975, p. 639); Chen (p. 325); Mal (3-46).

Biological Indicators of Environmental Quality: A Bibliography of Abstracts. **William A. Thomas, William H. Wilcox, and Gerald Goldstein.** Ann Arbor, MI: Ann Arbor Science, 1973.

A unique collection of abstracts on environmental monitoring. Aimed at aquatic biologists, plant physiologists, foresters, etc.
R: *ARBA* (1975, p. 692); Chen (p. 325); Mal (8-86).

Guide to the Indexes for Biological Abstracts and Bioresearch Index. Philadelphia, PA: Biosciences Information Service of Biological Abstracts, 1970.

Illustrated instructions to the format and use of the BASIC, author, biosystematic, and CROSS indexes incorporated in every issue of *Biological Abstracts* and *Bioresearch Index.* Explains the relationship between the four indexes and how they can be used in combination.
R: *MRW* S2, p. 13.

A Guide to the World's Abstracting and Indexing Services in Science and Technology: National Federation of Indexing and Abstracting Services Report Number 102. Washington, DC: Science and Technology Division, US Library of Congress, 1963. Repr. by Boston: Gregg Press, 1972.

Some 1,800 useful but dated services arranged by title.
R: *ARBA* (1974, p. 549); Chen (p. 325); Mal (3-45); Win (EA62).

An Index to Biographical Fragments in Unspecialized Scientific Journals. **E. Scott Barr.** University, AL: University of Alabama Press, 1973.

Designed as a guide to uncovering biographies and related material on pre-1920 scientists. Includes nearly 15,000 biographical references on nearly 8,000 scientists. Seven general scientific journals provide the name, dates, and appropriate source for each citation.
R: *MRW* S3, pp. 7, 47.

Survey of Abstracting Services and Current Bibliographical Tools in Agriculture, Forestry, Fisheries, Nutrition, Veterinary Medicine, and Related Subjects. **Sigmund von Frauendorfer, ed.** München, W Germany: BLV Verlagsgesellschaft, 1969.

International in scope, includes brief annotations; has subject and country indexes.
R: *Quarterly Bulletin of the International Association of Agricultural Libraries and Documentalists* 14: 138 (July 1969); Chen (p. 325); Wal (p. 397); Win (3EK5).

A World Bibliography of Bibliographies and of Bibliographic Catalogues, Calendars, Abstracts, Digests, Indexes, and the Like. 4th and final ed., rev. and greatly enl. 5 vols. Lausanne: Societas Bibliographica, 1965–1966.

The most comprehensive work of its kind.
R: Chen (p. 326); Jenkins (A11); Mal (3-36); Wal (p. 11).

GENERAL

Bioengineering Abstracts. Vols. 1–. New York: Engineering Index, 1974–. Monthly.

Service provides access to abstracts which appear in *Engineering Index* that are relevant to engineering in the life sciences. Weighted heavily in favor of research rather than clinical work. Conference proceedings, symposia, monographs, standards, and selected book reviews are included. Subject guide is given in preliminary pages.

Biological Abstracts. Vols. 1–. Philadelphia, PA: Biosciences Information, 1926–. Semimonthly.

The major abstracting service available on the biological sciences. Approximately 140,000 abstracts of articles from some 8,000 serials as well as books, reports, etc., are listed annually under 85 subject categories. Various indexes on colored paper: author; biosystemic or taxonomic; CROSS-referring abstract numbers to major categories and subheadings; and BASIC, or subjects in context based on titles. The computerized base is BA PREVIEW. From the BIOSIS data base several smaller abstracts such as *Abstracts of Entomology, Abstracts of Mycology,* etc., are generated. *BA* is supplemented by *Bioresearch Index.*
R: Chen (p. 332); Katz (p. 7); Jenkins (G7); Mal (9-4); Wal (p. 191; 194; 205; 222); Win (EC7).

Biological Abstracts/RRM. Vols. 18–. Philadelphia, PA: Biosciences Information, 1980–. Monthly.

Successor to *Bioresearch Index.* Consists of a "Content Summaries" section of indexed publications, including reports, reviews, and meetings; numerous indexes: author, biosystematic, generic, concept, and subject.

Biological Membrane Abstracts. London: Information Retrieval Ltd., 1973–. Monthly.

Monthly publication of 400 abstracts. Focuses on all aspects of transport across membranes. Papers range from membrane structure and function to role of membranes in immune response. Over 22,400 abstracts since 1973.
R: Chen (p. 332); Owen (p. 79).

Bioresearch Index. Philadelphia: Biosciences Information, 1967–. Monthly.
Original title: *Bioresearch Title,* 1965–1967.
Supplements *Biological Abstracts* by indexing life sciences research literature not included in *Biological Abstracts* such as theses, symposia, meetings, etc. Includes author and permuted-title indexes. Superceded by *Biological Abstracts/RRM,* 1980–.
R: Chen (p. 332); Jenkins (G8); *MRW* S1, p. 7; Wal (p. 191); Win (1EC1; 2EC3).

Bulletin of the Public Affairs Information Service. Vols. 1–. New York: Public Affairs Information Service, 1915–. Weekly.

An index which covers current literature pertaining to economic, social, and political issues; abstracts from books, pamphlets, documents, periodicals. Issued in weekly bulletins; cumulated five times yearly, the fifth issue cumulating the entire year. Useful for researching current legislation, government policy.
R: Sheehy (CA34).

Bulletin Signalétique. Paris: Centre National de la Recherche Scientifique, 1956–. Monthly for most sections.

Multiple sections, mostly monthly, carry about 400,000 abstracts per year from about 8,000 periodicals. Each issue of each part has an author index. Annual subject and author indexes.
R: Chen (p. 326); Wal (p. 5).

CBAC; Abstracts on the Chemical-Biological Activities of Chemical Substances. Vols. 13–. **American Chemical Society.** Easton, PA: American Chemical Society, 1971–. Semiweekly.

Continues *Chemical-Biological Activities.*
Semiweekly service abstracts over 600 biochemical journals. Indexes include subject, author, molecular formulae, registry numbers, and chemical substances.
R: *MRW* S2, pp. 12, 78.

Government Reports Announcements and Index. Springfield, VA: US National Technical Information Service, 1938–. Semimonthly.

Formerly *US Government Research and Development Reports Index.*
Announcements and *Index* sections combined into one publication in 1975. Abstracts of scientific and technical-report literature emanating from over 225 government organizations. Over 50,000 abstracts are produced annually. Entries arranged under 22 major subject categories, with numerous subdivisions. Index section includes subject, personal and corporate-author, contract-number, and accession report indexes.
R: Chen (p. 326); Katz (p. 14).

International Abstracts of Biological Sciences. Vols. 1–. London: Pergamon, 1954–. Monthly.

Original title, *British Abstracts of Medical Science.*
Focuses on crucial papers in experimental biology. Emphasizes anatomy, biochemistry, immunology, experimental pathology, microbiology, pharmacology, cytology, genetics and experimental zoology. Not all entries carry abstracts; all abstracts signed. Foreign-language titles translated into English. Includes author and subject indexes.
R: Win (EC9, ED16, EK64); Wal (p. 192).

Isotope Titles. Vols. 1–. Berlin: Isocommerz, 1967–. Monthly.

Monthly abstracting service covering 850 journals. Includes subject index (key word), author index, and list of abstracted periodicals.
R: *MRW* S1, p. 28.

Pandex Current Index to Scientific and Technical Literature. New York: Pandex, to 1969; CCM Information, 1967–. Biweekly.

A multidisciplinary index covering technical reports, books, and approximately 2,000 scientific journals. Arranged in two sections: subjects; and authors and permuted titles.
R: *American Documentation* 19: 357 (1968); *CRL* 29: 72 (1968); *Sci-Tech News* 23: 19 (1969); *SL* 58: 728 (1967); Chen (p. 326); Jenkins (A21); Mal (3-41); Wal (p. 8).

PHRA: Poverty and Human Resources Abstracts. Vols. 1–. Ann Arbor, MI: Institute of Labor and Industrial Relations, 1966–. Bimonthly.

A bimonthly abstract with author and subject index. Accompanied by *Annual Index to Poverty, Human Resources and Manpower Information,* a bibliography which can be used separately.
R: *MRW* S1, p. 32.

Referativnyi Zhurnal. Moscow: Akademiya Nauk, 1953–.

The most comprehensive abstracting service. In 1966, 21,000 periodicals as well as 6,000 monographs, etc., from 110 countries were covered. Over 1 million abstracts per year. There are 61 series.
R: Chen (p. 327); Wal (p. 8).

Repertorium Commentationum a Societatibus Litterariis Editarum . . . **Jeremias D. Reuss.** Gottingae: Dieterich, 1813–1821. Repr. by New York: B. Franklin, 1961.

T. 10–16, *Scientia et ars medica et chirurgica.*
An index to the publications of learned societies before 1800, with classified arrangement and author index for each section.
R: Win (EA27; EK50).

Science Abstracts. Vols.1–. London: Institution of Electrical Engineers, 1898–.

Originally issued in two sections: series A, *Physics Abstracts*; and series B, *Electrical and Electronics Abstracts.* Since 1966, series C, *Computer and Control Abstracts,* has been added.
The three abstract journals contain journal, patent, report, book, and conference information. Subject and author indexes. All abstracts are now part of the INSPEC (Information Service in Physics, Electrotechnical, and Control) system. For more information on each abstract, see under separate entry.
R: Chen (p. 327); Katz (p. 24); Wal (p. 9, 35); Win (EG12).

Science Citation Index. Vols. 1–. Philadelphia, PA: Institute for Scientific Information, 1961–. Quarterly.

The components of SCI are: *Citation Index, Source Index,* and *Permuterm Subject Index.* Five-year cumulations available.
A comprehensive computer-produced index that provides access to related articles by listing both cited and citing (source) authors and works. The vast majority of citations are from over 2,500 journals, though patents, reports, meetings, etc., are included. Critical in the sense that frequently cited material can be identified. Annual cumulations. The data base can also be accessed on-line through the use of SCISEARCH.
R: *Chemical and Engineering News* 42: 55–56 (Aug. 31, 1964); *Chemistry and Industry* 416 (March 6, 1965); *Journal of Documentation* 21: 139-141 (1965); *LJ* 89: 2735–2737 (1964); *LRTS* 9: 478 (1965); 12: 415 (1968); *LT* 16: 374 (1968); *Nature* 211: 556–557 (Aug. 6, 1966); 277: 1173 (Sept. 12, 1970); *Science* 145: 142 (1964); *ARBA* (1976, p. 640); Chen (p. 327); Jenkins (A20); Katz (p. 25); Mal (3-43); Wal (p. 10); Win (2EA15).

Science Research Abstracts. Vols. 1–. Riverdale, MD: Cambridge Scientific Abstracts, 1973–. 10/yr. for each pt.

Part A, "Superconductivity; Magnetohydrodynamics, Plasmas, Theoretical Physics and Superconductivity Research"; part B, "Laser and Electrooptic Reviews; Quantum Electronics." Approximately 32,000 abstracts annually. Subject and author indexes.
R: Chen (p. 327); Mal (6-12).

Sociological Abstracts. Vols. 1–. New York: Sociological Abstracts, 1952–. 5/yr.

Standard indexing service for sociological literature since 1952. Yearly cumulations.
R: *MRW* S1, p. 32.

SUBJECT TOOLS

The National Library of Medicine, through its computer-based MEDLARS (Medical Analysis and Retrieval System), produced the most important indexing tool of the medical literature, *Index Medicus* (*IM*), with its abridged version, *Abridged Index Medicus* (*AIM*). *IM* indexed over 2,400 medical and medical-related periodicals, while *AIM* indexed only the selected 100 periodicals from those included in *IM*. *AIM* is specially designed for use in hospital libraries.

Through MEDLARS, the National Library of Medicine also periodically produces lists of citations to journal articles in specialized biomedical fields. Most of these lists, termed "Recurring Bibliographies," are printed and distributed by nonprofit professional organizations and other government agencies with whom the Library cooperates. More detailed information on all these tools, together with *IM* and *AIM*, can be found either in the section following this listing of recurring bibliographies or in chapter 3, Bibliographies. However, for the convenience of the readers, all recurring bibliographies of the National Library of Medicine are listed here.

NATIONAL LIBRARY OF MEDICINE RECURRING BIBLIOGRAPHIES

Bibliography on Medical Education is included in the *Journal of Medical Education*, published monthly by the Association of American Medical Colleges, 1 Dupont Circle, Washington, DC 20036.

Index of Rheumatology, an annual, is available from the American Rheumatism Association Section of the Arthritis Foundation, 1212 Avenue of the Americas, New York, New York 10036.

Index to Dental Literature is a quarterly sold by the American Dental Association, 211 East Chicago Avenue, Chicago, Illinois 60611.

International Nursing Index is a quarterly sold by the American Journal of Nursing Company, 10 Columbus Circle, New York, New York 10019.

Kidney Disease and Nephrology Index is published bimonthly. Contact the Scientific Communications Officer, US National Institute of Arthritis, Metabolism, and Digestive Diseases, US National Institutes of Health, Bethesda, Maryland 20014.

Endocrinology Index is published bimonthly by the US National Institute of Arthritis, Metabolism, and Digestive Diseases, US National Institutes of Health, Bethesda, Maryland 20014.

Bibliography of Surgery of the Hand, annual, is published and distributed by the American Society for Surgery of the Hand. For information write: John A. Boswick, Jr., M.D., Secretary-Treasurer, American Society for Surgery of the Hand, 4200 East 9th Avenue, Denver, Colorado 80220.

Anesthesiology Bibliography, a quarterly, is published and distributed by the American Society of Anesthesiologists. For information write: Wood Library, Museum of Anesthesiology, American Society of Anesthesiologists, 515 Busse Highway, Park Ridge, Illinois 60068.

Current Bibliography of Plastic and Reconstructive Surgery, a bimonthly, is published and distributed by The Education Foundation of the American Society of Plastic and Reconstructive Surgeons, Incorporated. For information write: Plastic Surgery Executive Offices, 29 East Madison Street, Suite 807, Chicago, Illinois 60602.

Population Sciences: Index of Biomedical Research, is published monthly by the Center for Population Research of the National Institute of Child Health and Human Development, US National Institutes of Health, Bethesda, Maryland 20014.

Physical Fitness/Sports Medicine, a quarterly, is sponsored by the President's Council on Physical Fitness and Sports (Washington, DC 20201) and sold on subscription by the Superintendent of Documents.

Psychopharmacology Bibliography is published quarterly in the Psychopharmacology Bulletin by the US National Institute of Mental Health, US National Institutes of Health. For information write: Dr. Alice Leeds, National Institute of Mental Health, International Reference Center for Psychotropic Drugs, 5600 Fishers Lane, Room 9105, Rockville, Maryland 20852.

Neurosurgical Biblio-Index, a quarterly is published by the American Association of Neurological Surgeons. For information write to the Subscription Manager, *Journal of Neurosurgery*, 428 E. Preston Street, Baltimore, Maryland 21202.

Cranio-Facial—Cleft Palate Bibliography is published quarterly by the American Cleft Palate Association. For information write to the Dental Research Center, University of North Carolina, Chapel Hill, North Carolina 27514.

Index of Dermatology is published monthly by the US National Institute of Arthritis, Metabolism, and Digestive Diseases; US National Institutes of Health, Bethesda, Maryland 20014.

Recurring Bibliography of Hypertension is published bimonthly by the American Heart Association, Inc., 44 East 23rd Street, New York, New York 10010.

Recurring Bibliography on Education in the Allied Health Professions, an annual, is available from: Dr. John E. Burke, Director, Medical Communications Division. School of Allied Medical Professions, the Ohio State University, 1583 Perry Street, Columbus, Ohio 43210.

Parkinson's Disease and Related Disorders, Citations from the Literature, is published monthly by the US National Institute of Neurological and Communicative Disorders and Stroke, US National Institutes of Health, Bethesda, Maryland 20014.

Index of Tissue Culture is published annually by the Tissue Culture Association, Inc., W. Alton Jones Cell Science Center, P.O. Box 631, Lake Placid, New York 12946.

Annual Bibliography of Orthopaedic Surgery is published and distributed by The Journal of Bone and Joint Surgery, 10 Shattuck Street, Boston, Massachusetts 02115.

Current Citations on Strabismus, Amblyopia, and Other Diseases of Ocular Motility is published quarterly by the International Strabismological Association. For information write to: Robert D. Reinecke, M.D., Department of Ophthalmology, Albany Medical College, 47 New Scotland Avenue, Albany, New York 12208.

Interferon and Antiviral Substances Bibliography, is published annually by the US National Institute of Allergy and Infectious Diseases. For ordering information write to the National Technical Information Service, US Department of Commerce, 5285 Port Royal Road, Springfield, Virginia 22161.

Hepatitis Bibliography, is published annually by the US National Institute of Allergy and Infectious Diseases. For ordering information write to the National Technical Information Service, US Department of Commerce, 5285 Port Royal Road, Springfield, Virginia 22161.

Hospital Literature Index is published quarterly by the American Hospital Association, 840 N. Lake Shore Drive, Chicago, Illinois 60611.

Index of Audiovisual Serials in the Health Sciences is published quarterly by the Medical Library Association, 919 North Michigan Avenue, Chicago, Illinois 60611.

GENERAL—MEDICINE

Abridged Index Medicus. **US National Library of Medicine.** Washington, DC: US Government Printing Office, 1970–. Monthly.

Rapid access to 100 English-language journals of immediate interest to the practicing physician.
R: Chen (p. 331); Stearns & Ratcliff (*AJN*; NEJM, 1970).

Abstracts of World Medicine. Vols. 1–45. London: British Medical Association, 1947–1971. Monthly.

Continued *Bulletin of War Medicine*. Highlights outstanding journal articles on a monthly basis. Titles and abstracts listed in English. Includes signed abstracts. Subject and author indexes cumulated semiannually.
R: Win (EK59).

British Medical Abstracts and Therapeutic Progress. Vols. 1–. London: Medical Division, Haymarket Press, 1961–. Monthly.

Published monthly, abstracts from standard medical journals such as *Lancet, BMJ, JAMA*.
R: *MRW* S1, p. 1.

Computers in Medicine Abstracts. Vols. 1–. New York: Council for Interdisciplinary Communication in Medicine, 1968–. Bimonthly.

A bimonthly abstracting service.
R: *MRW* S1, p. 8.

Excerpta Medica. Vols. 1–. Princeton, NJ: Excerpta Medica, 1946–. Year of publication depends on sections.

A major indexing tool which screens 3,500 journals, publishes in 44 sections, 770 issues altogether each year, and adds about 250,000 references yearly. The 44 sections include 42 abstract journals in every aspect of health sciences and 2 literature indexes, *Adverse Reactions Titles* and *Drug Literature Index*. Each abstract journal features three individual index systems: classification, subject, and author. Pamphlets on the use of *Excerpta Medica, How to Use Excerpta Medica,* the *Excerpta Medica Abstract Journals: An Introduction* are useful guides.
The 42 abstract journals of *Excerpta Medica* are entitled *Anatomy, Anthropology, Embryology and Histology* (Section 1); *Anesthesiology* (24); *Arthritis and Rheumatism* (31); *Biophysics, Bio-engineering and Medical Instrumentation* (27); *Cancer* (16); *Cardiovascular Diseases and Cardiovascular Surgery* (18); *Chest Diseases, Thoracic Surgery and Tuberculosis* (15); *Clinical Biochemistry* (29); *Dermatology and Venereology* (13); *Developmental Biology and Teratology* (21); *Drug Dependence* (40); *Endocrinology* (3); *Environmental Health and Pollution Control* (46); *Epilepsy* (50); *Forensic Science* (49); *Gastroenterology* (48); *General Pathology and Pathological Anatomy* (5); *Gerontology and Geriatrics* (20); *Health Economics and Hospital Management* (36); *Hematology* (25); *Human Genetics* (22); *Immunology, Serology and Transplantation* (26); *Internal Medicine* (6); *Microbiology: Bacteriology, Mycology and Parasitology* (4); *Neurology and Neurosurgery* (8); *Nuclear Medicine* (23); *Obstetrics and Gynecology* (10); *Occupational Health and Industrial Medicine* (35); *Ophthalmology* (12); *Orthopedic Surgery* (33); *Otorhinolaryngology* (11); *Pediatrics and Pediatric Surgery* (7); *Pharmacology and Toxi-*

cology (30); *Physiology* (2); *Plastic Surgery* (34); *Psychiatry* (32); *Public Health, Social Medicine and Hygiene* (17); *Radiology* (14); *Rehabilitation and Physical Medicine* (19); *Surgery* (9); *Urology and Nephrology* (28); *Virology* (47).

Human Experimentation Abstracts. Vols. 1–. Ripon, England: Washington Publishing House, 1974–. Semiannual.

Annotated references to journal articles dealing with new research methods in human experimentation. International coverage. Entries arranged numerically. Includes author and subject indexes.
R: *MRW* S3, pp. 19, 30.

Index Medicus. **US National Library of Medicine.** Washington, DC: US Government Printing Office, 1960–. Monthly.

Cumulated annually under title *Cumulated Index Medicus.*
Produced by the National Library of Medicine's MEDLARS (Medical Literature Analysis and Retrieval System).
Nearly 3,000 journals with about 200,000 citations annually. Prior to 1976, coverage was limited to periodical literature. From 1976 on, conference publications, monographs, etc., are included. The most important indexing tool in the field of medicine. A must for every medical library.
R: Chen (p. 332).

Laser Abstracts for the Medical Profession. Vols. 1–. Evanston, IL: Lowry-Cocroft Abstracts, 1966–. Monthly.

Issued monthly. Loose-leaf format.
R: *MRW* S1, p. 28.

Medical Socioeconomic Research Sources. Vols. 1–. **American Medical Association, Division of Library and Archival Services.** Germantown, MD: Aspen Systems, 1971–. Quarterly. Annual cumulations.

Citations cover events and developments in the sociology and economics of medicine. Sources encompass medical and scientific journals, popular magazines, and newspapers.
Continues *Index to Medical Socioeconomic Literature* (1962-1970).
R: ARBA (1975, p.733); *MRW* S2, pp. 38, 96, 98; Sheehy (EK6).

ALLERGY AND IMMUNOLOGY

Allergy Abstracts. Vols. 1–. St. Louis, MO: C. V. Mosby, 1936–. Monthly.

A special section of the *Journal of Allergy,* 1936–1971; continued by *Journal of Allergy and Clinical Immunology,* 1971–.

Immunology Abstracts. London: Information Retrieval Ltd., 1976–. Monthly.

Nearly 1,450 abstracts fill each monthly issue. Covers all areas of immunology from chemical to clinical, such as antibodies and complement and their interactions, immunological methodology, and immunological aspects of transplantation and tumors. Over 41,500 abstracts since 1976.

BRAIN AND NERVOUS SYSTEM

Chemoreception Abstracts. London: Information Retrieval Ltd., 1973–. Quarterly.

Quarterly publication containing some 325 abstracts. Focuses on various disciplines dealing with taste, smell, and related forms of sensitivity. Ranges from animal and human physiology to internal chemoreceptors. Additional topics: animal behavior studies, psychophysics, and new legislation concerning substances in food and cosmetics. About 8,500 abstracts since 1973.

Electroencephalography and Clinical Neurology: Index to Current Electroencephalographic Literature. Vols. 1–. Amsterdam: Elsevier, 1967–.

Prepared by the Brain Information Service of the University of California at Los Angeles.

Index to Current Literature. Vols. 1–. Amsterdam, Holland: Elsevier, Feb. 1967–. Quarterly.

Deals with specialized topics in neurology. No indexes.
R: *MRW* S1, p. 19.

Neurosurgical Biblio-Index. **American Association of Neurological Surgeons.** Baltimore, MD: American Association of Neurological Surgeons. Quarterly.

Parkinson's Disease and Related Disorders, Citations from the Literature. **US National Institute of Neurological and Communicative Disorders and Stroke.** Bethesda, MD: US National Institute of Neurological and Communicative Disorders and Stroke, 1970–. Monthly.

DENTISTRY

Dental Abstracts. Vols. 1–6, Jan. 1945–Sept./Dec. 1950. New York: Columbia University, School of Dental and Oral Surgery, Dental Abstracts Society, 1945–1950.
R: Win (EK144).

Dental Abstracts: A Selection of World Dental Literature. Vols. 1–. American Dental Association, 1956–. Monthly.
R: Win (EK145).

Index of the Periodical Dental Literature Published in the English Language, 1839–1936/38. 15 vols. Chicago, IL: American Dental Association, 1921–1939.

Each volume consists of two parts: classified subject index using an extended Dewey Decimal Classification and author index.
R: Win (EK142).

Index to Dental Literature. Vols. 1–. **American Dental Association.** Chicago, IL: American Dental Association, 1939–. Quarterly, with annual cumulations.

Published 1939–1961 with title *Index to Dental Literature in the English Language*. Beginning in 1965 (vol. 35), the index has been produced through MEDLARS, thus page format has followed that of *Index Medicus*. Over 1,200 journals are indexed with 30 percent in foreign languages. Coverage includes nondental journals. Subject and name indexes.
R: *MRW* S1, p. 12; Win (EK143, 1EJ18).

Oral Research Abstracts. Vols. 1–. Chicago, IL: American Dental Association, 1966–. Monthly.

Abstracts in English of articles found in dental and related journals. Focuses on oral health research. International coverage. Some 7,200 noncritical abstracts written by professionals. Classified arrangement of entries. Annual author and subject indexes.
R: Win (EK146; 1EJ19).

DERMATOLOGY

Index of Dermatology. Vols. 3–. Bethesda, MD: US National Institute of Arthritis, Metabolism, and Digestive Diseases, US National Institutes of Health, 1971–. Monthly.

Culled from the current month's total MEDLARS input. Five main sections comprise the classification scheme: subject headings searched for the month, reviews, general (clinical), bio-science (research), and authors.
R: *MRW* S2, p. 27.

ENDOCRINOLOGY

Diabetes Literature Index: By Authors, Hierarchy, and By Keywords in the Title. Vols. 1–. Washington, DC: US Government Printing Office, 1966–. Monthly.

Computer-produced bibliography of worldwide literature on diabetes. In two sections: Diabetes mellitus, Endocrinology. Annual cumulations.
R: Win (EK54).

Endocrinology Index. Vols. 1–. Bethesda, MD: US National Institute of Arthritis and Metabolic Diseases, US National Institutes of Health, 1968–. Bimonthly.

Bimonthly index of endocrinology literature, including a review section. Provides full citation and brief annotation. Covers journals listed in *Index Medicus*. Contains subject, author, and review sections and subject and author indexes.
R: *MRW* S1, p. 13; Win (EK55).

Prostaglandin Abstracts: A Guide to the Literature, Volume 1: 1906–1970. **Richard M. Sparks, ed.** New York: Plenum, 1974.

Abstracts concerning prostaglandins for years 1906 to 1970. Range of citations covers journal articles, books, reviews, newspaper articles, and symposia. Coverage of world literature in chronological arrangement, with subject, author and

journal indexes. Appendix is directory of ongoing prostaglandin research throughout the world.
R: *MRW* S3, p. 42; *ARBA* (1975, p. 745).

GASTROINTESTINAL SYSTEM

Gastroenterology Abstracts and Citations. Vols. 1–. **US National Institute of Arthritis, Metabolism, and Digestive Diseases.** Washington, DC: US Government Printing Office, 1966–. Monthly.

Abstracts from all primary sources in gastroenterology. Arranged by subject, with subject and author indexes. Deals with all major subjects in the field.
R: Win (EK62, 1EJ7)

GENETICS

Genetics Abstracts. London: Information Retrieval Ltd., 1968–. Monthly.

Emphasizes bacterial, molecular, viral, algal, fungal, plant, animal, and human genetics in some 1,100 abstracts. Monthly publication includes papers on structure and properties of DNA and RNA, ribosomes, mutagenesis, extrachromosomal factors, radiation genetics, and population genetics. Over 124,600 abstracts since 1968.

HEALTH SERVICES ADMINISTRATION

Abstracts of Health Care Management Studies. Vols. 1–. Ann Arbor, MI: Cooperative Information Center for Hospital Management Studies, University of Michigan, 1964–. Quarterly.

International journal contains abstracts of studies of management, planning, and public policy related to delivery of health care. Material abstracted includes journal articles, books, reports, government publications, etc. Indexes are by author, locator, source of reference, subject, and microfilm. Each abstract has note indicating availability of document. Continues *Abstracts of Hospital Management Studies.*
R: Win (EK58).

Cumulative Index of Hospital Literature. 1945–. Chicago: American Hospital Association, 1950–.

Six five-year *Cumulative Index* cover the periods of 1945–1949, 1950–1954, 1955–1959, 1950–1964, 1965–1969, 1970–1974, and another cumulation covers the period of 1975–1977 (published 1979).
The major subject-author index lists citations to articles about health care from several hundreds of journals included in *Hospital Literature Index.* An essential tool for all medium and large hospital libraries. As of 1978 MeSH subject headings are used.
R: *ARBA* (1978, p. 722); Win (EK51).

Hospital Abstracts: A Monthly Survey of World Literature. Vols. 1–. London: Her Majesty's Stationery Office, 1961–. Monthly.

Focuses on the fields of administration, planning, and technology in hospitals. Excludes strictly medical matters. Presents abstracts of periodical articles and monographs, with roughly 1,800 entries appearing each year. Follows a detailed

classification scheme. International in coverage. Valuable companion to studies in nursing and management of health institutions.
R: Win (EK63).

Hospital Literature Index. Vols. 16–. **American Hospital Association.** Chicago, IL: American Hospital Association, 1960–. Quarterly. Annual and five-year cumulations.

Continues *Cumulative Index to Hospital Literature,* Vols. 1–15, 1945–1960. Published in cooperation with the National Library of Medicine. Basic author-subject index to hospital literature concerning administration, planning, and financing of hospitals and related health care institutions. Separate section lists journals indexed and recent acquisitions (books, monographs and journals) of the American Hospital Association Library. A must for any medical library.
R: Win (EK52); Stearns & Ratcliff (*AJN*).

INFECTIOUS DISEASES

Abstracts of Microbiological Methods. **V. B. D. Skerman, ed.** New York: John Wiley, 1969.

Abstracts describe techniques and methods of bacterial examination. Over 2,500 abstracts from selected English and French journals (1929–1967). Classified arrangement. Index of bacteria genera and specific tests.
R: *ARBA* (1970, p. 115); Mal (9-42); *MRW* S2, pp. 68, 102; Wal (p. 198).

Abstracts of Mycology. Vols. 1–. Philadelphia, PA: Biosciences Information Service of Biological Abstracts, 1967–. Monthly.

Monthly publication compiled from *Biological Abstracts* and *BioResearch Index.* Coverage includes cytology, genetics, microbiology, pathology, and fungi in biochemistry. Annual cumulative subject and author index.
R: *MRW* S1, p. 15.

Microbiology Abstracts. Vols. 1–. London: Information Retrieval Ltd., 1965–. Monthly.

In three sections: industrial microbiology; bacteriology; and algology, mycology and protozoology. Each section provides monthly coverage of specialized area, extensively reaching all applicable fields of microbiology. Indexes: patent, author, and subject. Annual cumulation since 1965.
R: Chen (p. 333); Jenkins (G175); Mal (9-41); *MRW* S1, p. 14; Wal (p. 198).

Tropical Diseases Bulletin. Vols. 1–. London: Bureau of Hygiene and Tropical Diseases, 1912–. Monthly.

Summaries of journal articles on tropical diseases, largely in English. Published in association with *Abstracts on Hygiene.* Monthly with annual index of subjects, authors, and sources.
R: Win (EK66).

Virology Abstracts. London: Information Retrieval Ltd., 1967–. Monthly.

Monthly listing of over 750 abstracts on all aspects of viruses. Topics covered: purification of viral components, cell-culture techniques, immune responses, and

infections of fungi, plants, animals, and man. Over 75,600 abstracts since 1967. Indexes: virus names, patents, author, subject.
R: *MRW* S1, p. 15; Wal (p. 200).

INTERNAL MEDICINE

Aerospace Medicine and Biology: A Continuing Bibliography With Indexes. Washington, DC: Scientific and Technical Information Division, US National Aeronautics and Space Administration, 1964–. Irregular.

Aviation Medicine, 1952–1953.
Includes abstracts of world literature on aviation and space medicine subjects. Literature coverage includes US and foreign books, periodicals, conference proceedings, and government reports with emphasis on applied research. Signed annotations in English. Subject and personal author indexes in each volume are cumulated annually. Corporate source index.
R: Win (EK60).

French's Index of Differential Diagnosis. 10th ed. **F. Dudley Hart, ed.** Baltimore, MD: Williams & Wilkins, 1973.
A handbook of symptoms arranged alphabetically. Provides comprehensive and succinct information helping physicians to make diagnoses. Contains close to 800 illustrations and an index; covers about 40,000 entries. Considered a detailed compendium, helpful in making bedside diagnoses.
R: *Lancet* 2: 132 (July 21, 1973); *ABL* 38: entry 500 (Sept. 1973); *ARBA* (1975, p. 740); Allyn.

Index of Tissue Culture. **Tissue Culture Association.** Lake Placid, NY: Tissue Culture Association. Annual.

Tissue Culture Abstracts. Vols. 1–. Grand Island, NY: Grand Island Biological Company, 1964–. Bimonthly.
Bimonthly abstracts from 30 to 40 English-language journals. No indexes.
R: *MRW* S1, p. 7.

NURSING

Cumulative Index to Nursing Literature. Vols. 1–. Glendale, CA: Seventh Day Adventist Hospital Association, 1956–. 5/yr.
Volume 19, 1974.
R: *Choice* 10: 1583 (Dec. 1973); *ARBA* (1971, p. 537; 1975, p. 745; 1977, p. 719); Win (EK162).

Cumulative Index to Nursing Literature: Nursing Subject Headings. 4th ed. **Seventh Day Adventist Hospital Association.** Glendale, CA: Seventh Day Adventist Hospital Association, 1970.
Lists subject headings used in the *Cumulative Index to Nursing Literature* with a format which follows that of the Library of Congress. Clear explanation may be found in the preface.
R: *ARBA* (1971, p. 537).

Index to Public Health Nursing Magazine, 1909–1952, NLN Pub. no. 21-1491. New York: National League for Nursing, 1974.

International Nursing Index. Vols. 1–. **American Journal of Nursing.** New York: American Journal of Nursing, 1966–. Quarterly with annual cumulation.

Published as a joint effort of the US National Library of Medicine and the American Journal of Nursing Company. Indexes some 200 US and foreign nursing journals and nursing articles from over 2,300 non-nursing journals presently covered in *Index Medicus.* Arranged in two sections: subject and name. Additional lists include: current-year nursing dissertations, journals and serials indexed, agency publications and nursing monographs published during the year. A must for all nursing libraries.

R: *The Canadian Nurse* 73: 55 (May 1977); Stearns & Ratcliff (*AJN*; *NEJM,* 1970); Win (EK163, 1EJ21).

Nursing Abstracts. Vols. 1–. Forest Hills, NY: Nursing Abstracts Co., 1979–.

Published quarterly with annual indexes. Subject arrangement of nonevaluative abstracts from selected nursing periodicals.

Nursing Studies Index; An Annotated Guide to Reported Studies, Research Methods, and Historical and Biographical Materials in Periodicals, Books, and Pamphlets Published in English. 4 vols. **Yale University. School of Nursing. Index Staff.** Philadelphia, PA: J. B. Lippincott, 1963–1972.

Volume 1, *1900–1929,* 1972; volume 2, *1930–1949,* 1970; volume 3, *1950–1956,* 1966; volume 4, *1957–1959,* 1963. Under the general direction of Virginia Henderson.

In four volumes, the index includes abstracts to reported studies, research methods, historical and biographical materials in periodicals, books, and pamphlets in English. It constitutes the only index to the nursing literature from 1900 to 1959.

R: *MRW* S2, p. 72; Win (EK164, 1EJ22); Stearns & Ratcliff (*AJN*; *NEJM,* 1970).

NUTRITION

Amino Acid Peptide and Protein Abstracts. London: Information Retrieval Ltd., 1972–. Monthly.

Surveys literature covering the major aspects of the subject. Arranged under broad subject areas. Includes author, peptide, and protein indexes and an annual subject index.

R: Chen (p. 333); Wal (p. 138).

Feeding, Weight and Obesity Abstracts. London: Information Retrieval Ltd., 1976–. Bimonthly.

Covers the energy balance in this bimonthly publication. Some 500 abstracts per issue dealing with the organism's response to the intake of calories, the use of metabolized food, causes and effects of weight disorders, etc. Over 6,200 abstracts since 1976.

Food Science and Technology Abstracts. Bucks, England: Commonwealth Agricultural Bureau, 1969–. Monthly.

Abstracts over 1,000 journals.
R: *Aslib Proceedings* 21: 505 (Dec. 1969); 23: 330 (July 1971); Chen (p. 342); Wal (p. 484).

Nutrition Abstracts and Reviews. **Prepared by Commonwealth Bureau of Animal Nutrition.** Farnham Royal, UK: Commonwealth Agricultural Bureau, 1931–. Quarterly to 1972; monthly from 1973.

International coverage of animal nutrition. Titles listed in original language and in English translation. Signed abstracts. Covers book reviews, symposia, congress reports, and government reports.
R: Chen (p. 333); Win (EK172).

ONCOLOGY AND NUCLEAR MEDICINE

Applied Health Physics Abstracts and Notes. Ashford, England: Nuclear Technology, 1975–. Quarterly.
R: Chen (p. 329).

Cancer Therapy Abstracts. Vols. 15–. Philadelphia, PA: Franklin Institute Press, 1975–. Monthly.

International coverage of the literature of cancer therapy. Supersedes *Cancer Chemotherapy Abstracts*, vols. 1–14, 1960–1974.

Carcinogenesis Abstracts. Bethesda, MD: US National Cancer Institute, 1962–. Monthly.

Publication suspended volumes 3–6, 1965–1968.
Worldwide abstracts of literature pertaining to cancer etiology. Covers journals not included in *Index Medicus*.

Oncology Abstracts. London: Information Retrieval Ltd., 1977–. Monthly.

Abstracts of experimental oncology; encompasses all related fields such as biochemistry, pathology, radiotherapy, etc. Monthly. Over 28,000 abstracts since 1977.

OPHTHALMOLOGY

Current Citations on Strabismus, Amblyopia, and Other Diseases of Ocular Motility. Vols. 1–. **International Strabismological Association.** Albany, NY: Albany Medical College, Department of Ophthalmology, 1971–. Quarterly.

Vision Index. Vols. 1–. Berkeley, CA: Visual Science Information Center, University of California, 1971–. Quarterly.

Abstracts from all primary sources beginning November 1970. Quarterly, with annual cumulations.
R: *MRW* S2, pp. 74, 107.

ORTHOPEDICS

The Annual Bibliography of Orthopaedic Surgery. **Subcommittee on Orthopedic Information Services of the Committee on the Skeletal System of the US National Research Council.** Washington, DC: US Government Printing Office, 1969.

Abstracts from the eighteen major journals of orthopedic surgery. *Index Medicus* format. Citations derived from National Library of Medicine computer tapes.
R: *MRW* S2, p. 75.

Calcified Tissue Abstracts. London: Information Retrieval Ltd., 1969–. Quarterly.

Includes nearly 680 abstracts per issue on bone structure, other mineralized systems in living organisms, and function. Covers the effects of various ions, hormones, vitamins, radiation, and diseases on calcium metabolism. About 22,300 abstracts since 1969.

PHARMACY AND PHARMACOLOGY

Adverse Reaction Titles. Vols. 1–. Amsterdam: Excerpta Medica Foundation, 1966–. Monthly. Section 37 of *Excerpta Medica.*

Annual cumulations of over 5,000 bibliographic items on adverse drug reactions. Citations from 3,400 biomedical journals published world wide.
R: Win (EK186).

Drug Literature Index. Vols. 1–. Amsterdam: Excerpta Medica Foundation, 1969 . Monthly. Section 38 of *Excerpta Medica.*

Indexes some 3,400 biomedical serials concerned with drugs and pharmaceutical products. International coverage. Access by generic name, drug classification, adverse reactions, authors, and manufacturers.
R: *MRW* S2, pp. 36, 78.

Index Guide to Drug Information Retrieval. **Hiroyuki Fukushima, Toshiro Okazaki, and Michiko Noguchi.** New York: Elsevier, North-Holland, 1979.

A combined index to eight drug information sources: *The Merck Index, PDR, Drug Effects in Hospitalized Patients, Handbook of Practical Pharmacology, Intravenous Medications, Handbook on Injectable Drugs, Extra Pharmacopoeia,* and *Side Effects of Drugs.* Quick reference tool to drug information for researchers, clinicians, pharmacists, and health science librarians.

Inpharma. Vols. 1–. New York: ADIS Press, 1975–. Weekly.

International coverage of drugs and drug treatment from some 1,700 selected English- and foreign-language journals.

International Pharmaceutical Abstracts. Vols. 1–. Washington, DC: American Society of Hospital Pharmacists, 1964–. Semimonthly.

Abstracts some 400 international pharmacy journals. Includes book reviews. Fea-

tures author and subject indexes issued semiannually and annually. Subject arrangement. Part of TOXLINE Data Base.
R: Win (EK187).

Psychopharmacology Abstracts. Vols. 1–. Bethesda, MD: Psychopharmacology Service Center, US National Institute of Mental Health, 1961–. Monthly, 1961–1971; quarterly since 1972. Annual cumulation.

A ready source for abstracts of recent information concerning development in psychopharmacological research. Covers journals, conference proceedings, government research.

Side Effects of Drugs. Vols. 1–. Amsterdam: Excerpta Medica, 1957–. Irregular.

Volume 1, 1955/1956; volume 2, 1956/1957; volume 3, 1958/1960; volume 4, 1963; volume 5, 1963/65. Monthly bibliography, *Adverse Reaction Titles,* since 1966.
Comprehensive and international coverage of review articles and citations concerning adverse drug reactions.
R: Win (EK188; 1EJ24).

PHYSICAL MEDICINE AND REHABILITATION

Rehabilitation Literature. Chicago, IL: National Society for Crippled Children and Adults, 1940–. Monthly.

Abstracts from all primary sources concerning the care and rehabilitation of handicapped children and adults. Monthly publication. For students and professionals involved in rehabilitation.

PSYCHIATRY AND PSYCHOLOGY

Abstracts for Social Workers. Vols. 1–. **National Association of Social Workers.** Albany, NY: National Association of Social Workers, 1965–. Quarterly.

Quarterly publication covers such areas as psychiatry and medicine and social psychology.
R: *MRW* S1, p. 32.

Abstracts on Criminology and Penology. Vols. 9–. Deventer, The Netherlands: Kluwer, 1969–. Bimonthly.

Bimonthly abstracts of journal articles and monographs which include material from psychiatric literature and criminological sources. Entries are arranged in classified order and indexed by author and subject.
R: *MRW* S2, pp. 24, 81, 96.

Behavioural Biology Abstracts. London: Information Retrieval, 1973–. Quarterly.

References and abstracts arranged under subject categories and subdivided by taxonomic groups. All abstracts in English, though foreign titles are included. International in scope.

R: Chen (p. 332); Owen (p. 69).

The Chicago Psychoanalytic Literature Index, 1920–1970. 3 vols. **Glenn E. Miller, ed.** Chicago, IL: Chicago Institute for Psychoanalysis, 1978.

———, *1971–1974,* 1979.
———, *1976,* 1977.
———, *1977,* 1978.
———, *1978,* 1979.

Child Development Abstracts and Bibliography. Vols. 1–. Chicago, IL: University of Chicago Press, 1927–. 3/yr.

Developmental Disabilities Abstracts. Vols. 1–. Bethesda, MD: US National Institute of Mental Health, 1964–. Quarterly.

Continues *Mental Retardation and Developmental Disabilities Abstracts.*
Besides abstracts, some issues include outlines of research in progress and specific mental retardation bibliographies.
R: Win (1EH5).

Mental Health Digest. Vols. 1–. Chevy Chase, MD: US National Clearinghouse for Mental Health Information, 1969–.

Volume 1 preceded by seven experimental issues, August 1967–July 1968. Abstracts of research reports, review articles, federal and state documents, and mental health laws.
R: *MRW* S1, p. 17.

Occupational Mental Health Notes. Chevy Chase, MD: US National Clearinghouse for Mental Health Information, 1965–. Irregular.

Computer generated. Numerical arrangement of abstracts. No indexes.
R: *MRW* S1, p. 27.

Psychological Abstracts. Vols. 1–. Lancaster, PA: American Psychological Association, 1927–. Monthly, with annual cumulations.

The standard abstracting service; covers all major sources since 1927. For literature earlier than 1927, see also *Psychological Index.*

———. *Author Index.* Compiled by the Psychological Library, Columbia University Libraries. Included in the *Author Index to Psychological Index,* 1894–1935, and its *Cumulative Author Index to Psychological Abstracts,* 1927–1958 and its supplements: Supplement 1, 1959–1963 (Boston: G. K. Hall, 1965); Supplement 2, 1964–1968 (Boston: G. K. Hall, 1970), 2 vols.; Supplement 3, 1969–1971 (American Psychological Association, 1973), 3 vols.

———. *Cumulative Subject Index.* Volumes 1–34, 1927–1960 (Boston: G. K. Hall, 1966), 2 vols; volumes 35–39, 1961–1965 (Boston: G. K. Hall, 1967), 1 vol.; volumes 40–42, 1966–1968 (Boston: G. K. Hall, 1970), 2 vols.; volumes 43–45, 1969–1971 (American Psychological Association, 1973), 3 vols.
R: Win (EH15; 1EH6; 1EH7).

Psychological Index, 1894–1935. 42 vols. Princeton, NJ: Psychological Review Co., 1895–1936.

Issued in connection with the *Psychological Review.* Continued by *Psychological Abstracts.*

An annual bibliography of the literature of psychology and cognate subjects.

PUBLIC HEALTH

Abstracts on Health Effects of Environmental Pollutants. Vols. 1–. Philadelphia, PA: Biosciences Information Service of Biological Abstracts, 1972–. Monthly.

Includes 1,000 abstracts per monthly issue; taken from *Biological Abstracts, Bioresearch Index,* and MEDLARS. Of interest to those involved in occupational and environmental health. Classified arrangement, key word index. Part of TOXLINE Data Base.

R: *MRW* S2, pp. 42, 56; Chen (p. 351).

Abstracts on Hygiene. Vols. 43–. London: Bureau of Hygiene and Tropical Diseases. 1968–. Monthly.

Volumes 1–42, *Bulletin of Hygiene,* 1926–1967.

Provides selective and critical abstracts of world literature on public health, with particular reference to regions outside the tropics. Classified arrangement includes annual index of sources, authors, and general subjects. Continues *Bulletin of Hygiene.*

R: Win (EK215).

Air Pollution Abstracts. Vols. 1–. Research Triangle Park, NC: Air Pollution Technical Information Center, 1970–. Subscriptions from US Government Printing Office. Monthly.

R: Chen (p. 351).

The Alcoholism Digest Annual. Vols. 1–. Rockville, MD: Information Planning Associates, 1972/1973–. Annual.

Annotated citations from books, journal articles, government documents, proceedings, and pamphlets, arranged topically. Given data for training and support programs includes objectives, eligibility, and authorization. Complete with author and subject indexes.

R: *MRW* S3, p. 2.

Biological Indicators of Environmental Quality: A Bibliography of Abstracts. **William A. Thomas, Gerald Goldstein, and William H. Wilcox.** Ann Arbor, MI: Ann Arbor Science Publishers, 1973.

Over 500 abstracts concerning the hazards of environmental pollution. Abstracts from European and American journals cover a wide spectrum of subjects, making this useful to medical and environmental researchers.

R: *Archives of Environmental Health* 27: 120 (1973).

Environment Abstracts. New York: Environment Information Center, 1974–. Monthly.

Lists articles, films, and books relating to environmental issues. Material arranged under 21 subject headings. Unfortunately, weak in areas related to the social sciences. Subject and author indexes as well as a list of keywords.
R: *ARBA* (1975, p. 706); Chen (p. 350).

Environment Index: A Guide to the Key Environmental Literature of the Year. New York: Environment Information Center, 1971–. Annual.

Over 70,000 citations (in 1973) each year from scientific and technical journals, government reports, conference papers, newspapers, books, and films in the environment area. Each entry is indexed by subject, industry, and author. Additional features include lists of federal and state environmental officials, and major federal legislation.
R: *ARBA* (1973, p. 580; 1975, p. 707); Chen (p. 350) Katz (p. 14); Mal (8-81).

Fluoride Abstracts. Cincinnati, OH: Kettering Laboratory in the College of Medicine, University of Cincinnati, 1955/1958–. Quarterly.

Supplements *Annotated Bibliography: The Occurrence and Biological Effects of Fluorine Compounds.* Volume 1, *The Inorganic Compounds.* Loose-leaf format.
R: *MRW* S1, p. 9.

Health and Crime Abstracts, 1960–1971. Houston, TX: School of Public Health, University of Texas at Houston, 1972.

English-language books, journal articles, government documents, papers, and reports comprise most of the 586 references. Intended as a comprehensive compilation of titles expressing the relationship between crime and health. Classified arrangement under eleven headings. Includes author and subject indexes.
R. *MRW* S2, pp. 24, 60, 66.

Health Aspects of Pesticides: Abstract Bulletin. Vols. 1–. Washington, DC: Pesticides Program, US Public Health Service, 1968–. Monthly.

Encompasses articles from over 500 US and foreign journals. Classified arrangement of abstracts.
R: Win (3EJ9; 3EJ32).

Index of Human Ecology. **J. Owen and Elizabeth A. Jones.** London: Europa. Distr. Detroit, MI: Gale Research, 1974.

A valuable index, given the cross-disciplinary nature of the field. Primarily a subject index to the abstracting journals that cover these subjects.
R: *RSR* 3: 25 (Apr./June 1975); *ARBA* (1975, p. 708); Chen (p. 333).

Occupational Safety and Health Abstracts. Vols. 1–. Geneva: International Occupational Safety and Health Information Centre, International Labour Office, 1963–.

Pesticide Index. 5th ed. **Entomological Society of America.** College Park, MD: Entomological Society of America, 1976.

Third edition, 1965; fourth edition, 1969.
Alphabetical listing of 5,800 chemical names of pesticides. Supplies serial number, names, structural formula, toxicity, physical properties. Appendixes contain

manufacturers directory and appropriate citations of publications.
R: *MRW* S2, p. 78.

Pesticides Abstracts. Vols. 1–. **US Public Health Service. Pesticides Program.** Washington, DC: US Government Printing Office, 1968–. Monthly.

A publication of the Environmental Protection Agency. Abstracts from over 1,000 foreign and domestic journals. Classified arrangement with author and subject indexes. Earlier title was *Health Aspects of Pesticides; Abstract Bulletin.*
R: Win (EK220).

Pollution Abstracts. Vols. 1–. La Jolla, CA: Pollution Abstracts, 1970–. Bimonthly.

Synthesizes published information on all forms of environmental pollution. Entries arranged alphabetically under topic. Index: key word, author. Contains publication list, cross-references.
R: *MRW* S2, pp. 4, 109.

Population Sciences; Index of Biomedical Research. Vols. 1–. **US National Institute of Child Health and Human Development, Center for Population Research.** Bethesda, MD: US National Institute of Child Health and Human Development, 1973–. Monthly.

Public Health Engineering Abstracts. Vols. 1–47. **US Public Health Service.** Washington, DC: US Government Printing Office, 1928–1967. Monthly.

Abstracts from more than 800 journals pertaining to environmental health. Arranged by subject. Annual subject and author index.
R: Win (EK216).

Speed: The Current Index to the Drug Abuse Literature. Vols. 1–. Madison, WI: Student Association for the Study of Hallucinogens, 1973–. Biweekly.

Biweekly abstracts from 4,000 journals, books, and unpublished papers. Interdisciplinary citations on drug abuse, covering the literature of pharmacology, psychology, law. Includes author directory.
R: *MRW* S3, p. 18.

Toxicology Abstracts. London: Information Retrieval Ltd., 1978–. Monthly, with annual cumulations.

Abstracts on the toxicity of household articles, heavy metals, industrial chemicals, etc. Over 9,000 abstracts since 1978. About 850 abstracts per monthly issue.

RHEUMATOLOGY

Index of Rheumatology. Vols. 1–. **American Rheumatism Association Section of the Arthritis Foundation.** New York: American Rheumatism Association, 1965–. Annual.

UROGENITAL SYSTEM

Kidney Disease and Nephrology Index. Vols. 1–. **US National Institute of Arthritis, Metabolism, and Digestive Diseases.** Bethesda, MD: US National Institute of Arthritis, Metabolism, and Digestive Diseases, 1975–. Bimonthly.

The Searle Review of Obstetric & Gynecologic Literature. **E. A. Banner and A. V. Greeley, eds.** New York: Science & Medicine Publishing, 1971–. Annual.

Contains citations from all significant English-language articles on clinical obstetrics and gynecology during the preceding year. Classified arrangement, author and subject index.
R: *MRW* S2, pp. 50, 74.

VETERINARY MEDICINE

Index Veterinarius. Vols. 1–. Farnham Royal, Slough, England: Commonwealth Agricultural Bureaux, 1933–. Monthly.

A subject-author index to articles dealing with veterinary literature. Encompasses several languages. Prepared by the Commonwealth Bureau of Animal Health.
R: Win (EK229).

CURRENT-AWARENESS SERVICES

GENERAL

Current Contents. Philadelphia: Institute for Scientific Information, 1957–. Weekly.

A current-awareness table-of-contents service. Sections relevant to science and technology are the following: *Physical and Chemical Sciences,* 1961–; *Life Sciences,* 1958–; *Engineering and Technology,* 1970–; *Agricultural, Food, and Environmental Sciences,* 1970–; *Clinical Practice,* 1973–; *Social and Behavior Sciences,* 1974–. Each section covers upwards of about 1,000 journals, or some 200 journals per week.
R: Chen (p. 353); Jenkins (G11); Katz (p. 12; supp., p. 3); Mal (3-44); *MRW* S2, p. 46, 96, 107; Wal (p. 6; 92; 116; 192; 284; 396); Win (3EA12).

Weekly Government Abstracts. Springfield, VA: National Technical Information Service. Weekly.

Weekly newsletters describe most unclassified federally funded research as it is completed. The abstracts are issued under the following sections: *Administration; Behavior; Building Technology; Business and Economics; Computer, Control, and Information Theory; Energy; Environmental Pollution and Control; Industrial Technology; Library and Information Sciences; Material Sciences; Medicine and Medical Services; Transportation;* and *Urban Technology.*
R: Chen (p. 353).

SUBJECT

Chemical-Biological Activities. Vol. 1, nos. 1–. Columbus, OH: American Chemical Society, 1965–. Biweekly.

Computer-based abstracting service covering literature on biological aspects of organic compounds. Indexed by authors, molecular formulas, and KWIC.
R: *Chemical and Engineering News* 42: 64–65 (Nov. 16, 1974); *Journal of Chemical Documentation* 3: 81–85 (1963); Chen (p. 353); Wal (p. 201); Win (1EC12).

Drug Abuse Current Awareness System (DACAS). **US National Institute on Drug Abuse. National Clearinghouse for Drug Abuse Literature.** Washington, DC: US Government Printing Office. Biweekly.

Comprehensive listing of citations under 21 subject categories, abstracted from all major publication media, including journals, popular magazines, newspapers, books, and government reports.
R: *RSR* 4: 108 (Oct.–Dec. 1976).

FDA Consumer. **US Food and Drug Administration.** Washington DC: US Government Printing Office. Monthly.

Current-awareness publication of FDA, citing legislation, legal decisions, and governmental processes affecting drugs and their usage.

FDA Reports, "The Pinksheet". **US Food and Drug Administration.** Washington DC: US Government Printing Office. Weekly.

A government publication intended for pharmaceutical and related industry. Covers legal, economic, and scientific development.

Insta-dex to 140 Medical-Surgical Journals (A Browsing Tool). Vols. 1–. Chico, CA: Windward Press, 1968–. Monthly.

Monthly subject index. Cumulates annually. An asterisk signifies pediatric papers. Supersedes *Physicians' Basic Index*.
R: *MRW* S1, p. 1.

Pharmaceutical News Index. Vols. 1–. Louisville, KY: Data Courier, 1975–. Monthly.

Loose-leaf issues with indexes, quarterly index cumulated on microfiche, and binder.

Supplies current information concerning the pharmaceutical industry. Available on-line. Covers *Drug Research Reports,* the Blue Sheet; *FDC Reports,* the Pink Sheet; *Medical Devices, Diagnostics, and Instrumentation Reports,* the Gray Sheet; *PMA Newsletter; Quality Control Reports,* the Gold Sheet; *Washington Drug and Device Letter; Weekly Pharmacy Reports,* the Green Sheet. Starting from 1980, it will include *SCRIP World Pharmaceutical News,* a British publication.

INFORMATION SERVICES

For information services on microform formats, see chapter 22, Nonprint Materials. Certain commercial companies provide information services, including actual copies of articles. For example, the service entitled *Grassroots* is provided by STASH, 1185 Bedford St., Madison, WI 53703. It is a monthly subscription service furnishing copies of articles on drug abuse to be filed in a three-ring binder under twenty subject headings. Sample copies of various newsletters are included from time to time.

CHAPTER 17 PERIODICALS

REFERENCE SOURCES

Periodicals, unquestionably, are the most important primary-information sources for health scientists. In this chapter, only a limited number of major-subject journals are listed. Readers should consult the comprehensive serial bibliographic source, *Ulrich's International Periodical Directory*, for more detailed information on the journals listed and for further pertinent journal titles.

The following are a few sample tools that can provide general and specific reference information on medical periodicals:

Directory of Canadian Scientific and Technical Periodicals. **Canada, National Science Library.** Ottawa: National Research Council of Canada, 1969.
R: *Aslib Proceedings* 22: 185 (May 1970); Chen (p. 356); Wal (p. 39).

Directory of Japanese Scientific Periodicals, 1967. Tokyo: National Diet Library, 1967.
Earlier edition, 1964.
Some 5,000 periodicals in a classified arrangement.
R: Chen (p. 356); Win (2EA12).

Guides to Scientific Periodicals; An Annotated Bibliography. **Maureen J. Fowler.** London: Library Assoc., 1966.
Contains 1,018 items in classed arrangement.
R: *Journal of Documentation* 23: 84 (1967); *LJ* 92: 2541 (1967); Chen (p. 356); Jenkins (A192); *MRW* S1, p. 30; Wal (p. 36); Win (1EA8).

A History of Scientific and Technical Periodicals: The Origins and Development of the Scientific and Technical Press, 1665–1790. 2d ed. **David A. Kronick.** Metuchen, NJ: Scarecrow Press, 1976.
R: Chen (p. 356).

International Bibliography of Medicolegal Serials 1736–1967. **Jaroslav Nemec.** Reference Services Division, US National Library of Medicine. Washington, DC: US Government Printing Office, 1969.
Lists 333 annotated citations to medicolegal periodicals within the NLM's collection. Begins with an historial introduction and includes a chapter on current trends in medicolegal serials. Contains six indexes: title; editors; publishers and sponsors; subject; geographic and chronological.
R: *MRW* S2, pp. 11, 47, 77.

N. W. Ayer and Sons Directory of Newspapers and Periodicals. Philadelphia, PA: Ayer Press, 1973.

Periodicals Relevant to Microbiology and Immunology; A World List, 1968. **Goesta Tunevall.** New York: Wiley-Interscience, 1969.

Includes 750 periodicals alphabetically listed. Complete bibliographic data, availability of abstracts, etc.
R: *Aslib Proceedings* 21: 389 (Oct. 1969); Chen (p. 356); Mal (9-43); Wal (p. 199).

The Scientific Journal: Editorial Policies and Practices; Guidelines for Editors, Reviews, and Authors. **Lois DeBakey et al.** St. Louis: C. V. Mosby, 1976.
R: Chen (p. 356).

Scientific Periodicals: Their Historical Development, Characteristics and Control. **Bernard Houghton.** London: Bingley; Hamden, CT: Linnet Books, 1975.
The book covers the history of scientific periodicals, provides a bibliography of bibliographies, and discusses the problem of identifying the "core" journals in the various branches of science.
R: *ARBA* (1976, p. 631); Chen (p. 356).

Ulrich's International Periodicals Directory 1977–1978. 17th ed. New York: Bowker, 1977.
Fifteenth edition, 1973.

World List of Scientific Periodicals Published in the Years 1900–1960. 4th ed. 3 vols. London: Butterworths, 1963–1965.
A major tool for locating scientific and technical periodicals. It is continued in *British Union-Catalogue of Periodicals, Incorporating World List of Scientific Periodicals. New Periodical Titles,* 1964–, quarterly with annual cumulations.
R: Chen (p. 357).

ABBREVIATIONS

Periodicals frequently are indicated by codes of journal titles for machine entry or are cited by abbreviated titles in references. The following few sample tools demonstrate how information on standard periodical abbreviations can be obtained.

Abbreviated Titles of Biological Journals: A List Culled with Permission from "The World List of Scientific Periodicals," with Indications of the Abbreviations Recommended by the USA Standards Institute Where These Differ from the "World List." 3d ed. **P. C. Williams, comp.** London: Biological Council, 1968.
Second edition, 1954.
More than 1,400 titles.
R: Chen (p. 357); Mal (9-8); Wal (p. 194); Win (3EC1).

Chemical Abstracts Service Source Index. 2 vols. Columbus, OH: Chemical Abstracts Service, 1907–1974. Cumulative.

CODEN for Periodical Titles: An Aid to the Storage and Retrieval of Information and to Communication Involving Journal References. 2 vols. **American**

Society for Testing and Materials. Philadelphia: ASTM, 1967. Also, supps. 1968–.

Supersedes the 1963 edition.
An A–Z list of four-letter codes (CODEN) for titles of scientific periodicals designed for information retrieval. Covers over 40,000 periodical titles.
R: *American Documentation* 4: 54 (1953); Chen (p. 357); Wal (p. 33).

List of Journals Indexed in Index Medicus. **US National Library of Medicine.** Washington, DC: US Government Printing Office, 1960–. Annual.

Lists more than 2,400 journals indexed for MEDLARS and indicates those that are only selectively indexed. This annual publication includes abbreviations, title, subject, and geographic listings. A must for medical libraries.
R: *ARBA* (1972, p. 614); Win (EK34a).

List of Serials with Coden, Title Abbreviations, New, Changed, and Ceased Titles. Philadelphia, PA: Biosciences Information Service. Annual.

Includes significant serial publications covered by BIOSIS. International in scope. Contains 8,000 serial titles published in 107 countries.

Source Index Quarterly. Vols. 1–. Columbus, OH: Chemical Abstracts Service, 1970–. Quarterly.

Provides complete identification of over 10,000 source publications included in *Chemical Abstracts* that are generally cited by abbreviated titles. Identifies libraries at which original documents are available. Various notes are provided with complete bibliographical information. Supersedes *Access*.
R: Chen (p. 357); Mal (7-1?)

SELECTIVE TITLES

Since over 2,400 periodicals are included in *Index Medicus,* it is impossible to include all of them in this chapter. The following are the 100 journals included in *Abridged Index Medicus* and a selected few others.

GENERAL

American Journal of Law and Medicine. Vols. 1–. 1975–. Quarterly.

American Journal of Medicine. Vols. 1–. 1946–. Monthly.

American Journal of the Medical Sciences. Vols. 1–. 1820–. Bimonthly.

British Medical Journal. Vols. 1–. 1832–. Weekly.

Canadian Medical Association Journal. Vols. 1–. 1911–. Semimonthly.

Hastings Center Report. Vols. 1–. 1971–. Bimonthly.

Journal of Behavioral Medicine. Vols. 1–. 1978–. Quarterly.

Journal of Medical Education. Vols. 1–. 1926–. Monthly.

JAMA; Journal of the American Medical Association. Vols. 1–. 1848–. Weekly.

Lancet. Vols. 1–. 1823–. Weekly.   1960 +

Mayo Clinic Proceedings. Vols. 1–. 1926–. Monthly.

Medicine. Vols. 1–. 1922–. Bimonthly.

Nature. 1869–. Weekly.
In 3 weekly editions: *Nature; Nature Physical Sciences; Nature New Biology.*

New England Journal of Medicine. Vols. 1–. 1812–. Weekly. 1828

Postgraduate Medicine. Vols. 1–. 1947–. Monthly.

Science. 1880–. Weekly. 1883

Scientific American. 1845–. Monthly.

Southern Medical Journal. Vols. 1–. 1906–. Monthly.

ALLERGY AND IMMUNOLOGY

Clinical Immunology & Immunopathology. Vols. 1–. New York: Academic Press, 1972–.
Volumes 1–8, 1972–1977, bimonthly; volume 9–, 1978–, monthly.

Clinical Immunology Newsletter. Vols. 1–. Boston, MA: G. K. Hall, 1980–. Biweekly.

Journal of Allergy and Clinical Immunology. Vols. 1–. 1929–. Monthly.

Journal of Immunology. Vols. 1–. 1916–. Monthly.

ANATOMY

American Journal of Anatomy. 1901–. Monthly.

American Journal of Physiology. 1898–. Monthly.

Journal of Applied Physiology. 1948–. Monthly.

Journal of General Physiology. 1918–. Monthly.

Journal of Physiology. 1878–. 8/yr. 1926 +

ANESTHESIOLOGY AND GENERAL SURGERY

American Journal of Surgery. Vols. 1–. 1891–. Monthly.

Anaesthesia. Vols. 1–. 1946–. 10 issues/year.

Anesthesia and Analgesia. Vols. 1–. 1922–. Bimonthly.

Anesthesiology. Vols. 1–. 1940–. Monthly.

Annals of Surgery. Vols. 1–. 1885–. Monthly.

Archives of Surgery. Vols. 1–. 1920–. Monthly.

British Journal of Surgery. Vols. 1–. 1913–. Monthly.

Current Problems in Surgery. Vols. 1–. 1964–. Monthly.

Plastic and Reconstructive Surgery. Vols. 1–. 1946–. Monthly. 1970-1976

Surgery. Vols. 1–. 1937–. Monthly.

Surgery, Gynecology and Obstetrics. Vols. 1–. 1905–. Monthly.

Surgical Clinics of North America. Vols. 1–. 1920–. Bimonthly.

BRAIN AND NERVOUS SYSTEM

Archives of Neurology. Vols. 1–. 1959–. Monthly.

Brain. Vols. 1–. 1878–. Quarterly. 1962 +

Chemical Senses & Flavour. 1974–. Quarterly.

Journal of Neurosurgery. Vols. 1–. 1944–. Monthly.

Neurology. Vols. 1–. 1951–. Monthly.

CARDIOVASCULAR SYSTEM

American Heart Journal. Vols. 1–. 1925–. Monthly.

American Journal of Cardiology. Vols. 1–. 1958–. Monthly.

Annals of Thoracic Surgery. Vols. 1–. 1965–. Monthly.

British Heart Journal. Vols. 1–. 1939–. Monthly.

Heart and Lung. Vols. 1–. 1972–. Bimonthly.

Journal of Thoracic and Cardiovascular Surgery. Vols. 1–. 1931–. Monthly.

Progress in Cardiovascular Diseases. Vols. 1–. 1958–. Bimonthly.

DENTISTRY

Bulletin of the History of Dentistry. Vols. 1–. 1953–. Semiannual.

Journal of Oral Surgery. Vols. 1–. 1943–. Monthly.

Journal of Preventive Dentistry. Vols. 1–. 1973–. Bimonthly.

Dermatology

Archives of Dermatology. Vols. 1–. 1920–. Monthly.

International Journal of Dermatology. Vols. 1–. 1962–. 10 issues/year.

Endocrinology

Diabetes. Vols. 1–. 1952–. Monthly.

Endocrinology. Vols. 1–. 1917–. Monthly.

Journal of Clinical Endocrinology and Metabolism. Vols. 1–. 1941–. Monthly.

Journal of the American Dietetic Association. Vols. 1–. 1925–. Monthly.

Gastrointestinal System

Diseases of the Colon and Rectum. Vols. 1–. 1958–. 8 issues/year.

Gastroenterology. Vols. 1–. 1943–. Monthly.

Gut. Vols. 1–. 1960–. Monthly.

Genetics

Biochemical Genetics. 1973–. Monthly.

Genetical Research. 1960–. Bimonthly.

Genetics. 1916–. Monthly.

Heredity. 1947–. Bimonthly.

Journal of Heredity. 1910–. Bimonthly.

Gerontology

Geriatrics. Vols. 1–. 1946–. Monthly.

Journal of Gerontology. Vols. 1–. 1946–. Bimonthly.

Health Services Administration

Hospital Practice. Vols. 1–. 1966–. Monthly.

Hospital Progress. Vols. 1–. 1920–. Monthly.

Hospitals. Vols. 1–. 1936–. Monthly.

Hematology

Blood. Vols. 1–. 1946–. Monthly.

Circulation. Vols. 1–. 1950–. Monthly.

Seminars in Hematology. 1964–. Quarterly.

HISTORY

Bulletin of the History of Medicine. Vols. 1–. 1933–. Quarterly.

Journal of the History of Medicine and Allied Sciences. Vols. 1–. 1946–. 4 issues/year.

INFECTIOUS DISEASES

American Journal of Tropical Medicine and Hygiene. Vols. 1–. 1921–. Bimonthly.

Applied Microbiology. 1953–. Monthly.

Clinical Microbiology Newsletter. Vols. 1–. Boston, MA: G. K. Hall, 1979–. Biweekly.

CRC Critical Reviews in Microbiology. 1971–. Quarterly.

Journal of Bacteriology. 1916–. Monthly.

Journal of General Microbiology. 1947–. Bimonthly.

Journal of Infectious Disease. Vols. 1–. 1904–. Monthly.

INTERNAL MEDICINE

American Family Physician. Vols. 1–. 1950–. Monthly.

Annals of Internal Medicine. Vols. 1–. 1922–. Monthly.

Archives of Internal Medicine. Vols. 1–. 1908–. Monthly.

Critical Care Medicine. Vols. 1–. 1973–. Bimonthly.

Dm. Disease-A-Month. Vols. 1–. 1954–. Monthly.

Jacep. Vols. 1–. 1972–. Monthly.

Journal of Clinical Investigation. Vols. 1–. Monthly.

Journal of Family Practice. Vols. 1–. 1974–. Quarterly.

Journal of Laboratory and Clinical Medicine. Vols. 1–. 1915–. Monthly.

Journal of Trauma. Vols. 1–. 1961–. Monthly.

Medical Clinics of North America. Vols. 1–. 1916–. Bimonthly.

Modern Healthcare. Vols. 1–. 1974–. Monthly.

Nursing

- *Advances in Nursing Science.* Vols. 1–. 1978–. Quarterly.
- *American Journal of Nursing.* Vols. 1–. 1900–. Monthly. 1924 +
- *Canadian Nurse.* Vols. 1–. 1905–. Monthly. 1966 +
- *Journal of Nursing Administration.* Vols. 1–. 1971–. Monthly.
- *Nurse Practitioner.* Vols. 1–. 1975–. Bimonthly.
- *Nursing Clinics of North America.* Vols. 1–. 1966–. Quarterly. +
- *Nursing Outlook.* Vols. 1–. 1953–. Monthly. +
- *Nursing Research.* Vols. 1–. 1952–. Bimonthly. +
- *Nursing Times.* Vols. 1–. 1905–. Weekly.

Nutrition

- *American Journal of Clinical Nutrition.* Vols. 1–. 1952–. Monthly. +
- *British Journal of Nutrition.* 1947–. Bimonthly. +
- *Food and Nutrition.* 1971–. Bimonthly. 1975 +
- *Food and Nutrition News.* 1929–. 9 issues/yr.
- *Journal of Applied Nutrition.* 1973–. Semiannually.
- *Journal of Nutrition.* 1928–. Monthly. +
- *Journal of Nutrition Education.* 1969–. Quarterly. +
- *Nutrition News.* 1937–. Quarterly.

Oncology and Nuclear Medicine

- *Ca. Cancer Journal for Clinicians.* Vols. 1–. 1961–. Bimonthly.
- *Cancer.* Vols. 1–. 1947–. Monthly.
- *Clinical Nuclear Medicine.* Vols. 1–. 1976–. Monthly.
- *Seminars in Nuclear Medicine.* 1971–. Quarterly.
- *Seminars in Oncology.* 1974–. Quarterly.

Ophthalmology

- *American Journal of Ophthalmology.* Vols. 1–. 1884–. Monthly.
- *Archives of Ophthalmology.* Vols. 1–. 1869–. Monthly.

Orthopedics

Clinical Orthopaedics and Related Research. Vols. 1–. 1953–. 8 issues/year.

Journal of Bone and Joint Surgery. American Volume. Vols. 1–. 1903–. 8 issues/year.

Journal of Bone and Joint Surgery. British Volume. Vols. 1–. 1903–. 4 issues/year.

Orthopedic Clinics of North America. Vols. 1–. 1970–. Quarterly.

Otorhinolaryngology

Annals of Otology, Rhinology and Laryngology. Vols. 1–. 1892–. Bimonthly.

Archives of Otolaryngology. Vols. 1–. 1925–. Monthly. 1970 +

Journal of Laryngology and Otology. Vols. 1–. 1887–. Monthly.

Pathology

American Journal of Clinical Pathology. Vols. 1–. 1931–. Monthly. +

American Journal of Pathology. Vols. 1–. 1924–. Monthly.

Archives of Pathology and Laboratory Medicine. Vols. 1–. 1926–. Monthly.

Journal of Clinical Pathology. Vols. 1–. 1947–. Monthly.

Pediatrics

American Journal of Diseases of Children. Vols. 1–. 1911–. Monthly. 1918 +

Archives of Disease in Childhood. Vols. 1–. 1926–. Monthly.

Clinical Pediatrics. Vols. 1–. 1962–. Monthly. +

Journal of Pediatrics. Vols. 1–. 1932–. Monthly. 1936 +

Pediatric Clinics of North America. Vols. 1–. 1954–. Quarterly.

Pediatrics. Vols. 1–. 1948–. Monthly. 1978 +

Seminars in Perinatology. 1977–. Quarterly.

Pharmacy and Pharmacology

American Journal of Hospital Pharmacy. Vols. 1–. 1943–. Monthly.

American Journal of Pharmaceutical Education. Vols. 1–. 1937–. Quarterly.

American Pharmacy. Vols. 1–. 1978–. Monthly.

British Journal of Pharmacology. Vols. 1–. 1946–. Monthly. 1946 +

Bulletin on Narcotics. Vols. 1–. 1949–. Quarterly.

Clinical Pharmacokinetics. Vols. 1–. 1976–. Bimonthly.

Clinical Pharmacology and Therapeutics. Vols. 1–. 1960–. Monthly.

Contemporary Pharmacy Practice. Vols. 1–. 1978–. Quarterly.

Drug and Therapeutics Bulletin. Vols. 1–. 1963–. Biweekly.

Drug Intelligence and Clinical Pharmacy. Vols. 1–. 1967–. Monthly.

Drugs: International Journal of Current Therapeutics and Applied Pharmacology Reviews. Vols. 1–. 1971–. Monthly.

Hospital Pharmacy. Vols. 1–. 1966–. Monthly.

Journal of Clinical Pharmacology. Vols. 1–. 1961–. 8 issues/year.

Journal of Pharmaceutical Sciences. Vols. 1–. 1912–. Monthly.

Journal of Pharmacokinetics and Biopharmaceutics. Vols. 1–. 1973–. Bimonthly.

Journal of Pharmacology and Experimental Therapeutics. Vols. 1–. 1909–. Monthly.

Journal of Pharmacy and Pharmacology. Vols. 1–. 1949–. Monthly. 1958+

Medical Letter on Drugs and Therapeutics. Vols. 1–. 1959–. Fortnightly.

Pharmacological Reviews. Vols. 1–. 1949–. Quarterly.

Pharmacology, Biochemistry and Behavior. Vols. 1–. 1973–. Monthly. +

Pharmacy in History. Vols. 1–. 1955–. Quarterly.

Psychopharmacology. Vols. 1–. 1959–. Irregular. 1963+

Psychopharmacology Bulletin. Vols. 1–. 1965–. Quarterly. 1964+ ??

Rational Drug Therapy. Vols. 1–. 1967–. Monthly.

Therapeutic Drug Monitoring. Vols. 1–. 1979–. Quarterly.

PHYSICAL MEDICINE AND REHABILITATION

American Journal of Physical Medicine. Vols. 1–. 1921–. Bimonthly. 1972+ 1979

Archives of Physical Medicine and Rehabilitation. Vols. 1–. 1921–. Monthly. 1971+

Physical Therapy. Vols. 1–. 1921–. Monthly. 1968–1980

Rheumatology and Rehabilitation. Vols. 1–. 1952–. Quarterly.

PSYCHIATRY AND PSYCHOLOGY

American Journal of Psychiatry. Vols. 1–. 1844–. Monthly.

Archives of General Psychiatry. Vols. 1–. 1959–. Monthly.

Journal of Nervous and Mental Disease. Vols. 1–. 1874–. Monthly. 1958+

PUBLIC HEALTH

American Journal of Public Health. Vols. 1–. 1911–. Monthly. 1923+

Archives of Environmental Health. Vols. 1–. 1950–. Bimonthly.

Clinical Toxicology. Vols. 1–. 1968–. 2 vols./year.

Public Health Reports. Vols. 1–. 1896–. Bimonthly. 1908+

Toxicology and Applied Pharmacology. Vols. 1–. 1959–. Monthly.

World Health. Vols. 1–. 1948–. Monthly. 1972+

RADIOLOGY

American Journal of Roentgenology. Vols. 1–. 1906–. Monthly.

British Journal of Radiology. Vols. 1–. 1896–. Monthly.

Radiologic Clinics of North America. Vols. 1–. 1963–. 3 issues/year.

Radiology. Vols. 1–. 1915–. Monthly.

Seminars in Roentgenology. 1966–. Quarterly.

RESPIRATORY SYSTEM

American Review of Respiratory Disease. Vols. 1–. 1917–. Monthly.

Chest. Vols. 1–. 1935–. Monthly.

Respiratory Care. Vols. 1–. 1956–. Monthly.

RHEUMATOLOGY

Arthritis and Rheumatism. Vols. 1–. 1958–. Monthly.

Seminars in Arthritis and Rheumatism. 1971–. Quarterly.

UROGENITAL SYSTEM

American Journal of Obstetrics and Gynecology. Vols. 1–. 1920–. Semimonthly.

British Journal of Obstetrics and Gynaecology. Vols. 1–. 1902–. Monthly.

Journal of Urology. Vols. 1–. 1917–. Monthly.

Obstetrics and Gynecology. Vols. 1–. 1952–. Monthly.

Sexually Transmitted Diseases. Vols. 1–. 1974–. Quarterly.

Urologic Clinics of North America. Vols. 1–. 1974–. 3 issues/year.

VETERINARY MEDICINE

Journal of Veterinary Pharmacology and Therapeutics. Vols. 1–. 1978–. Quarterly.

Journal of Veterinary Surgery. Vols. 6–. 1977–. Quarterly.

Journal of the American Veterinary Medical Association. Vols. 1–. 1915–. Monthly.

CHAPTER 18 TECHNICAL REPORTS AND GOVERNMENT DOCUMENTS

TECHNICAL REPORTS

Since World War II, technical-report literature has become an indispensable aspect of medical and scientific communication. The literature itself is generally the result of research supported by governmental grants and contracts, and may be issued in various formats including individual-author reprints, corporate-proposal reports, progress reports, state-of-the-art surveys, and the final report of a technical contract.

The majority of the literature emanating from certain agencies is issued in technical-report format. Among these are the National Aeronautics and Space Administration, the Energy Research and Development Administration, and the Defense Documentation Center. The major abstracting tools of the agencies (which are discussed in more detail elsewhere) such as *Scientific and Technical Aerospace Reports* (*STAR*) and *Nuclear Science Abstracts* (*NSA*), now *Atomindex,* are indispensable aids in accessing report literature. Although these tools include mainly technical reports in the fields of science and technology, they also include medical reports and reports of interest to the health science professional. Of specific importance to medical scientists are the technical reports from agencies such as the National Institutes of Health and its mother organization, the US Department of Health, Education, and Welfare (HEW). Frequently the reader can locate information sources included in various chapters of this work with technical report numbers at the end of the bibliographic listing, such as DHEW-Technical Report No. –.

It is the responsibility of the National Technical Information Service, Springfield, Virginia, to act as a clearinghouse for all unclassified reports of federally sponsored research and development. Librarians should consider that because NTIS must remain fiscally self-sufficient, there are frequent price increases for NTIS publications.

From the international scene, international health organizations such as World Health Organization are also major producers of technical report literature in the health sciences. Lists of their publications, including technical reports, can be obtained directly from these organizations.

The following list provides current and retrospective sources for accessing technical reports, as well as a source designed to promote a better understanding of this type of literature. Chapter 24, Data Bases, contains on-line information from technical reports and document sources.

GENERAL REFERENCE TOOLS

Correlation Index: Document Series and PB Reports. **Special Libraries Council of Philadelphia and Vicinity.** New York: Special Libraries Association, 1953.

Alphanumerical listing of technical-report numbers and corresponding Publication Board accession numbers needed for searching early issues of *Bibliography of Technical Reports.*
R: Chen (p. 370).

Dictionary of Report Series Codes. 2d ed. **Lois E. Godfrey and Helen F. Redman, eds.** New York: Special Libraries Association, 1973.

First edition, 1962.
Comprehensive guide to the alphanumeric codes used in identifying technical report literature. The work is divided into three color-coded sections: explanations of series designations or assigners methods in expanding on a series designation; list of report series code by letter, with corresponding agency; corporate entries with corresponding report series codes. Also includes a bibliography of articles on technical codes. Indispensable for anyone needing control over the vast array of report literature.
R: *ARBA* (1974, p. 547); Chen (p. 370).

Government Reports Announcement and Index. Vol. 75, nos. 7–. Springfield, VA: US National Technical Information Service, Apr. 1975–.

Announcement and *Index* sections published separately, 1971 to 1975.
Lists and indexes available reports from NTIS under 22 subject fields. Subject, personal-author, corporate-author, report-number, and accession-number indexes.
R: Chen (p. 371).

Government Wide Index to Federal Research and Development Reports. 71 vols. Washington, DC: US Clearinghouse for Federal Scientific and Technical Information, 1965–1971.

A subject, author, report-number, and accession-number index to the following publications: *US Government Research and Development Reports; Technical Abstract Bulletin; Scientific and Technical Aerospace Reports; Nuclear Science Abstracts.* This information is currently available in *Government Reports Announcement and Index.*
R: Chen (p. 371).

Guidelines for Format and Production of Scientific and Technical Reports. **American National Standards Institute.** New York: American National Standards Institute, 1974.
R: Chen (p. 371).

NTIS Data Base
See chapter 24, Data Bases.

Technical Abstract Bulletin. **US Defense Documentation Center, Defense**

Supply Agency. Springfield, VA: Clearinghouse for Federal Scientific and Technical Information, 1946–. Semimonthly.

Lists classified scientific research. Restrictions on availability and use.
R: Chen (p. 371).

US Government Research and Development Reports. 71 vols. Washington, DC: US Clearinghouse for Federal Scientific and Technical Information, 1946–. 1971.

Superseded by *Government Reports Announcement and Index.* Picked up reports not included in *Nuclear Science Abstracts* and *STAR.*
R: Chen (p. 371).

Use of Reports Literature. **Charles P. Auger, ed.** Hamden, CT: Archon Books, 1975.

A systematic guide deals with the nature and development of reports; the acquisition, bibliographical control, organization, etc., of reports. Two appendixes provide keys to reports, series code, and trade literature. Invaluable reference for librarians and researchers.
R: *ARBA* (1976, p. 631); Chen (p. 371).

Weekly Government Abstracts. Springfield, VA: US National Technical Information Service. Weekly.

See chapter 16, Abstracts and Indexes, and Current-Awareness Services.
R: Chen (p. 371).

SUBJECT REFERENCE TOOLS

The following is only a sample list of both private and governmental sources that bear on the report literature of a specific subject. As far as private sources are concerned, professional societies are essential ones. Readers are well advised to contact each professional society in a specialized field for a list of this type of publication.

Abstracts of Published Reports. **American Hospital Association.** Chicago, IL: American Hospital Association, 1979.

A 64-page publication which abstracts the published AHA reports.

Cancer Chemotherapy Reports. **National Cancer Institute.** Bethesda, MD: National Cancer Institute, 1959–. Bimonthly.

Catalog of the Clearinghouse for Hospital Management Engineering: A Listing of Case Studies and Technical Reports Designed to Increase Productivity and Efficiency in Hospital Department. **American Hospital Association.** Chicago, IL: American Hospital Association, 1979.

A 48-page catalog that lists AHA case studies and technical reports by subjects which are pertinent for hospital management engineering.

Indexed Bibliography of Office of Research and Development Reports, Updated to

January 1975, EPA-600/9-74-001. **US Environmental Protection Agency.** Washington, DC: US Government Printing Office.

List of reports to the EPA arranged by report number under major series. Similar information may be gleaned from *Government Research Reports*, but not so quickly. Quarterly supplements are planned.
R: *ARBA* (1976, p. 697); Chen (p. 372).

Public Health Reports. **Health Resources Administration, US Public Health Service, US Department of Health, Education, and Welfare.** Washington, DC: US Government Printing Office, 1978–. Bimonthly.

Official journal of US Public Health Services.
R: Stearns & Ratcliff (*AJN*).

Union Internationale Centre le Cancer (UICC) Technical Report Series. **International Union Against Cancer/Union Internationale Centre le Cancer.** Geneva: International Union Against Cancer, 1968–. Irregular.

GOVERNMENT DOCUMENTS

Both the international and national governments and their contractors write and print numerous publications intended for use by health scientists, professionals, and the general public. For example, World Health Organization and the US Department of Health, Education, and Welfare, with its National Institutes of Health and National Library of Medicine, are major producers of medical literature. Throughout this book, we find government publications. In fact, most of the significant indexing and abstracting tools in the fields of health sciences are products of governmental agencies and/or professional societies.

While access to such information is generally considered a complex matter, there are numerous bibliographical tools that provide access to unclassified and general government publications as listed in General Major Bibliographic Sources. Medical government documents are generally more readily accessible through the numerous tools available from the National Library of Medicine.

Technical reports may formally be considered government documents, but their nature and importance is such that they are discussed separately in the earlier section of this chapter.

The following sources, published by both government and commercial publishers, are the most significant titles for both determining the availability of documents and providing a sound understanding of the scope and use of government publications in general. A small selected subject guide to medical government publications follows the general listing.

GENERAL MAJOR BIBLIOGRAPHICAL SOURCES

Bibliographic Guide to Government Publications-Foreign: 1978. **The Research Libraries of the New York Public Library and the US Library of Congress.** Boston, MA: G. K. Hall, 1979.

Bibliographic Guide to Governmental Publications-US: 1978. **The Research Libraries of the New York Public Library and the US Library of Congress.** Boston, MA: G. K. Hall, 1979.

British Official Publications. 2d ed. **John E. Pemberton.** New York: Pergamon, 1973.

Updates and revises the 1971 edition, including a new chapter on non-HMSO publications.
R: *SL* 65: 252 (May/June 1974); Chen (p. 373).

Catalog of the Public Documents of the Congress and of all Departments of the Government of the United States for the Period from March 4, 1893–Dec. 31, 1940 (Document Catalog). Washington, DC: US Government Printing Office, 1896–1945.

This major retrospective guide is an analytic dictionary catalog of significant congressional and departmental publications. Of historical interest to scientists.
R: Chen (p. 373).

Checklist of Major US Government Series. **John Andriot.** McLean, VA: Documents Index, 1973–.

Volume 1, *Department of Agriculture.*
Projected 30 volumes covering major series published by government departments and independent agencies.
R: Chen (p. 373).

Cumulative Subject Index to the Monthly Catalog of US Government Publications, 1900–1971. **William W. Buchanan and Edna M. Kanely.** Washington, DC: Carrollton Press, 1973–.

Projected completion in 15 volumes.
R: Chen (p. 373)

Government Publications and Their Use. 2d rev. ed. **Laurence F. Schmeckebier and Roy B. Eastin.** Washington, DC: The Brookings Institution, 1969.

A now somewhat dated analysis of US governmental organizations and their publications.
R: Chen (p. 374).

Government Publications Reviews. Vols. 1–. Elmsford, NY: Microforms International, July 1973–. Quarterly.

Covers the field of documents distribution, library handling, and use of documents produced by all levels of government—federal, state, and municipal—and by the UN, international agencies, and other countries.
R: Chen (p. 374).

Government Reference Books 74/75: A Biennial Guide to US Government Publications. Littleton, CO: Libraries Unlimited.

Earlier biennials since 1968.

A comprehensive annotated bibliography of works published by the US government. Personal-author, title, and subject indexes.
R: Chen (p. 374).

A Guide to Popular Government Publications: For Libraries and Home Reference. **Linda C. Pohle.** Littleton, CO: Libraries Unlimited, 1972.

The new guide describes some 2,000 government publications, covering more than 100 topics of popular interest, that include consumer education, environment, etc. Indexed by subject.
R: *Choice* (Jan. 1973); *LJ* (Feb. 1, 1973); *RQ* (Winter 1972); *WLB* (Oct. 1972); Chen (p. 374).

Guide to US Government Publications. **John Andriot.** McLean, VA: Documents Index. Annual.

Fundamental information for over 2,000 agencies that issue series or periodicals. Annotated entries arranged by SUDOCS classification number.
R: Chen (p. 374).

Guide to US Government Statistics. 4th ed. **John Andriot.** McLean, VA: Documents Index, 1973.

Third edition, 1961.
An annotated guide to more than 1,700 recurring government publications and 3,000 titles in statistical numbered series.
R: Chen (p. 374).

Introduction to United States Public Documents. **Joe Morehead.** Littleton, CO: Library Unlimited, 1975.

This is the first textbook designed for use in library-school government-documents courses. The usefulness of this text is enhanced by many illustrations and a detailed index.
R: *CRL* (July 1975); *RQ* (Summer 1975); Chen (p. 374).

MEDOC: A Computerized Index to U.S. Government Publications in the Medical and Health Sciences. VI (1968–1974)–. Quarterly, with annual cumulations.

See chapter 24, Data Bases.

Monthly Catalog of US Government Publications. **US Superintendent of Documents.** Washington, DC: US Government Printing Office, 1895–.

Most comprehensive bibliography of US government publications. Does not include much of the material issued as technical reports and contracted for by such agencies as NIH, NASA, ERDA, and DOD. Does include significant publications from agencies such as the Bureau of Mines, National Bureau of Standards, etc. Monthly indexes with annual cumulations.
R: Chen (p. 374).

Monthly Checklist of State Publications. Washington, DC: US Government Printing Office, 1910–. Monthly.

State documents do not figure to be of overwhelming importance to scientists, but this source is the most complete bibliographical tool available.
R: Chen (p. 375).

Publications of the UN Systems: A Reference Guide. **Harry Winton.** New York: Bowker, 1972.
R: Chen (p. 375).

State Government Reference Publications: An Annotated Bibliography. **David Parish.** Littleton, CO: Libraries Unlimited, 1974.
Covers only selected publications.
R: Chen (p. 375).

Subject Guide to Government Reference Books. **Sally Wynkoop.** Littleton, CO: Libraries Unlimited, 1972.
Concentrates on pre-1968 reference material published by the GPO and various government agencies. Part 3 devoted to fields of science, technology, and medicine. Includes brief annotations.
R: *MRW* S2, pp. 50, 88.

United Nations Documents Index. **UN Document Index Unit.** New York: United Nations, 1950–.
Covers only United Nations documents and publications. Checklist and subject index cumulate annually.
R: Chen (p. 375).

US Government Manual. Washington, DC: US Government Printing Office, 1935–. Annual.
Standard reference and guide to government agencies and internal structure.
R: Chen (p. 375).

Subject Bibliographical Sources

Cancer: Publications of the World Health Organization and the International Agency for Research on Cancer. **World Health Organization and the International Agency for Research on Cancer.** Geneva: World Health Organization and the International Agency for Research on Cancer, 1978.
Catalog lists and annotates about 100 in-print publications on cancer issued by the World Health Organization and the International Agency for Research on Cancer.
R: IBID 7: 48 (1979).

National Institutes of Health Publications List, DHEW Pub. no. (NIH) 78-6. **Editorial Operations Branch, US National Institutes of Health.** Bethesda, MD: Editorial Operations Branch, Division of Public Information, Office of the Director, US National Institutes of Health, US Public Health Service, US Department of Health, Education, and Welfare, 1978.

Publications: Catalogue 1947–1971. **World Health Organization.** Geneva: World Health Organization, 1971.
A catalog of all WHO publications, arranged according to subject and agency. Includes author and subject index.
R: *MRW* S2, p. 85.

Publications of the World Health Organization, 1947–1957: A Bibliography. **World Health Organization.** Geneva: World Health Organization, 1958.

———, *1958–1962: A Bibliography,* 1964.
———, *1963–1967: A Bibliography,* 1969.
———, *1968–1972: A Bibliography,* 1974.
Subject bibliography covers work published by the World Health Organization. Contains technical articles and publications as well as administrative and general publications grouped by subject. Includes author and country index. Supplementary volumes are issued on a five-year basis.
R: *IBID* 3: 57 (Mar.–June 1975); *MRW* S2, p. 85; *ARBA* (1970, p. 140); Win (EK213; 3EJ33).

Selected Publications of the Division of Nursing, DHEW Pub. no. (NIH) 72-83. **US Department of Health, Education, and Welfare, Health Manpower Education Bureau.** Washington, DC: US Government Printing Office, 1972.

NATIONAL LIBRARY OF MEDICINE (NLM) PUBLICATIONS

As mentioned several times in this book, NLM is probably the most important producer and disseminator of medical literature. While many of its publications are listed in numerous chapters of this book according to types of publications, they are all government documents, which are available through the US Government Printing Office and the National Technical Information Service. The NLM *NEWS* announces new titles and prices, and an annual supplement, published in December, provides current ordering information for the library's publications. Inquiries about the *NEWS* and its supplement should be addressed to the National Library of Medicine, 8600 Rockville Pike, Bethesda, MD 20209. Attention: Mrs. Beckwith. Or call Mrs. Beckwith at (301) 496-6308.

CHAPTER 19 CONFERENCE PROCEEDINGS, TRANSLATIONS, DISSERTATIONS, AND RESEARCH IN PROGRESS, PREPRINTS, AND REPRINTS

CONFERENCE PROCEEDINGS

As a primary source of information, conferences and their proceedings can be of considerable value to the health sciences professional. The conferences, congresses, and symposia themselves may range from small meetings of professional societies to elaborate international medical and scientific conventions. The papers that are called for and presented at the events very often provide access to original research months before it appears in periodical literature. The comments and rebuttals generated by such presentations also play important roles in scientific and technical communication. Adequate bibliographical control of such information is contingent on both prior notification of meetings and details of the publications arising from them. The following are the major tools in the area:

CALENDARS AND FORTHCOMING MEETINGS

GENERAL

Forthcoming International Scientific and Technical Conferences. London: Aslib. Quarterly.

Lists conferences in chronological order with date, title, location, and address. Subject, location, and sponsoring-organization indexes.
R: Chen (p. 378); Wal (p. 44).

International Congress Calendar. Brussels: Union of International Associations, 1961–. Annual. Monthly supplement.
R: Chen (p. 378).

Scientific Meetings. Vols. 1–. New York: Special Libraries Association, 1956–.

Alphabetical list of scientific and technical organizations and universities that are sponsoring regional, national, and international meetings and institutes. Subject index.
R: Chen (p. 378).

World Meetings Outside USA and Canada. Newton Centre, MA: Technical Meetings Information, 1968–. Quarterly.

A two-year registry, revised and updated each quarter, of future medical, scientific, and technical meetings. Indexed by sponsor, date, keyword, location, and deadline for papers.
R: Chen (p. 379).

World Meetings: United States and Canada. Newton Centre, MA: Technical Meetings Information, 1963–. Quarterly.
R: Chen (p. 378).

SUBJECT
Some of the best sources for information on medical and scientific meetings in specific subject fields would probably be the "meeting" sections of medical journals since they can provide the most up-to-date and complete information and listing. Samples of these journals are:

Journal of the American Medical Association. Vols. 1–. 1848–. Weekly.

Nature. 1869–. Weekly.

New England Journal of Medicine. Vols. 1–. 1812–. Weekly.

Science. 1880–. Weekly.

Official news journals of each specialty of the health sciences, such as *American Journal of Nursing.*

PUBLISHED PROCEEDINGS

MAJOR BIBLIOGRAPHICAL TOOLS

Bibliographic Guide to Conference Publications: 1978. **The Research Libraries of the New York Public Library and the US Library of Congress.** Boston, MA: G. K. Hall, 1979.

Computext Book Guides: Conference Publications. Vols. 1–. Boston: G. K. Hall, 1974–. Monthly.
R: *ARBA* (1976); Chen (p. 379).

Current Index to Conference Papers in Engineering. Vol. 1, nos. 1–. New York: Crowell Collier, 1969–.
Indexed by subject, author, and meeting.
R: Chen (p. 379); Wal (p. 288).

Current Index to Conference Papers: Science and Technology. Vols. 2–. New York: CCM Information, 1971–. Monthly.
Combines and supersedes the following publications: *Current Index to Conference Papers in Chemistry,* 1969; *Current Index to Conference Papers in Engineering,* 1969;

Current Index to Conference Papers in Life Sciences. Lists conferences and papers presented. Subject and author indexes.
R: Win (3EA25); Chen (p. 379).

Current Programs. Vols. 1–. Chestnut Hill, MA: World Meetings Information Center, 1973–.

A monthly current-awareness service that provides the titles of some 120,000 scientific and technical papers presented at about 1,200 worldwide meetings annually. Covers the life sciences, chemistry, physical sciences, geosciences, and engineering. Subject, author, and meetings indexes.
R: Chen (p. 380).

Directory of Published Proceedings, Series SEMT—Science/Engineering/Medicine/Technology. Vols. 1–. White Plains, NY: Inter Dok, 1965–. Annual cumulation.

A monthly chronological listing of proceedings, meetings, symposia, congresses, etc.
R: *ARBA* (1971, p. 477); Chen (p. 380); Jenkins (A 136); Wal (p.45); Win (IEA29).

Index of Conference Proceedings Received. Boston Spa, England: British Lending Library, 1973–. Monthly.

Formerly *Index of Conference Proceedings Received by the NLL,* 1964–1973.
An accession list of conference proceedings with brief annotations and a key word subject index.
R: Chen (p. 380).

International Meeting Reports. Brussels: Union of International Associations. Annual.
R: Chen (p. 380).

Medi-KWOC Index: An Index to the Published Proceedings of Conferences and Symposia on Biomedicine. Vols. 1–. St. Louis, MO: School of Medicine Library, Washington University, 1974–. 3 issues/yr.

A key word, out-of-context index of papers presented at biomedical meetings, conferences, symposia, and congresses. Includes only papers written in English, papers received at the Washington University School of Medicine Library, nonjournal publications, and papers that are not indexed by major indexing services. Arranged in three sections: register of conferences (lists full bibliographical information), personal names (authors and editors); and key word index. Papers must be presented during five years prior to index publication. Fills a need not met by major services.

NATO Advanced Study Institutes Series. New York: Plenum, 1975–.

Series A, *Life Sciences,* Vols. 1–. Volume 23, *The Molecular Biology of the Picornaviruses,* 1979; volume 24, *Humoral Immunity in Neurological Diseases,* 1979; volume 25, *Synchrotron Radiation Applied to Biophysical and Biochemical Research,* 1979; volume 30, *Human Physical Growth and Maturation,* 1980.

NATO Conference Series. New York: Plenum, 1962–.

Series III, *Human Factors*: volume 6, *Language Interpretation and Communication*, 1978; volume 9, *Human Evoked Potentials: Applications and Problems*, 1979.

Nobel Symposia. New York: Raven Press, 1966–.

Vols. 1–22 published by Halsted Press; from vol. 24 publisher will vary. Number 37, *Substance P*, Ivon Euler and B. Pernow, eds., 1977.

Proceedings in Print. Vols. 1–. Arlington, MA: Proceedings In Print, 1964–. Bimonthly.

Volume 1, numbers 1, 2; volume 3, number 2, published by the Aerospace Division, Special Libraries Association. Originally meant as an index to conference proceedings related to aerospace technology, but beginning with volume 3, number 3, an index to all published conference proceedings regardless of subject. A subject and agency index.

R: Chen (p. 380); Win (1EA30).

Yearbook of International Congress Proceedings: Bibliography of Reports Arising Out of Meetings Held by International Organizations During the Year, 1960– 67–, Union of International Associations, Pub. no. 211, etc. **Eyvind S. Tews, ed.** Brussels, Belgium: Union of International Associations, 1969–.

Conference reports are listed in English, German, Spanish, French and are arranged chronologically. Includes an index of organizations plus an author-editor index.

R: Chen (p. 380); *MRW* S2, pp. 23, 59.

It is necessary to state the importance of abstracting and indexing journals as location tools for conference publications. Most of the major sources listed in chapter 16 under abstracts and indexes cover conference publications extensively. Some current-awareness services are also very helpful. For example, *Biological Abstracts/RRM* is specifically devoted to reports, reviews, and meetings.

CONFERENCE PUBLICATIONS

Besides the above general bibliographical tools for locating information on conference publications, information on the actual contents of specific-subject conferences can be obtained from various sources, such as professional organizations' conference proceedings series, symposium series issued either by commercial publishers or conference sponsoring organizations, and periodicals devoted to providing either abstracts or full contents of papers presented at various meetings. The following are some of these types of sources, arranged by subject:

GENERAL

CIBA Foundation Symposia. Nos. 1–. New York: Elsevier, 1973–.
Number 61, 1979.

The CIBA Foundation sponsors numerous symposia. Sample titles are *Outcome of Severe Damage to the Central Nervous System,* no. 34; *Health and Disease in Tribal Societies,* no. 49; *The Control of Cerebral Vascular Smooth Muscles,* no. 56.

Cold Spring Harbor Laboratory. Symposia on Quantitative Biology. Vols. 1–. 1933–. Annual.
A publication of the proceedings of the symposia, covering the texts of all papers delivered. Arranged by subject.
R: Chen (p. 382).

Excerpta Medica. International Congress Series. Nos. 1–. Amsterdam: Excerpta Medica Foundation, 1952–.
Number 471, 1978.
R: *Brain* 98: 186 (Mar. 1975); *Journal of Neurosurgery* 43: 380 (Sept. 1975).

Federation Proceedings. Federation of American Societies for Experimental Biology, 1942–. Monthly.
R: Chen (p. 382).

Hahnemann Medical College and Hospital of Philadelphia Symposia. Proceedings. 1st–. New York: Grune & Stratton, 1962–.
Sample symposia publications: *Arteriosclerosis and Coronary Heart Disease; Cardiac Arrythmias; Emergency Medical Management; Epithelial-Mesenchymal Interactions; Hypertension: Mechanisms and Management; New Concepts in Endocrinology and Metabolism; Pulmonary Care; Sex and the Life Cycle; Psychosomatic Medicine; The Stomach;* forty-sixth symposium, *Cancer Chemotherapy III,* Isadore Brodsky, Sigmund B. Kahn, and James F. Conroy, eds., 1979.
R: *BMJ* 2: 436 (Aug. 18, 1979).

Manual For the Organization of Scientific Congresses. **Helena B. Lemp.** Basel: S. Karger, 1979.
Step-by-step guide to the organization and management of congresses. Offers expert advice on procedures ranging from the structuring of committees to on-site management of a congress. Includes a complete subject index and 30-page appendix of sample forms. Based on the author's extensive experience in managing large international congresses as Director of the Office of Scientific Meeting, Federation of American Societies for Experimental Biology (FASEB).

Royal Society of Medicine International Congress and Symposium Series. Nos. 1–. New York: Academic Press, 1967–.
Number 18, 1980.

Symposia of the Society for Experimental Biology. Vols. 1–. Cambridge, England: University Press, 1947–. Annual.
R: Chen (p. 382).

ALLERGY AND IMMUNOLOGY

Progress in Immunology. Proceedings, International Congress of Immunology.
First Congress, New York: Academic Press, 1971.
Second Congress, New York: American Elsevier, 1974.
Third Congress, Amsterdam: North Holland, 1977.
R: Allyn.

ANESTHESIOLOGY AND GENERAL SURGERY

Symposium on Basic Science in Plastic Surgery. St. Louis, MO: C. V. Mosby.
Volume 15, 1976.
A series of symposia sponsored and published by the Foundation of the American Society of Plastic and Reconstructive Surgeons.
R: *JAMA* 237: 2425 (May 30, 1977).

Transplantation Proceedings. New York: Grune and Stratton. Annual.
Official publication of the Transplantation Society and the American Association of Clinical Histocompatibility Testing. Each issue is a proceedings of one or more international conferences.

BRAIN AND NERVOUS SYSTEM

Clinical Neurosurgery. Vols. 1–. Baltimore, MD: Williams & Wilkins, 1953–.
Volume 24, 1977.
Proceedings of the annual conference of the Congress of Neurological Surgeons. Covers diverse subjects which vary from year to year.
R: *Journal of Neurosurgery* 41: 115 (July 1974); *JAMA* 232: 75 (Apr. 7, 1975); 239: 651 (Feb. 13, 1978); 239: 1912 (May 5, 1978).

Sleep. Vols. 1–. Basil: S. Karger, 1972–.
Consists of proceedings of the European Congress on Sleep Research; state-of-the-art presentations of current international research.

World Congress of Neurology. Proceedings. 3d Congress. Amsterdam: Excerpta Medica Foundation, 1939–.
Previous titles: International Neurological Congress and International Congress of Neurology.
Eleventh Congress, *Neurology*, W. A. den Hartog Jager, G. W. Bruyn, and A. P. J. Heijstee, eds., 1978. (International Congress Series no. 434).
R: *Brain* 102: 232 (Mar. 1979).

ENDOCRINOLOGY

Proceedings of the Congress of the International Diabetes Federation. 1st Congress–. New York: American Elsevier, 1966–.
Eighth Congress, *Diabetes*, W. J. Malaisse and J. Pirart, eds., 1974.
R: *Annals of Internal Medicine* 82: 445 (Mar. 1975).

GASTROINTESTINAL SYSTEM

Frontiers of Gastrointestinal Research. Vols. 1–. **L. van der Reis, ed.** Basel: S. Karger, 1960–. Irregular.

Formerly *Bibliotheca Gastroenterologica.*
Volume 4, *Gastrointestinal Cancer: Advances in Basic Research,* 1979 (selected papers from the International Conference on Gastrointestinal Cancer, Tel Aviv, Nov. 1977); volume 5, *Gastrointestinal Cancer: Advances in Diagnostic Techniques and Therapy,* 1979 (selected papers from the International Conference on Gastrointestinal Cancer, Tel Aviv, Nov. 1977).
Text in English.

Wine and the Digestive System: The Effects of Wine and Its Constituents on the Organs and Functions of the Gastrointestinal Tract. **Salvatore P. Lucia.** San Francisco, CA: Fortune House, 1970.

Approximately 500 references concerning the digestive effects of wine; covers time period from the fourth century through 1969. Topically arranged by gastrointestinal tract function. Author index.
R: *MRW* S2, pp. 48, 110.

GENETICS

Chromosomal Variation in Man: A Catalog of Chromosomal Variants and Anomalies. 2d ed. **D. S. Borgaonkar.** Baltimore, MD: Johns Hopkins University Press, 1977.

First edition, 1975.
Bulk of the volume consists of a listing of published reports on structural and numerical chromosomal variations. Also includes abstracts submitted to meetings of the *American Society of Human Genetics* and to the Birth Defects Conferences of the National Foundation-March of Dimes. A final section, entitled "Chromosomal Breakage Syndrome," outlines significant literature by providing two key citations to the genetic disorders frequently associated with chromosomal breakage. Catalog information simultaneously stored on magnetic tape, resulting in continuous updating. Despite some inconsistencies in data, the catalog will be a welcome reference tool for clinical and experimental cytogeneticists.
R: *American Journal of Human Genetics* 28: 195 (Mar. 1976); *Quarterly Review of Biology* 52: 460 (1976); 54: 83 (Mar. 1979).

Chromosomes Today. Vols. 1–. Edinburgh: Oliver & Boyd, 1966–.

Volume 6, *Chromosomes Today,* 1977. Sixth International Chromosome Conference, Helsinki, Aug. 12, 1977.
R: *American Journal of Human Genetics* 30: 668 (1978).

INFECTIOUS DISEASES

International Symposium on Influenza Immunization. Proceedings. **International Association of Biological Standardization.** Basel: S. Karger, 1972–.

Fourth symposium, 1977.

Presents a series of symposia on influenza held by the International Association of Biological Standardization since 1972. Up to date and of high standard. R: *BMJ* 35: 95 (Jan. 1979).

Proceedings of International Symposium on Infectious Antibiotic Resistance. 1st Symposium–. New York: Springer-Verlag, 1972–.

First Symposium, *Bacterial Plasmids and Antibiotic Resistance,* V. Krcmery, L. Rosival, and T. Watanabe, eds., 1972.

NURSING

Communicating Nursing Research. **Marjorie V. Batey, ed.** Boulder, CO: Western Interstate Commission for Higher Education, 1968–. Annual.

Papers presented at the Annual Western Interstate Commission for Higher Education conferences on nursing research.

Nursing Research Conference. 1st–. **American Nurses Association.** Kansas City, MO: American Nurses Association, 1965–.

Nursing Theory Conference. **University of Kansas Medical Center. Department of Nursing Education.** Kansas City, KS: University of Kansas Medical Center, 1968–. Annual.

NUTRITION

Health and Sugar Substitutes. **B. Guggenheim, ed.** Basel: S. Karger, 1979.

Consists of 48 original papers on sugar substitutes given at the ERGOB Conference on Sugar Substitutes in Geneva. All six sections stress specific issues of health. Comprehensive coverage of this controversial topic.

ONCOLOGY AND NUCLEAR MEDICINE

Antibiotics and Chemotherapy. Vols. 1–. Basel: S. Karger, 1954–. Irregular.

Volume 26, *New Developments in Immunoassays,* 1979 (Proceedings of the International Conference on New Developments in Immunoassays, Dusseldorf, Nov. 1977, and Chicago, Dec. 1977); volume 28, *Design of Cancer Chemotherapy,* 1980. Text in English.

Antimicrobial Agents and Chemotherapy. Detroit, MI: American Society for Microbiology, 1961–1971. Annual.

Volumes for 1961–1971 constitute the *Proceedings of the 1st–10th Interscience Conference on Antimicrobial Agents and Chemotherapy.* Continued by *Antimicrobial Agents and Chemotherapy,* 1971–. Monthly.

Cancer Chemotherapy: Fundamental Concepts and Recent Advances. **M. D. Anderson Hospital and Tumor Institute.** Chicago, IL: Year Book Medical Publishers, 1975.

Proceedings from the nineteenth annual clinical conference on cancer; presents an in-depth review of current methods of chemotherapy, which is both factual

and critical. Covers a range of subjects from drug interactions to postoperative situations. A useful book for oncologists.
R: *Lahey Clinic Foundation Bulletin* 25: 96 (Apr.–June 1976).

IARC Scientific Publications. Nos. 1–. Lyon, France: International Agency for Research on Cancer, 1971–.
Number 8, 1973; number 19, 1978.
R: *Archives of Environmental Health* 30: 520 (1975); *Journal of Clinical Pathology* 28: 166 (1975).

Progress in Chemotherapy. 3 vols. Athens, Greece: Hellenic Society for Chemotherapy, 1974.
Proceedings of the International Congress of Chemotherapy.
R: *Archives of Internal Medicine* 135: 1410 (Oct. 1975).

Symposia on Fundamental Cancer Research. Proceedings. New York: Raven Press. Annual.
Thirtieth symposium, *Cell Differentiation and Neoplasia,* Grady F. Saunders, ed., 1978.
R: *Quarterly Review of Biology* 54: 79 (Mar. 1979).

ORTHOPEDICS

The Hip. **The Hip Society.** St. Louis, MO: C. V. Mosby, 1973–.
Proceedings of the open meetings of the Hip Society. First Proceedings, 1973; Fifth Proceedings, 1977.
Focus on total hip replacement, bioengineering, and arthritis of the hip. Major source for orthopedic surgeons.
R: *Physical Therapy* 57: 469 (1977).

PATHOLOGY

Cold Spring Harbor Conferences on Cell Proliferation. Vols. 1–. Cold Spring Harbor, NY: Cold Spring Harbor Laboratory, 1974–.
Volume 1, *Control of Proliferation in Animal Cells,* Bagard Clarkson and Renato Baserga, eds., 1974; volume 2, *Proteases and Biological Control,* E. Reich, D. B. Rifkin, and E. Shaw, eds., 1975; volume 3, *Cell Motility,* R. Goldman, T. Pollard, and J. Rosenblum, eds., 1976; volume 4, *Origins of Human Cancer,* H. H. Hiatt, J. D. Watson, and J. A. Winsten, eds., 1977; volume 5, *Differentiation of Normal and Neoplastic Hematopoietic Cells,* Baynard Clarkson, Raul A. Marks, and James E. Till, eds., 1978.
R: *Nature* 273: 688 (June 22, 1978); 274: 194 (July 13, 1978).

PEDIATRICS

Modern Problems in Paediatrics. **F. Falkner, N. Kretchmer, and E. Rossi, eds.** Basel: S. Karger, 1954–.
Volume 18, *Pediatric Neurosurgery,* 1977; volume 20, *Pediatric Dermatology: Internal and External Medicine,* 1978.
The basis for the individual volumes consists of international symposia or of the

collaborative of international work authorities. Each volume is a problem-oriented collection of contemporary knowledge on a specific aspect of pediatrics.
R: *Archives of Neurology* 36: 526 (Aug. 1979).

PHARMACY AND PHARMACOLOGY

Topics in Therapeutics. Vols. 1–. Boston, MA: G. K. Hall, 1979–.
Based on annual conferences held at the Royal College of Physicians, London, England. Brings together new information and research on drugs, patient care, treatment schedules, and medicinal therapy.

PSYCHIATRY AND PSYCHOLOGY

Bibliotheca Psychiatrica. Nos. 1–. **P. Berner and E. Gabriel, eds.** Basel: S. Karger, 1917–. Irregular.
Number 159, *The Teaching of Psychosomatic Medicine and Consultation-Liaison Psychiatry,* 1979 (4th Congress of the International College of Psychosomatic Medicine, Kyoto, Sept. 1977).
Text in English and German.

TRANSLATIONS

While much of the world's medical and scientific literature is in English and thus presents no great problems to the American health scientist, the years since World War II have seen a considerable increase in significant scientific contributions in languages not generally known by American and British health scientists. To facilitate medical and scientific investigation, numerous translation services have been devised to keep English-speaking scientists informed about the work of their foreign counterparts. On the other hand, non-English-speaking scientists' needs for translations from foreign languages to their native languages are much more obvious. The following tools are essential to people in search of both information on translations and individual translations themselves:

GENERAL SOURCES

BLLD Announcement Bulletin: A Guide to British Reports, Translations, and Theses. London: Her Majesty's Stationery Office, 1971–. Monthly.
Formerly *NLL Announcement Bulletin.*
R: Chen (p. 384).

Bulletin des traductions-CNRS. Paris: Centre National de la Recherche Scientifique.
Leading source for French translators.
R: Chen (p. 384).

Consolidated Index of Translations Into English. **National Translations Center, The John Crerar Library.** New York: Special Libraries Association, 1969.

A guide to translations, including translation bibliographies, selective translation journals, etc.
R: Chen (p. 385).

Cumulative Index to English Translations 1948–68. Boston: G. K. Hall, 1973.
R: Chen (p. 385).

Directory of Technical and Scientific Translators and Services. **Patricia Millard.** London: Lockwood; Hamden, CT: Archon Books, 1968.
A directory of individual translators and translation services in Great Britain.
R: Chen (p. 385); Win (2EA9).

Index Translationum. Paris: International Institute of Intellectual Cooperation. Paris: Unesco, 1949–.
Previous volumes, 1932–1940.
Arranged by country and subdivided under ten universal decimal classification classes. Covers books and monographs.
R: Chen (p. 385).

International Directory of Translators and Interpreters. **B. Pond.** London: Pond Press, 1967.
R: Chen (p. 385).

Monthly Catalog. **US Superintendent of Documents.** Washington, DC: US Government Printing Office, 1895–.
Lists members of Joint Publication Research Service series that are primarily translations of Russian and Chinese scientific literature.
R: Chen (p. 385).

Nachweise von Vebersetzungen. Hanover, W. Germany: Technische Informationslibliothek der Technischen Universitat.
Leading tool for German translations.
R: Chen (p. 385).

Transdex. Bibliography and Index to the US Joint Publications Research Service Translations. New York: Macmillan, 1970–.
Translations generated by the Joint Publications Research Service.
R: Chen (p. 385).

Translations Register-Index. New York: National Translations Center, 1967–. Semimonthly.
Succeeds *Technical Translations,* Washington, DC, Clearinghouse for Federal Scientific and Technical Information, 1959–1967.
Lists accessions of the translations center and thus provides the scientist with unpublished translations into English from the world literature in the natural, physical, medical and social sciences.
R: Chen (p. 385); *MRW* S1, p. 31.

Translators and Translations; Services and Sources in Science and Technology. 2d ed. **F. F. Kaiser.** New York: Special Libraries Association, 1965.

R: Chen (p. 385).

World Index of Scientific Translations. Delft, Netherlands: European Translations Centre, 1967–. Monthly.

Translations acquired by ETC listed by subject and citation index.
R: Chen (p. 385); *MRW* S1, p. 31.

ABSTRACTING AND INDEXING SOURCES

Like conference publications, abstracting and indexing tools are essential for obtaining access to translations of research reports, conference papers, and other sources of both primary and secondary information. All titles listed in the conference proceedings section also cover translation information. Government agencies have heavy translation activities, thus sources such as *Government Reports Announcements and Index, Nuclear Science Abstracts* (now *Atomindex*), and *Scientific and Technical Aerospace Abstracts* are major tools covering the government's translation report series, such as AEC-tran-, and NASA-TT-.

COVER-TO-COVER TRANSLATIONS

The "cover-to-cover" translation is a phenomenon dating back only to the late 1940s. Publications chosen for such treatment are generally primary-research journals, though some secondary sources of information are also available. As the labor involved in undertaking such a translation is often not justified by the worth of many of the articles themselves, the process has in recent years been modified to include the translations of only selected articles from foreign journals and selected articles that are composites of several originals. The following is an example of a useful bibliographic source for the identification of both cover-to-cover and selected translations of scientific and technical journals:

A Guide to Scientific and Technical Journals in Translation. 2d ed. **Carl J. Himmelsbach and Grace E. Brociner, comps.** New York: Special Libraries Association, 1972.

First edition, 1968.
Lists some 278 cover-to-cover translations and 53 miscellaneous journals. Primary emphasis on Russian journals. Titles are transliterated and arranged alphabetically.
R: *CRL* 30: 83 (1969); *LJ* 93: 2790 (1968); *ARBA* (1974, p. 548); Chen (p. 387); Jenkins (A155); Wal (p. 39); Win (2EA8).

DISSERTATIONS AND RESEARCH IN PROGRESS

DISSERTATIONS

As primary sources of information, theses and dissertations can play a vital role in medical and scientific communication. While they are rarely used with such frequency as is the journal article, patent, or technical report, satisfactory bibliographic control over such items is nevertheless essential. For practical purposes, the following list will include major tools that attempt to provide information on completed dissertations as well as theses and research in progress:

GENERAL TOOLS

American Doctoral Dissertations. Ann Arbor, MI: University Microfilms. Annual.

Complete listing of all doctoral dissertations accepted by American and Canadian universities.
R: Chen (p. 387).

BLLD Announcement Bulletin: A Guide to British Reports, Translations, and Theses. London: Her Majesty's Stationery Office, 1971–. Monthly.

Formerly *NLL Announcement Bulletin.*
R: Chen (p. 387).

Comprehensive Dissertation Index, 1861–1972. 37 vols. Ann Arbor, MI: Xerox University Microfilms, 1973.

Succeeds *Dissertation Abstracts International Retrospective Index,* 1970. Some 417,000 entries from US and foreign universities. Eliminates the need for retrospective compilations such as H. W. Wilson's *Doctoral Dissertations Accepted by American Universities, 1933/34–1954/55.*
R: Chen (p. 388).

Comprehensive Dissertation Index: Five Year Cumulation, 1973–1977. 19 vols. Ann Arbor, MI: University Microfilms International, 1978.

Comprehensive Dissertation Index. 1978 Supplement. 5 vols. Ann Arbor, MI: University Microfilms International, 1978.

Volume 1, *Sciences* (Agriculture; Biological, Chemical, and Environmental Sciences; Health Sciences); volume 2, *Sciences* (Astronomy; Engineering; Geology; Mathematics and Statistics; Physics); volume 3, *Social Sciences and Humanities* (Psychology; Fine Arts; Music; Education; Library and Information Science); volume 4, *Social Sciences and Humanities* (History; Sociology; Language and Literature; Business and Economics; Law; Philosophy; Religion); volume 5, *Author Index.* Five-volume reference source to some 42,000 doctoral dissertations that were accepted for academic degress in 1978 by United States and Canadian institutions. Entries list title, author, degree and year, institution, number of pages, and reference to *Dissertation Abstracts International.*

DATRIX (Direct Access to Reference Information, a Xerox Service).

A university microfilms service that provides title-key word searches back to 1938. Covers some 275,000 dissertations.
See chapter 24, Data Bases.
R: Chen (p. 388).

Dissertation Abstracts International. Ann Arbor, MI: University Microfilms International, 1969–.
Volume 1–11, 1938–1951, as *Microfilm Abstracts*; volumes 12–29, 1952–1969, as *Dissertation Abstracts*.
Primary emphasis on theses emanating from US academic institutions. Section B is entitled *The Sciences & Engineering*. For earlier French thesis, consult *Catalogue des theses de doctorat en sciences naturelles soutenues à Paris de 1891 à 1954*. Paris: Person, 1956. Sections A and B available separately in microfiche or hard copy since 1977.
For German theses, consult *Jahresverzeichnes der Deutschen Hochschulschriften*.
R: Chen (p. 388); Jenkins (A2); Wal (p. 31).

Doctoral Dissertations in the Health and Behavioral Sciences. Ann Arbor, MI: University Microfilms International. Irregular.
Available free.

Guide to Theses and Dissertations: An Annotated, International Bibliography of Bibliographies. **Michael M. Reynolds, ed.** Detroit, MI: Gale Research, 1974.
Identifies and annotates more than 2,000 bibliographies of theses and dissertations in the US and throughout the world. Indexed by institution, name and title, and subject. A key source for academic librarians and researchers.
R: *LJ* (Nov. 1, 1975); Chen (p. 388).

Index to Theses Accepted for Higher Degrees in the Universities of Great Britain and Ireland. London: Aslib, 1953–. Annual.
Emphasizes theses relating to science and engineering. Arranged by school and subarranged by subject and author.
R: Chen (p. 388).

Master Abstracts. Ann Arbor, MI: University Microfilms International, 1962–. Quarterly.
Covers only selected universities. Cumulative author and subject index.
R: Chen (p. 388).

University of London Theses and Dissertations Accepted for Higher Degrees. London: University of London. Annual.
R: Chen (p. 389).

SUBJECT GUIDES
List of subject theses are often available on a regular basis from the institutions granting the degrees.

A Bibliography of Doctoral Research on Ecology and the Environment, 1938–1970. Ann Arbor, MI: University Microfilms International, 1971.
R: Chen (p. 389).

Energy: A Key-Phrase Dissertation Index. Ann Arbor, MI: University Microfilms International, 1976. Annual supps.
Over 5,000 citations are selected from the University Microfilm's over .5-million-dissertation data base. Arranged by a key-phrase system with author index.
R: Chen (p. 389).

International Directory of Nurses with Doctoral Degrees. Kansas City, MO: American Nurses Foundation, 1973.
Until a supplement or updated edition is available, more recent nursing dissertations may be identified by using the Nursing Dissertation appendix in the *International Nursing Index* from 1973 to date.

Nursing Theses 1932–1961: An Alphabetical Listing and Keyword Index. **Catholic University of America.** Washington, DC: Catholic University of America Press, 1970.
Indexes nearly 1,000 masters' theses accepted by the School of Nursing. Divided into two main sections: alphabetical listing by author, with biographical data; computer-produced key word index (KWOC) to the theses and dissertations.
R: *ARBA* (1971, p. 536).

Readers should keep in mind that subject abstracting and indexing journals, such as those listed in the sections on conference proceedings, are also important sources for subject thesis information.

Research in Progress

GENERAL

Annual Register of Grant Support, 1969–. Los Angeles: Academic Media, 1969–. Annual.
Supersedes *Grant Data Quarterly.* One of four major sections is devoted to science and as such describes grant-support programs of government agencies, foundations, business, and professional organizations.
R: Chen (p. 390); Mal (3-59).

Federal Funds for Research Development and Other Scientific Activities. **US National Science Foundation.** Washington, DC: US Government Printing Office, 1974. Annual.
R: Chen (p. 390).

Grant and Awards; Fiscal Year 1976. **US National Science Foundation.** Washington, DC: US Government Printing Office, 1977. Annual.
R: Chen (p. 390).

Grant Data Quarterly. Vols. 1–. Los Angeles, CA: Academic Media, 1967–. Quarterly.

Each issue devoted to a specific type of grant support (e.g. Government Support Programs; Foundation Support Programs). Entries include the following data: type, purpose, eligibility, financial data, duration, application information, deadlines, etc. Includes organization and subject indexes.
R: *MRW* S1, p. 30.

Guide to Science and Technology in the USA. St. Peter Port, Guernsey, England: Hodgson, 1974.
R: Chen (p. 390).

Guide to Science and Technology in the USSR; A Reference Guide to Science and Technology in the Soviet Union. **Sarah White, ed.** St. Peter Port, Guernsey, England: Hodgson, 1971.

An extensive guide to Soviet science and technology.
R: Chen (p. 390).

Medical Research Index: A Guide to World Medical Research, Including Dentistry, Nursing, Pharmacy, Psychiatry, and Surgery. 4th ed. 2 vols. Guernsey, England: Hodgson, 1971.

Volume 1, Afghanistan-Puerto Rico; volume 2, Rhodesia-Zambia.
A directory of research institutions in 135 countries. Entries, alphabetical by name under countries, include addresses and scope of interests of establishments as well as key personnel. Indexes of names in original language and in English.
R: *MRW* S2, pp. 2, 89, 97.

National Patterns of R&D Resources: Funds and Manpower in the United States 1953–1972. **US National Science Foundation.** Washington, DC: US Government Printing Office, 1972.
R: Chen (p. 390).

1980–1981 National Biomedical Research Directory. Bethesda, MD: National Health Directory, 1980.

Provides information on biomedical research organizations, research institutions, publications, research/medical libraries, and key NIH personnel. Useful for every person engaged in biomedical research or administration.

Research and Development in the Federal Budget: FY 1977. **Willis N. Shapley.** Washington, DC: American Association for the Advancement of Science, 1976.
R: Chen (390).

Research Contracts in the Life Sciences. **US Energy and Research Development Agency (ERDA).** Springfield, VA: National Technical Information Service. Annual.

Listing of ERDA-funded research projects.
R: Chen (p. 391).

Research Grant Index, DHEW Pub. no. 76-200. 2 vols. **US National Institutes of Health.** Washington, DC: US Government Printing Office. Annual.

Fifteenth, 1976.
The first volume contains approximately 9,000 subject headings under which appear the identification numbers of pertinent projects. The second volume contains project identification date, etc.
R: Chen (p. 389).

Research in Biological and Medical Sciences; Annual Progress Report. Vols. 1–. **Walter Reed Army Institute of Research.** Washington, DC: US Government Printing Office, 1975/1976–.

Includes research relating to biochemistry, communicable diseases and immunology, internal medicine, physiology, psychology, surgery, and veterinary medicine.

Science and Technology Research in Progress 1972–1973. 7 vols. Orange, NJ: Academic Media, in cooperation with Smithsonian Science Information Exchange, 1973. Also updates annually.

Volume 1, *Engineering Sciences*; volume 2, *Chemistry and Chemical Engineering*; volume 3, *Earth and Space Sciences*; volume 4, *Electronics and Electrical Engineering*; volume 5, *Materials;* volume 6, *Mathematics;* volume 7, *Physics.*
Provides current and accurate information on research in progress. Contains investigator index, research-organization index, funding-organization index, and subject index.
R: Chen (p. 390).

Science Research in Progress. **US National Science Foundation.** Washington, DC: Smithsonian Institution, 1949–. Annual.

Printout of unpublished but planned research and research in progress.
R: Chen (p. 390).

Scientific Research in British Universities and Colleges. **Great Britain Department of Education and Science.** London: Her Majesty's Stationery Office, 1973–1974.

R: Chen (p. 390).

SSIE Science Newsletter. Vols. 1–. Washington, DC: Smithsonian Science Information Exchange, 1971–.

Volume 8, no. 9, August 1979.
Outlines information on some 200,000 ongoing and recently completed projects in all fields of basic and applied research active during the present and past two years. Project information gleaned from over 1,300 organizations that support research: federal, state and local government agencies; nonprofit associations and foundations; colleges and universities; and foreign research organizations. Contains extensive section on medical sciences research. Also available on-line.
R: Chen (p. 390).

Unique 3-in-1 Research and Development Directory. Washington, DC: Government Data Publications, 1976.
R: Chen (p. 391).

SUBJECT

Active Research Grants of the National Cancer Institute. **Statistics and Analysis Branch, Division of Research Grants, US National Institutes of Health, comp.** Bethesda, MD: US National Cancer Institute, 1965–. Annual.

Three volumes: grant number; name of investigator; and state and institution. An annual publication.
R: *MRW* S1, p. 16.

Dental Research in the United States, Canada, and Great Britain, DHEW Pub. no. (NIH) 74-450, etc. **US National Institute of Dental Research.** Bethesda, MD: US National Institute of Dental Research, 1972–.

Yearly listing of biomedical dental research projects by project title, researcher, institution, source of support, amount, and summary. No research in dental education care, delivery systems, and manpower is included. Indexed by investigator, institution, and agency.
R: *MRW* S3, pp. 13, 46.

Directory of On-Going Research in Cancer Epidemiology, 1978, IARC Scientific Publications, 26. **C. S. Muir et al., eds.** Lyon, France: International Agency for Research on Cancer, 1978. Annual updates.

Abstracts of over 1,000 research projects in cancer epidemiology. Coverage is international. Indexes by site of cancer, subject term, chemical, types of study, and country. Produced in collaboration with the International Cancer Research Data Bank Program.
R: *Quarterly Review of Biology* 54: 219 (June 1979); *IBID* 6: 68 (Mar. 1978); 7:48 (1979); *WHO Chronicle* 31: 531 (Dec. 1977).

Directory of On-going Research in Smoking and Health. 1st ed.–. Arlington, VA: US National Clearinghouse for Smoking and Health, 1967–.

Second edition, 1968; fifth edition, 1974; sixth edition, 1978, compiled by Informatics, Inc.
Contains research resumes on current research related to smoking and health from about forty countries. Indexed by principal investigator, organization, and subject.
R: *RSR* 4: 110 (Oct.–Dec. 1976); *MRW* S1, p. 24.

Environmental Pollution: A Guide to Current Research. Produced from data gathered by Science Information Exchange, Smithsonian Institution, Washington, DC. New York: CCM Information, 1971–.

Materials on projects are classified by subjects. For each project, information on name, organization, and address, brief description of objectives, progress, and supporting organization are given.
R: Chen (p. 393); Mal (8-79).

Environmental Protection Agency Research Catalog. **US Environmental Protection Agency, Office of Research and Monitoring.** Washington, DC: US Government Printing Office, 1972.
A two-volume set covering ongoing and projected research.
R: Chen (p. 393).

International Review of Connective Tissue Research. Vols. 1–. New York: Academic Press, 1963–.
Volume 8, 1979.

Laboratory and Research Methods in Biology and Medicine. Vols. 1–. New York: Alan R. Liss, 1977–.

Medicinal Research: A Series of Monographs. Vols. 1–. New York: Marcel Dekker, 1967–.
Volume 9, 1978.

Pollution Research Index: A New Reference Guide. Guernsey, England: Hodgson, 1975.
R: Chen (p. 393).

Progress in Respiration Research. Vols. 1–. Basel: S. Karger, 1963–.
Volume 12, 1979.

A Review of the US EPA Environmental Research Outlook FY 1976–1980. **US Congress, Office of Technology Assessment,** Washington, DC: US Government Printing Office, 1976.
R: Chen (p. 393).

Skeletal Research: An Experimental Approach. **David J. Simmons and Arthur S. Kunin, eds.** New York: Academic Press, 1979.
Well referenced review of experimental research of hard tissue.

Toxicology Research Projects Directory, DHEW Pub. no. (OS). Vols. 1–. **US Department of Health, Education, and Welfare.** Toxicology Information Subcommittee of the DHEW Committee to Coordinate Toxicology and Related Programs. Springfield, VA: National Technical Information Service, 1976–. Quarterly.
Inventory of ongoing research projects in toxicology and related fields, selected from the files of the Smithsonian Science Information Exchange.

Tox-tips: Notices of Research Projects. 1977–. Monthly.
Publication of the United States National Library of Medicine. Lists ongoing publications of toxicology information progress.

PREPRINTS

Current use of the term *preprints* implies a broad range of documents from informal communications to finished manuscripts awaiting publication in a journal. While bibliographic control is often troublesome, those preprints that more closely resemble advance copies of journal articles or transaction papers are often adequately controlled by the issuance of preprint series by professional organizations. For a more complete listing of preprint series consult

Directory of Engineering, Scientific and Management Document Sources, **D. Simonton.** Newport Beach, CA: Global Engineering Documentation Services, 1974.
R: Chen (p. 394).

REPRINTS

REFERENCE TOOLS

Out-of-print or discontinued publications are commonly acquired through reprint services and microreprography. Reprinted material is available from various institutes and organizations as well as from more familiar reprint publishers.

The useful tools for locating these reprints are catalogs of reprint publishers, such as Johnson's, and the following general sources:

Encyclopedia Reprints Series. 5 vols. **N. M. Bikales, ed.** New York: Wiley-Interscience, 1971.
R: Chen (p. 395).

Guide to Reprints. **Carol Wade, ed.** Washington, DC: NCR Microcard Editions, 1967–. Annual.
Lists books, journals, and various materials available as reprints from US and foreign publishers. Includes a directory of publishers. Supplemented by *Announced Reprints,* Washington, DC: NCR Microcard Editions, 1969–, quarterly.
R: Chen (p. 395).

SUBJECT TOOLS

On the other hand, it should be kept in mind that scientists are generally concerned with "reprints" of current publications (most popular journal articles) obtained from publishers at the time of publication for ready dissemination purposes. These play an important role in the scientific and technical communication process. In addition, research centers and laboratories, professional organizations, and governmental agencies also frequently issue reprint series of papers produced by their staff scientists. The following are sample publications:

Contemporary Nursing Series. **American Journal of Nursing.** New York: American Journal of Nursing, 1972–.
Series consists of articles from American Journal of Nursing journals on various important topics in nursing. Sample titles are *The Nurse in Community Mental Health,* 1972; *The Expanded Role of the Nurse,* 1973; *Human Sexuality,* 1973; *Mater-*

nal and Newborn Care: Nursing Interventions, 1973; Nursing and the Cancer Patient, 1973; The Nursing Process in Practice, 1974; Advances in Cardiovascular Nursing, 1975; Dying and Grief: Nursing Interventions, 1976; Nursing in Neurological Disorders, 1976; Nursing of Children and Adolescents, 1976; Nursing in Respiratory Diseases, 1977; Psychotherapeutic Nursing Practice, 1977; Nursing: Critically Ill Patients, 1978; Nursing: The Older Adult, 1978; Nursing in Community Health Settings, 1978.

Karger Highlights. Basel: S. Karger, 1978–.

Cardiology 1; Exercise Cardiology (1976–1978), 1978; *Gerontology 1; Experimental Studies* (1976–1978), 1979; *Medical Imaging 1* (1977–1978), 1979; *Nephrology 1* (1976–1977), 1978; *Oral Science 1* (1977), 1979; *Oncology 1* (1976–1978), 1979; *Oncology 2; Cancer Chemotherapy* (1976–1978), 1979.

A new series designed to provide physicians with ready access to prominent articles from Karger publications. Each volume consists of timely articles. A helpful series, assembles much essential information. Recommended to those concerned with keeping abreast of basic, current information in specialized fields.

Nursing Resources Series. Wakefield, MA: Contemporary Publishing, Inc., 1974–.

Subject compilations of articles which appeared in the *Journal of Nursing Administration* and *Nursing Digest*.

CHAPTER 20 CLASSIFICATIONS, STANDARDS, AND PATENTS

CLASSIFICATIONS

For standardized medical nomenclatures, readers are referred to chapter 5, Dictionaries.

GENERAL

A Guide to International Recommendations on Names and Symbols for Quantities and on Units of Measurement. **D. Armstrong Lowe.** Geneva: World Health Organization, 1975.

Summarizes international recommendations on the nomenclature of physical quantities. Part I is a dictionary of quantities, which establishes preferred quantity name, symbol, and appropriate SI unit. Recognizes the source of the recommendation and references to original literature. Part II lists measurement units along with correct symbol and conversion factors from non-SI units to correct SI units. Practical annexes describe SI units, new ionizing radiation units, and clinical chemistry conversion values.
R: *IBID* 3: 266 (Dec. 1975).

The International Classification of Diseases: 9th Revision, Clinical Modification 1CD.9.CM. 3 vols. **Commission on Professional and Hospital Activities.** Ann Arbor, MI: Commission on Professional and Hospital Activities, 1978.

International Classification of Procedures in Medicine. 2 vols. **World Health Organization.** Geneva: World Health Organization, 1978.
R: *IBID* 6: 306 (1978); 7: 48 (1979).

Manual of the International Statistical Classification of Diseases, Injuries, and Causes of Death. 2 vols. **World Health Organization.** Geneva: World Health Organization, 1977–1978.

Physicians' Current Procedural Terminology for Naming, Coding, and Reporting Medical Services. 3d ed. **Burgess L. Gordon, ed.** American Medical Association. Chicago, IL: American Medical Association, 1973.

First edition, 1966; second edition, 1970.
Codes various services provided by physicians. Establishes a uniform language among doctors, patients, and third party payers. Medicine, surgery, radiology, pathology, and anesthesia comprise the five sections of terminology.
R: *MRW* S3, p. 37.

World Health Organization Eighth Revision International Classification of Diseases, Adapted for Use in the United States. 2 vols. **US National Center for**

Health Statistics. Washington, DC: US National Center for Health Statistics, 1967–1968.

Volume 1, Tabular List, 1967; volume 2, Alphabetical List, 1968.

DENTISTRY

Application of the International Classification of Diseases to Dentistry and Stomatology. 2d ed. **World Health Organization.** Geneva: World Health Organization, 1978.

First edition, 1973.
Draws on the ninth revision of the *International Classification of Diseases* (ICD) of 1975. Outlines classification scheme in terms of oral and dental disorders. Numeric tables and alphabetical index add to its reference value.
R: *Journal of Oral Surgery* 37: 451 (1979); *IBID* 7: 49 (1979); *MRW* S3, pp. 35, 53.

HEALTH SERVICES ADMINISTRATION

H-ICDA: Hospital Adaptation of ICDA. 2d ed. 2 vols. **Commission on Professional and Hospital Activities.** Ann Arbor, MI: Commission on Professional and Hospital Activities, 1973.

First edition, 1968.
Arranges diagnostic and surgical codes as used by North American hospitals for medical records indexed according to classified system. Includes new and revised section on surgery. Based on *International Classification of Diseases* (1965 revision).
R: *MRW* S3, p. 11.

Hospital Adaptation of ICDA, H-ICDA (International Classification of Diseases, Adapted), US Public Health Service Pub. no. 1693. 2 vols. **Commission on Professional and Hospital Activities.** Ann Arbor, MI: Commission on Professional and Hospital Activities, 1973.

First edition, 1968.

ONCOLOGY AND NUCLEAR MEDICINE

A Coded Compendium of the International Histological Classification of Tumours. **L. H. Sobin et al., eds.** International Histological Classification of Tumours. Geneva: World Health Organization, 1978.

Compendium of histological tumor classifications. Includes diagnostic terms, international classification of diseases for oncology, and systematized nomenclature of medicine.
R: *IBID* 7: 48 (1979).

Cytology of the Female Genital Tract: International Histological Classification of Tumours No. 8. **G. Riotton and W. M. Christopherson.** Geneva: World Health Organization, 1973.

Concentrates on the standardization of nomenclature and classification of female genital tract cytology. Based on the findings of a panel of experts in conjunction with the World Health Organization. Second half of text is essentially a color

atlas. Features almost 200 photomicrographs of excellent quality. Does not achieve its intended purpose of being the authoritative text.
R: *BMJ* 2: 286 (May 4, 1974).

International Classification of Diseases for Oncology. **World Health Organization.** Geneva: World Health Organization, 1976.

Amplifies chapter II (Neoplasms) of Ninth Revision of *International Classification of Diseases.* Contains two numeral lists: topographical, according to anatomical site; and morphological, according to histological type of neoplasm. Includes alphabetical index as well as list of tumorlike lesions.
R: *Quarterly Review of Biology* 52: 335 (1976); *IBID* 5: 153 (June 1977).

TNM Classification of Malignant Tumours. 3d ed. **M. H. Harmer, ed.** Geneva: International Union Against Cancer, 1978.

Second edition, 1968.
Two-part edition deals with the classification of tumor sites. Main booklet presents the proposals of the Union Internationale Centre le Cancer (UICC). Supplement deals with the classification agreement between UICC and the American Joint Committee on Cancer Staging and End Results Reporting. Total agreement will lead to a single volume. TNM classification scheme is standard and deserves continued use.
R: *British Journal of Radiology* 47: 428 (1974).

Psychiatry and Psychology

Definition and Measurement of Mental Health, Public Health Service Pub. no. 1873. **Saul B. Sells, ed.** National Center for Health Statistics. Washington, DC: US Government Printing Office, 1968.

A Multi-Axial Classification of Child Psychiatric Disorders. **Michael Rutter, David Shaffer, and Michael Shepherd.** Geneva: World Health Organization, 1975.

Consists of clinical studies and implications of multi-axial disease; aims to revise international classification of these disorders.
R: *RSR* 4: 107 (July–Sept. 1976).

Veterinary Medicine

Tumors in Domestic Animals. 2d ed. **Jack E. Moulton, ed.** Berkeley, CA: University of California Press, 1978.

Summarizes general biology of tumors for pathologists, teachers, and oncologists.

STANDARDS

Standardization, for our purposes, applies to the rules, regulations, techniques, and various conditions which must be adhered to in medical practices, care, units of measurement, instrument and equipment design and manufacturing, terminology, drug application, safety design, and so on. Standards may be voluntary or mandatory, a condition that varies from specialty to specialty, country to country. Some standards are generally accepted either internationally and nationally. Interestingly enough, standardization is defined by the American Society for Testing and Materials as "a democratic procedure for evolving accepted rules of behaviour." Hence the rules and regulations for insuring the quality, the standard, and/or the performance of activities, services, practices, and so on in an orderly way are contingent on the cooperation of all concerned, be they producers of medical products, providers of medical care and services, medical practitioners, medical service consumers, or general-interest groups.

In the field of medicine, while general standards developed and recommended by general standard organizations, such as the International Organization for Standardization, American National Standards Institute, American Society for Testing and Materials, and US National Bureau of Standards, are essential, it is fair to say that medical professionals have their own specialized standards in the fields of health sciences. In the following sections, the listed tools will show that governmental organizations, whether international, national, or local, professional societies and associations, medical trade and industry, and many other organizations are involved in providing standards and recommending practices. Of all these, the organizations which develop health-related standards and regulations of general and international interest, thus of the widest implications for health professionals, are World Health Organization and the International Association of Biological Standardization.

Guides to Standards

Directory of United States Standardization Activities, NBS Special Publication, no. 417. **US National Bureau of Standards.** Washington, DC: US Government Printing Office, 1975.
R: Chen (p. 402).

The Guide to Biomedical Standards. **Allan F. Pacela, and Hans A. von der Mosel.** Diamond Bar, CA: Quest Publications, 1971.
Concentrates on US, international, and foreign standards for the regulation of medical care centers and equipment. Alphabetical arrangement of 250 references are within three sections: United States, international, and foreign.
R: *MRW* S2, p. 43.

Guide to Specifications and Standards of the Federal Government. **US General Services Administration.** Washington, DC: US Government Printing Office, 1963.
A general guide to the many specifications and standards set by the federal government.
R: Chen (p. 402).

Lists of International Biological Standards and International Biological Refer-

ence Preparations, 1975. **World Health Organization.** Geneva: World Health Organization, 1975.

Main entry is by substance and supplies name. International unit of standard in milligram form. Also includes duration of standardization and references. Indexed.
R: *RSR* 4: 46 (Jan.–Mar. 1976).

Standards and Specifications Information Sources, MIG No. 6. **Erasmus J. Struglia.** Detroit, MI: Gale Research, 1965.

Annotated bibliography of literature of standardization, catalogs and indexes of standards and specifications, and guides to periodical indexes that include material on standards. Author-title and subject indexes.
R: *SL* 57: 260 (1966); Chen (p. 402); Jenkins (K206); Mal (3-58); Win (2EA42).

Technical Information Sources: A Guide to Patent Specifications, Standards and Technical Reports Literature. 2d ed. **Bernard Houghton.** Hamden, CT: Shoe String Press, 1972.

First edition, 1967.

Five chapters on patents, three on standards, and two on technical-report literature for the library student and professional. Emphasizes British publications but presents suitable coverage of US sources. Useful bibliographies.
R: *AL* 3: 926 (Sept. 1972); *ARBA* (1973, p. 626); Chen (p. 403); Jenkins (pp. 2, 23); Wal (p. 240); Win (2EA40).

Major Bibliographical Tools—General

ANSI Catalog. New York: American National Standards Institute, 1923–. Annual.

Latest edition, 1976. Present name since 1969.

Supplemented by the *Listing of New and Revised American National Standards,* alternate months. More than 6,000 American and 4,000 international standards approved by ANSI. The 1977 catalog will start a new format by issuing two catalogs: one listing American National Standards and a second, international standards and recommendations. Both catalogs list standards by subject and by the sponsor's designation.
R: Chen (p. 403).

Book of ASTM Standards. Philadelphia, PA: American Society for Testing Materials, 1939–. Annual.

While the adoption of ASTM standards is purely voluntary, they do represent a common ground between producers and consumers. The 48 parts contain current ASTM standards and tentative specifications, test methods, recommended practices, definitions, proposed methods, etc. Each annual supersedes the previous edition. Essential material for the engineer.
R: *ARBA* (1976, p. 761; 1971, p. 545); Chen (p. 403); Jenkins (K201); Wal (p. 534, 537); Win (EA204).

British Standards Yearbook. London: British Standards Institution, 1937–. Annual.

Complete annotated list of British standards, plus handbooks and codes of practice. Kept up to date by *B&I News*.
R: Chen (p. 403).

Canadian Standards Association. Catalogue of Standards. Rexdale, Ontario: Canadian Standards Association. Annual.
R: Chen (p. 403).

Federal Information Processing Standards Index, US National Bureau of Standards FIPS-Pub-12-1. **US National Bureau of Standards.** Washington, DC: US Government Printing Office, 1972.
A bibliography, directory, and handbook in one package.
R: Chen (p. 403).

Index of Federal Specifications and Standards. **US General Services Administration.** Washington, DC: US Government Printing Office, 1952–. Monthly.
A guide to the standards and specifications to which suppliers of goods to the US government must conform. Arranged by subject. Does not include military suppliers.
R: Chen (p. 404); Mal (11-28).

An Index of International Standards. **Sophie Cnumas, ed.** Prepared for the US National Bureau of Standards. Washington, DC: US Government Printing Office, 1974.
Computer-produced index containing almost 3,000 standard titles of the ISO, IEC, CEE, OIML, and CISPR.
R: *ARBA* (1975, p. 770); Chen (p. 404).

MEDICAL STANDARDS

As stated earlier, governmental organizations and professional societies at all levels are major sponsoring bodies of numerous standards in medical subject areas. On the other hand, journals, particularly official news publications of those professional societies that are involved in standardization activities, are essential information sources of current standards. For example, *Journal of the American Medical Association,* monthly journals of the American Hospital Association, and many other associations, have columns on standards in their issues.

Besides the subject guides to standards mentioned earlier, the works in this section are indicative of titles that are available on particular applications of health sciences related standards. The American Society for Testing and Materials has advanced the concept that most of the applications of standards fit frequently into four major categories: units of measurement, terminology and symbolic representation, products and processes, and safety of persons and goods. Some of the standards related to units of measurement and terminology and nomenclature can be found in tools included in chapter 5, Dictionaries, while some others are included in either this section or in the classifications section of this chapter. Those standards related to products and processes and safety are included here, with a subject breakdown:

GENERAL

Biological Substances: International Standards and Reference Preparations 1975. **World Health Organization.** Geneva: World Health Organization, 1975.

Highlights the revisions of the 26th WHO Expert Committee on Biological Standardization. Includes new proposals and discontinued standards and preparations.
R: *IBID* 3: 266 (Dec. 1975).

Developments in Biological Standardization. Vol. 23. **International Association of Biological Standardization, ed.** Basel: S. Karger, 1974–.

Volume 41, 1978; volume 43, 1979.
Formed by the Union of Progress in Immunological Standardization and Symposia Series in Immunobiological Standardization and assumes the volume numbering of the latter.
All volumes represent congress proceedings. For example, volume 41, *Vaccinations in the Developing Countries,* 1979, is the proceedings of the fifteenth IABS International Congress for Biological Standardization, Le Gosier, Guadeloupe, April 1978.

International Health Regulations. 2d annotated ed. **World Health Organization.** Geneva: World Health Organization, 1974.

First annotated edition, 1971.
These regulations replace International Sanitary Regulations last published in 1966. Diseases which are discussed are cholera, plague, smallpox, and yellow fever. Notification procedure, requirements for port and airport health measures, description of required health measures and procedures, and a section on each disease are included.
R: *British Medical Bulletin* 30: 289 (1974).

WHO Expert Committee on Biological Standardization Report. **World Health Organization.** Geneva: World Health Organization. Annual.

Twenty-ninth report, 1978.
Report on Committee's reviews of antibiotics, antigens, blood products, and endocrinological substances. Sets requirements for the collection, processing, and quality control of biological substances.
R: *IBID* 7: 48 (1979).

ANATOMY

Report of the Task Group on Reference Man, International Commission on Radiological Protection Report no. 23. **International Commission on Radiological Protection, Task Group of Committee 2.** New York: Pergamon, 1975.

This work synthesizes anatomical standards of man. Provides physiological, gross and elemental, and anatomical data. These statistics are then related to radiation protection and hazards of each body system. Deals with metabolism of trace elements, takes into account variations in populations. This manual comprises an enormous amount of data and detailed information. It is highly recommended as a source of reference for physicians, health physicists, and biomedical researchers.
R: *British Journal of Radiology* 49: 576 (1976); *Health Physics* 30: 152 (Jan. 1976).

CARDIOVASCULAR SYSTEM

Standards for Cardiopulmonary Resuscitation and Emergency Cardiac Care. **American Heart Association.** New York: American Heart Association, 1973.

A guide for the standard training and performance of cardiopulmonary resuscitation (CPR) and emergency cardiac care (ECC). Based on recommendations of leading authorities. Outlines principles, techniques, training, and certification related to basic and advanced life support and approved by the American Heart Association. Recommended to all oral surgeons.
R: *Journal of Oral Surgery* 33: 311 (Apr. 1975).

GASTROINTESTINAL SYSTEM

Diseases of the Liver and Biliary Tract: Proceedings of the 5th Quadranial Meeting of the International Association for the Study of the Liver, Acapulco 1974. **C. M. Leevy, ed.** Basel: S. Karger, 1976.

Collection of 44 papers dealing with experimental and clinical hepatology. Papers result from the 1974 meeting of the IASL. Special emphasis on the standardization of a common scientific language for diseases of the liver and biliary tract. A must for every gastroenterologist.
R: *Digestion* 17: 278 (1978).

HEALTH SERVICES ADMINISTRATION

Hospital Medical Records: Guidelines for Their Use and the Release of Medical Information. Chicago, IL: American Hospital Association. 1972.

Intended for hospital administrators and medical records supervisors. Concentrates on maintenance, legal aspects, release of information, and common administrative practices.

JCAH Accreditation Manual for Hospital. **Joint Commission on Accreditation Hospitals.** Chicago, IL: Joint Commission on Accreditation Hospitals, 1971, 1973 and 1975. Loose-leaf updates.

Based on *JCAH Standards for Hospital Accreditation*. A major tool for every hospital.

Standards for Library Services in Health Care Institutions. **Hospital Library Standards Committee, Association of Hospital and Institution Libraries.** Chicago, IL: American Library Association, 1970.

Outlines administrative principles and methods yielding positive results in libraries connected with health care institutions. Useful appendix lists standard physical requirements; 22 references and glossary.
R: *MRW* S2, p. 62.

NURSING

How to Write Meaningful Nursing Standards. **E. J. Mason.** New York: John Wiley, 1978.
A practical guide to defining, writing, and implementing effective standards in all areas of nursing care. Necessary reference tool for students and administrators.

The JCAH Standards; A Journal of Nursing Administration Reader. **Marjorie M. Cantor, ed.** Wakefield, MA: Contemporary Publishing, 1974.

Nursing Care Evaluation: Concurrent and Retrospective Review Criteria. **Sharon Van Sell Davidson et al.** St. Louis, MO: C. V. Mosby, 1977.
Provides criteria to be used as models for nursing care audits and quality assurance programs. Sections devoted to complications related to specific diagnosis and synopsis of quality assurance and means by which to achieve it. Step-by-step procedure for nursing care audit is presented.
R: *American Journal of Nursing* 78: 1267 (July 1978).

Nursing Care Staffing Requirements in Nursing Homes. **National Geriatrics Society.** Milwaukee, WI: National Geriatrics Society, 1979.
The first national survey of nursing care staff requirements. Enables professional associations to compare requirements by state.
R: *Hospitals* 53: 32 (Aug. 16, 1979).

National League For Nursing. Various publications regularly revised by the NLM on accreditation include *Criteria for the Appraisal of Baccalaureate and Higher Degree Programs in Nursing,* 1977; *Criteria for the Evaluation of Diploma Programs in Nursing,* 1978; *Criteria for the Evaluation of Educational Programs in Nursing Leading to an Associate Degree,* 1976; *Criteria for the Evaluation of Educational Programs in Practical Nursing,* 1976.

Standards for Accreditation of Extended Care Facilities, Nursing Care Facilities and Resident Care Facilities. **Joint Commission on Accreditation of Hospitals.** Chicago, IL: Joint Commission on Accreditation of Hospitals, 1968 and updates.

Standards of Nursing Practice. Kansas City, MO: American Nurses Association.
Frequent revisions. In addition to these general standards for nursing practice, the ANA has standards for specific areas such as Medical-Surgical, Gerontological, Community Health, and others.

NUTRITION

Laboratory Indices of Nutritional Status in Pregnancy. **Committee on Nutrition of the Mother and Preschool Child, Food and Nutrition Board, US National Research Council.** Washington, DC: US National Academy of Sciences, 1978.
Scientific review of current state of knowledge regarding laboratory indices reflecting nutritional and metabolic status during normal pregnancy. Seven chapters written by experts cover such topics as physiological adjustments, hematologic indices, and electrolytes. Abnormal or diseased states are not considered. Timely publication for research scientist.
R: *American Journal of Public Health* 68: 911 (Sept. 1978); 68: 913 (Sept. 1978); *Lancet* 2: 242 (July 29, 1978); *Nutrition Reviews* 36: 160 (May 1978).

An Outline of Food Law: Structure, Principles, Main Provisions, Legislative Studies, 7. **Alain Gerard, prep.** Rome: Food and Agriculture Organization, 1975.
Contents include such topics as the nature, domain, and general forms of food law, food standardization, food additives, and regulation of food labeling. Appendix includes a bibliography.
R: *IBID* 3: 165 (Sept. 1975).

Specifications for the Identity and Purity of Some Food Colours, Flavour Enhancers, Thickening Agents, and Certain Food Additives, WHO Food Additives Series, No. 7. **World Health Organization.** Geneva: World Health Organization, 1976.
Material is a result of World Health Organization meeting held in June 1974. Describes fourteen food colors, ten flavor enhancers, five thickening agents, and twenty food additives.
R: *RSR* 4: 107 (July–Sept. 1976).

PHARMACY AND PHARMACOLOGY

British Herbal Pharmacopoeia. **Scientific Committee, British Herbal Medicine Association.** London: British Herbal Medicine Association, 1971.
Alphabetical listing of herbs possessing some medicinal value. Includes herbs excluded from official British pharmacopoeias. Descriptions include definition, synonyms, microscopic and macroscopic physical details, and relevant therapeutic data.
R: *MRW* S2, p. 47.

British National Formulary. 10th ed. **Joint Formulary Committee.** London: British Medical Association and the Pharmaceutical Society of Great Britain, 1974–1976.
First edition, 1949.
Comprehensive guide to prescribing of medications. Includes detailed index and index of proprietary preparations and their nonproprietary equivalents.

British Pharmaceutical Codex, 1973. **Pharmaceutical Society of Great Britain.** London: Pharmaceutical Press, 1973.

First edition, 1907.
Descriptive source of drugs, pharmaceutical substances, and related products. Also sets standards of identity and purity for substances not covered by the *British Pharmacopoeia*.
R: *Journal of Pharmaceutical Sciences* 63: 478 (Mar. 1974); Win (EK205, 3EJ27).

British Pharmacopeia 1977. 13th ed. London: Pharmaceutical Press, 1977.

Eleventh edition, 1968; twelfth edition, 1973.
An extensive compilation of some 1,000 monographs, providing descriptions and specifications for the quality of chemical, physical, and biological compounds used in medical practice. Two addendum volumes include further descriptive data. Necessary reference tool for any medically related library.
R: *Journal of Pharmaceutical Sciences* 63: 1176 (July 1974); Win (EK203, 3EJ28).

Code of Federal Regulations. Title 21. *Food & Drugs.* Washington, DC: US Government Printing Office.

Updates can be found in *Federal Register*.

Compilation of OTC Drug Regulations. Washington, DC: Proprietary Association, 1977–. Loose-leaf binding.

A convenient source available for all federal regulations affecting OTC medicines, including all OTC review documents and other relevant regulations from FDA, FTC, and CPSC. Reproduced directly from the *Federal Register*. Divided in three parts: Part I, *OTC Review Regulations*; Part II, *FDA Regulations other than the OTC Review*; Part III, *Miscellaneous Documents*.

FDA Drug and Device Product Approvals. Washington, DC: National Technical Information Service, 1978–. Monthly.

A successor to *New Drug Applications,* lists new drugs approved for marketing by the Food and Drug Administration.

Homeopathic Pharmacopeia of the U.S. 8th ed. Falls Church, VA: American Institute of Homeopathy, 1979–.

First edition, 1897.
Volume 1, 1979.
Alphabetical list by scientific name of material from which the drug is made. Gives common name, chemical symbol, description, parts used, preparations, etc.

National Drug Code Directory, FDA no. 77-3037. 2 vols. and suppl. **United States Department of Health, Education, and Welfare; Bureau of Drugs, Food and Drug Administration; Drug Listing Branch.** Washington, DC: US Government Printing Office, 1978.

Alphabetical list by product name; numerical index, alphabetical index by short name.

National Drug Code Index 1978–79. New York: Ext. Pharm. Data, Inc., 1979.

In three sections: manufacturers products, alphabetical list of product name, list of manufacturers address. Includes about 50,000 NDC numbers. New edition contains information on thousands of new products.

1980 United States Pharmacopeia XX—National Formulary XV (The United States Pharmacopeia). Easton, PA: United States Pharmacopeial Convention, 1980–.

This edition combines the *United States Pharmacopeia,* 1820–1976, and the *National Formulary,* 1888–1975. Contains information on 2,300 active and 200 pharmaceutical ingredients, updating supplements available from publisher.
R: *Journal of Pharmaceutical Sciences* 64: 1084 (June 1975); 64: 1266 (July 1975); *Pharmaceutical Journal* 214: 577 (1975); 219: 523 (1977); *ARBA* (1976, p. 740); Win (EK204; EK206).

Specifications and Criteria for Biochemical Compounds. 3d ed. **US National Academy of Sciences.** Washington, DC: US National Academy of Sciences, 1972.

Government recommended standardization of organic compounds important to the pharmaceutical industry. Includes a bibliography on each item.

Specifications for the Quality Control of Pharmaceutical Preparations: Second Edition of the International Pharmacopoeia. **World Health Organization.** Geneva: World Health Organization, 1967.

———, Supplement, 1971.

Collection of recommended specifications in accordance with the resolutions of the Third World Health Assembly. Serves as a reference so that national specifications can be established on a similar basis.

Standards and Planning Guide for Pharmacy Library Service. **Martha J. K. Zachert, ed.** Bethesda, MD: American Association of Colleges of Pharmacy, 1975.

Standards accompanied by a self-study workbook for assessing adequacy of pharmacy college library services.

PHYSICAL MEDICINE AND REHABILITATION

Fitness, Health, and Work Capacity; International Standards for Assessment. **Leonard A. Larson, ed.** International Committee for the Standardization of Physical Fitness Tests. New York: Macmillan, 1974.

Well-organized text covers theoretical aspects of physical fitness as well as procedures for assessment of fitness. Reference contains reliable data regarding fitness, health, and work capacity. Interdisciplinary approach; useful to researchers, coaches, physical therapists, and students.
R: *Physical Therapy* 55: 89 (1975).

PUBLIC HEALTH

A Guide to Electrical Hazards and Safety Standards. **The Hospital Physicists' Association.** London: The Hospital Physicists' Association, 1977.

Focuses on two electrical safety standards: *National Health Service Hospital Technical Memorandum Number 8—Safety Code for Electromedical Apparatus* (1969 revision) and the *Draft Standard of the International Electrotechnical Commission* (Document 62A, 1976). Bulk of text is a comparison of the recommendations of these two standards. Compares equipment classification, insulation, equipment temperatures, etc. Geared towards British-physicists involved with safety standards. Less useful in the United States and other countries where different standards apply.
R: *Physics in Medicine & Biology* 23: 530 (May 1978).

Occupational Safety, Health and Fire Index. Vol. 1 **David E. Miller, ed.** New York: Marcel Dekker, 1976.

Computer-generated listing of thousands of safety, health, and fire codes, standards, guides, and publications. Also identifies sources of information like US Department of Labor, American Petroleum Institute, National Safety Council, etc. Formal results in easy retrieval.
R: *Archives of Dermatology* 112: 1624 (Nov. 1976).

OSHA Compliance Guide. Chicago, IL: Commerce Clearing House, 1978.

Nontechnical explanation of OSHA and OSHA standards. One volume covers standards, variances from standards, OSHA record keeping, OSHA inspections etc. Also summarizes state OSHA controls. Monthly newsletter updates standards and relates new developments.

RADIOLOGY

Alphabetical Index of Roentgen Diagnoses and Procedures. **Gerhart S. Schwarz and Henry Powsner.** Springfield, IL: Charles C. Thomas, 1966.

An alphabetical guide to the coding system for X-rays used by the American College of Radiology (ACR). Includes explanatory pages, appendixes dealing with different retrieval methods, and anatomical sketches of the body indicating ACR coding.

A Practitioner's Guide to the Diagnostic X-ray Equipment Standard, DHEW Pub. no. (FDA) 78-8050. **US Food and Drug Administration, Bureau of Radiological Health.** Washington, DC: US Government Printing Office, 1978.

Reports the new Federal X-ray standard. Issued by the Food and Drug Administration in an effort to reduce unnecessary patient exposure to X-rays. Available free to physicians.
R: *Journal of Oral Surgery* 33: 150 (Feb. 1975).

Radiation Protection Standards. **Lauriston S. Taylor.** Cleveland, OH: Chemical Rubber Company, 1971.

Reviews contributions of individuals, institutions, and committees in many countries, with special attention to 39 reports issued by US National Committee on Radiation Protection and Measurements and 14 reports from International Commission on Radiological Protection. Written by an authority on radiation protection standards. Provides a readable history of radiation for health physicists.
R: *Health Physics* 25: 615 (Dec. 1973).

Radiation Science at the National Physical Laboratory, 1912–1955. **E. E. Smith.** London: Her Majesty's Stationery Office, 1975.

Relates historical progress in the field of radiation standards research dating from the 10th Roentgen Congress in 1905, covering the growth of industrial and commercial use of radiation technology. Well recommended to physicians, university libraries as an interesting source on the history of radiology.

R: *Physics in Medicine & Biology* 20: 1037 (Nov. 1975).

PATENTS

Patents are a significant part of technical literature for health scientists and engineers engaged in research and development. Accurate knowledge of existing and pending patents saves the researcher from the possibility of duplicating the efforts of other scientists and, more importantly, reduces the possibility of legal complications resulting from infringement upon a patent belonging to another party. In certain fields, such as chemical research, no literature search is complete without an examination of existing patents. *Chemical Abstracts* provides a patent index and concordance for such purposes.

The patent itself is a document that represents a contract between a government and inventor or patentee. As patents are honored only in the country in which they are issued, necessary tools have been developed to provide international coverage of patent literature. These tools will be listed with those that provide coverage of the US patent system. The Patent Office Search Center in Arlington, Virginia, maintains files of issued patents and their supporting records. Interested parties may order copies of original patents or consult them at regional patent copy depository libraries.

As patents may present considerable complications for the science librarian and scientist or engineer who have no access to patent attorneys or agents, the following list of sources is intended to provide a fundamental understanding of patent classification, procedure, and practice.

See chapter 24, Data Bases, for on-line patent information.

Mainly on Patents: The Use of Literature of Industrial Property and Its Literature. **Felix Liebesny, ed.** Hamden, CT: Archon Books, 1973.

Emphasis on British publications.

R: *ARBA* (1974, p. 545); Chen (p. 396).

Manual of Classification of Patents. **US Patent Office.** Washington, DC: US Government Printing Office, 1974–. Irregular.

There are some 3,000 major classes and approximately 60,000 subclasses under which a patent may be placed. This tool explains the system and provides class and subclass numbers that facilitate the use of the *Official Gazette*.

R: Chen (p. 396); Mal (2-14).

Manual of Patent Examining Procedures. 3d ed. **US Patent Office.** Washington, DC: US Government Printing Office, 1969.

First edition, 1949.
Material pertaining to all practices and procedures used by examiners at the Patent Office.
R: *ARBA* (1970, p. 146); Chen (p. 396).

Technical Information Sources: A Guide to Patent Specification, Standards, and Technical Reports Literature. 2d ed. **Bernard Houghton.** Hamden, CT: Shoe String Press, 1972.
Primarily a guide to British patent information for librarians.
R: Chen (p. 397).

INDEXES TO US AND INTERNATIONAL PATENTS

Abstracting and indexing journals can be valuable sources of patent information. Unquestionably *Chemical Abstracts* is the most important one. Journals often also include abstracts or notes on new patents. In the fields of health sciences, specific attention also should be paid to the numerous trade journals and publications which include invaluable information on new patents, such as those in the field of pharmacy and medical instrumentation and equipments.

The most important guides to the patent literature are various indexes issued either by government patent offices or commercial firms. The following list is indicative of the range of these tools. Some of the data bases on these indexes are machine searchable, and readers should consult the chapter on data bases for further information. In the field of pharmaceutical sciences, *Merck Index* provides excellent patent information.

SOURCES ABOUT PATENTS

About Patents; Patents as a Source of Technical Information. **Great Britain: The Patent Office, Department of Trade and Industry.** London: Her Majesty's Stationery Office, n.d.
R: *Engineering* (Oct. 14, 1971); Chen (p. 397).

Development and Use of Patent Classification Systems. **US Patent Office.** Washington, DC: US Government Printing Office, 1966.
R: Chen (p. 397).

The Encyclopedia of Patent Practice and Invention Management. **Robert Peyton Calvert, ed.** New York: Van Nostrand Reinhold, 1964.
A two-volume encyclopedia that presents comprehensive statements of principles and procedures in many phases of patent practice and invention management.
R: *Choice* 2: 567 (1966); Chen (p. 397), Win (1EA40).

Foreign Patents: A Guide to Official Patent Literature. **Francis J. Kase.** Dobbs Ferry, NY: Oceana, 1973.
Foreign patent material arranged alphabetically by country, including informa-

tion on foreign patent offices, English translations of printed specifications, patent journals, data on trademarks, etc. Primarily for use by searchers in the US.
R: *Choice* 10: 946 (Sept. 1973); *LJ* 98: 2325 (Aug. 1973); *ARBA* (1974, p. 548); Chen (p. 397).

General Information Concerning Patents: A Brief Introduction to Patent Matters. Washington, DC: US Government Printing Office, 1973.
Practical information on the general subject of patents. Intended for company and private-inventor use.
R: Chen (p. 397).

How to Find Out About Patents. **Frank Newby.** New York: Pergamon Press, 1967.
Practical information on typical patents.
R: *NTB* 52: 267 (1967); Chen (p. 398); Jenkins (A182); Wal (p. 240).

International Classification of Patents. **Council of Europe.** West Wickham, England: Morgan-Grampian, 1968.
R: Chen (p. 398).

The Inventor's Patent Handbook. Rev. ed. **Stacy V. Jones.** New York: Dial Press, 1969.
Earlier edition, 1969.
Practical information on obtaining a patent, selling patents, contract agreements, etc.
R: *Choice* 4: 400 (1967); *RQ* (Fall 1970); *ARBA* (1971, p. 545); Chen (p. 398); Jenkins (A181); Win (2EA41).

Understanding Chemical Patents. **John T. Maynard.** Washington, DC: American Chemical Society, 1978.

US Patents

Index of Patents. **US Patent Office.** Washington, DC: US Government Printing Office, 1920–. Annual.
Two main sections: part I, an alphabetical list of patentees, persons or companies with new or reissued patents; part II, index of subjects of inventions arranged according to Patent Office classification.
R: Chen (p. 398).

Index of Trademarks Issued from the United States Patent Office. **US Patent Office.** Washington, DC: US Government Printing Office, 1927–. Annual.
R: Chen (p. 398).

Index to Classification. **US Patent Office.** Washington, DC: US Government Printing Office, 1947–.
Index to classification by subject descriptors.
R: Chen (p. 398); Mal (2-15).

Official Gazette of the United States Patent Office. **US Patent Office.** Washington, DC: US Government Printing Office, 1872–. Weekly.

Lists and briefly describes patents on a weekly basis. Includes sections on notices, suits, and reissues of former patents. Numerical listing under four groups: general and mechanical, chemical, electrical, and design. Includes numbers, title, inventor, and assignees. Patentee, classified, and geographical indexes. Most comprehensive US source.
R: Chen (p. 398); Mal (2-12).

US Patent Previews. New York: Bowker, 1965–70.

Lists 60,000 patent applications.
R: Chen (p. 398).

INTERNATIONAL PATENTS

Only major international sources of patent information have been included here. For information on the patent offices of the major industrial countries and their official journals, consult the front section of the patent index in *Chemical Abstracts.*

Chemical Abstracts Patent Index and Concordance. Columbus, OH: American Chemical Society.

One of the number of indexes issued annually in *Chemical Abstracts.* A major tool to chemical patent literature.
R: Chen (p. 399).

IINPADOC (International Patent Documentation Center). Arlington, VA: IFI/Plenum.

A microfiche service offered in collaboration with World Intellectual Property Organization, covering patent family, classification, and applicant services.
R: Chen (p. 399).

The International Index of Patents. Williamsport, PA: Bro-Dart Books, 1964–.

Not limited to general science.
R: Chen (p. 399).

Derwent Publications Ltd. Documentation Services. London.

This firm is the publisher of the most important current-awareness services for worldwide patent literature. The data base contains patent specifications from 24 countries and is added to at the rate of some 12,000 weekly. For machine-readable data bases see the chapter on data bases.

The following are Derwent's most significant publications in the field:

Central Patents Index—CPI. 1970–. Weekly.

Two "Alerting Bulletins," arranged by country and by systematic classification. Includes patent number, CPI class, patentee, and basic number or patent concordance indexes.

R: Chen (p. 399).

General Patents Index—GPI. 1970–. Weekly.

Contains three printed abstracts journals; *P, General, Q, Mechanical, R, Electrical.* Also issued on cards and microfilm.
R: Chen (p. 399).

World Patents Index. 1974–. Weekly.

General, electrical, mechanical, and chemical sections. Easy access through numerous indexes.
R: Chen (p. 399).

Some publishers, such as Noyes Data Corporation, provide reviews of patent information on a specific subject area. Each looks like a monographic publication but is actually a publication on patents.

CHAPTER 21 TRADE LITERATURE

Trade literature, while often a useful source of health science information, is often ignored by many science librarians. As the quality of such publications increases, however, librarians would do well to appreciate such literature for its information value rather than denigrate it for its commercial overtones. Often it is highly specialized, as in the case of the literature of pharmacy and pharmacology, where trade publications are likely to provide detailed information on the biochemical properties and chemical structure of drugs.

While organizations are naturally amenable to providing details of their products to potential customers, an individual undertaking a deliberate collection of trade literature would start by consulting buyers' guides such as *Thomas' Register of American Manufacturers*. Such sources are available in various formats, including comprehensive listings of manufacturers' names and addresses, specific subject area directories, and directories that include examples of trade literature for each concern.

Also common is the compendium of individual brochures and pamphlets that are reissued as manufacturers' catalogs and distributed to allied health professionals. As an ample listing of directories is included elsewhere in this book, the reader is advised to consult these works for appropriate companies and manufacturers.

The literature itself takes various forms, including that of journals, bulletins, monographs, audiovisual presentations, and similar publications. However, certain health fields offer specialized publications aimed primarily at their own professionals. For example, Eli Lilly & Company publishes specialized literature for the pharmacist. Much of this literature is free for the asking. The following sections will include examples of significant trade literature as well as a guide to sources of other free and inexpensive materials.

GUIDE TO TRADE LITERATURE

Free and Inexpensive Materials. **Robert Monahan.** Belmont, CA: Fearon, 1973.
R: Chen (p. 412).

Gebbie House Magazine Directory. Sioux City, IA: House Magazine, 1946–. Triennial.
Latest edition, 1974.
Alphabetical, title, geographic, and printers listings. Also arranged by standard industrial classification numbers.
R: Chen (p. 412).

Magazines for Libraries. 2d ed. **Bill Katz.** New York: Bowker, 1972.
Free-magazines section.

R: Chen (p. 412).

Vertical File Index: A Subject and Title Index to Selected Pamphlet Material. New York: Wilson, 1932–. Monthly.
R: Chen (p. 412).

TRADE REFERENCE TOOLS

Publications of manufacturers concerning their products, devices, and equipment include all types of information sources, such as handbooks, manuals, catalogs, buyers' guides, etc. Many of these reference sources can be found in the chapters on handbooks, manuals, directories, guides, and so on, in this book. For example, one such publication is the *Hospital Purchasing Guide 1978.* Although intended as a trade reference tool, it is cited in the chapter on directories. Numerous pharmaceutical manufacturers publish their own price catalogs; however, a cumulation of price lists are available from the following two sources:

American Druggist Blue Book. 50th ed. New York: Hearst Publications, 1978.

Drug Topics Red Book. New York: Medical Economics Co. Annual.

These two publications (see chapter 11 for further information) contain an index to drug manufacturers as well as price lists, which are arranged by trademark. All other pertinent information, such as National Drug Code number, packaging, drug indentification, etc., is included.

Other than drug manufacturers, many other firms in the allied health sciences publish their own price catalogs. The following is a sample listing:

Alcon Laboratories Wholesale Price List. Alcon Laboratories.

Central Processing Sterilizer Products and Nursing Products General Catalog. AMSC (American Sterilizer Company).

Colson Equipment Division Binder and Price List.

Dermatological Price List. Owen Laboratories.

Emergency Medical Supply Catalog. South Shore Medical Supply Company.

General Reference Catalog of Health Care Products. Searle-Will Ross, Inc.

Hill-Rom Hospital Furnishing Binder. Hill-Rom Company, Inc.

Hospital Reference File. Castle Sybron Corporation.

Hotpack Controlled Environmental Equipment. Hotpack Corporation.

Macbick Catalog. Macbick Company.

Metro Healthcare Products. Metropolitan Wire Corporation.

Physicians Catalog Equipment and Supplies. General Medical.

Price Book and Product Reference for Community Pharmacy. 53d ed. Canadian Pharmaceutical Association, 1977 (final ed.).

Product Information and Identification. Roerig Company.

Surgical Equipment Catalog. AMSCO (American Sterilizer Company).

Teaching Hospital Price List. Allergan.

West-ward Catalog. West-ward, Inc.

Aside from the traditional types of reference tools, trade literature also appears in some unique formats. Occasionally, well-established pharmaceutical companies collect in-house documents of significant scientific importance. For example, Parke, Davis & Company published its *Scientific Contributions from the Laboratories 1866–1966*. Its historical value to health professionals warrants its inclusion in the chapter on history. Audiovisual presentations are also useful trade reference tools available to allied health professionals and students. One such audiovisual presentation, *Functional Anatomy of the Human Kidney* by Smith, Kline & French Laboratories, can be found in the chapter on nonprint material.

SAMPLE TRADE PERIODICALS

Action in Pharmacy. Sponsored by National Pharmaceutical Council. 1968–. Monthly, Sept.–May.

Chemist Analyst. J. T. Baker. Frequency varies.

Ciba-Geigy Journal. 1957–. Quarterly.

Cutter Laboratories Annual Report. 1959–.

Focal Point. Will-Ross, Inc. 1979–.

Guidelines to Metabolic Therapy. Upjohn Company. 1972–. Quarterly.

Guidelines to Professional Pharmacy. Upjohn Company. Quarterly.

Lilly Digest. Eli Lilly & Company. 1933–. Annual.

M & B Pharmaceutical Bulletin. 1952–. 4/year.

NACDS—Lilly Digest, a Survey of Chain Pharmacy Operations. Eli Lilly & Company. 1971–. Annual.

PMA Annual Report. Pharmaceutical Manufacturers Association.

PMA Bulletin. Pharmaceutical Manufacturers Association.

PMA Newsletter. Pharmaceutical Manufacturers Association. 1959–. Weekly.

PMA News Releases. Pharmaceutical Manufacturers Association.

Psychiatric Spectator. Sandoz Pharmaceuticals. 1963–.

Rohm and Haas Reporter. 1943–. Quarterly.

Tile and Till. Eli Lilly & Company. 1915–. Quarterly.

Triangle. Sandoz Pharmaceuticals. 1952–. 3/year.

Wellcome Trends in Pharmacy. Burroughs Wellcome Company. 1973–. Quarterly. There is also a hospital pharmacy edition.

White Sheet; Hospital Pharmacy. Philips Roxane Laboratories. 1967–. Monthly.

MONOGRAPHS

Pharmaceutical firms also publish monographic material. One such example is *Scope Monographs,* published by the Upjohn Company in Kalamazoo, Michigan, since 1958. This series of monographs covers such health related topics as cytology, nutrition, vitamins. Another example of monographic publication by a pharmaceutical company is the *Ciba Symposium Series.* This prolific series is available to libraries directly through Ciba. For more information see chapter 19.

CHAPTER 22 NONPRINT MATERIALS

Various types of information sources are currently available in nonprint formats. Numerous current reports, documents, journals, and so on are now also available as microforms, for a broad range of reasons, including the convenience of storage, accessibility, economy, and durability. Nonprint materials of all kinds are enjoying an increasingly important role in the development and dissemination of medical and scientific information. They have also been considered an important adjunct to the conventional materials in the process of medical education and continuing education. In the fields of health sciences, National Medical Audiovisual Center (NMAC, part of the National Library of Medicine) has been the most important organization for coordinating all the activities related to medical audiovisual materials. The most essential tool for health sciences professionals from NMAC is the following:

National Medical Audiovisual Center Catalog; Audiovisuals for the Health Scientists, 1977, DHEW Pub. no. (NIH) 75-506. **US National Medical Audiovisual Center.** Washington, DC: US Government Printing Office, 1977.

First edition, 1968. Earlier title: *National Medical Audiovisual Center Motion Picture and Videotape Catalog.*
An alphabetical listing of audiovisuals available for loan to professional educational programs; geared toward the health scientist. Includes full bibliographic information in the name/title section. Annotated description on technical quality, currency, educational level, accuracy, etc., is also available. MeSH headings are used in the subject section. All titles are available through AVLINE. A major tool for all medical libraries.
R: *ARBA* (1978, p. 708); MRW S1, p. 13; MRW S3, pp. 4, 27, 32; Win (EK31).

To better understand the activities and services of NMAC, readers are referred to:

National Medical Audiovisual Center of the National Library of Medicine; Overview. Atlanta, GA: NMAC, current.

NMAC has extensive publication programs. Some of their specific catalogs and guides are included in the subject sources listed in the later section of this chapter. Readers are reminded of their training programs and some of the more general publication series, such as the *Case Studies Series* and *Monograph Series.*

NMAC and the Association of American Medical Colleges, aided by the American Association of Dental Colleges, developed the Audio-Visuals On-line (AVLINE) (see chapter 24, Data Bases). The AVLINE data base now has more than 7,000 titles of multimedia educational materials in the health sciences.

Besides NMAC and its publications and services, the following sources, both general and specific, are intended as a selective guide to the nonprint materials.

GENERAL REFERENCE SOURCES

Basic US Government Micrographic Standards and Specifications. **National Microfilm Association.** Silver Spring, MD: NMA, 1976.

This book contains 464 pages providing copies of 23 standards and specifications, in effect all federal government standards and specifications.
R: Chen (p. 417).

Educational Film Locator. **The Consortium of University Film Centers.** New York: Bowker, 1978.

A large 2,178-page volume which provides complete access to educational films, includes 37,000 titles and provides bibliographic information, translated titles, major subject groupings, brief annotations, rental and buying information, and holdings of film libraries. Indexed by author, title, audience level, and foreign title. Useful to educators as a media bibliography.
R: *Previews* 8: 2 (1979).

Educational Media Catalogs on Microfiche. 2 pts. New York: Olympic Media Information, 1978.

Subscription includes updates twice a year. Collection of supplier catalogs, films, filmstrips, audiocassettes.

The Evaluation of Micropublications; A Handbook for Librarians. **A. B. Veaner.** Chicago: American Library Association, 1971.
R: Chen (p. 415).

Guide to Microforms in Print. Washington, DC: NCR Microcard Editions, 1961–. Annual.

Books, journals, etc., available on microforms from US publishers. Does not cover theses and dissertations. For subject approach use *Subject Guide to Microforms in Print.* Washington, DC: NCR Microcard Editions, 1962–1963–, biennial.
R: Chen (p. 415).

Guide to Searching the Biological Literature. **Michael M. King and Linda S. King.** Boca Raton, FL: J. Huley Associates, 1978.

A practical, audiovisual guide to practical aspects of searching the biological literature. A set of 78 visuals in slide format (35mm), including two audio cassettes.
R: *Nature* 276: 538x (Nov. 30, 1978).

International Index to Film Periodicals. New York: Bowker, 1973.
R: Chen (p. 416).

International Index to Multimedia Information. **Audio-Visual Association.** Monterey Park, CA: AVA.

Formerly *Film Review Index.*
R: Chen (p. 416).

Library of Congress Catalog: Motion Pictures and Filmstrips. **US Library of Congress.** Washington, DC: US Government Printing Office. Annual.
R: Chen (p. 416).

Media: Indexes and Review Sources. **Margaret Chisholm.** College Park, MD: University of Maryland Press, 1972.
R: Chen (p. 416).

Media Review Digest. Ann Arbor, MI: Pierian Press. Annual.
Formerly *Multi Media Reviews Index.*
R: Chen (p. 416).

Microfilm Source Book. 1973–1974 ed. New Rochelle, NY: Microfilm Publishing, 1973.
A single-source reference guide to the microfilm industry, including products and services. Gives the sources of supply for every important microfilm service and piece of equipment. Also included are an industrywide name and address section; trademark/trade name reference guide; guide to consultants; list of microfilm publishers and their products; directory of associations and officers; listings of service companies and their services; storage centers; employment services; bibliographies; etc.
R: Chen (p. 416).

Microform Review. Weston, CT: Microform Review, 1972–. Quarterly.
Critical analysis of many new publications, including an abundance of scientific material.
R: Chen (p. 416).

Microforms: The Librarians' View, 1978–79. 2d ed. **Alice H. Bahr.** White Plains, NY: Knowledge Industry, 1978.
First edition, 1976.
A useful update to trends in microforms. Explains the proposed American National Standards Institute (ANSI) microforms standards and their implications for librarians. Covers the five different methods for handling micromaterials. Profusely illustrated.
R: *Journal of Academic Librarianship* (Mar. 1979).

The 1980–81 International Micrographics Source Book. New York: Microfilm Publishing, 1980.
A single-volume directory of international sources for micrographic products, service bureaus, dealers, trade names, publishers, storage centers, etc. Includes bibliography and key word index. A major reference tool for librarians.

Practical Video: The Manager's Guide to Applications. **John A. Bunyan, James C. Crimmins, and N. K. Watson.** White Plains, NY: Knowledge Industry, 1978.
A practical guide on the day-to-day application of video. Case histories and actual user experience are included.

Previews: Audiovisual Software Reviews. Vols. 1–. New York: Bowker, 1972–. Monthly.

A monthly publication which reviews audiovisual materials. Multidisciplinary, the reviews are separated by subject such as consumer education, holidays, etc. Also reviews films and slide tapes related to health and medicine. Useful for medical and undergraduate libraries; provides pertinent annotations indicating audience level.

Princeton Guide to Microforms: Serials. Princeton, NJ: Microfilm Corporation. Annual.

R: Chen (p. 416).

Princeton Telephone Guide to Microforms. Princeton, NJ: Princeton Microfilm Corporation. 1975–1976.

R: Chen (p. 416).

A Reference Guide to Audiovisual Information. **James Limbacher.** New York: Bowker, 1972.

R: Chen (p. 416).

Science Books & Films. **American Association for the Advancement of Science.** Washington, DC: AAAS. Quarterly.

Quarterly review magazine which each year gives reviews of 1,000 new science trade/text books and 250 new 16mm science films. The reviews are both descriptive and critical. Ordering information, nine explicit level designations (kindergarten through professional), and four ratings (highly recommended to not recommended) are also given.

Television and Management: The Manager's Guide to Video. **John Bunyan and James Crimmins.** White Plains, NY: Knowledge Industry, 1977.

The User's Guide to Standard Microfiche Formats. **National Microfilm Association.** Silver Spring, MD: NMA, 1975.

A 16-page illustrated booklet providing accurate descriptions of all standard microfiche formats. Includes the latest NMA, ANSI, DOD, and ISO standards in one publication. A glossary is also provided.

R: Chen (p. 417).

Video in Libraries: A Status Report, 1979–80. 2d ed. **Alice H. Bahr.** White Plains, NY: Knowledge Industry, 1979.

Highlights the current status of library involvement with video and the rationale for offering video services. A helpful guide for any library using or planning to use video.

R: *Computers and the Humanities* (Sept./Oct. 1977); *Video Systems* (Sept. 1977).

The Video Programs Index. 4th ed. **Ken Winslow, ed.** Syosset, NY: The National Video Clearinghouse, 1979.

Covers subjects, formats, and rental/purchase information for some 400 major video program distributors.

The Video Register, 1979–80. White Plains, NY: Knowledge Industry, 1979.

Lists major users in business, government, health, education, with names, addresses; manufacturers of nonbroadcast video gear; dealers, production/post-production houses and other service companies; and video producers/publishers/distributors who have programs for sale or rent.

The Video Source Book. Syosset, NY: The National Video Clearinghouse, 1979.

Lists some 15,000 video titles and their descriptions, producers, casts, ratings, and awards. Includes directory information on distributors. Indexed by subject and title.
R: *LJ* 105: 601 (March 1, 1980).

AV EQUIPMENT

The Audio-Visual Equipment Directory. Fairfax, VA: National Audio-Visual Association. Annual.

Twenty-second edition, 1976–1977.
The only comprehensive, up-to-date AV equipment guide. Contains information on over 2,000 currently available audiovisual equipment items. There are over 1,500 photographs.
R: Chen (p. 417).

Audiovisual Market Place: A Multimedia Guide. 9th ed. New York: Bowker, 1979. Annual.

Now an annual, quick reference guide. Consists of three major areas: AV software, hardware, and reference sources. Listings provide company names, addresses, and product lines. Contains 5,000 entries arranged within 25 sections. Classified indexes.
R: Chen (p. 417).

Buyer's Guide to Microfilm Equipment, Products, and Services, 1979. Silver Spring, MD: National Microfilm Association, 1979. Annual.
R: Chen (p. 417).

Buyer's Guide to Micrographic Equipment, Products, and Services. Silver Spring, MD: National Microfilm Association, 1979. Annual.

A listing of sustaining members of NMA by product and service. Designed as a concise introduction and continuing reference for present and potential users of micrographic equipment, products, and services.
R: Chen (p. 417).

A Guide to Microforms and Microform Retrieval Equipment. **M. McKay.** Washington, DC: Applied Library Resources, 1972.
R: Chen (p. 417).

Guide to Micrographic Equipment. 6th ed. 3 vols. **National Microfilm Association.** Silver Spring, MD: NMA, 1975.

Volume 1, *Production Equipment* (cameras, processors, duplicators, and inspection apparatus); volume 2, *User Equipment* (readers, reader-printers, enlargers, and automatic retrieval units); volume 3, *COM Recorders.*
Illustrated directories provide specifications, prices, and pictures of micrographic equipment.
R: Chen (p. 417).

Index to Producers and Distributors. **National Information Center for Educational Media.** Los Angeles: NICEM, 1971.
R: Chen (p. 417).

The International File of Micrographics Equipment & Accessories 1979–1980. **William Saffady, comp.** Westport, CT: Microform Review, 1979.
A vendor catalog of micrographic equipment providing information on micrographic equipment, from automated storage and retrieval systems to fiche readers. Contains complete information, an index for easy access to information. A detailed source, listing all significant micrographic equipment worldwide.

MICROFORM INFORMATION SERVICES

There are numerous firms and institutions which provide information services on microforms, such as the following listed sources from Micromedex, Inc. in Englewood, Colorado, and others:

Drugdex. Englewood, CO: Micromedex, Inc.
Monographs on drugs and groups of drugs. Available in microfiche. Subscription service provides most up to date information.

Iowa Drug Information Service. **University of Iowa, College of Pharmacy.** Iowa City, IO: University of Iowa. Annual.
In microfiche format.

Paul deHaen Information Systems. Englewood, CO: Micromedex, Inc.
A subscription, current awareness service, provides up-to-date information on new drugs, adverse drug effects, drug research. Comprehensive monthly updates, available in microfiche.

Poisindex. Englewood, CO: Micromedex, Inc.
A computer-generated index which provides up-to-date information on toxic plants and products. Available in microfiche.

SUBJECT SOURCES

General

AAAS Audiotape Cassette Album Series. Washington, DC: American Association for the Advancement of Science.
R: Chen (p. 418).

AAAS Science Books and Films. Washington, DC: American Association for the Advancement of Science. Quarterly.

Reviews approximately 1,000 new science books as well as over 250 new science films produced by commercial firms, universities, and government agencies each year. A quick and reliable source for the evaluation of the latest science books and films.
R: Chen (p. 418).

AAAS Science Film Catalog. **Ann Seltz-Petrash, ed.** New York: Bowker, 1975.

Comprehensive listing of some 5,600 films devoted to the pure, applied, and social sciences that can be bought, related, or borrowed from 150 US producers and distributors.
R: Chen (p. 418).

Bibliography of Audiotapes and Tape-Slide Programs Applicable to Undergraduate Medical Education. **Helene Zubkoff, comp.** Washington, DC: George Washington University, 1973.

A bibliography of slide tape and audiotape materials of undergraduate education, covering a wide range of topics and listing material on each topic. A handy reference source, identifying all appropriate sources; a good aid for instructors. Indexed.
R: *ARBA* (1975, p. 736).

Health: A Multimedia Source Guide. **Joan Ash.** New York: Bowker, 1976.

Some 650 sources for the acquisition of print and nonprint materials.

Health Educator's International Guide to Free and Low Cost Audiovisual Teaching/Training Aids. Long Island City, NY: Pharmaceutical Communications, 1977/1978–. Annual.

More than 600 entries in the first edition. Divided into two sections: lists of advanced and technical items that will be of interest to postgraduate teaching; and lists of those items which appeal more to paramedical groups.

Health Policy Cassette Series. Vols. 3–5. **Science and Health Publications.** Washington, DC: Science and Health Publications, 1973.

Volume 3, *Impoundment of Health Funds in the Nixon Administration*; volumes 4 and 5, *The Administration's Views on Health Policy.*
Cassette tapes of interviews with health organization leaders and their attorneys as they discuss the impoundment of health funds in the Nixon Administration. Explains political, legal, and constitutional issues surrounding the impoundment.

The Health Sciences Video Directory 1977. **Lawrence Eidelberg, ed.** New York: Shelter Books, 1977. Also quarterly supplements in 1978 by Esselte Video, New York.

From 1979, superceded by *Videolog: Programs for the Health Sciences.* Annual.
A catalog of video programs in the health sciences. Includes material from a wide range of topics such as dentistry, nursing, psychology, public health, patient

education. Includes 4,400 programs, listed alphabetically by title, producer name, subscription service, and subject. Each title is cross-referenced with the mesh. A useful reference work intended for college and graduate level programs.
R: *Journal of Allied Health* 6: 68 (Spring 1977); *BL* 74: 636 (Dec. 1, 1977); *Choice* 14: 513 (June 1977); *LJ* 102: 902 (Apr. 15, 1977); *ARBA* (1978, p. 715); Sheehy (EK5).

Helpis-Medical: A Catalogue of Audio-Visual and Other Educational Materials in Medicine and Allied Fields Produced by Institutions of Higher Education in the United Kingdom. **Higher Education Learning Programmes Information Service.** London: Council for Educational Technology for the United Kingdom, 1974.
Lists films and other audiovisual educational materials for medical institutions. Supplies producer name and all other pertinent information. Considered useful in Great Britain and the United States.
R: *RSR* 3: 31 (Apr.–June 1975).

Index of Audiovisual Serials in the Health Sciences. **Medical Library Association.** Chicago, IL: Medical Library Association. Quarterly. On microfiche.

The Management of 35mm Medical Slides. **Alfred Strohlein.** New York: United Business Publications, 1975.
Discusses all aspects of slide collection management.
R: *Special Libraries* 66: 610 (1975).

Medical-Health Film Library. **American Medical Association.** Chicago, IL: American Medical Association, 1972.
A subject listing of films for medical schools, hospitals, and professional societies.
R: Win (EK29).

Multi-Media Medicine. Vols. 1–. **American College of Physicians.** Philadelphia, PA: American College of Physicians, 1979–. Monthly.
This is the upgraded, expanded sequel to ACP's popular *Self-Learning Series*. A flexible teaching/learning tool with the choice of microfiche or 35mm slides to accompany the monograph and cassette. Each component communicates a whole topic independently. Some of the topics covered are *Update on Mycotic Infections; Common Hepatic Disorders; Noninvasive Cardiac Diagnosis; Changing Concepts of Platelet Function;* and *Congestive Heart Failure.*

NICEM Index to Health and Safety Education—Multimedia. 4th ed. **National Information Center for Educational Media** (NICEM). Los Angeles, CA: National Information Center for Educational Media, 1979.
Alphabetical guide to titles and series; subject guide directory of producers and distributors. Covers eight different media forms.

1970 Film Reference Guide for Medicine and Allied Sciences. **Federal Advi-**

sory Council on Medical Training Aids, comp. **US National Library of Medicine.** Washington, DC: US Government Printing Office, 1971.

Alphabetically arranged by title; a list of films useful in medical education. Contains subject index. Supplies full information and physical description of film.
R: *ARBA* (1972, p. 612); Win (EK30).

Non-Print Resources; A Union List of Health Science Materials in Connecticut. **Carol Thomsen, project coordinator.** Farmington, CT: University of Connecticut, Health Center, Department of Biomedical Communications, 1974–.

Reviews of Medical Motion Pictures. **American Medical Association.** Chicago, IL: American Medical Association, 1968.

Sources of Medical Motion Pictures. **American Medical Association.** Chicago, IL: American Medical Association, 1968.

Videolog: Programs for the Health Sciences. **Lawrence Eidelberg, ed.** New York: Esselte Video, 1979.

Walter Reed Army Medical Center Television Videotape Catalog. 4th ed. **Walter Reed Army Medical Center, US Department of Defense.** Washington, DC: US Government Printing Office, 1975.

Consists of 350 videotape programs that deal with medical and dental problems. Subject arrangement; covers all cogent matters related to health care.
R: *RSR* 4: 107 (Oct.–Dec. 1976).

ANATOMY

Stereoscopic Atlas of Human Anatomy. **David L. Bassett.** St. Louis, MO: C. V. Mosby, 1978.

Eight sections comprised of 23 volumes. A stereoscopic atlas with 3,318 pages of labeled drawings and explanatory text. It covers all regions of the body. The 1,554 stereoscopic color photographs in AV formats can be viewed through different viewing equipment.

ANESTHESIOLOGY AND GENERAL SURGERY

Audio Journal Review: General Surgery. Vol. 8. **Robert N. McClelland, ed.** New York: Grune & Stratton, 1979.

A monthly audio tape service that reviews medical literature of specific fields. Provides balanced, critical accounts in an hour-long cassette which has twelve to fifteen abstracts. Useful for busy physicians and surgeons in helping them keep abreast of medical literature.

Davis and Geck Surgical Film Catalog, 1969–1970. Danbury, CT: Davis and Geck, 1969.

Medical and Surgical Motion Pictures: A Catalog of Selected Films. **American Medical Association.** Chicago, IL: American Medical Association, 1969.

Motion Picture Library, 1971–1972. **American College of Surgeons.** Chicago, IL: American College of Surgeons, n.d. Updates.

BRAIN AND NERVOUS SYSTEM

Neurological and Sensory Disease Film Guide, 1966. **US Public Health Service. Audiovisual Facility.** Washington, DC: US Neurological and Sensory Disease Service, 1966.

DENTISTRY

Audiovisual Materials in Dentistry: A Film Catalog. **American Dental Association.** Chicago, IL: American Dental Association, 1969.

HEALTH SERVICES ADMINISTRATION

AHA Film Catalog. **American Hospital Association.** Chicago, IL: American Hospital Association, 1974, and updates.

Hospital/Health Care Training Media Profiles, Volume One. Rev. ed. New York: Olympic Media Information, 1975.
A loose-leaf volume of reviews of audiovisual aids. Covers many topics, including nursing, anatomy, physiology, management, public health, medical ethics, etc. Reviews are informative, well written, and include full information. Intended for health educators.
R: *ARBA* (1976, p. 732).

Media Handbook: A Guide to Selecting, Producing, and Using Media For Patient Education. **American Hospital Association.** Chicago, IL: American Hospital Association, 1978.
For hospital staff; helps to guide in selecting programs for patient education. Covers a wide range of situations in educational programs.
R: *Hospitals* 53: 44 (May 16, 1979).

INFECTIOUS DISEASES

Drugs and Microbes. **US Food and Drug Administration.** Released by Washington, DC: National Audiovisual Center, 1972.
Sixty-two color slides and taped narrations provide an introduction to microorganisms. Deals with personal hygiene and cleaning of equipment.

Topics in Clinical Microbiology. **Richard R. Clark, ed.** Baltimore, MD: Williams & Wilkins, 1976.
An audiovisual training program in microbiology. Covers gram negative and positive bacteria, acid-fast bacteria, disease agents. A manual accompanies the thirty-minute cassettes and color slides. Highly recommended for medical technologists.

NURSING

Audio-Visual Color Films from the Frances Payne Bolton School of Nursing.

Case Western Reserve University. Chicago, IL: Year Book Medical Publishers.

Lists both 8mm and 16mm films; covers all levels of nursing.

Audiovisuals. **American Journal of Nursing Company. Educational Services Division.** New York: American Journal of Nursing Company. Annual.

American Journal of Nursing Company is a major company supplying nursing audiovisual materials. Many of them are used for patient care and education, and nursing education and continuing education. Some of the sample series are *Critical Care Nursing* (eight video cassettes), *Current Drug Therapy: Nursing Focus* (six audiocassettes); and *Dimensions of Leadership in Nursing* (five course series on 16mm or videotape.)

The Comprehensive Nursing Audiovisual Resource List: 1979. 3 vols. **Marian K. Adrich et al., eds.** Farmington, CT: University of Connecticut Health Center, 1979.

Volume 1, *Subject Index*; volumes 2–3, *Title Index*.

The National Survey of Audiovisual Materials for Nursing, 1968–1969. **American Nurses Association.** New York: American Journal of Nursing Company, 1970.

Nursing Media Index 16mm Films. **Marilynne Sequin, ed.** Toronto, Ontario: Mission Press, 1974.

Nursing Skills and Techniques Film Series. **Luis E. Folgueras and Crystal M. Lange.** Delta College, Department of Nursing. Englewood Cliffs, NJ: Prentice-Hall, 1969.

Single-concept film loops packaged in super 8mm technicolor magi-cartridges. Over 750 brief films (2½ to 4½ minutes) which aim to acquaint nursing students with basic skills and procedures. Series comprehensively illustrates all major procedures. Since 1969, over 500 junior colleges, universities, hospitals, schools of nursing have used the films.

Oncology and Nuclear Medicine

Cancer Film Guide. **US Public Health Service. Cancer Control Board.** Washington, DC: US Public Health Service, Cancer Control Branch.

Ophthalmology

Sights and Sounds in Ophthalmology. Vol. 1. **Arnall Patz, Stuart Fine, and David Orth.** St. Louis, MO: C. V. Mosby, 1976.

Volume 1, *Diseases of the Macula.*
A combined presentation of slides, audiotapes, and text concerning the diseases of the macula. Contains concise information; considered a well-illustrated teaching guide. Also provides self-assessment quizzes for the reader.
R: *American Journal of Ophthalmology* 83: 427 (Mar. 1977).

Orthopedics

Visual Aids Index. **American Academy of Orthopaedic Surgeons.** Chicago, IL: American Academy of Orthopaedic Surgeons, 1970.

Pediatrics

The Pediatric Examination: Art and Process. 2 parts. Videocassettes. **Walter Tunnesson.** Philadelphia, PA: J. B. Lippincott, 1978.

Part 1, *Pre-school: Douglas 4 years, Maria 5 years*; part 2, *School Age: Anne 9 years, Kevin 7 years.*

Pharmacy and Pharmacology

Guide to Films (16 mm) About the Use of Dangerous Drugs, Narcotics, Alcohol and Tobacco (With a Separate Section on Filmstrips). **Daniel Sprecher.** Alexandria, VA: Serina Press, 1971.

An alphabetical arrangement of approximately 300 films and filmstrips; supplies all necessary pertinent data.

R: *MRW* S2, pp. 5, 9, 33, 34, 95.

Psychiatry and Psychology

Current Audiovisuals for Mental Health Education. 2d ed. **Mental Health Materials Center, ed.** Indianapolis, IN: Marquis Academic Media, 1979.

A comparative guide to more than 700 filmstrips and other audiovisuals. Information on evaluations and comparative ratings are given by the Mental Health Materials Center staff. Subject and title index.

Drug Abuse Films. 3d ed. **National Coordinating Council on Drug Education.** Washington, DC: National Coordinating Council on Drug Education, 1973.

A well-organized volume that critically evaluates films, audio recordings, and kits related to drug abuse. Materials named are for professionals who work with drug education; the book is a useful tool for those who need access to these films and audio materials.

R: *ARBA* (1975, p. 750).

Film Reviews in Psychiatry, Psychology and Mental Health: A Descriptive & Evaluative Listing of Educational & Instructional Films. **Robert E. Froelich, ed.** Ann Arbor, MI: Pierian Press, 1974.

R: *RQ* 15: 73 (Fall 1975).

A Guide to Drug Abuse Education & Information Materials, DHEW Pub. no. (HSM) 71-9077. **US National Institute of Mental Health, US Department of Health, Education, and Welfare.** Washington, DC: US Government Printing Office, 1972.

A guide to nonprint materials concerning drug abuse education. Arranged topically; intended for use as an ordering guide and a catalog. Includes directory of lending libraries.

R: *MRW* S3, pp. 17, 18, 26.

Guide to Films on Mental Handicap: A List of Films on All Aspects of Mental Handicap, Classified by Subject and Suggested Audiences. **Thomas A. Pilkington.** London: National Society for Mentally Handicapped Children, 1973.

A catalog of close to 175 16mm films concerning the mentally handicapped. Films are available in Great Britain. Volume includes list of distributors and full description of each film.
R: *MRW* S3, pp. 33, 34.

Mental Health Film Guide. **National Medical Audiovisual Center.** Atlanta, GA: US National Medical Audiovisual Center, 1969.

Lists approximately 400 films alphabetically by title. Includes full data and description of films which were compiled by the International Index of Medical Film Data. Includes annotation.
R: *MRW* S2, pp. 66, 69.

Mental Retardation Film List. **US National Medical Audiovisual Center.** Washington, DC: US Social and Rehabilitation Service, 1967.

Films for professional and nonprofessional audiences; annotated listing.
R: *MRW* S1, p. 19.

A Selected Guide to Audiovisual Materials on Alcohol and Alcoholism. **US National Institute on Alcohol Abuse and Alcoholism, US Department of Health, Education, and Welfare.** Washington, DC: US Government Printing Office, 1974.

A list of films since 1960 on drug abuse and alcoholism. Supplies sale prices, rental fees, distributors.
R: *RSR* 3: 101 (July–Dec. 1975).

Selected Mental Health Audiovisuals. **US National Institute of Mental Health, US Department of Health, Education, and Welfare.** Washington, DC: US Government Printing Office, 1975.

Annotated abstracts of over 2,000 audiovisuals pertaining to mental health. Covers such subjects as delinquency, death and suicide, religion, and aging. Includes sources of film rental, rental libraries, and order information.
R: *RSR* 4: 110 (Oct.–Dec. 1976).

PUBLIC HEALTH

Buyer's Guide to Environmental Media: A Directory of Books, Magazines, Films, and Information Sources. No. 1. New York: Environment Information Center, 1973.

Sources are listed under 21 headings. Broad in coverage.
R: *ARBA* (1975, p. 699); Chen (p. 2).

The Environment Film Review: A Critical Guide to Ecology Films. New York: Environment Information Center, 1972–.

A comprehensive guide to environmental films; basic information on each film, such as length, color or B/W, cost, where to obtain, intended audience, etc. are given. Materials are organized by EIC's 21 major environmental subject classifications. Highly recommended.
R: Chen (p. 418).

Urogenital System

Film Guide on Reproduction and Development. **US National Institute of Child Health and Human Development.** Washington, DC: US Government Printing Office, 1969.

Films listed and evaluated under six main topics in reproduction and developmental biology. Guide supplies full information such as distributor, purchase information, accompanying materials, etc.
R: *ARBA* (1970, p. 135).

Functional Anatomy of the Human Kidney. Smith Kline & French Laboratories.

CHAPTER 23   PROFESSIONAL SOCIETIES AND THEIR PUBLICATIONS

Professional organizations are generally one of the most valuable sources of information for medical subject. Whether as publishers of abstracting and indexing journals, periodicals, monographs, reports or symposia, standards, and so on, or sponsors of conferences, producers of audiovisual materials, etc., professional organizations remain a vital link in medical communication. Useful sources of information on societies and associations and their publications, and sample listing of the names of some major societies themselves are included here for the reader's convenience. It is impossible to list any of the professional societies' and associations' publications since they are so diversified in nature and so numerous in volume. Throughout every chapter of this work, readers will frequently notice the informations sources of this category. They should serve as good illustrations of the importance and value of this type of publication. Readers are advised to request for complete and up-to-date (current-year) catalogs of appropriate societies and associations for appropriate information.

DIRECTORIES

Directory of British Associations. 4th ed. **G. P. and S. P. A. Henderson, eds.** Distr. Detroit, MI: Gale Research, 1974.
R: Chen (p. 420).

Directory of European Associations. **I. G. Anderson, ed.** London: CBD Research, 1971–1975. Distr. Detroit, MI: Gale Research, 1975.
Volume 1, *National Industrial, Trade, and Professional Associations*, 1971; volume 2, *National Learned, Scientific, and Technical Societies*, 1975.
Covers learned, scientific, and technical societies in all countries, excluding Great Britain and Ireland. The latter are included in *Directory of British Associations.*
R: Chen (p. 420).

Directory of National Trade and Professional Associations of the United States, and Buyer's Guide, 1972. Washington, DC: Columbia Books, 1972.
R: Chen (p. 420).

Encyclopedia of Associations. 13th ed. 3 vols. Detroit, MI: Gale Research, 1979.
Volume 1, *National Organizations of the U.S.*; volume 2, *Geographic and Executive Index*; volume 3, *New Associations and Projects.*
A key to "inside" information of 13,589 national organizations of the United States. Organizations are arranged in seventeen subject categories. Information

given in each entry includes the organization's name, address, chief executive, telephone number, purpose and activities, membership, publications, convention schedule, and other pertinent information. Further indexed by geographic area and the executives mentioned. A major directory of organizations.
R: *Food Technology* (Sept. 1977); *Medical Meetings* (Oct. 1977); *American Libraries* (Dec. 1970); *ASLIB Proceedings* (June 1975); *BL* (Oct. 15, 1975); *Choice* (1976); *Herald of Library Science* (Oct. 1974); *LJ* (Dec. 15, 1956); *RQ* (Spring 1973); *RSR* (Jan.–Mar. 1975); *SL* (July 1975); *ARBA* (1971, 1973, 1977).

Guide to World Science Series. 25 vols. St. Peter Port, Guernsey, England: Hodgson, 1974.

Good source to associations and services on international level.
R: Chen (p. 421).

Health Organizations of the United States, Canada and Internationally: A Directory of Voluntary Associations, Professional Societies and Other Groups Concerned With Health and Related Fields. 4th ed. **Paul Wasserman and Jane K. Bossart, eds.** Ann Arbor, MI: Anthony T. Kruzas, 1977.

First edition, 1961; second edition, 1965; third edition, 1974.
Expanded fourth edition of directory which lists about 1,300 societies, foundations, associations, and other nongovernmental organizations in health field. Each entry provides address, telephone number, founding date, principal official, and information on finances, meetings, purposes, activities, and publications. Subject index of 29 pages lists organizations by field, interest or form of association.
R: *American Journal of Public Health* 64: 921 (1974); *BL* 72: 925 (May 1, 1975); *Choice* 3: 19 (Mar. 1966); *RSR* 6: 67 (1978); *WLB* 45: 854 (June 1974); 52: 348 (Dec. 1977); *ARBA* (1976, p. 734); Win (EJ140; EK218; 1EJ26).

Medical and Health Information Directory: A Guide to State, National and International Organizations, Government Agencies, Educational Institutions, Hospitals, Grant-Award Sources, Health Care Delivery Agencies, Journals, Newsletters, Review Serials, Abstracting Services, Publishers, Research Centers, Computerized Data Banks, Audiovisual Services, and Libraries and Information Centers. **Anthony T. Kruzas, ed.** Detroit, MI: Gale Research, 1977.

Reference source contains over 12,000 entries providing basic data on agencies, institutions, companies, and associations concerned with medicine and health care at state and national level. Material is arranged in 32 subject sections and includes biomedical journals, abstracts, books, and computerized information services. Introduction outlines scope and selection criteria for each section. Indexes and references are given. Recommended for public, academic, and medical libraries.
R: *Radiology* 128: 600 (1978); *LJ* 102: 2421 (Dec. 1, 1977); 103: 510 (Mar. 1, 1978); *WLB* 52: 649 (Apr. 1978); *ARBA* (1978, p. 716).

National Trade and Professional Associations of the United States and Canada and Labor Unions. **Craig Colgate, Jr., ed.** Washington, DC: Columbia Books, 1976. Annual.

Complete and up-to-date source of names, addresses, telephone numbers, conference dates, etc. Alphabetical arrangement.
R: Chen (p. 421).

Scientific, Technical, and Related Societies of the United States. 9th ed. Washington, DC: US National Academy of Sciences, 1971.
Seventh edition, 1961; eighth edition, 1968.
Entries include only those membership societies devoted to particular scientific, engineering, and technical disciplines. Descriptive rather than evaluative information.
R: *Choice* 4: 88 (1968); *ARBA* (1972, p. 548); Chen (p. 421); Jenkins (A127); Mal (3-54); Wal (p. 44); Win (EA159; 2EA31).

World Guide to Scientific Associations/Verbande und Gesellschaften der Wisenschaft: Ein internationales Verzeichnis. Munich: Verlag Dokumentation. Distr. New York: Bowker, 1974.
Over 10,000 associations and groups, from all five continents, concerned with scientific research.
R: *Choice* 11: 1459 (Dec. 1974); *LJ* 99: 3124–3125 (Dec. 1, 1974); *ARBA* (1975, p. 641); Chen (p. 421).

World Guide to Trade Associations. (Internationales Verzeichnis der Wirtschaftsverbande). 2 vols. **Michael Zils, ed.** New York: Bowker, 1973.
Information on 26,000 trade and industry-related organizations throughout the world. Detailed subject index.
R: Chen (p. 421).

SOCIETY PUBLICATIONS

Guides

Scientific, Engineering and Medical Societies Publications in Prints, 1978–79. 3d ed. **James M. Matarazzo and James M. Kyed, eds.** New York: Bowker, 1979.
First edition, 1974; second edition, 1976.
A one-stop reference intended to provide coverage of published materials of over 350 US scientific and engineering societies. Provides ordering information.
R: *Choice* 11: 1458 (Dec. 1974); *LJ* 99: 1927 (Aug. 1974); *ARBA* (1975, p. 638); Chen (p. 424).

SELECTIVE LIST OF PROFESSIONAL ORGANIZATIONS

General

American Academy of Family Physicians
1740 W. 92nd Street
Kansas City, MO 64114
(816) 333-9700

American Association for the Advancement of Science (AAAS)
1515 Massachusetts Avenue, NW
Washington, DC 20005

American Association of Medical Assistants
One Wacker Drive
Chicago, IL 60601

American Chemical Society
1155 16th Street NW
Washington, DC 20036
(202) 872-4600

American Institute of Biological Sciences (AIBS)
104 Wilson Boulevard
Arlington, VA 22209

American Medical Association
535 N. Dearborn Street
Chicago, IL 60610
(312) 944-2722

American Medical Students Association
14650 Lee Road
Chantilly, VA
(703) 968-7920

Association for the Advancement of Medical Instrumentation
1901 N. Ft. Myer Drive
Suite 602
Arlington, VA 22209
(103) 525-4890

Federation of American Societies for Experimental Biology (FASEB)
9650 Rockville Pike
Bethesda, MD 20014

International Union of Biological Sciences (IUBS)
51 Boulevard de Montmorecy
F-75016 Paris
France

National Health Federation
PO Box 688
Monororia, CA 91016
(213) 357-2181

National Resident Matching Program
1603 Orrington Avenue
Evanston, IL 60201
(312) 328-3440

Pan American Medical Association
2601 North Flagler Drive
West Palm Beach, FL
(305) 832-4105

Society for Experimental Biology and Medicine
630 West 168th Street
New York, NY 10032
(212) 927-6914

ALLERGY AND IMMUNOLOGY

American Academy of Allergy
611 East Wells Street
Milwaukee, WI 53202
(414) 272-6071

ANESTHESIOLOGY AND GENERAL SURGERY

American Academy of Facial Plastic and Reconstructive Surgery
2800 North Lakeshore Drive
Chicago, IL

American College of Surgeons
55 Erie Street
Chicago, IL 60611
(312) 664-4050

American Society of Abdominal Surgery
675 Main Street
Melrose, MA 02176
(617) 665-6102

American Society of Anesthesiologists
515 Busse Highway
Park Ridge, IL 60060
(312) 825-5586

American Society of Plastic and Reconstructive Surgeons
29 East Madison, Suite 807
Chicago, IL 60602

International Anesthesia Research Society
3645 Warrensville Center Road
Cleveland, OH 44122
(216) 295-1124

International College of Surgeons
1516 North Lake Shore Drive
Chicago, IL 60610
(312) 642-3555

Brain and Nervous System

American Academy of Neurology
4015 West 65th Street, Suite 3024
Minneapolis, MN 55435
(612) 920-3636

United Parkinson Foundation
220 South State Street
Chicago, IL 60604
(312) 922-9734

World Federation of Neurological Society
c/o Dr. Willem Ivyendyk
Academic Hospital
Leiden, Netherlands

Cardiovascular System

American College of Cardiology
911 Old Georgetown Road
Bethesda, MD 20014
(301) 897-5400

American Heart Association
7320 Greenville Avenue
Dallas, TX 75231
(214) 750-5300

American Society of Electroencephalographic Technologists
2997 Moon Lake Drive
West Bloomfield, MI 48033

Dentistry

American Dental Association
211 East Chicago Avenue
Chicago, IL 60611
(312) 440-2500

Dermatology

American Academy of Dermatology
820 Davis Street
Evansville, IL 60201
(312) 869-3954

Endocrinology

American Diabetes Association
600 Fifth Avenue

New York, NY 10020
(212) 541-4310

Gastrointestinal System

American Digestive Disease Society
420 Lexington Avenue
New York, NY 10017

American Gastroenterological Association
6900 Grove Road
Thorofare, NJ
(609) 848-1000

Gerontology

American Geriatrics Society
Ten Columbus Circle
New York, NY 10019
(212) 582-1333

Health Services Administration

American College of Hospital Administration
American Hospital Association
840 North Lake Shore Drive
Chicago, IL 60611
(312) 645-9400

American Hospital Association
840 North Lake Shore Drive
Chicago, IL 60611
(312) 645-9400

Catholic Hospital Association
1438 South Grand Boulevard
St Louis, MO 63104
(314) 773-0646

Hospital Institution and Educational Food Service Society
4410 West Roosevelt Road
Hillside, IL 60167
(312) 644-2770

National Registry of Emergency Medical Technicians
PO Box 29233
Columbus, OH 43229
(614) 888-4484

Hematology

American Association of Blood Banks
1828 L Street, NW
Washington, DC 20036
(202) 872-8333

International Society of Hematology
AP Postal 47-11
Mexico 10 DF
Mexico

National Hemophilia Foundation
25 West 39th Street
New York, NY 10018
(212) 869-9740

Infectious Diseases

Society for Epidemiological Research
811 Vermont Avenue
Washington, DC 20420
(202) 275-1780

Internal Medicine

American Burn Association
New York Hospital, Cornell Medical Center
525 East 68th Street
Room F0758
New York, NY 10021

International Federation of Sportive Medicine
Farnham Park Rehabilitation Center
Farnham Royal
Slough SL2 3LR
England

Nursing

American Academy of Nursing
2420 Pershing Road
Kansas City, MO 64108
(816) 474-5720

American Association of Critical Care Nurses
P.O. Box c-19528
Irvine, CA 92713

American Association of Occupational Health Nursing
575 Lexington Avenue
New York, NY 10022
(212) 355-7733

American Nurses Association
2420 Pershing Road
Kansas City, MO 64108
(816) 474-5620

American Society of Nurse Anesthetists
111 East Wacker Drive
Chicago, IL 60601
(312) 644-3093

National Federation of Licenced Practical Nurses
888 7th Avenue
New York, NY 10019
(212) 246-6629

National League For Nursing
10 Columbus Circle
New York, NY 10019
(212) 582-1022

Nutrition

American Dietetic Association
430 North Michigan Avenue
Chicago, IL 60611
(312) 822-0330

Oncology and Nuclear Medicine

American Cancer Society
777 Third Avenue
New York, NY
(212) 371-2900

American Society of Cytology
Health Sciences Center
130 South Ninth Street
Suite 1006
Philadelphia, PA 19107
(215) 922-3880

National Foundation for Cancer Research
7315 Wisconsin Avenue
Suite 851 W
Bethesda, MD 20014
(301) 654-1250

Society of Nuclear Medicine
475 Park Avenue South
New York, NY 10016
(212) 889-0717

Ophthalmology

American Academy of Ophthalmology and Otolaryngology
15 2nd Street
Rochester, MI
(507) 288-7444

American Optometric Association
2000 Chippewa Street
St Louis, MO 63119
(314) 832-5770

Orthopedics

American Academy of Orthopedic Surgeons
444 North Michigan Avenue
Chicago, IL 60611
(312) 822-0970

Otorhinolaryngology

American Council of Otolaryngology
1100 17th Street, NW
Suite 602
Washington, DC 20036
(202) 659-4591

Pathology

American Society of Clinical Pathologists
2100 West Harrison
Chicago, IL 60612
(312) 738-1336

Pediatrics

American Academy of Pediatrics
1801 Hinman Avenue
Evanston, IL 60204
(312) 869-4255

Pharmacy and Pharmacology

American Pharmaceutical Association
2215 Constitution Avenue, NW
Washington, DC 20037
(202) 628-4410

American Society of Hospital Pharmacists
4630 Montgomery Avenue
Washington, DC 20014
(301) 657-3000

PHYSICAL MEDICINE AND REHABILITATION

American Academy for Cerebral Palsy
1255 New Hampshire Avenue, NW
Washington, DC 20036
(202) 659-8251

American Foundation for the Blind
15 West 16th Street
New York, NY 10011
(212) 924-0420

American Physical Therapy Association
1156 15th Street, NW
Washington, DC 20005
(202) 466-2070

Association for Education of the Visually Handicapped
919 Walnut Street
4th Floor
Philadelphia, PA 19107
(215) 923-7555

National Association for the Deaf
814 Thayer Avenue
Silver Spring, MD 20910
(301) 587-1788

National Federation of the Blind
PO Box 4422
Baltimore, MD 21223
(301) 727-6166

National Foundation-March of Dimes
1275 Mamaroneck Avenue
White Plains, NY 10605
(914) 428-7100

PSYCHIATRY AND PSYCHOLOGY

American Association on Mental Deficiency
5101 Wisconsin Avenue
Washington, DC 20016
(202) 686-5400

American Psychiatric Association
1700 18th Street, NW
Washington, DC 20009
(202) 797-4900

National Society for Autistic Children
169 Tampa Avenue
Albany, NY 12208
(518) 489-7375

PUBLIC HEALTH

American Occupational Medical Association
150 North Wacker Drive
Chicago, IL 60605
(312) 782-2166

American Public Health Association
1015 18th Street, NW
Washington, DC 20036
(202) 467-5000

Health Physics Society
4720 Montegomery Lane
Bethesda, MD 20014
(301) 654-3080

National Environmental Health Association
1200 Lincoln Street
Suite 704
Denver, CO 80203
(313) 861-9090

RADIOLOGY

American College of Radiology
20 North Wacker Drive
Chicago, IL 60605
(312) 236-4963

RESPIRATORY SYSTEM

American Lung Association
1740 Broadway
New York, NY 10019
(212) 245-8000

RHEUMATOLOGY

American Rheumatism Association
The Arthritis Foundation
3400 Peachtree Road NE
Atlanta, GA
(404) 226-0795

Urogenital System

American College of Obstetricians and Gynecologists
One Wacker Drive
Chicago, IL 60601
(312) 222-1600

International Childbirth Education Association
PO Box 20852
Milwaukee, WI 53220
(612) 381-9194

Veterinary Medicine

American Society for Laboratory Animal Science
2317 West Jefferson Street
Suite 208
Joliet, IL 60435

American Veterinary Medical Association
930 North Meachem Road
Schaumburg, IL 60196
(312) 885-8070

Other Organizations

Aerospace Medical Association
Washington National Airport
Washington, DC 20001
(703) 892-2240

American Chiropractic Association
2200 Grand Avenue
Des Moines, IA 50312
(515) 243-1121

American Osteopathic Association
212 East Ohio Street
Chicago, IL 60611
(312) 944-2713

CHAPTER 24   DATA BASES

There is no need to elaborate the importance of data bases for those who are concerned with medical information. The following are good examples of sources of information data bases:

DIRECTORY SOURCES

Computer-Readable Data Bases: A Directory and Data Sourcebook, 1979 ed. **Martha E. Williams, ed.** White Plains, NY: Knowledge Industry, 1979.
Earlier edition, 1976.
List more than 500 data bases worldwide. Each entry contains the name and producer of the data base, its coverage, year of origin, number of items in the base, availability in batch or on-line mode, pricing, and other information. Indexed by subect, producer, processor, and data base name. Useful tool for users of data bases, producers of data bases, and information suppliers, students, and teacher.
R: Chen (p. 428).

The Directory of On-Line Data Bases. Vols. 1–. Santa Monica, CA: Cuadra, 1979–. Quarterly.
Includes six types of data bases: bibliographic, referral, numeric, numeric-textual, chemical, and physical properties. Describes producer, content, availability, and frequency of update.

EVALUATION OF DATA BASES

For information on the evaluation of data bases, and information retrieval systems, the following sources should be consulted:

Information Retrieval: On Line. **F. Wilfrid Lancaster.** Los Angeles: Melville, 1973.
R: Chen (p. 428).

Information Retrieval Systems; Characteristics, Testing, and Evaluation. **F. Wilfrid Lancaster.** New York: John Wiley, 1968.
R: Chen (p. 428).

NATIONAL LIBRARY OF MEDICINE

The most important medical information organization dealing with the organization and dissemination of medical information is the National Library of Medicine (NLM). NLM is both the producer and processor of a great many on-line data bases of vital importance not only to researchers in medicine but also to those in related scientific fields.

To familiarize the readers with its computerized literature retrieval services, the following information is taken from DHEW Pub. no. (NIH) 79-1286 (revised January 1979), entitled *MEDLARS: The Computerized Literature Retrieval Services of the National Library of Medicine.* This brochure describes for potential users the Library's computer-based literature retrieval services. These services represent but one of the Library's many information programs for the benefit of the health community.

Brief Introduction of the National Library of Medicine

The National Library of Medicine (NLM) is a part of the National Institutes of Health, one of the six health agencies of HEW's Public Health Service. The Library was established in 1836 as the Library of the Army Surgeon General's Office and it remained in the military until 1956, when it was transferred to the Department of Health, Education, and Welfare and upgraded to be the National Library of Medicine.

NLM is the world's largest research library in a single scientific and professional field. Its holdings include over 2,500,000 books, journals, technical reports, theses, microfilms, and pictorial and audiovisual materials. Housed in the Library is one of the nation's largest medical history collections, with contents dating from the eleventh to the mid-nineteenth century.

Computerized Literature Retrieval Services of the National Library of Medicine

Persons studying or working in the health sciences have access to the professional literature by means of a computerized system known as MEDLARS (a registered acronym for Medical Literature Analysis and Retrieval System). Based at the National Library of Medicine in Bethesda, Maryland, MEDLARS is available through a nationwide NLM network of centers at more than 900 universities, medical schools, hospitals, government agencies, and commercial organizations.

MEDLARS contains some 4,500,000 references to journal articles and books in the health sciences published after 1965. Most of these references have been published via MEDLARS in *Index Medicus* or in other printed NLM indexes and bibliographies. This same computer system also makes it possible for an individual user to search the store of references and to produce a list of them pertinent to a specific question.

Terminals (keyboard devices that look like typewriters) at each of the 900 institutions are connected via commercial networks of telephone lines to the Library's IBM 370/158 computers. To retrieve references, a user carries on a "dialog" with the computer, refining the search by typing in successive queries until the needed references are identified and printed out at the terminal. Such an "online" search, as it is called, usually takes about ten to fifteen minutes.

There are a number of online data bases available through the online network, such as MEDLINE (MEDLARS online), the largest and most frequently used.

References may be retrieved by searching on one or a combination of the 14,000 designated Medical Subject Headings (MeSH®) used by NLM in indexing and cataloging materials. It is also possible to search for references by using words appearing in titles and abstracts. The computer's ability to search rapidly through a large number of references to see which meet the specified criteria results in an individualized bibliography that would not be possible except by the most laborious and time-consuming manual search.

The requestor may ask that the complete record be printed out for each reference retrieved—including the subject headings and abstract—or that a less detailed format include only the elements necessary to locate the item: author, title, and publication source.

Articles or books identified by computer search at the online center may be requested through that institution's library. Requests for items not available locally are routed through an established network of eleven Regional Medical Libraries (see list). The National Library of Medicine provides copies or original loans of material that cannot be found in local or Regional Medical Libraries.

The online search service is available to health practitioners, researchers, educators, sutdents—anyone faced with the difficult task of searching through the scientific and professional literature related to health. At many online centers the librarian will do the search for the requestor; at others, users may be encouraged to do their own searches after some preliminary instruction. Complicated or difficult searches are best left to the center's specialists who have been trained in the techniques of searching.

The charge for a search varies among centers. Some absorb all or most of the costs, others levy a modest fee to recover the communication cost they incur for time connected to the NLM computers and for staff time. If a search results in an extensive bibliography that would be time-consuming (and therefore expensive) to print out at the terminal, it can be printed less expensively offline at NLM and mailed the next morning. The online center may recover the per page charge for offline prints from the requestor.

Regional Medical Libraries

Eleven Regional Medical Libraries, each responsible for a geographic area, coordinate NLM's online search services in the United States. These libraries also handle requests for health literature not available locally, passing on to NLM requests they cannot fill. To find out the nearest Online Center, or how your institution can become a Center, write to the Regional Medical Library for your area.

Region I
New England Regional Medical Library Service (Connecticut, Massachusetts, Maine, New Hampshire, Rhode Island, and Vermont)
Francis A. Countway Library of Medicine
Harvard University
10 Shattuck St, Boston, MA 02115

Online Centers with Access to NLM Data Bases

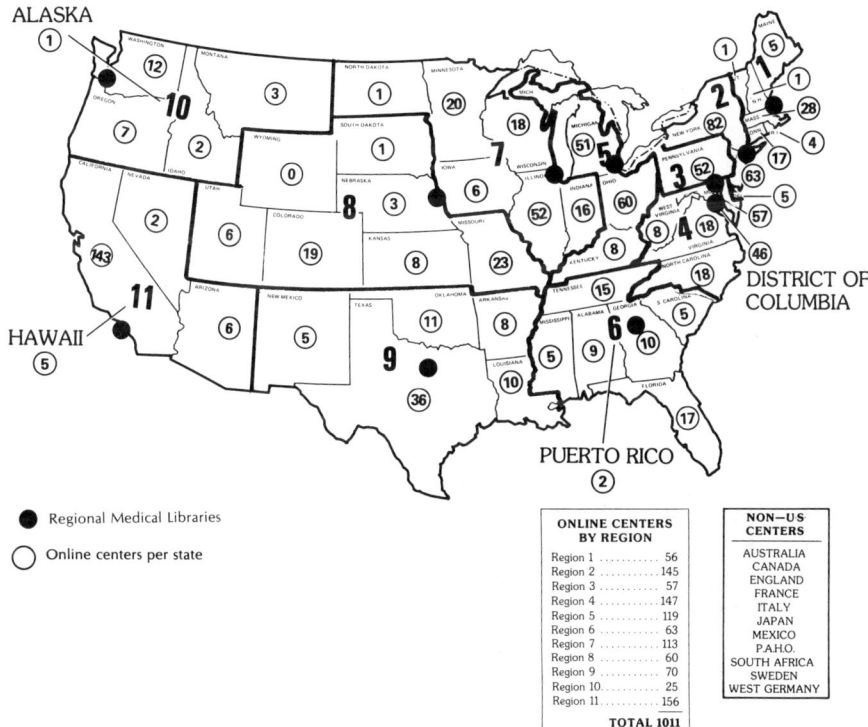

Region II
New York and New Jersey Regional Medical Library
New York Academy of Medicine Library
2 E 103 St, New York, NY 10029

Region III
Mideastern Regional Medical Library Service (Delaware and Pennsylvania)
Library of the College of Physicians
19 S 22 St, Philadelphia, PA 19103

Region IV
Mid-Atlantic Regional Medical Library (District of Columbia, Maryland, North Carolina, Virgina, and West Virginia)
National Library of Medicine
8600 Rockville Pike, Bethesda, MD 20014

Region V
Kentucky-Ohio-Michigan Regional Medical Library Program
Wayne State University
Shiffman Medical Library
4325 Brush St, Detroit, MI 48201

Region VI
Southeastern Regional Medical Library Program (Alabama, Florida, Georgia, Mississippi, South Carolina, Tennessee, and Puerto Rico)
AW Calhoun Medical Library
Emory University, Atlanta, GA 30322

Region VII
Midwest Health Sciences Library Network (Iowa, Illinois, Indiana, Minnesota, North Dakota, and Wisconsin)
John Crerar Library
33 W 33 St, Chicago, IL 60616

Region VIII
Midcontinental Regional Medical Library Program (Colorado, Kansas, Missouri, Nebraska, South Dakota, Utah, and Wyoming)
Library of Medicine
University of Nebraska Medical Center
Omaha, NB 68105

Region IX
South Central Regional Medical Library Program (Arkansas, Louisiana, New Mexico, Oklahoma, and Texas)
University of Texas Health Science Center
5323 Harry Hines Blvd, Dallas, TX 75235

Region X
Pacific Northwest Regional Health Sciences Library (Alaska, Idaho, Montana, Oregon, and Washington)

University of Washington Health Sciences Library
Seattle, WA 98195

Region XI
Pacific Southwest Regional Medical Library Service (Arizona, California, Hawaii, and Nevada)
Biomedical Library
Center for the Health Sciences
University of California at Los Angeles
Los Angeles, CA 90024

NLM ONLINE SERVICES PROGRAM POLICY STATEMENT

Consistent with its legislative mandate and recommendations of the Board of Regents, the National Library of Medicine (NLM) is committed to the development and operation of a domestic online services network. The objectives of the network are to provide rapid and efficient delivery of bibliographic and other literature-based information; cost effective online services complemented by efficient document delivery through participating members; equal network access, to the extent practicable, while serving the basic purpose of support to health services delivery, education, and research.

Service Policies

General
  The NLM exercises overall management and provides supporting services such as training and assistance to users. The Regional Medical Libraries (RML) plan and support online and network services in their regions.

Qualified Users
  Qualified institutional users include Regional Medical Libraries and Resource Libraries; hospitals and institutions with health-science education and training programs; health-related research organizations, government agencies, universities, and library and information science schools; other organizations with health-related needs that can be accommodated within the system's capacity.
  Individuals are encouraged to use the system through established institutional centers, but may apply for access codes in unusual cases.
  In the case of an overload of the system, service may be limited and the addition of new users suspended by NLM management.

Responsibilities of Members
  Online centers agree to send at least one individual for training in the use of NLM's online system. NLM reserves the right to waive training

for qualified individuals who demonstrate significant online experience or on-the-job training.

Service costs may be passed on to the individual requester. Where charges are imposed, they must clearly distinguish that portion which is a result of NLM connect-hour and page costs from the charges levied by the network participants.

Prices

Consistent with the National Library of Medicine Act, the Board of Regents has established a domestic pricing policy permitting NLM to recover costs associated with the direct provision of services. Such costs include communications, back-up computer services, and the use fees for data bases from other organizations. The Board of Regents has delegated to the Director of the National Library of Medicine the authority to set prices at the level required to ensure effective and efficient management of the system. To the extent practicable, such costs recovered from member institutions will be independent of their geographic location.

Data Bases Available on the Online Network

AVLINE (Audiovisuals Online) contains citations to some 6,000 audiovisual teaching packages used in health sciences education at the college level and for the continuing education of practitioners. All titles in AVLINE are screened for technical quality; all but lecture-type recordings are also reviewed for currency, content accuracy, and teaching effectiveness. AVLINE may be searched by words in abstracts, medical subject headings, titles, names, source, and elements of physical description such as medium and playing time. Entry date: 1970–.

BIOETHICSLINE is a file of about 6,500 references to materials on bioethical topics such as euthanasia, human experimentation, and abortion. They are selected from the literature of the health sciences, philosophy, law, religion, psychology, and from the popular media. BIOETHISCLINE is produced in cooperation with the Kennedy Institute of Ethics, Center for Bioethics, at Georgetown University. Entry date: 1973–.

CANCERLIT (Cancer Literature), formerly called CANCERLINE, is sponsored by NIH's National Cancer Institute (NCI) and contains more than 140,000 references dealing with various aspects of cancer. All references have English abstracts. Over 3,000 US and foreign journals, as well as selected monographs, meeting papers, reports, and dissertations are abstracted for inclusion in CANCERLIT. Entry date: 1977.

CANCERPROJ (Cancer Research Projects), also sponsored by NCI, contains 20,000 descriptions of ongoing cancer research projects from the current and two preceding years. The descriptions are provided by cancer researchers in many countries and are collected for NCI by the Smithsonian Science Information Exchange. Entry date: 1977–.

CATLINE® (Catalog Online) contains about 200,000 references to books and serials cataloged at NLM since 1965. CATLINE gives medical libraries in the network immediate access to authoritative cataloging information, thus reducing the need for these libraries to do their own original cataloging. Libraries also find this data base a useful source of information for ordering books and journals and for providing reference and interlibrary loan services. Entry date: 1965–.

CHEMLINE® (Chemical Dictionary Online) is a file of 760,000 names for chemical substances, representing 380,000 unique compounds. CHEMLINE, created by NLM in collaboration with Chemical Abstracts Service (CAS), contains such information as CAS Registry Numbers, molecular formulas, preferred chemical nomenclature, and generic and trivial names. The file may be searched by any of these elements and also by nomenclature fragments, making chemical structure searches possible. Entry date: 1977–.

CLINPROT (Clinical Cancer Protocols) is another NCI-sponsored data base. It contains summaries of clinical investigations of new anticancer agents and treatment techniques. Entry date: 1976.

EPILEPSYLINE is sponsored by NIH's National Institute of Neurological and Communicative Disorders and Stroke. The file contains about 25,000 references and abstracts to articles on epilepsy that have been abstracted by Excerpta Medica.

Two subsidiary online files that support the bibliographic data bases are the Name Authority File (an authority list of about 100,000 personal names, corporate names, and decisions on how monographic series are classed), and the MeSH Vocabulary File (information on 14,000 Medical Subject Headings—main headings and qualifiers—used for indexing and retrieving references). Entry date: 1977–.

HEALTH PLANNING & ADMIN (Health Planning and Administration) contains about 100,000 references to literature on health planning, organization, financing, management, manpower, and related subjects. The references are from journals indexed for MEDLINE, *Hospital Literature Index,* and other journals selected for their emphasis on health care matters. This data base will eventually also contain references to nonserial items such as books and technical reports.

HISTLINE (History of Medicine Online) contains some 35,000 references to articles, monographs, symposia, and other publications dealing with the history of medicine and related sciences. This data base is the source of NLM's annual *Bibliography of the History of Medicine*. Although there are selected references back to 1964, most of the material cited in the HISTLINE file was published after 1970. Entry date: 1970–.

MEDLINE contains approximately 600,000 references to biomedical journal articles published in the current and two preceding years. An English abstract, if published with the article, is frequently included. The articles are from 3,000 journals published in the United States and 70 foreign countries; MEDLINE also includes a limited number of chapters and articles from selected monographs. Coverage of previous periods (back to 1966) is provided by backfiles that total some 2,250,000 references.

MEDLINE can also be used to update a search periodically. The search formulation is stored in the computer and each month, when new references are added to the data base, the search is processed automatically and the results mailed from NLM. Entry date: Last 2–3 years; backfiles 1966–.

RTECS (*Registry of Toxic Effects of Chemical Substances,* formerly the *Toxic Substances List*) is an annual compilation prepared by the National Institute for Occupational Safety and Health. RTECS contains toxicity data for approximately 31,600 substances. Threshold limit values, recommended standards in air, and aquatic toxicity data are also included in this file. Entry date: 1977–.

SERLINE (Serials Online) contains bibliographic information for about 30,000 serial titles, including all journals which are on order or cataloged for the NLM collection. For one-fifth of these, SERLINE has locator information for the user to determine which US medical libraries own a particular journal. SERLINE is used by librarians to obtain information needed to order journals and to refer interlibrary loan requests. Entry date: 1965–.

TDB (Toxicology Data Bank) contains chemical, pharmacological, and toxicological information and data on approximately 1,000 substances. Information on an additional 1,500 substances is being prepared. Data for the TDB are extracted from handbooks and textbooks and reviewed by a peer review group of subject specialists.

TOXLINE® (Toxicology Information Online) is a collection of 520,000 references from the last five years on published human and animal toxicity studies, effects of environmental chemicals and pollutants, and adverse drug reactions. Older material (400,000 references) is in TOXBACK. Almost all references in TOXLINE have abstracts or indexing terms, and most chemical compounds mentioned in TOXLINE are further identified with Chemical Abstracts Service Registry Numbers. The references are from five major published secondary sources and five special literature collections maintained by other organizations. Entry date: 1970–.

TOOLS FOR THE USE OF NLM DATA BASES

Medical Subject Headings, Annotated Alphabetic List, 1979, PB-285 356. **US National Library of Medicine.** Washington, DC: US Government Printing Office, 1979. Annual update.

Expanded version of *Medical Subject Headings,* currently used by indexers, catalogers, and seachers of the NLM computer data bases. Highly recommended to all MEDLINE users.
R: *RSR* 6: 55 (Apr.–June 1978).

Medical Subject Headings, Three Structures, 1979, PB-270 945, DHEW Pub. no. (NIH) 79-265. **US National Library of Medicine.** Washington, DC: US Government Printing Office, 1978. Annual update.

Lists all medical subject headings currently used by indexers, catalogers, and searchers at the National Library of Medicine. Arrangement by hierarchy, showing relationships between broader and narrower terms.
R: *RSR* 6: 55 (Apr.–June 1978).

SELECTIVE DATA BASES

There are numerous commercial vendors of data bases. The largest are Lockheed Information Systems (Lockheed), which provides access to more than 35 data bases, and System Development Corporation (SDC) Search Service, with access to about 30 data bases. Since the rates for these data bases vary greatly from one to another and change substantially over time, readers are advised to write to these vendors directly for detailed and up-to-date information.

In January 1977, a new data base vendor called Bibliographic Retrieval Service (BRS) in Schenectady, New York, started as a "low-cost" competitor of SDC and Lockheed. BRS provides initial access to 11 data bases.

The following is an extensive list of data bases of interest to health sciences professionals:

DATA BASES

Data Base Name	Subject and Source	Entry Date	Items (Approx.)	Vendors
AGRICOLA (formerly CAIN)	Worldwide coverage of journal and monographic literature on agriculture and related subjects prepared by US National Agricultural Library.	1970	1,150,000	Lockheed BRS SDC
APTIC	Covers air pollution, including legal, administrative, social, and political aspects. Data base covers effects on human health, plants, livestock, etc.	1966	89,000	Lockheed
ASI (American Statistics Index)	Index of government statistical indexes and abstracts covering all types of periodicals and reports. Comprehensive coverage of statistics.	1973	55,000	Lockheed SDC
BIOSIS PREVIEWS	Contains citations from *Biological Abstracts* and *Bioresearch Index*. Worldwide coverage of research in the life sciences from 8,000 primary journals. Prepared by Biological Sciences Information Services.	1969	2,735,000	Lockheed BRS
CAB ABSTRACTS	A comprehensive file of agricultural and biological information. Covers several abstracts, including *Index Veterinarius, Nutrition Abstracts and Reviews*, etc.	1973	635,000	Lockheed

DATA BASES

CA CONDENSATES	Corresponds to *Chemical Abstracts* prepared by Chemical Abstracts Services.	1972	585,000	Lockheed BRS SDC
CA PATENT CONCORDANCE	Covers all chemically related patents received by CAS from 1972 to the present.	1972	132,300	Lockheed
CA SEARCH	Expanded data base which is the merger of two files: *CA Condensates* and *CASIA*, which contains CA general subject headings and controlled vocabulary from *CAS Registry* numbers.	1972	2,580,000	Lockheed BRS SDC
CHEMNAME	Contains a listing of chemical substances in dictionary, nonbibliographic file. Provides *CAS Registry* number, molecular formula, and other pertinent data.	1972	434,000	Lockheed
CHILD ABUSE AND NEGLECT	Ongoing research, bibliographic references, service programs. Includes US documents. For social workers, planners, legal researchers. Prepared by DHEW.	1965	7,000	Lockheed
CIS/INDEX	Covers US Congress publications. Prepared by Congressional Information Service.	1970	110,000	Lockheed SDC

cont'd.

DATA BASES

Data Base Name	Subject and Source	Entry Date	Items (Approx.)	Vendors
CLAIMS/CHEM	Chemical and chemically related patents. Eighty percent US and 20 percent foreign patents.	1950–1970	265,000	Lockheed
CLAIMS/CLASS	Classification code and title dictionary of the US Patent Classification System.		15,000	Lockheed
CLAIMS/US PATENTS	Patents listed in *Official Gazette* of the US Patent Office.	1971	550,000	Lockheed
COMPENDEX	Corresponds to *Engineering Index* (monthly/annual). Prepared by Engineering Index.	1970	700,000	Lockheed SDC
COMPREHENSIVE DISSERTATION ABSTRACTS CDI	Dissertations accepted for academic doctoral degrees granted by United States and Non-US universities. Contents from *Dissertation Abstracts*. Prepared by University Microfilms International.	1861	600,000	Lockheed BRS SDC
CONFERENCE PAPERS INDEX	Covers international scientific and technical conferences in such areas as pharmacology, biology, animal science, clinical and experimental medicine, biochemistry. Prepared by Data Courier.	1973	714,000	BRS SDC Lockheed

Name	Description	Year	Records	Vendor
CURRENT RESEARCH INFORMATION SYSTEM	Current awareness in agriculture research. Encompasses biological sciences, food and nutrition, environmental projects, consumer health and safety.	1974	29,000	Lockheed
DRUGDOC	Corresponds with *Drug Literature Index* and *Adverse Reaction Titles*. Produced by Excerpta Medica.	1968	60,000	BRS
DRUGINFO	Pharmacy and pharmacology.	1968		BRS
ENVIROLINE	Produced by the Environment Information Center. Covers the world's environmental information in all formats from over 5,000 primary and secondary publications.	1971	65,600	Lockheed SDC
Environmental Impact Statements	Environmental problems and issues and their impacts.	1977		BRS
EPB Environmental Periodical Bibliography	Covers fields of general human ecology, nutrition, health, and others. Indexes almost 250 periodicals.	1973	108,000	Lockheed
EXCEPTIONAL CHILD EDUCATION RESOURCES	Published and unpublished literature on the education of handicapped and gifted children.	1966	28,000	Lockheed

cont'd.

Data Base Name	Subject and Source	Entry Date	Items (Approx.)	Vendors
EXCERPTA MEDICA	Abstracts and citations from over 3,500 biomedical journals worldwide, covering the entire field of human medicine. Includes 43 speciality journals. Also covers pharmaceutical literature, environmental literature, environmental health, hospital management. Prepared by Excerpta Medica.	1974	700,000	Lockheed
FSTA (Food Science and Technology Abstracts)	Covers all literature related to human food commodities. Includes information on basic food science, microbiology, nutrition, laws, standards.	1969	17,000	SDC Lockheed
FOUNDATION DIRECTORY	Describes over 3,000 foundations. Prepared by the Foundation Center.	1973	3,000	Lockheed
FOUNDATION GRANTS INDEX	Cumulation of grants records of more than 400 US philanthropic foundations. Prepared by the Foundation Center.	1973	53,000	Lockheed
GRANTS	Over 1,500 grant programs in all fields offered by federal, state, and local governments, private foundations, and other sources. Prepared by Oryx Press.	Current	1,500 per update	SDC

INTERNATIONAL PHARMACEUTICAL ABSTRACTS	Abstracts from over 500 pharmaceutical, medical, and related journals, covering all aspects of pharmacology. Prepared by the American Society of Hospital Pharmacists.	1970	48,000	Lockheed
LISA	Source material from the British Library and ASLIB Library. Covers all phases of library service, information storage and retrieval. Prepared by the Library Association (London).	1976	20,000	Lockheed SDC
MEDOC	All areas of medicine (government documents).	1976		BRS
NATIONAL FOUNDATIONS	Provides records of foundations, including smaller ones excluded from the *Foundation Directory*.	1975	20,000	Lockheed
NICSEM/NIMIS National Instructional Materials Information System	Audiovisual materials and devices for use with handicapped children. Subject areas are of wide range, including health.	1974–1977	35,000	Lockheed BRS
NIMH	Covers citations from over 1,000 journals worldwide, as well as monographs, reports, nonprints produced by the National Clearing House for Mental Health.	1969–	360,000	BRS

cont'd.

Data Base Name	Subject and Source	Entry Date	Items (Approx.)	Vendors
NTIS	Corresponds to the *Weekly Government*.	1964	695,000	Lockheed SDC BRS
NUTRITION DATA BANK	Food composition values.			*Swift and Co.
PAIS INTERNATIONAL	Corresponds to printed *PAIS Bulletin* and *Foreign Language Index*. Covers Congressional hearings and government documents.	1976	71,000	Lockheed
PANDEX	Science, technology, medicine.			*Macmillan Information
PNI (Pharmaceutical News Index)	Index to *Drug Research*, *FDC Reports*, *PMA Newsletter*, *Washington Drug and Device Letter*. Prepared by Data Courier.	1974	42,000	BRS Lockheed SDC
POLLUTION ABSTRACTS	Corresponds to printed abstracts. Covers human health effects, statistics, environmental law. Prepared by Data Courier.	1970	67,000	BRS Lockheed SDC
POPULATION BIBLIOGRAPHY	Covers monographs, journals, technical reports, government documents, proceedings. A principal source of information on abortion, demography, fertility studies.	1966	41,000	Lockheed

DATA BASES

PSYCHOLOGICAL ABSTRACTS	Worldwide coverage of the literature in psychological and behavioral sciences, from periodicals, monographs, reports.	1967	266,000	Lockheed BRS SDC
RINGDOC	Covers pharmaceutical literature. Prepared by Derwent Publications.	1964	50,000	SDC
SABIR	Medicine, cancer, virology, immunology, radiobiology.			*Institute Gustave-Roussy
SAFETY SCIENCE ABSTRACTS	Covers occupational safety, environmental safety and law, radiation, drug dosages, epidemics. Prepared by Cambridge Scientific Abstracts.	1975	15,000	SDC
SCISEARCH	Corresponds to *Science Citation Index*. From the Institute for Scientific Information.	1974	2,060,000	Lockheed
SOCIOLOGICAL ABSTRACTS	Worldwide coverage of literature in sociology from over 1,200 journals, reports, monographs.	1963	95,000	SDC Lockheed
SSIE CURRENT RESEARCH	Describes current research in agricultural, behavioral, biological, chemical, medical, and physical sciences.	1976	253,000	Lockheed BRS SDC

* Producer of the data base.

cont'd.

DATA BASES

Data Base Name	Subject and Source	Entry Date	Items (Approx.)	Vendors
TOXITAPES	Industrial and pharmaceutical toxicology literature.			*Bioscience Information Service
UNION CATALOG OF MEDICAL PERIODICALS	Medicine and health-related fields. Periodicals and scientific literature.			*Medical Library Center of New York
VETDOC	Veterinary science.			*Derwent Publications
WPI	Covers pharmaceuticals, agricultural and other chemicals worldwide.	1963	264,000	SDC *Derwent Publications

* Producer of the data base.

REFERENCE LIST

The reference list in *Scientific and Technical Information Sources* (Cambridge, MA: MIT Press, 1977), the companion volume of this book, provides extensive bibliographies on numerous topics regarding the characteristics and use of the scientific and technical literature. Many of these citations should be pertinent to health science professionals, as they are related to the nature and use of medical information. This list includes only references that are highly relevant to health sciences.

In addition, readers are referred to Ching-chih Chen's *Sourcebook on Health Sciences Librarianship* (Metuchen, NJ: Scarecrow Press, 1977), which supplies extensive references on all aspects of the field. One book is a citation bibliography consisting of approximately 3,500 entries.

ABSTRACTS AND INDEXES
See also INDEX MEDICUS; INDEXING AND ABSTRACTING

Adams, S., and Baker, D. B. "Mission and Discipline Orientation in Scientific Abstracting and Indexing Services." *Library Trends* 16: 307–322, 1967.

Ashwroth, W. "Abstracting." In *Handbook of Special Librarianship and Information Work,* 3d ed., pp. 453–481. London: Aslib, 1967.

Bourni, C. P. "Evaluation of Indexing Systems." *Annual Review of Information of Science and Technology* 1: 180, 1966.

Brandon, Alfred N. "Subject List of Journals Indexed in *Index Medicus*." *Bulletin of the Medical Library Association* 50: 353–406, July 1962.

Burkett, J. "Published Indexing and Abstracting Services." *Trends in Special Librarianship,* pp. 35–72. London: Bingley, 1968.

Day, Philip E. "The *International Nursing Index*." *American Journal of Nursing* 66: 783–786, April 1966.

Dorr, H. A., and Sher, I. H. "The *Science Citation Index* System and Pharmaceutical Education." *American Journal of Pharmaceutical Education* 32: 177–188, 1968.

Drage, J. R. "User Preferences in Published Indexes, a Preliminary Test." *Information Scientist* 2: 111–114, Nov. 1968.

Elliott, C. K. "Abstracting Services in Psychology: A Comparison of Psychological Abstracts and Bulletin Signaletique." *Library Association Record* 71: 280–283, September 1969.

Garfield, E. "*Science Citation Index*—A New Dimension in Indexing." *Science* 144: 649–654, 1964.

Gould, A. M. "User Preference in Published Indexes." *Journal of the American Society for Information Science* 25: 279–286, Sept. 1974.

Jacobus, David P., et al. "Direct User Access to the Biological Literature through Abstracts: A Cooperative Experiment in Customized Service." *BioScience* 16: 599–603, September 1966.

Keenan, Stella. "Abstracting and Indexing Services in Science and Technology." In *Annual Review of Information Science and Technology*, vol. 4, pp. 273–303. Chicago: Encyclopaedia Britannica, 1969.

Keenan, S. V., and Elliot, M. "World Inventory of Abstracting and Indexing Services," *Special Libraries* 64: 145–150, Mar. 1973.

Lancaster, F. W. "The Evaluation of Published Indexes and Abstract Journals: Criteria and Possible Procedures." *Bulletin of the Medical Library Association* 59: 479–494, 1971.

Parkins, P. V. "*BioScience*'s Information Service of Biological Abstracts." *Science* 152 (3724): 889–894, 1966.

Ring, Malvin E. "Fifty Years of the *Index to Dental Literature*: A Critical Appraisal." *Bulletin of the Medical Library Association* 59: 463–478, July 1971.

Schultz, Louise. "New Developments in Biological Abstracting and Indexing." *Library Trends* 16: 337–352, 1967–1968.

Stavely, Ronald. "Periodicals: Indexes and Abstracts." In *Introduction to Subject Study*, edited by Ronald Stavely. Deutsch, 1967.

Sutherland, F. M. "Indexes, Abstracts, Bibliographies, and Reviews." In *Use of Medical Literature*. 2d ed., pp. 39–61. London: Butterworth & Co., 1977.

Thompson, C. W. N. "Functions of Abstracts in the Initial Screening of Technical Documents by the User." *Journal of the American Society for Information Science* 24: 270–276, July 1973.

Torr, D. V.; Fried, C.; and Prevel, J. J. *Program of Studies on the Use of Published Indexes*. Bethesda, MD: General Electric Company, Information Systems Operation, 1964.

Truelson, Stanley D., Jr. "What the *Index Medicus* Indexes, and Why." *Bulletin of the Medical Library Association* 54: 329–336, October 1966.

Wilkinson, D., and Hollander, S. "Comparison of Drug Literature Coverage by *Index Medicus* and *Drug Literature Index*." *Bulletin of the Medical Library Association* 61: 431–432, Oct. 1973.

Wood, J. L.; Flanagan, C.; and Kennedy, H. E. "Overlap among the Journal Articles Selected for Coverage by 'Biosis,' *Chemical Abstracts Service*, and *Engineering Index*." *Journal of the American Society for Information Science* 24: 25–28, Jan. 1973.

Wood, J. L.; Flanagan, C.; and Kennedy, H. E. "Overlap in the Lists of

Journals Monitored by 'Biosis,' *Chemical Abstracts Service,* and *Engineering Index.*" *Journal of the American Society for Information Science.* 23: 36–38, Jan. 1972.

BIBLIOGRAPHY

Baer, K. A. "Bibliography in the Special Libraries of the United States: A Non-statistical Survey." *International Library Review* 2: 85–100, Jan. 1970.

Bottle, R. T. "Information Obtainable from Analyses of Scientific Bibliographies." *Library Trends* 22: 60–71, July 1973.

Brodman, Estelle. *The Development of Medical Bibliography.* Baltimore: Medical Library Association, 1954.

Buckland, M. K., et al. "Methodological Problems in Assessing the Overlap Between Bibliographical Files and Library Holdings." *Information Processing and Management* 11: 89–105, Aug. 1975.

Parr, T. "Automation of Cartobibliography: Review of MARC for Map Library Information Retrieval and Cartographic Bibliography." *SLA Geography and Map Division Bulletin* 100: 26–73, June 1975.

Postell, William Dosite. *An Introduction to Medical Bibliography.* New Orleans, 1951.

Price, K. "Defining Death and Dying: A Bibliographic Overview." *Law Library Journal* 71: 49–67, Feb. 1978.

Ruhl, Mary Jane. "Development of a Medical Specialty Recurring Bibliography—*Index of Rheumatology.*" *Bulletin of the Medical Library Association* 55: 70–74, January 1967.

Sanders, E. "Indexing an Annotated Bibliography: Step-by-Step Procedure." *Special Libraries* 64: 86–90, February 1973.

Shilling, C. W. "Development of Specialized Scientific Bibliographies." In *Acquisition of Latin American Library Materials.* 14th Seminar, San Juan, 1969. Vol. 2, Organization of American States, General Secretariat, 1970.

Simon, H. R. "Outlook-Analyses of Bibliographies in the Future." *Library Trends* 22: 72, 1973.

Sutherland, F. M. "Indexes, Abstracts, Bibliographies, and Reviews." In *Use of Medical Literature,* 2d ed., pp. 39–61. London: Butterworth & Co., 1977.

Velleman, R. A. "Rehabilitation Information: A Bibliography." *Library Journal* 98: 2971–2976, October 15, 1973.

BIOGRAPHY

Damerau, F. J. "Automatic Compilation of Biographic Dictionaries." *Information Storage and Retrieval* 8: 315, 1972.

Holton, G. "Lessons of Intellectual Biography of Science." *Science* 170: 933, 1970.

BOOK REVIEWS

Chen, Ching-chih. *Biomedical, Scientific, and Technical Book Reviewing.* Metuchen, NJ: Scarecrow Press, 1976.

_____. "Current Status of Biomedical Book Reviewing: Part II. Time Lag in Biomedical Book Reviewing." *Bulletin of the Medical Library Association* 62: 113–119, April 1974.

_____. "Current Status of Biomedical Book Reviewing: Part III. Duplication Patterns in Biomedical Book Reviewing." *Bulletin of the Medical Library Association* 62: 296–301, July 1974.

_____. "Current Status of Biomedical Book Reviewing: Part IV. Major American and British Biomedical Book Publishers." *Bulletin of the Medical Library Association* 62: 302–308, July 1974.

_____. "Current Status of Biomedical Book Reviewing: Part V. A List of Most Frequently Reviewed Biomedical Books in 1970." *Bulletin of the Medical Library Association* 62: 309–313, July 1974.

Chen, Ching-chih, and Wright, Arthuree M. "Current Status of Biomedical Book Reviewing: Part I. Key Biomedical Reviewing Journals with Quantitative Significance." *Bulletin of the Medical Library Association* 62: 105–112, April 1974.

CITATION INDEXING AND CITATIONS

Garfield, Eugene. "Citation Analysis as a Tool in Journal Evaluation." *Science* 178: 471–479, Nov. 3, 1972.

Martyn, J. "Citation Analysis." *Journal of Documentation* 31: 290–297, 1975.

Price, D. J. de Solla. "Citation Measures of Hard Science, Soft Science, Technology, and Nonscience." In *Communication Among Scientists and Engineers,* edited by C. E. Nelson and D. K. Pollack, pp. 3–22. Lexington, MA: Heath, Lexington Books, 1970.

Weinstock, M. "Citation Indexes. In *Encyclopedia of Library and Information Science,* vol. 5, pp. 16–40. New York: Marcel Dekker, 1971.

CLASSIFICATION AND INDEXING

Aitchison, T. M.; Hall, A. M.; Lavalle, K. H.; and Tracy, J. M. *Compara-*

tive Evaluation of Index Languages, Part II: Results. Report R70/2. London: INSPEC, Institution of Electrical Engineers, 1970.

American Standards Association. *American Standard Basic Criteria for Indexes.* New York: ASA, 1959.

Anderson, David C. CATLINE: "Use and Costs at the Health Sciences Library, University of California, Davis." *Bulletin of the Medical Library Association* 64 (3): 328–331, July 1976.

Bock, Rochelle, and Braude, Robert M. "Cataloging costs with CATLINE: A followup study." *Bulletin of the Medical Library Association* 63: 414–415, October 1975.

Boston Medical Library. *Boston Medical Library Medical Classification,* 3d ed., 2d rev. Boston: Boston Medical Library, 1955.

British Standards Institution. *BS 1000c. Guide to the Universal Decimal Classification (UDC).* 1963.

Butkovich, Margaret, and Braude, Robert M. "Cost-Performance Analysis of Cataloging and Card Production in a Medical Center Library." *Bulletin of the Medical Library Association* 63: 29–34, January 1975.

"Cunningham Classification into Greek." *Bulletin of the Medical Library Association* 56: 201, April 1968.

Cunningham, Eileen R. *Classification for Medical Literature,* 4th ed. rev. and enl. With the collaboration of Eleanor G. Steinke. Nashville, TN: Vanderbilt University Press, 1967.

Jones, M. Irene. "Classification." In Medical Library Association *Handbook of Medical Library Practice.* 2d ed., rev. and enl., edited by Janet Doe and Mary Louise Marshall, p. 150. Chicago: American Library Association, 1956.

Kennedy, Jean, and Kossmann, Charles E. "Nomenclatures in Medicine." *Bulletin of the Medical Library Association* 61: 238–252, April 1973.

Messinger, K., and Flood, B. "Recent Advances in Indexing." *Drexel Library Quarterly* 8: 113–208, Apr. 1972.

Ramsden, M. J. "Some Basic Considerations in Subject Indexing." *Australian Library Journal* 24: 10–16, Feb. 1975.

Saracevic, T. "Comparative Effects of Titles, Abstracts, and Full Texts on Relevance Judgments." *Proceedings of the American Society for Information Science* 6: 293–299, 1969.

Scheerer, George, and Hines, Lois E. "Classification Systems Used in Medical Libraries." *Bulletin of the Medical Library Association* 62: 273–280, July 1974.

Swanson, D. R. "Tests for Indexing Performance Factors." *Library Quarterly* 41: 223, 1971.

US National Library of Medicine. *Catalog.* Washington, DC, 1948–1965.

US National Library of Medicine. *Current Catalog.* Washington, DC, January 1–14, 1966–.

US National Library of Medicine. *Current Catalog Proof Sheets.* Chicago: Medical Library Association, 1971–.

US National Library of Medicine. *Index Medicus. Medical Subject Headings.* Part 2 of the January *Index Medicus.* Washington, DC: US Government Printing Office, annual.

US National Library of Medicine. *National Library of Medicine Classification: A Scheme for the Shelf Arrangement of Books in the Field of Medicine and Its Related Sciences,* 3d ed. Public Health Service Pub. no. 1108. Bethesda, MD: US Department of Health, Education, and Welfare, Public Health Service, National Library of Medicine, 1964 (with 1969 supplementary pages added). Washington, DC: US Government Printing Office, 1969.

Wellisch, H. "Flow Chart for Indexing with a Thesaurus." *Journal of the American Society for Information Science* 23: 185–194, May 1972.

Wright, K. C. "Trends in Modern Subject Analysis with Reference to Text Derivative Indexing and Abstracting Methods: The State of the Art." *Information*; pt. 2: *Reports/Bibliographies* 1: 1–18, Sept. 1972.

COLLECTION DEVELOPMENT
See also REVIEWS

For citation analyses and use studies, see also sections below on citation indexing and citations and on use and users.

Broadus, Robert N. *Selecting Materials for Libraries.* New York: H. W. Wilson, 1973.

Bastille, J. D., and Mankin, C. J. "Report on Subsequent Demand for Journal Titles Dropped in 1975." *Bulletin of the Medical Library Association* 66: 346–349, July 1978.

Chen, Ching-chih. *Application of Operations Research Models to Libraries.* Cambridge, MA: MIT Press, 1976.

———. *Biomedical, Scientific, and Technical Book Reviewing.* Metuchen, NJ: Scarecrow Press, 1976.

Drott, M. C., and Griffith, B. C. "Empirical Examination of Bradford's Law and the Scattering of Scientific Literature." *Journal of the American Society of Information Science* 29: 238–246, Sept. 1978.

Goffman, William, and Morris, Thomas G. "Bradford's Law and Library Acquisitions." *Nature* 226: 922–923, June 6, 1970.

Kraft, M. "An Argument for Selectivity in the Acquisition of Materials for Research Libraries." *Library Quarterly* 37: 284–295, July 1967.

Schad, Jasper G. "Allocating Book Fund: Control or Planning." *College and Research Libraries* 31: 155–159, May 1970.

Seymour, C. A. "Weeding the Collection: A Review of Research on Identifying Obsolete Stock Monographs." *Libri* 22: 137–148, 1972.

Spiller, David. *Book Selection: An Introduction to Principles and Practice.* Hamden, CT: Linnet Books, 1971.

———. "The Use Patterns of Physics Journals in a Large Academic Research Library." *Journal of the American Society for Information Science* 23: 254–270, July/August 1972.

———. "Trends in Biophysical Research and Their Implications for Medical Libraries." *Bulletin of the Medical Library Association* 61: 214–224, April 1973.

CONFERENCE PROCEEDINGS

Agranovs, A. I. "Proceeding of Major International Conferences: Source of Scientific Information." *Nauchno-tekhnicheskaia Information* 22: 1, 1973.

Baum, Harry. "Scientific and Technical Meeting Papers: Transient Value or Lasting Contribution." *Special Libraries* 56: 651–653, 1965; *Journal of Chemical Documentation* 13: 187–189, 1973.

Cermakova, Jirina. "International Scientific Congresses and Conferences: Calendars, Bibliographies of Congress Proceedings, and Conference Technique Handbooks." *Annals of Library Science and Documentation* 19: 104–113, 1972.

"Flow of Information from International Scientific Meetings." *Unesco Bulletin for Libraries* 24: 88–97, 1970.

Garfield, Eugene. "Of Conferences and Reviews." *Current Contents* No. 48, December 1, 1975.

Garvey, W. D. *Role of the National Meeting in Scientific and Technical Communication,* PB-202-367. Baltimore, MD: Johns Hopkins University, Center for Research in Scientific and Technical Communication, 1970.

Haigh, P. A. "Conferences and Their Proceedings." *National Lending Library Review* 2: 7–10, 1972.

Meakin, F. A., and Lewis, R. F. "Bibliographic Fugitives: Papers Presented at Meetings." In *3rd International Congress of Medical Librarianship,* Amsterdam, 1969, pp. 239–246.

Mills, P. R. "Characteristics of Published Conference Proceedings." *Journal of Documentation* 29: 36–50, March 1973.

"Papers and Proceedings of Professional Meetings on Microfiche." *Microform Review* 3: 15–21, 1974.

Peters, B. "International Scientific Meetings: Why Go? Who Profits?" *R&D Management* 5: 139–147, 1975.

Weinman, J. "Medical and Biological Engineering: Plea for New Pattern in International Scientific Congresses. *Medical and Biological Engineering* 12: 396, 1974.

CORE LISTS

Allyn, Richard. "A Library for Internists Recommended by the American College of Physicians." *Annals of Internal Medicine* 84: 346–373, 1976.

Allyn, Richard, and Stearns, Norman S. "A Library for Internists Recommended by the American College of Physicians." *Annals of Internal Medicine* 79: 293–322, September 1973.

Brandon, Alfred N., and Dorothy R. Hill. "Selected List of Books and Journals for the Small Medical Library." *Bulletin of the Medical Library Association* 67: 185–211, April 1979.

Brandon, Alfred N., and Dorothy R. Hill. "Selected List of Nursing Books and Journals." *Nursing Outlook* 27: 672, Oct. 1979.

Duncan, Howertine Farrell. "Selected Reference Aids for Small Medical Libraries." *Bulletin of the Medical Library Association* 58: 134–158, April 1970. (Single reprint free from the National Library of Medicine.)

Graber, T. M. "Books for the Dentist." *Journal of American Dental Association* 88: 1322–1342, June 1974.

Library Association. Medical Section. *Books and Periodicals for Medical Libraries in Hospitals*. 4th ed. London: The Association, 1973.

Onsager, L. W. "Bibliography of Recommended Lists of Books and Journals for Health Sciences Libraries." *Bulletin of the Medical Library Association* 66: 338–339, July 1978.

Raskin, Robert B., and Hathorn, Isabel V. "Selected List of Books and Journals for a Small Dental Library. *Bulletin of the Medical Library Association* 64 (3): 265–271, July 1976.

Stearns, Norman S., and Ratcliff, Wendy W. "A Core Medical Library for Practitioners in Community Hospitals." *New England Journal of Medicine* 280: 474–480, February 27, 1969.

Stearns, Norman S., and Ratcliff, Wendy W. "An Integrated Health Science Core Library for Physicians, Nurses and Allied Health Practitioners in Community Hospitals." *New England Journal of Medicine* 283: 1489–1498, December 31, 1970.

Stearns, Norman S.; Ratcliff, Wendy W.; Getchell, Marjorie E.; and

Zeller, Karen. "A Core Nursing Library for Practitioners." *American Journal of Nursing* 70: 818–823, 1970.

Timour, John A. "Selected Lists of Journals for the Small Medical Library: A Comparative Analysis. *Bulletin of the Medical Library Association* 59: 87–93, January 1971.

US Veterans Administration. Central Office Library. *Basic List of Books and Journals for Veterans Administration Medical Libraries.* 1971 revision. (G-14, M-2, Part XIII, July 31, 1972). Available upon request from US Veterans Administration, H Street and Vermont Avenue, NW, Washington, DC 20420. (Eleven parts were published from September 1968 through September 1970: Urology; Pathology; Surgery; Radiology; Psychiatry; Internal Medicine; Neurology and Neurosurgery; Dermatology; Gastroenterology; Anesthesiology; and Physical Medicine, Rehabilitation and Orthopedics. These are available upon request from the US Veterans Administration.)

Yast, Helen T. "90 Recommended Journals for the Hospital's Health Science Library." *Hospitals* 41: 59–62, July 1967.

CURRENT-AWARENESS SERVICES

Barker, Frances H., et al. "Report on the Evaluation of an Experimental Computer-Based Current Awareness Service for Chemists." *Journal of the American Society for Information Science* 23: 85–99, March–April 1972.

Bloomfield, M. "Current Awareness Publications: An Evaluation." *Special Libraries* 60: 514–520, October 1969.

Gaffney, Inez. "CAN/SDI: Experience with Multi-source Computer Based Current Awareness Services in the National Science Library, Ottawa." *Medical Library Association Bulletin* 61: 309–313, July 1973.

Wente, Van A., and Young, Clifford A. "Current Awareness and Dissemination." *Annual Review of Information Science and Technology* 5: 259–295, 1970.

DATA BASES
See also INFORMATION RETRIEVAL

Science Information Exchange (SIE). "A National Registry of Research in Progress." *Scientific Information Notes* 1: 43–46, 1969.

Tagliacozzo, R. "The Consumers of New Information: A Survey of the Utilization of MEDLINE." *Journal of the American Society for Information Science* 26: 294–304, October 1975.

Williams, Martha E. "Use of Machine-readable Data Bases." *Annual Review of Information Science and Technology* 9: 221–284, 1974. Avail. Washington, DC: American Society for Information Science.

DICTIONARIES

Callard, J. C., and Freuhauf, E. L. "Comparison of American Medical Dictionaries." *Bulletin of the Medical Library Association* 66: 327–330, July 1978.

Gardner, A. L. "Technical Translating Dictionaries." *Journal of Documentation* 6: 25–31, 1950.

DIRECTORIES

Dickson, W. M., and Redowska, C. A. "Determination of Feasibilities of Establishing a Pharmacy Continuing Education Resource Directory." *American Journal of Pharmaceutical Education* 39: 43–48, 1975.

Garfield, E. "Does ISIS International Directory of R&D Authors and Organizations Perpetrate Alphabetical Discrimination?" *Current Contents Life Sciences* 14: 4, 1971.

Tauber, S. J.; Elias, A. W.; and Schneider, J. H. "Production of a Comprehensive Research Directory from Multiple Secondary Sources," *Journal of Chemical Information* 15: 109–115, 1975.

DISSERTATIONS, THESES, AND RESEARCH IN PROGRESS

Armstrong, Robert P. "The Qualities of a Book, the Wants of a Dissertation." *Scholarly Publishing* 3: 99–109, January 1972.

Boyer, Calvin James. *The Doctoral Dissertation.* Metuchen, NJ: Scarecrow Press, 1973.

Cobb, Mary M. "Publication of Medical Research Reports in Scientific Journals." *Bulletin of the Medical Library Association* 41: 154–155, April 1953.

Urquhart, D. J. "Doctoral Theses." *NLL Review* 1: 8–9, 1971.

ENCYCLOPEDIAS

Kochen, M. "Wise World Information Synthesis and Encyclopedia." *Journal of Documentation* 28: 322, 1972.

GUIDES TO LITERATURE

Beatty, William K. "Keys to the Medical Literature." *The New Physician* 18: 634–641, August 1969.

Cornelius, E. H. "The Provision of Bio-Medical Literature: The Present Position and Future Possibilities. *Postgraduate Medical Journal* 42: 1–4, January 1966.

Ingelfinger, Franz J. "Medical Literature: The Campus without Tumult." *Science* 169: 831–837, August 28, 1970.

Miller, Lois B., and Rathbun, Edith N. "Growth and Development of

Nursing Literature." *Bulletin of the Medical Library Association* 52: 420–426, 1964.

Narin, Francis; Pinski, Gabriel; and Gee, Helen H. "Structure of the Biomedical Literature." *Journal of the American Society for Information Science* 27 (1): 25–45, January–February 1976.

Orr, Richard H., and Leeds, Alice A. "Biomedical Literature: Volume, Growth, and Other Characteristics." *Federation Proceedings* 23: 1310–1331, November/December 1964.

Wyatt, H. V. "Paper Epidemic: A Guide to the Use of the Biomedical Literature." *American Journal of Epidemiology* 87: 509–519, 1968.

HANDBOOKS

International Council of Scientific Unions. "Selected Sections from Study on the Problems of Accessibility and Dissemination of Data for Science and Technology." *Information: News and Sources* 7: 169–177, July 1975.

Mountstephens, Brenda, et al. *Quantitative Data in Science and Technology.* Aslib Occasional Publications, no. 7. London: Aslib, 1971.

Sarett, L. H. "Scientist and Scientific Data." *American Documentation* 19: 299–304, July 1968.

Wendt, R. E. "Handbook Prescription." *Instrumentation Technology* 18: 37, 1971.

HISTORY

Billings, John Shaw. "The Medical Journals of the United States." *Boston Medical and Surgical Journal* 100: 1–4, 108, 1879.

Cantu, Jane Q. "American Medical Literary Firsts, 1700–1820, in the Countway Library." *Bulletin of the Medical Library Association* 54: 48–61, January 1966.

Garrison, Fielding H. "The Medical and Scientific Periodicals of the 17th and 18th Centuries, with a Revised Catalogue and Check List. *Bulletin of the History of Medicine* 2: 285–343, in *Bulletin of Johns Hopkins Hospital* July 1934.

Gnudi, Martha Teach. "Building a Medical History Collection," *Bulletin of the Medical Library Association* 63: 42, January 1975.

Olch, Peter D. "Oral History and the Medical Librarian." *Bulletin of the Medical Library Association* 57: 1–4, January 1969.

Poynter, F. N. L. "Medicine and the Historian." *Bulletin of the History of Medicine* 30: 420–435, September–October 1956.

Temkin, Owsei. "An Essay on the Usefulness of Medical History for Medicine." *Bulletin of the History of Medicine* 19: 9–47, January 1946.

INDEX MEDICUS

Dolcourt, Joyce L., and Braude, Robert M. "Determination of Overlap in Coverage of *Excerpta Medica* and *Index Medicus* through SERLINE." *Bulletin of the Medical Library Association* 64 (3): 324–325, July 1976.

Wildinson, Doris, and Hollander, Stephen. "A Comparison of Drug Literature Coverage by *Index Medicus* and *Drug Literature Index*." *Bulletin of the Medical Library Association* 61: 431–432, October 1973.

INDEXING AND ABSTRACTING
See also ABSTRACTS AND INDEXES

Charen, Thelma. "Gynecology: An Etymological Note." *Bulletin of the Medical Library Association* 59: 585–588, October 1971.

Doe, Janet. "Methods for Medical Indexing." *Bulletin of the Medical Library Association* 39: 23–27, January 1951.

Gordon, B. L. "Biomedical Language and Format for Manual and Computer Applications." *Diseases of the Chest* 53: 38–42, January 1962.

Pings, Vern M. *A Plan for Indexing the Periodical Literature of Nursing.* New York: The American Nurses Foundation, 1966.

A Proposed System for the Automated Production of a KWOC Index of Medical Conference Proceedings, Symposia, etc. Proposed by Frances Lim, William Loughner, Stanley Moreo, and Helena Zekveld. St. Louis, Washington University School of Medicine Library, 1972.

Taine, Seymour I. "New Program for Indexing at the National Library of Medicine." *Bulletin of the Medical Library Association* 47: 117–123, April 1959.

US National Library of Medicine. *Principles of Indexing.* Videotapes and 18-page syllabus. Available from National Medical Audiovisual Center, Atlanta, Georgia.

Welt, Isaac D. "Abstracting and Indexing in the Medical Sciences." *Methods of Information in Medical Science* 3: 100–104, July 1962.

West, K. M. "Using Literature Indexes in Clinical Practice." *Journal of the Oklahoma Medical Association* 59: 393–395, 1966.

INFORMATION RETRIEVAL

Adams, Scott. "The Way of the Innovator: Notes toward a Prehistory of MEDLARS." *Bulletin of the Medical Library Association* 60: 523–533, October 1972.

Adams, S., and Taine, S. "Searching the Medical Literature. Information Retrieval (MEDLARS) at the National Library of Medicine." *Journal of the American Medical Association* 188: 251–254, April 20, 1964.

Birnbaum, H. "PESTDOC and VETDOC: A Description of 2 Documentation Services." *International Association of Agricultural Librarian and Documentalists Quarterly Bulletin* 19: 133–147, 1974.

Broaduf, H., et al. "Searching the Literature of Veterinary Science; A Comparative Study of 10 Different Information Systems for Retrospective Searches from January 1972 to December 1974." *Veterinary Record* 101: 461–463, Dec. 1977.

Foreman, Gertrude, and Baldwin, Carol. "Use of Multiple Data Bases in Bibliographic Services." *Bulletin of the Medical Library Association* 64: 55–57, January 1976.

Hitchingham, Eileen E. "MEDLINE Use in a University without a School of Medicine." *Special Libraries* 67 (4): 188–194, April 1976.

Lancaster, F. W. Evaluation and testing of information retrieval systems. In *Encyclopedia of Library and Information Science,* vol. 8, pp. 234–259. New York: Marcel Dekker, 1972.

Lancaster, F. W. *Information Retrieval Systems: Characteristics, Testing and Evaluation* 2d ed. New York: John Wiley, 1979.

McCarn, D. B., and Leiter, J. "On-Line Services in Medicine and Beyond." *Science* 181: 318–324, July 27, 1973.

Miller, J. K. "Mechanization of Library Procedures in the Medium Sized Library: XI. Two Methods of Providing Selective Dissemination of Information to Medical Scientists." *Bulletin of the Medical Library Association* 58: 378–397, July 1970.

Mitchell, P. C.; Richman, J. T.; and Walden, W. E. "Solar: A Storage and On-Line Automatic Retrieval System." *Journal of the American Society for Information Science* 24 (5): 347–358, 1973.

Moll, W. "MEDLINE Evaluation Study." *Bulletin of the Medical Library Association* 62: 1–5, January 1974.

Sodergren, Linnea. "MEDLARS II: A Review." *Bulletin of the Medical Library Association* 61: 400–407, October 1973.

Swanson, D. R. "Selective Dissemination of Biomedical Information." *Library Quarterly* 44: 189, 1974.

Werner, G. "Use of On-Line Bibliographic Retrieval Services in Health Sciences Libraries in the United States and Canada." *Bulletin of the Medical Library Association* 67: 1–14, January 1979.

Williams, Martha E. "Criteria for Evaluation and Selection of Data Bases and Data Base Services," *Special Libraries* 66 (12): 561–569, December 1975.

INFORMATION SERVICES AND SOURCES
See also INFORMATION RETRIEVAL

Bartlett, Marjorie H., et al. "Dial Access Library—Patient Information Service." *New England Journal of Medicine* 288: 994–998, May 10, 1973.

"Biomedical Literature and Information Services." *Federation Proceedings* 33: 1693–1723, June 1974.

Davies, G., and Gregory, M. W. "Study of the Creation of a System for Providing Information on the Prevalence and Cost of Animal Disease." *IAALD Quarterly Bulletin* 23: 49–56, Fall–Winter 1978.

Elwin, C. E. "Some Apects on Integration of Information Services in Medicine, Biology, and Chemistry at a Multidisciplinary Documentation Center." *Information Storage and Retrieval* 8: 49–56, April 1972.

Foster, Willis R. "Reference Books and Computerized Information Services: Partners in Librarianship." *Bulletin of the Medical Library Association* 60: 439–444, July 1972.

Friedlander, J. "Clinician Search for Information." *Journal of the American Society for Information Science* 24: 65–69, January–February 1973.

Lehman, L. J., and Wood, M. S. "Effect of Fees on an Information Service for Physicians." *Bulletin of the Medical Library Association* 66: 58–61, January 1978.

MEDICAL COMMUNICATION

Basu, R. N. "Barriers to Effective Communication in the Scientific World." *IEEE Transactions on Professional Communication* 15: 30–33, 1972.

Crane, Diana. *Invisible Colleges: Diffusion of Knowledge in Scientific Communities.* Chicago, IL: University of Chicago Press, 1972.

Fox, Sir Theodor. *Crisis in Communication: The Functions and Future of Medical Journals.* Athlone Press, 1965.

Garvey, W. D., and Griffith, B. C. "Communication and Information Processing within Scientific Disciplines: Empirical Findings for Psychology." *Information Storage and Retrieval* 8: 123–136, June 1972.

Knox, William T. "Systems for Technological Information Transfer." *Science* 181: 415–419, August 3, 1973.

Korfhage, R. R. "Informal Communication of Scientific Information." *Journal of the American Society for Information Science* 25: 25–32, January 1974.

Price, D. J. de Solla. *Little Science, Big Science.* New York: Columbia University Press, 1963.

Sengupta, I. N. "Impact of Scientific Serials on the Advancement of

Medical Knowledge: An Objective Method of Analysis." *International Library Review* 4: 169–195, April 1972.

Tschirgi, Robert D. "Should Scientists Communicate—and If So, with Whom?" *Bulletin of the Medical Library Association* 61: 1–3, January 1973.

US National Academy of Sciences. *Scientific and Technical Communication.* Report of the Committee of the Scientific and Technical Communication (SATCOM Report). Washington, DC: NAS, 1969.

US National Academy of Sciences. National Research Council. Division of Medical Sciences. *Communication Problems in Biomedical Research: Report of a Study.* Washington, DC, October 1963; Supplement, March 1964.

Yokote, Gail, and Utterback, Robert A. "Time Lapses in Information Dissemination: Research Laboratory to Physician's Office." *Bulletin of the Medical Library Association* 62: 251–257, July 1974.

NONPRINT MATERIALS

Beauchamp, Sister E. A. "Breathing Manikin Facilitates Teaching of Respiratory Care." *Heart and Lung* 1: 621–625, 1972.

Bell, J. A. H. "Microform: Uses and Potential." *Bulletin of the Medical Library Association* 66: 232–238, April 1978.

Brantz, Malcolm H. "Bibliographic Controls for Audio-Visuals: Recommendations Based on Response to a Questionnaire in the Field of Nursing Education." *Bulletin of the Medical Library Association* 64: 57–60, January 1976.

Dwyer, Thomas F. "Telepsychiatry: Psychiatric Consultation by Interactive Television." *American Journal of Psychiatry* 130: 865–869, 1973.

Kronick, David A. "Nonprint Media as Information Resources: Software and Hardware." *Bulletin of the Medical Library Association* 62: 19–24, January 1974.

Meiboom, Esther R. "Conversion of the Periodical Collection in a Teaching Hospital Library to Microfilm Format." *Bulletin of the Medical Library Association* 64: 36–40, January 1976.

Raymond, Sue L., and Algermissen, Virginia L. "A Retrieval System for Biomedical Slides Using MeSH." *Bulletin of the Medical Library Association* 64: (2): 233–235, April 1976.

Sequin, Marilynne, ed. *Nursing Media Index 16mm Films.* Toronto: Mission Press, 1974.

Veaner, Allen. *The Evaluation of Micropublications: A Handbook for Librarians.* Chicago: American Library Association, 1971.

PATENTS

Asher, Gordon. "International Patent Cooperation." *Journal of Chemical Documentation* 11: 14–18, 1971.

Clark, C. V. "Obsolescence of Patent Literature." *Journal of Documentation* 32: 32, 1976.

Malcolm, M. E. "Patents and Their Place in Technology." *New Zealand Libraries* 37: 85–88, April 1974.

Schwartz, J. H. "What Has Been Published—More Patents Than Journal Literature." *Journal of Chemical Education* 53: 57, 1976.

PERIODICALS

Arndt, K. "Science, Information Crisis, and Journal." *Chemische Technik* 25: 745, 1973.

Garfield, E. "Is There a Future for the Scientific Journal?" *Sci-Tech News* 29 (2): 42–44, April 1975.

Herschman, A. "The Primary Journal: Past, Present, and Future." *Journal of Chemical Documentation* 10: 37–43, February 1970.

Kuney, J. H. "New Developments in Primary Journal Publication." *Journal of Chemical Documentation* 10: 42–46, February 1970.

Maddox, John. "Journals and the Literature Explosion." *Nature* 221: 128–130, 1969.

Narin, F., et al. "Interrelationship of Scientific Journals." *Journal of the American Society for Information Science* 23: 323–331, September 1972.

Raisig, L. Miles. "World Bio-Medical Journals, 1951–1960: A Study of the Relative Significance of 1,388 Titles Indexed in *Current List of Medical Literature*." *Bulletin of the Medical Library Association* 54: 108–125, 1966.

Sengupta, I. N. "Impact of Scientific Serials on the Advancement of Medical Knowledge: An Objective Method of Analysis." *International Library Review* 4: 169–195, April 1972.

Sengupta, I. N. "Recent Growth of the Literature of Biochemistry and Changes in Ranking of Periodicals." *Journal of Documentation* 29: 192–211, June 1973.

Staiger, D. L. "Separate Article Distribution as an Alternate to Journal Publication." *IEEE Transactions on Professional Communication* 16: 107–112, 1973.

PRIMARY LITERATURE

Cross, L. C. "Primary Scientific Literature in the Next Few Years." *Aslib Proceedings* 26: 425–429, November 1974.

Dannatt, R. J. "Primary Sources of Information." In *Use of Medical Literature,* edited by L. T. Morton, pp. 12–33. Hamden, CT: Shoe String Press, 1974.

Gannett, Elwood K. "Primary Publication Systems and Services." *Annual Review of Information Science and Technology* 8: 243–275, 1973.

Moore, J. A. "An Inquiry on New Forms of Primary Publications." *Journal of Chemical Documentation* 12: 75–78, May 1972.

REVIEWS OF PROGRESS

Burke, M. S., and Graf, F. "Review Sources: Health Sciences." *Serials Review* 3: 36–37, Oct. 1977.

Burke, M. S., and Graf, F. "Review Sources: Medicine." *Serials Record* 3: 38–40, July 1977.

Manten, A. A. "Scientific Review Literature." *Scholarly Publishing* 5: 75–89, October 1973.

Sutherland, F. M. "Indexes, Abstracts, Bibliographies, and Reviews." In *Use of Medical Literature.* 2d ed., pp. 39–61. London: Butterworth & Co., 1977.

Virgo, J. A. "Review Article: Its Characteristics and Problems." *Library Quarterly* 41: 275–291, 1971.

Woodward, A. M. "Review Literature Characteristics, Sources, and Output in 1972," *Aslib Proceedings* 26: 367, 1974.

STANDARDS

Houghton, Bernard. *Standardization for Documentation.* London: Bingley. 1969.

———. *Technical Information Sources: A Guide to Patent Specification, Standards, and Technical Reports Literature.* 2d ed. Hamden, CT: Shoe String Press, 1972.

Hudson, S. "International Documentation Standards." *Aslib Proceedings* 20: 553–564, 1968.

Reck, D., ed. *National Standards in a Modern Economy.* New York: Harper, 1956.

Sanders, T. R. B. *Aims and Principles of Standardization.* International Organization for Standardization, 1972.

TECHNICAL REPORTS

Auger, C. P. *Use of Report Literature.* Hamden, CT: Shoe String Press, 1975.

"Do Technical Reports Belong to Literature?" *Nature* 236: 275, 1972.

Van Deusen, A. "Unavailability of Technical Reports of Government and Government Sponsored Research: The Effect on Science and Technology." Research paper, SUNY Albany, 1971.

TRADE LITERATURE

Bailery, J. L. "Trade Literature, Its Nature, Significance, and Treatment." *Business Archives*, pp. 19–23, December, 1969.

Brand, R. "Documentation of Trade Literature." *Nachrichten fur Dockumentation* vol. 24, April 1973.

Cosma, M. "The Trade Catalog File; an Important Source of Information in an Enterprise." *Probleme de informare si documentare* 5(7), July 1971.

Drott, M. C.; Bearman, T. C.; and Griffith, B. C. "Hidden Literature—Scientific Journals of Industry." *Aslib Proceedings* 27: 376–384, 1975.

Drott, M. C., and Griffith, B. C. "Characteristics of Technically Oriented House Journals." *IEEE Transactions on Professional Communication* PC-18: 45–49, 1975.

Ford, M. "The Technical Indexes System for the Control of Trade Literature," *Aslib Proceedings* 24: 284–292, 1972.

Lakie, M. H. "Surgical Instruments and Dressings Information Service." *British Medical Journal* 4: 448, 1975.

Smith, E. B. "Trade Literature; Its Value, Organization and Exploitation." In *The Provision and Use of Library and Documentation Services*, edited by W. Saunders, pp. 29–54. New York: Pergamon Press, 1966.

TRANSLATIONS

Abrams, F. A. "A Market Survey: Translation of Foreign Language Biomedical Periodicals." *RQ* 10: 321–324, Summer 1971.

Bishop, David, and Pukteris, Sophie. "English Translations of Biomedical Literature: Availability and Control." *Bulletin of the Medical Library Association* 61: 24–28, January 1973.

Chillag, J. P. "Translations and Their Guides." *NLL Review* 1: 46–53, April 1971.

Lufkin, J. M. "What Everybody Should Know About Translation," *Special Libraries* 60: 74–81, 1969.

Scott, P. H. "Technical Translations: Meeting a Need." *Aslib Proceedings* 23: 89–99, 1971.

US Office of Technical Services. *Bibliography of Medical Translations; January 1959–June 1962*. Bethesda, MD: US Public Health Service, National Library of Medicine, 1962.

USES AND USERS

Ash, J. "Library Use of Public Health Materials: Description and Analysis." *Bulletin of the Medical Library Association* 62: 95–104, April 1974.

Basile, Victor A., and Smith, Reginald W. "Evolving the 90% Pharmaceutical Library." *Special Libraries* 61: 81–88, February 1970.

Bowden, Charles L., and Bowden, Virginia M. "A Survey of Information Sources Used by Psychiatrists." *Bulletin of the Medical Library Association* 59: 603–608, October 1971.

Brodman, E. "Users of Health Sciences Libraries." *Library Trends* 23: 63–72, 1974.

Chen, Ching-chih. "How do Scientists Meet Their Information Needs?" *Special Libraries* 65: 272–280, July 1974.

_____. "The Use Patterns of Physics Journals in a Large Academic Research Library." *Journal of the American Society for Information Science* 23: 254–270, May/June 1972.

Fleming, Thomas P., and Kilgour, Frederick G. "Moderately and Heavily Used Biomedical Journals." *Bulletin of the Medical Library Association* 52: 234–241, January 1964.

Gomes, Stella S. "The Nature of the Use and Users of the Midwest Regional Medical Library." *Bulletin of the Medical Library Association* 58: 559–577, October 1970.

Kilgour, Frederick C. "Use of Medical and Biological Journals in the Yale Medical Library: Part I. Frequently used Journals." *Bulletin of the Medical Library Association* 50: 429–443, July 1962.

Kilgour, Frederick G. "Use of Medical and Biological Journals in the Yale Medical Library: Part II. Moderately Used Journals." *Bulletin of the Medical Library Association* 50: 444–449, July 1962.

Kovacs, H. "Analysis of One Year's Circulation at the Downstate Medical Center Library." *Bulletin of the Medical Library Association* 54: 42–47, January 1966.

Lloyd, H. A., and Fraser, M. D. E. "Information Needs of Physiotherapists in the Atlantic Provinces with Suggested Physiotherapy Working Collections for Small Hospitals." Halifax: Dalhousie University, School of Library Service, 1977.

McMurtray, H. F., and Ginski, J. M. "Citation Patterns of the Cardiovascular Serial Literature." *Journal of the American Society for Information Science* 23: 172–175, May–June 1972.

Mick, C. K., et al. "Periodical Use by Medical Students: An Unobtrusive Study." *Journal of Medical Education* 47: 825–827, October 1972.

Oseasohn, Robert. "Borrower Use of a Modern Medical Library by Practicing Physicians." *Bulletin of the Medical Library Association* 58: 58–59, January 1970.

Raisig, L. M. "Statistical Bibliography in the Health Sciences." *Bulletin of the Medical Library Association* 50: 450–461, July 1962.

Rees, A. M. "Medical Libraries and the Assessment of User Needs." *Bulletin of the Medical Library Association* 54: 99–103, April 1966.

Smith, Joan M. B. "A Periodical Use Study at Children's Hospital of Michigan." *Bulletin of the Medical Library Association* 58: 65–67, January 1970.

Stangl, Peter, and Kilgour, Frederick G. "Analysis of Recorded Biomedical Book and Journal Use in the Yale Medical Library." *Bulletin of the Medical Library Association* 55: 290–315, 1967.

Tibbetts, Pamela. "A Method for Estimating the In-House Use of the Periodical Collection in the University of Minnesota Bio-Medical Library." *Bulletin of the Medical Library Association* 62: 37–48, January 1974.

Wood, D. N., and Bower, C. A. "The Use of Biomedical Literature at the National Lending Library for Science and Technology." *Methods of Information Medicine* 9: 46–53, January 1970.

Wood, G. C. "Serving the Information Needs of Physicians." *New England Journal of Medicine* 286: 603–604, March 16, 1972.

TITLE INDEX

AAAS Audiotape Cassette Album Series, 592
AAAS Reviews of Science, 373
The AAAS Science Book List: A Selected and Annotated List of Science and Mathematics Books for Secondary School Students, College Undergraduates, and Non-specialists, 3
AAAS Science Books and Films, 593
AAAS Science Film Catalog, 593
AAMC Curriculum Directory, 292
Abbreviated Titles of Biological Journals: A List Culled with Permission from "The World List of Scientific Periodicals," with Indications of the Abbreviations Recommended by the USA Standards Institute Where These Differ from the "World List", 525
Abbreviations and Acronyms in Medicine and Nursing, 63
Abbreviations Dictionary, 63
Abbreviations in Medicine, 64
The ABC of Acid-Base Chemistry, 394
Abdominal Operations, 255
Abdominal Surgery: An Atlas of Operative Techniques, 255
Abhandlungen Aus Der Augenheilkunde und Ihren Grenzgebieten, 361
Abortion Bibliography, 50
Abortion in America: The Origins and Evolution of National Policy, 1800–1900, 343
About Patents; Patents as a Source of Technical Information, 579
Abridged Index Medicus, 504, 507, 526
Abstracting Scientific and Technical Literature, 499
Abstracting Services, 499
Abstracts and Indexes in Science and Technology: A Descriptive Guide, 499
Abstracts for Social Workers, 517
Abstracts of Health Care Management Studies, 511
Abstracts of Microbiological Methods, 512
Abstracts of Mycology, 512
Abstracts of Published Reports, 538
Abstracts of The Standard Edition of The Complete Psychological Works of Sigmund Freud, 338
Abstracts of World Medicine, 507
Abstracts on Criminology and Penology, 517
Abstracts on Health Effects of Environmental Pollutants, 519
Abstracts on Hygiene, 519
Accepted Dental Therapeutics, 211
Accident and Emergency Paediatrics, 121
Accident Prevention Manual for Industrial Operations, 182
Accidents and Emergencies: A Practical Handbook for Personal Use, 111
Acid-Base Balance, 394
The Acid-Base Status of the Blood, 429
Acne: Morphogenesis and Treatment, 416
Acronym Handbook, 63
Acronyms, Initialisms, and Abbreviations Dictionary, 63
Action in Pharmacy, 585
Activation and Decay Tables of Radioisotopes, 140
Active Research Grants of the National Cancer Institute, 561
Acupuncture: A Research Bibliography, 30
Acupuncture: An International Bibliography, 30
Acupuncture and Moxibustion: A Handbook for the Barefoot Doctors of China, 111
Acupuncture Anesthesia in the People's Republic of China: A Trip Report of the American Acupuncture Anesthesia Study Group, 401
Acupuncture Directory: Yellow Pages, 297
Acute Coronary Care, 439

TITLE INDEX

Acute Drug Abuse Emergencies: A Treatment Manual, 168
Adler's Physiology of the Eye, 455
Administration in Nursing, 439
Administrator's Collection, 27
Admission Requirements of US and Canadian Dental Schools, 1977–1978, 291
Adolescence: A Select Bibliography, 36
Adolescents in Health and Disease, 465
Adult Assessment: A Source Book of Tests and Measures of Human Behavior, 128
The Advance of American Nursing, 335
An Advanced Atlas of Histology, 268
Advanced Concepts in Clinical Nursing, 439
Advances and Technical Standards in Neurosurgery, 349
Advances in American Medicine, 344
Advances in Applied Microbiology, 357
Advances in Behavioral Biology, 367
Advances in Biochemical Engineering, 344
Advances in Biochemical Psychopharmacology, 365
Advances in Biological and Medical Physics, 344
Advances in Biological Psychiatry, 367
Advances in Biology of Skin, 353
Advances in Biomedical Engineering, 344
Advances in Biomedical Engineering and Medical Physics, 345
Advances in Cancer Research, 360
Advances in Cardiology, 352
Advances in Cardiopulmonary Diseases, 352
Advances in Cardiovascular Surgery, 408
Advances in Cell and Molecular Biology, 345
Advances in Cell Biology, 345
Advances in Cerebral Angiography: Anatomy, Stereotaxy, Embolization, Computerized Axial Tomography, 370

Advances in Chromatography, 345
Advances in Clinical Chemistry, 358
Advances in Clinical Child Psychology, 367
Advances in Diagnosis and Therapy, 349
Advances in Drug Research, 365
Advances in Electrocardiography, 352
Advances in Environmental Science and Technology, 368
Advances in Enzymology and Related Areas of Molecular Biology, 353
Advances in Experimental Medicine and Biology, 345
Advances in Food Research, 359
Advances in Forensic and Clinical Toxicology, 369
Advances in General and Cellular Pharmacology, 365
Advances in Genetics, 355
Advances in Heart Disease, 352
Advances in Human Genetics, 355
Advances in Human Psychopharmacology, 367
Advances in Immunology, 346
Advances in Internal Medicine, 358
Advances in Lipid Research, 358
Advances in Mass Spectrometry in Biochemistry and Medicine, 365
Advances in Mental Handicap Research, 367
Advances in Microcirculation, 352
Advances in Modern Nutrition, 359
Advances in Modern Toxicology, 369
Advances in Nephrology from the Necker Hospital, 371
Advances in Neurochemistry, 349
Advances in Neurology, 349
Advances in Neurosurgery, 350
Advances in Noninvasive Diagnostic Cardiology, 352
Advances in Nursing Science, 531
Advances in Nutritional Research, 359
Advances in Obstetrics and Gynecology, 492
Advances in Ophthalmology, 361
Advances in Oral Surgery, 353
Advances in Oto-Rhino-Laryngology, 362

Advances in Pain Research and Therapy, 348
Advances in Parasitology, 357
Advances in Pediatrics, 364
Advances in Pharmaceutical Sciences, 365
Advances in Pharmacology and Chemotherapy, 365
Advances in Prostaglandin Research, 371
Advances in Psychobiology, 367
Advances in Psychosomatic Medicine, 367
Advances in Radiation Biology, 370
Advances in Radiation Chemistry, 370
Advances in Radiation Research, 370
Advances in Radiation Research: Biology and Medicine, 485
Advances in Reproductive Physiology, 347
Advances in Sex Hormone Research, 371
Advances in Sleep Research, 367
Advances in Surgery, 348
Advances in Teratology, 355
Advances in the Biosciences, 345
Advances in the Study of Behavior, 367
Advances in Tuberculosis Research, 371
Advances in Uveal Surgery, Vitreous Surgery, and the Treatment of Endophthalmitis, 361
Advances in Veterinary Science and Comparative Medicine, 372
Advances in Virus Research, 351
Adventures in Medical Research: A Century of Discovery at Johns Hopkins, 322
Adverse Effects of Oral Contraceptives, 50
Adverse Reaction Titles, 516
Aerospace Medicine and Biology: A Continuing Bibliography with Indexes, 513
Age Changes in the Neuromuscular System, 491
Aging, 383
Aging and Mental Health: Positive Psychosocial Approaches, 478

The Aging of Connective Tissue, 491
Aging: The Process and the People, 426
AGRICOLA, 624
Agriculture Handbook: Food Yields Summarized by Different Stages of Preparation, 94
AHA Film Catalog, 596
Aids for the Severely Handicapped, 231
Ainsworth and Bisby's Dictionary of the Fungi, 85
Air Pollution Abstracts, 519
Air Pollution Publications: A Selected Bibliography, 46
Alcohol Education Materials: An Annotated Bibliography, 41
Alcoholism: A Handbook, 132
The Alcoholism Digest Annual, 519
Alexander's Care of the Patient in Surgery, 401
Algal Physiology and Biochemistry, 147
Alimentary Tract Roentgenology, 485
Allergy Abstracts, 508
Allergy in Children: A Guide to Practical Management, 207
Allergy Management in Clinical Practice, 157
Allied Medical Education Directory, 291
The Alpha Syllabus: A Handbook of Human EEG Alpha Activity, 23
Alphabetical Index of Roentgen Diagnoses and Procedures, 577
Alphabetical Index of Roentgen Diagnoses and Procedures, with Code Numbers of the American College of Radiology, 237
AMA Drug Evaluations, 179
Ambulatory Care Manual for Nurse Practitioners, 172
Ambulatory Obstetrics: A Clinical Guide, 239
American Academy of Ophthalmology and Otolaryngology Directory, 299
American College of Physicians Directory, 297
American Dental Directory, 294
American Doctoral Dissertations, 556

American Drug Index, 123
American Druggist Blue Book, 300, 584
American Family Physician, 530
American Handbook of Psychiatry, 128
American Heart Journal, 528
American Hospital Association Guide to the Health Care Field; 1979 edition, 295
American Hospital Association Resource Catalog, 27
American Hospital Formulary Service, 179
American Journal of Anatomy, 527
American Journal of Cardiology, 528
American Journal of Clinical Nutrition, 531
American Journal of Clinical Pathology, 532
American Journal of Diseases of Children, 532
American Journal of Hospital Pharmacy, 532
American Journal of Law and Medicine, 526
American Journal of Medicine, 526
American Journal of Nursing, 531, 545
American Journal of Obstetrics and Gynecology, 534
American Journal of Ophthalmology, 531
American Journal of Pathology, 532
American Journal of Pharmaceutical Education, 532
American Journal of Physical Medicine, 533
American Journal of Physiology, 527
American Journal of Psychiatry, 534
American Journal of Public Health, 534
American Journal of Roentgenology, 534
American Journal of Surgery, 527
American Journal of the Medical Sciences, 526
American Journal of Tropical Medicine and Hygiene, 530
American Medical Association Directory of National Voluntary Health Organizations, 288
American Medical Bibliography, 1639–1783, 322
American Medical Directory, 288
American Medical Education: The Formative Years, 1765–1910, 322
American Medical Ethnobotany: A Reference Dictionary, 66
American Men and Women of Science, 315
American Men and Women of Science: Agricultural, Animal and Veterinary Sciences 1974, 321
American Men and Women of Science: Medical and Health Sciences 1977, 316
American Men and Women of Science: The Medical Sciences 1975, 316
American Nursing; History and Interpretation, 335
American Optometric Association Directory, 300
American Pharmaceutical Association Drug Names, 08
American Pharmacy, 532
American Physicians in the Nineteenth Century: From Sects to Science, 322
American Red Cross Advanced First Aid and Emergency Care, 111
American Red Cross Standard First Aid and Personal Safety, 111
American Review of Respiratory Disease, 534
American Self-Dosage Medicines: An Historical Perspective, 337
American Society for Microbiology: Directory and Constitution, 297
American Society of Parasitologists Directory of Members, 297
American Statistics Index; A Comprehensive Guide and Index to the Statistical Publications of the United States Government, 148
Amino Acid Peptide and Protein Abstracts, 514
Amino-Acids, Peptides, and Proteins, 345

TITLE INDEX

Anaerobic Bacteria in Human Disease, 432
Anaerobic Bacteria: Role in Disease, 432
Anaesthesia, 527
Analgesic Drugs, 402
An Analysis of Health Care Delivery, 394
Analysis of Roentgen Signs in General Radiology, 485
Analytical Profiles of Drug Substances, 365
Analytical Toxicology Methods Manual, 198
Analyzer of Medical-Biological Words, 73
Anatomic Guide for the Electromyographer: The Limbs, 227
Anatomical Correlates of Clinical Electromyography, 242
Anatomical Dictionary With Nomenclatures and Explanatory Notes, 66
Anatomy: A Regional Atlas of the Human Body, 242
Anatomy and Physiology: Workbook and Laboratory Manual, 187
Anatomy of the Central Nervous System in Review, 99
Anatomy of the Orbit, 176
Anesthesia and Analgesia, 527
The Anesthesiologist's Handbook, 98
Anesthesiology, 528
Anesthesiology: A Manual of Concept and Management, 158
Anesthesiology Bibliography, 22, 505
Angina Pectoris, 408
Animal Agents and Vectors of Human Disease, 497
Animal Cytology and Evolution, 61
Animal Health Yearbook: Annuaire de la Sante Animale: Annuario de Sanidad Animal, 315
Animal Science, 497
Animals for Research: A Directory of Sources of Laboratory Animals, Equipment and Materials, 308
Annals of Internal Medicine, 530
Annals of Otology, Rhinology and Laryngology, 532
Annals of Surgery, 528
Annals of Thoracic Surgery, 528
An Annotated Bibliography of Induced Abortion, 50
An Annotated Bibliography on Diving and Submarine Medicine, 30
Annotated Bibliography on Maternal Nutrition, 33
An Annotated Glossary of the Terms Used in Electroretinography, 88
An Annotated International Bibliography of National Education: Materials, Research Personnel, and Agencies, 33
Annual Bibliography of Orthopaedic Surgery, 36, 506, 516
The Annual Handbook for Group Facilitators, 129
The Annual of Psychoanalysis, 314
Annual Progress in Child Psychiatry and Child Development, 368
Annual Register of Grant Support, 281, 558
Annual Report of the Council on Environmental Quality, 150
Annual Reports in Medicinal Chemistry, 366
Annual Review of Allergy, 346
Annual Review of Clinical Biochemistry, 345
Annual Review of Genetics, 355
Annual Review of Medicine, 345
Annual Review of Microbiology, 357
Annual Review of Neuroscience, 350
Annual Review of Pharmacology, 366
Annual Review of Physiology, 348
Annual Review of Psychology, 368
Annual Statistics of Medical School Libraries in the United States and Canada, 1978–1979, 151
ANSI Catalog, 569
Antibiotics, 390
Antibiotics: A Critical Review, 473
Antibiotics and Chemotherapy, 551
The Antibody Molecule, 398
The Antigens, 375
Antimicrobial Agents and Chemotherapy, 551
Antique Medical Instruments, 334
Aphasia Therapy Manual, 160

Application of the International Classification of Diseases to Dentistry and Stomatology, 566
Applied Health Physics Abstracts and Notes, 515
Applied Microbiology, 530
Applied Physiology of Respiratory Care, 238
Applied Statistics for Food and Agricultural Scientists, 151
Applied Surgical Pathology, 462
APTIC, 624
Archives of Dermatology, 529
Archives of Disease in Childhood, 532
Archives of Environmental Health, 534
Archives of General Psychiatry, 534
Archives of Internal Medicine, 530
Archives of Neurology, 528
Archives of Ophthalmology, 531
Archives of Otolaryngology, 532
Archives of Pathology and Laboratory Medicine, 532
Archives of Physical Medicine and Rehabilitation, 533
Archives of Surgery, 528
Archives of the International Congress and Society of Neuropathology, 1952–1977, 330
Army Medical Department Handbook of Basic Nursing, 115
Arthritis: A Comprehensive Guide, 239
Arthritis and Allied Conditions: A Textbook of Rheumatology, 239, 491
Arthritis and Rheumatism, 534
Artificial Insemination, 492
Artificial Kidney Bibliography, 50
The Artificial Larynx Handbook, 120
Artificial Organs, 436
Asbestos and Disease, 482
Asbestosis: A Bibliography of the World's Literature Abstracted and Indexed 1960–1968, 46
ASI[American Statistics Index], 624
Asimov's Biographical Encyclopedia of Science and Technology: The Lives and Achievements of 1,195 Great Scientists from Ancient Times to the Present Chronologically Arranged, 316
ASLIB Book List, 2
Assessing Quality in Health Care, 395
Assessment of Medical Care for Children, 465
An Assessment of the Community Mental Health Movement, 338
Association for Research in Nervous and Mental Disease (ARNMD) Research Publications, 368
Atherosclerosis—Is it Reversible?, 161
Atlas and Dissection Guide for Comparative Anatomy, 242
Atlas der Rectoskopie und Coloskopie, 256
Atlas of Abdominal Ultrasonography in Children, 272
Atlas of Adult Echocardiography, 251
Atlas of Aesthetic Plastic Surgery, 246
An Atlas of Anatomy Basic to Radiology, 242
Atlas of Anatomy of the Hand, 242
Atlas of Aquatic Dermatology, 254
Atlas of Arterial Histology, 208
An Atlas of Artifacts: Encountered in the Preparation of Microscopic Tissue Sections, 268
Atlas of Brain Anatomy for EMI Scans, 242
Atlas of Cancer Mortality for U.S. Countries: 1950–1969, 264
An Atlas of Cardiology: Electrocardiograms and Chest X-Rays, 251
Atlas of Carotid Angiography, 251
Atlas of Cataract Surgery, 265
Atlas of Cell Biology, 268
Atlas of Cerebrospinal Fluid Cells, 248
Atlas of Cerebrovascular Disease, 248
An Atlas of Children's Surgery, 272
Atlas of Clinical Anatomy, 243
An Atlas of Clinical Neurology, 248
Atlas of Coloscopy, 256
Atlas of Colposcopy, 256
Atlas of Computed Body Tomography: Normal and Abnormal Anatomy, 274
Atlas of Cross Section Anatomy of the

TITLE INDEX

Brain: Guide to the Study of the Morphology and Fiber Tracts of the Human Brain, 248
An Atlas of Cross-Sectional Anatomy, 243
Atlas of Dermatology, 254
Atlas of Diagnostic and Therapeutic Procedures for Emergency Personnel, 274
Atlas of Diagnostic Cytology, 269
Atlas of Diagnostic Microbiology, 262
An Atlas of Diseases of the Eye, 264
Atlas of Diseases of the Jaws, 253
Atlas of Echocardiography, 252
Atlas of Electroencephalography in Coma and Cerebral Death, 248
Atlas of Enteroscopy, 256
An Atlas of Examination, Standard Measurements and Diagnosis in Orthopedics and Traumatology, 266
Atlas of External Diseases of the Eye, 265
Atlas of Eye Surgery and Related Anatomy, 265
Atlas of Gastrointestinal Surgery, 256
Atlas of Gray Scale Ultrasonography, 274
Atlas of Gross Neurosurgical Pathology, 269
An Atlas of Gynecological and Obstetric Pathology, 278
Atlas of Haematology, 260
Atlas of Hand Radiographs, 266
Atlas of Hand Surgery, 266, 267
An Atlas of Head and Neck Surgery, 246
An Atlas of Histology, 269
Atlas of Human Anatomy, 243
Atlas of Human Embryos, 243
Atlas of Human Histology, 269
Atlas of Infertility Surgery, 278
Atlas of Liver Biopsies, 257
An Atlas of Mammalian Chromosomes, 258
Atlas of Medical Anatomy, 243
Atlas of Medical Helminthology and Protozoology, 262
An Atlas of Medical Microbiology: Common Human Pathogens, 262
Atlas of Medical Parasitology, 262
Atlas of Men: A Guide for Somatotyping the Adult Male at All Ages, 258
Atlas of Microscopic Anatomy: A Companion to Histology and Neuroanatomy, 269
Atlas of Neonatal Histopathology, 270
Atlas of Neuropathology, 249
An Atlas of Non-Invasive Techniques: Sound and Pulse Tracings—Echograms, 274
An Atlas of Normal Roentgen Variants That May Stimulate Disease, 275
Atlas of Nuclear Medicine, 264
Atlas of Orthopaedic Surgery, 267
Atlas of Orthotics: Biomechanical Principles and Application, 267
An Atlas of Otolaryngologic Radiology, 268
Atlas of Pathologic Anatomy, 270
Atlas of Pediatric Echocardiography, 272
Atlas of Pediatric Surgery, 272
Atlas of Plaster Cast Techniques, 273
Atlas of Practical Proctology, 257
An Atlas of Primate Gross Anatomy: Baboon, Chimpanzee, and Man, 244
Atlas of Protein Sequence & Structure, 1967–68, 259
An Atlas of Radiation Histopathology, 275
Atlas of Radical Pelvic Surgery, 246
An Atlas of Radiological Anatomy, 275
Atlas of Roentgen Anatomy of the Newborn and Infant Skull: Including Illustrations of Some Pathologic Changes and Congenital Variations with Emphasis on Fetal Radiology, 272
Atlas of Roentgenographic Measurement, 275
Atlas of Roentgenographic Positions and Standard Radiologic Procedures, 275
Atlas of Scanning Electron Microscopy in Medicine, 270
Atlas of Small Animal Surgery; Thoracic, Abdominal and Soft Tissue Techniques, 280

Atlas of Surgery, 246
Atlas of Surgery in the First Six Months of Life, 273
Atlas of Surgical Operations, 247
Atlas of Technics in Surgery, 247
An Atlas of the Anatomy of the Ear, 244
Atlas of the Arteries of the Human Brain, 249
An Atlas of the Blood and Bone Marrow, 260
Atlas of the Face in Genetic Disorders, 259
Atlas of the Human Brain and the Orbit for Computed Tomography, 276
An Atlas of the Human Brain for Computerized Tomography, 276
Atlas of the Newborn, 273
Atlas of the Ultrastructure of Human Breast Diseases, 270
An Atlas of the Ultrastructure of Human Skin: Development, Differentiation, and Post-Natal Features, 254
Atlas of Topographical Anatomy of the Domestic Animals, 280
Atlas of Tumor Pathology, 264
Atlas of Tumor Radiology, 276
An Atlas of Tumors Involving the Central Nervous System, 249
Atlas of Tumors of the Skin, 254
Atlas of Vaginal Surgery, 278
Atlas of Vaginal Surgery: Surgical Anatomy and Technique, 278
Atlas of Vascular Surgery, 260
Atomindex, 536, 555
Attachment and Loss, 390
Audio Journal Review: General Surgery, 595
Audiological Handbook of Hearing Disorders, 120
Audio-Visual Color Films from the Frances Payne Bolton School of Nursing, 596
Audio-Visual Equipment Directory, 591
Audiovisual Market Place: A Multimedia Guide, 591
Audiovisual Materials in Dentistry: A Film Catalog, 596
Audiovisuals, 597

Audio-Visuals On-Line [AVLINE], 587, 620
Author Catalog of the New Academy of Medicine, 6
Autopsy Pathology, Procedure and Protocol, 177
Avian Physiology, 497
Aviation Medicine, 513
Awards, Honors and Prizes: A Source Book and Directory, 281

Babies: Human Development During the First Year, 465
Baby and Child Care, 228
Back to Nursing: A Guide to Current Practice for Active and Inactive Nurses, 221
Backache, 459
Bacterial and Mycotic Infections of Man, 432
Bacteriological Reviews, 373
Bacteriology Illustrated, 263
Bacteriology, Virology and Immunity for Students of Medicine, 432
Bailey and Scott's Diagnostic Microbiology: A Textbook for the Isolation and Identification of Pathogenic Microorganisms, 432
Bailey's Textbook of Histology, 462
Bailliere's Nurses Dictionary, 86
The Barbara Kraus Dictionary of Protein, 87
A Barefoot Doctor's Manual, 169
Barron's Guide to Medical, Dental, and Allied Health Science Careers, 205
Basic and Clinical Immunology, 399
Basic Arithmetic Review and Drug Therapy, 172
A Basic Atlas of the Human Nervous System, 249
Basic Book and Periodical List, Nursing School and Small Medical Library, 3
Basic Dental Reference Works, 13
Basic Electrocardiography Handbook, 102
Basic Handbook of Child Psychiatry, 129

Basic Human Neuroanatomy: An Introductory Atlas, 250
Basic List of Books and Journals for Veterans Administration Medical Libraries, 3
Basic List of Guides and Information Sources for Professional and Patient's Libraries in Hospitals, 3
Basic Medical Statistics, 395
Basic Medical-Surgical Nursing, 194
Basic Nursing Techniques: A Programmed Introduction to Nursing Fundamentals, 439
Basic Pathology, 462
Basic Pediatrics for the Primary Health Care Provider, 466
Basic Statistics for Nurses, 439
Basic Steps in Planning Nursing Research: from Question to Proposal, 221
Basic Texts of the Food and Agriculture Organization of the United Nations, 4
Basic US Government Micrographic Standards and Specifications, 588
The Battered Child, 478
Becker-Shaffer's Diagnosis and Therapy of the Glaucomas, 456
Beck's Obstetrical Practice and Fetal Medicine, 466
Bedside Cardiology, 161
Bedside Diagnosis, 169
Bedside Diagnostic Examination, 169
A Beginner's Handbook in Biological Electron Microscopy, 120
Behavior and Adaptation in Late Life, 478
Behavior Disorders of Childhood and Adolescence, 466
Behavioral Pediatrics and Child Development: A Clinical Handbook, 129
Behavioural Biology Abstracts, 517
Benchmark Papers in Genetics, 355
Benchmark Papers in Human Physiology Series, 348
Benchmark Papers in Microbiology, 357
Benzodiazepines in Clinical Practice, 473

Bergey's Manual of Determinative Bacteriology, 190
Best and Taylor's Physiological Basis of Medical Practice, 436
Beverage Literature: A Bibliography, 33
Beyond the Best Interests of the Child, 479
Bibliographic Control of the Literature of Oncology, 1800–1960, 35
Bibliographic Guide for Editors and Authors, 154
Bibliographic Guide to Conference Publications: 1978, 545
Bibliographic Guide to Government Publications-Foreign: 1978, 539
Bibliographic Guide to Governmental Publications-US: 1978, 540
Bibliographic Guide to Technology: 1978, 18
Bibliographica Genetica Medica, 1930–1970 with Technical Assistance of Martine De Boel, 26
Bibliography of Animal Venoms, Envenomations, and Treatments Period 1500–1968, 51
Bibliography of Audiotapes and Tape-Slide Programs Applicable to Undergraduate Medical Education, 593
Bibliography of Bioethics, 19
A Bibliography of Books on Death, Bereavement, Loss, and Grief, 1935–1968, 41
Bibliography of Child Psychiatry and Child Mental Health with a Selected List of Films, 41
A Bibliography of Chinese Sources on Medicine and Public Health in the People's Republic of China, 1960–1970, 46
A Bibliography of Dentistry in America, 1790–1840, 331
A Bibliography of Doctoral Research on Ecology and the Environment, 1938–1970, 558
A Bibliography of Drug Abuse, Including Alcohol and Tobacco, 41
Bibliography of Drug Dependence and Abuse, 1928–1966, 41

TITLE INDEX

Bibliography of Interlingual Scientific and Technical Dictionaries, 68
Bibliography of Medical Bibliographies, 18
Bibliography on Medical Education, 504
Bibliography of Medical Reviews, 372
A Bibliography of Noise, 1965–1970, 46
A Bibliography of Nursing Literature, 1859–1960, 32
Bibliography of Nursing Monographs, 32
Bibliography of Pharmaceutical Reference Literature, 37
Bibliography of Reproduction: A Classified Monthly Title List Compiled from the World's Research Literature, Vertebrates, Including Man, 51
A Bibliography of Scientific, Technical and Specialized Dictionaries, Polyglot, Bilingual, Unilingual, 68
Bibliography of Society, Ethics, and the Life Sciences, 19
Bibliography of Statistical Bibliographies, 148
Bibliography of Statistical Literature, 148
Bibliography of Surgery of the Hand, 23, 505
Bibliography of the History of Medicine, 322, 622
Bibliography of the History of Medicine of the United States and Canada, 1939–1960, 323
Bibliography of the Socioeconomic Aspects of Medicine, 27
Bibliography of Translations in the Neural Sciences, 1950–1966, 23
Bibliography on Early Childhood, 36
Bibliography on Medical Education, 19
Bibliography on Nuclear Medicine, 35
Bibliography on Smoking and Health, 46
Bibliography on Speech, Hearing, and Language in Relation to Mental Retardation, 1900–1968, 26
Bibliography on Suicide and Suicide Prevention: 1897–1957, 1958–1970, 41

Bibliotheca Anatomica, 348
Bibliotheca Haematologica, 356
Bibliotheca Nutritio et Dieta, 359
Bibliotheca Psychiatrica, 553
Bibliotheca Radiologica, 370
Bibliotherapy: Methods and Materials, 129
Bing's Local Diagnosis in Neurological Diseases, 403
BIO-BASE, 316
Biochemical Genetics, 529
Biochemical Methods in Medical Genetics, 105
Biochemical Values in Clinical Medicine: The Results Following Pathological or Psychological Change, 55
The Biochemistry and Physiology of Bone, 388
Biochemistry: The Molecular Basis of All Structure and Function, 395
Bio-Energy Directory, 288
Bioengineering Abstracts, 500
BIOETHICSLINE, 620
The Biofeedback Syllabus: A Handbook for the Psychophysiologic Study of Biofeedback, 129
A Biographical Dictionary of Scientists, 316
Biographical Directory of the American College of Physicians, 319
Biographical Directory of the American Psychological Association, 320
Biographical Directory of the American Public Health Association, 321
Biographical Directory of the Fellows and Members of the American Psychiatric Association, 321
A Biographical History of Medicine: Excerpts and Essays on the Men and Their Work, 316
Biographical Memoirs, 317
Biographical Memoirs of Fellows of the Royal Society, 319
Biological Abstracts, 501
Biological Abstracts/BIOSIS: The First Fifty Years: The Evolution of a Major Science Information Service, 323
Biological Abstracts/RRM, 501, 547
Biological and Biomedical Resource Literature, 11

Biological Aspects of Lead; An Annotated Bibliography, 46
The Biological Basis of Medicine, 390
Biological Effects of Microwaves, 47
Biological Indicators of Environmental Quality: A Bibliography of Abstracts, 499, 519
Biological Laboratory Data, 141
Biological Membrane Abstracts, 501
Biological Nomenclature, 65
Biological Research Method: A Practical Guide, 241
Biological Sciences: A Bibliography of Bibliographies, 18
Biological Substances: International Standards and Reference Preparations 1975, 571
Biology Data Book, 141
Biology: Its Historical Development, 323
The Biology of Aging, 426
The Biology of Alcoholism, 391
Biology of Cancer, 451
Biomedical Electronics: Marketing Guide and Company Directory for Patient Care Systems and Laboratory Equipment, 295
Biomedical Instrumentation and Measurements, 395
Biomedical Physics and Biomaterials Science, 395
Biomedical, Scientific and Technical Book Reviewing, 1
Biomedical Subject Headings: A Reconciliation of National Library of Medicine and Library of Congress Subject Headings, 11
Biomedical Thesaurus and Guide to Classification, 65
Biomedical Ultrasonics, 485
Biomembranes, 346
Biometrika Tables for Statisticians, 151
Bioresearch Index, 501
Bioscientific Terminology: Words from Latin and Greek Stems, 74
BIOSIS PREVIEWS, 624
Biosynthetic Products for Cancer Chemotherapy, 360
Birth Defects Compendium, 259
Birth Defects: Original Article Series, 382

The Birth of the Clinic—An Archaeology of Medical Perception, 334
Black's Medical Dictionary, 77
Black's Veterinary Dictionary, 93
Blakiston's Gould Medical Dictionary: A Modern Comprehensive Dictionary of the Terms Used in All Branches of Medicine and Allied Sciences; With Illustrations and Tables, 77
Blakiston's Pocket Medical Dictionary, 77
BLLD Announcement Bulletin: A Guide to British Reports, Translations, and Theses, 553, 556
Blood, 529
Blood and Other Body Fluids, 109
Blood Disorders Due to Drugs and Other Agents, 109
Blood Groups in Man, 429
Blue Book of Optometrists: A Directory of Legally Registered Optometrists of the U.S., 300
Blueprint for Medical Care, 214
Bone Marrow and Bone Tissue: Color Atlas of Clinical Histopathology, 260
Bone Marrow Interpretation, 261
Bone Tumors, 451
Bonney's Gynaecological Surgery, 493
Book of ASTM Standards, 569
The Book of Health: A Medical Encyclopedia for Everyone, 52
Books and Periodicals for Medical Libraries in Hospitals, 4
Braille Book Review, 5
Brain, 528
Brain Control, 330
Brain Metastasis, 451
Brain's Clinical Neurology, 404
Brain's Diseases of the Nervous System, 404
Breast Cancer: Advances in Research and Treatment, 360
A Brief Atlas of Histology, 244, 270
British Books in Print, 2
British Health Centres Directory, 295
British Heart Journal, 528
British Herbal Pharmacopoeia, 574
British Initials and Abbreviations, 63
British Journal of Nutrition, 531

British Journal of Obstetrics and Gynaecology, 534
British Journal of Pharmacology, 532
British Journal of Radiology, 534
British Journal of Surgery, 528
British Medical Abstracts and Therapeutic Progress, 507
British Medical Journal, 526
British Medicine, 19
British National Formulary, 574
British Official Publications, 540
British Pharmaceutical Codex, 1973, 575
British Pharmacopeia 1977, 575
British Standards Yearbook, 569
Brock's Injuries of the Brain and Spinal Cord and Their Coverings, 404
Bronchial Asthma: Mechanisms and Therapeutics, 61
Bronchial Carcinoma, 488
Bulletin des traductions-CNRS, 533
Bulletin of the History of Dentistry, 528
Bulletin of the History of Medicine, 530
Bulletin of the Public Affairs Information Service, 501
Bulletin on Narcotics, 533
Bulletin Signalétique, 501
Burger's Medicinal Chemistry, 473
Burket's Oral Medicine: Diagnosis and Treatment, 414
Butterworths Medical Dictionary, 77
Buyer's Guide to Environmental Media: A Directory of Books, Magazines, Films, and Information Sources, 599
Buyer's Guide to Microfilm Equipment, Products, and Services, 1979, 591
Buyer's Guide to Micrographic Equipment, Products, and Services, 591

Ca. Cancer Journal for Clinicians, 531
CA CONDENSATES, 625
CA PATENT CONCORDANCE, 625
CA SEARCH, 625
CAB ABSTRACTS, 624

CAIN, 624
Calcified Tissue Abstracts, 516
Canadian Medical Association Journal, 526
Canadian Medical Diectory, 288
Canadian Nurse, 531
Canadian Nurses' Association Bibliographies, 32
Canadian Standards Association, Catalogue of Standards, 570
Cancer, 531
Cancer: A Comprehensive Treatise, 386
Cancer: A Manual for Practitioners, 175
Cancer Chemotherapeutic Agents: Handbook of Clinical Data, 118
Cancer Chemotherapy, 452
Cancer Chemotherapy; Fundamental Concepts and Recent Advances, 551
Cancer Chemotherapy Reports, 538
Cancer Chemotherapy III, 452
Cancer: Diagnosis, Treatment, and Prognosis, 452
Cancer, Epidemiology and Prevention: Current Concepts, 152
Cancer Film Guide, 597
Cancer Handbook of Epidemiology and Prognosis, 118
Cancer in Children: Clinical Management, 466
CANCERLIT [Cancer Literature], 620
Cancer Medicine, 452
Cancer Mortality, England and Wales 1911–1970, 149
Cancer of the Lung, 488
Cancer of the Skin: Biology, Diagnosis, Management, 416
CANCERPROJ [Cancer Research Projects], 620
Cancer: Publications of the World Health Organization and the International Agency for Research on Cancer, 542
Cancer Therapy Abstracts, 515
Canine Neurology; Diagnosis and Treatment, 497
Cannabis and Health, 473
Cannabis '71, 37
Carcinogenesis Abstracts, 515

Cardiac and Vascular Diseases, 409
Cardiac Arrest and Resuscitation, 200
Cardiac Catheterization and Angiocardiography: An Introductory Manual, 161
Cardiac Catheterization and Angiography, 409
Cardiac Diagnosis and Treatment, 409
Cardiac Mechanics: Physiological, Clinical, and Mathematic Consideration, 409
Cardiovascular Care Unit: A Guide for Planning and Operation, 210
Cardiovascular Clinics Series, 380
Cardiovascular Disease: Epidemiology, Prevention, and Rehabilitation: A Guide to Literature, 25
Cardiovascular Diseases: Guidelines for Prevention and Care, 210
Cardiovascular Dynamics, 102
Cardiovascular Nursing: Prevention, Intervention, Rehabilitation, 440
Cardiovascular Physiology, 409
Cardiovascular Therapy: A Systematic Approach, 210
Care of the Adult Patient, 440
The Care of the Sick: The Emergence of Modern Nursing, 335
The Careful Writer: A Modern Guide to English Use, 154
Carini and Owen's Neurological and Neurosurgical Nursing, 440
The Case for Consultation in Nursing: Designs for Professional Practice, 440
Case Studies in Clinical Nutrition: A Workbook and Study Guide for Students of Nursing and Dietetics, 196
Case Studies Series, 587
Catalog of Biographies, 317
Catalog of Teratogenic Agents, 105, 145
Catalog of the Clearinghouse for Hospital Management Engineering: A Listing of Case Studies and Technical Reports Designed to Increase Productivity and Efficiency in Hospital Department, 538
Catalog of the Library of the American Hospital Association, 6
Catalog of the National Library of Medicine, 1948–1965, 6
Catalog of the Public Documents of the Congress and of all Departments of the Government of the United States for the Period from March 4, 1893–Dec. 31, 1940 (Document Catalog), 540
Catalog of the Sophia F. Palmer Memorial Library, 7
Catalog of Works in the Neurological Sciences Collected by Cyril Brian Courville, M.D., 7
Catalogs of the F. B. Power Pharmaceutical Library, School of Pharmacy, University of Wisconsin, Madison, 7
Catalogue of Arthropod-Borne Viruses of the World: A Collection of Data on Registered Arthropod-Borne Animal Viruses, 109
A Catalogue of Incunabula and Manuscript in the Army Medical Library, by Dorothy M. Schullian and Francis E. Sommer, 323
A Catalogue of Printed Books in the Wellcome Historical Medical Library, 323
A Catalogue of Sixteenth Century Printed Books in the National Library of Medicine, 323
Catalogue of Strains, 147
Cataract Surgery and its Complications, 456
CATLINE [Catalog Online], 621
CBAC; Abstracts on the Chemical-Biological Activities of Chemical Substances, 502
CBE Style Manual, 154
Cecil-Loeb Textbook of Medicine, 436
Cell Biology, 120
Cell Fine Structure: An Atlas of Drawings of Whole-Cell Structure, 270
Centennial Anniversary Volume of the American Neurological Association, 330
A Centennial Bibliography of Huntington's Chorea, 1872–1972, 23
The Central Nervous System of Vertebrates, 378

Central Patents Index—CPI, 581
A Century of DNA: A History of the Discovery of the Structure and Function of the Genetic Substance, 332
Cerebral Arterial Disease, 409
Cerebral Computed Tomography: A Text-Atlas, 277
Cerebral Palsy and Related Development Disabilities Prevention and Early Care: An Annotated Bibliography, 40
C. G. Jung: Letters 1906–1961, 338
Chagas's Disease: (South American Tryanosomiasis): A Bibliography Compiled From Sleeping Sickness Bureau Bulletin, 1908–1912, and Tropical Diseases Bulletin, 1912–1270, 29
Chambers Dictionary of Science and Technology, 75
Checklist of Major US Government Series, 540
Chem Sources Europe, 282
Chem Sources U.S.A., 282
ChemBuyDirect, the International Chemical Buyers Directory, 282
Chemical Abstracts, 578, 579
Chemical Abstracts Patent Index and Concordance, 581
Chemical Abstracts Service Registry Handbook, 94
Chemical Abstracts Service Source Index, 525
Chemical-Biological Activities, 522
Chemical Carcinogens, 452
Chemical Dictionary (American and British Usage), 75
Chemical, Medical and Pharmaceutical Books Printed Before 1800, in the Collection of the University of Wisconsin Libraries, 337
Chemical Mutagenesis: A Survery of the Literature, 16
Chemical Mutagens, 355, 383
Chemical Senses and Flavour, 528
Chemical Synonyms and Trade Names: A Dictionary and Commercial Handbook, 75
Chemist Analyst, 585

A Chemist's Guide to Regulatory Drug Analysis, 229
CHEMLINE [Chemical Dictionary Online], 621
CHEMNAME, 625
Chemoreception Abstracts, 509
Chemotherapy of Cancer, 453
Chest, 534
Chest, Heart, and Vascular Disorders for Physiotherapists, 409
Chest Injuries: A Guide for the Accident Departments, 238
Chest Roentgenology, 488
The Chicago Psychoanalytic Literature Index, 1920–1970, 518
CHILD ABUSE AND NEGLECT, 625
Child Care Issues for Parents and Society: A Guide to Information Sources, 15
Child Development Abstracts and Bibliography, 518
Child Health Encyclopedia: The Complete Guide for Parents, 57
Child Health in the Community: A Handbook of Social and Community Paediatrics, 129
Child Health Maintenance: A Guide to Clinical Assessment, 440
Child Health Maintenance: Concepts in Family Centered Care, 440
The Child Protection Team Handbook: A Multidisciplinary Approach to Managing Child Abuse and Neglect, 130
The Child With a Chronic Medical Problem—Cardiac Disorders, Diabetes, Haemophilia: Social, Emotional and Educational Adjustment: An Annotated Bibliography, 36
The Child with Disabling Illness: Principles of Rehabilitation, 476
Childbearing: A Nursing Perspective, 440
Chinese Herbs: Their Botany, Chemistry, and Pharmacodynamics, 180
Chiropractic: An International Bibliography, 30
Cholera 1832, 333
Chromatography: A Laboratory Hand-

book of Chromatographic and Electrophoretic Methods, 94
Chromosomal Variation in Man; A Catalog of Chromosomal Variants and Anomalies, 550
Chromosome Techniques: Theory and Practice, 383, 423
Chromosomes Today, 550
Chronicles of Pharmacy, 338
CIBA Foundation Symposia, 547
Ciba-Geigy Journal, 585
Ciba Symposium Series, 586
Circulation, 529
Circulatory Physiology, 380
CIS/INDEX, 625
CIS Thesaurus, 66
CLAIMS/CHEM, 626
CLAIMS/CLASS, 626
CLAIMS/US PATENTS, 626
Classics and Other Selected Readings in Medical Librarianship, 12
Classics of Orthopaedics, 459
Classification and Nomenclature of Viruses: 2nd Report of the International Committee on Taxonomy of Viruses, 66
Cleft Lip and Palate: Surgical, Dental, and Speech Aspects, 414
Clinical and Biochemical Analysis Series, 112
Clinical Anesthesia Procedures of the Massachusetts General Hospital, 158
Clinical Aspects of Aging, 426
Clinical Aspects of Immunology, 399
Clinical Atlas of Human Chromosomes, 259
Clinical Cancer Medicine: Treatment Tactics, 453
Clinical Cardiac Radiology, 485
Clinical Cardiovascular Physiology, 410
Clinical Chemistry: Conversion Scales for SI Units with Adult Normal Reference Values, 192
Clinical Concepts in Infectious Disease, 433
Clinical Dental Anesthesia: A Manual of Principles and Practice, 163
Clinical Dermatology, 381
Clinical Diagnosis of Mental Disorders: A Handbook, 130

Clinical Disorders of the Heart Beat, 410
Clinical Education in the Health Professions: An Annotated Bibliography, 20
Clinical Gastroenterology, 420
Clinical Gastroenterology Monographs, 355
Clinical Genetics: A Source Book for Physicians, 200
Clinical Geriatrics, 426
Clinical Guide to Behavior Therapy, 232
Clinical Guide to Undersirable Drug Interactions, 229
Clinical Handbook of Psychopharmacology, 123
Clinical Hematology, 109, 429
Clinical Immunobiology, 375
Clinical Immunology & Immunopathology, 527
Clinical Immunology Newsletter, 527
Clinical Laboratory Tests: A Manual for Nurses, 194
Clinical Management of Seizures: A Guide for the Physician, 209
Clinical Microbiology, 433
Clinical Microbiology Newsletter, 530
Clinical Neurology, 378
Clinical Neurosurgery, 378, 549
Clinical Nuclear Medicine, 531
Clinical Nursing, 440
Clinical Nursing and Techniques, 172
Clinical Nutrition, 449
Clinical Oncology: A Manual for Students and Doctors, 176
Clinical Ophthalmology, 387
Clinical Orthopaedics and Related Research, 532
Clinical Paediatric Surgery, 466
Clinical Pediatric Oncology, 466
Clinical Pediatrics, 532
Clinical Perinatology, 467
Clinical Perspectives in Nursing Research, 440
Clinical Pharmacokinetics, 533
Clinical Pharmacology and Therapeutics, 533
Clinical Phonocardiography and External Pulse Recording, 410

Clinical Physiology Series, 348
Clinical Radioassay Procedures: A Compendium, 193
Clinical Scalar Electrocardiography, 410
Clinical Scintillation Imaging, 453
Clinical Sexuality: A Manual for the Physician and the Professions, 185
Clinical Surgery, 55
Clinical Toxicology, 534
Clinical Toxicology of Commercial Products: Acute Poisoning, 180, 182
Clinical Tropical Diseases, 217
Clinical Urography: An Atlas and Textbook of Roentgenologic Diagnosis, 278
Clinical Vectorcardiography, 410
Clinics in Developmental Medicine, 364
Clinics in Endocrinology and Metabolism, 354
Clinics in Gastroenterology, 355
Clinics in Haematology, 356
CLINPROT [Clinical Cancer Protocols], 621
The CNS Depressant Withdrawal Syndrome and Its Management. An Annotated Bibliography: 1950–1973, 23
Coal Workers' Pneumonoconiosis: A Critical Review, 482
Cocaine, 473
A Cocaine Bibliography—Nonannotated, 37
Code of Federal Regulations, 575
A Coded Compendium of the International Histological Classification of Tumors, 566
CODEN for Periodical Titles: An Aid to the Storage and Retrieval of Information and to Communication Involving Journal References, 525
Cold Spring Harbor Conferences on Cell Proliferation, 552
Cold Spring Harbor Laboratory Symposia on Quantitative Biology, 548
The Cole Library of Early Medicine and Zoology: Catalogue of Books and Pamphlets, 323
The Collaborative Study on Cerebral Palsy, Mental Retardation, and Other Neurological and Sensory Disorders of Infancy and Childhood Bibliography no. 8, July 1974–June 1975, 24
The Collected Works of C. G. Jung, 339
Colleges of Pharmacy, Accredited Programs, 300
Colon, Rectum and Anus, 382
The Colonial Physician and Other Essays, 335
Color Atlas and Textbook of Diagnostic Microbiology, 263
Color Atlas and Textbook of Human Anatomy, 244
Color Atlas and Textbook of Macropathology, 270
Color Atlas and Textbook of Oral Anatomy, 253
Color Atlas of Cardiac Pathology, 252
Color Atlas of Cytodiagnosis of the Prostate, 279
Color Atlas of Dermatology, 255
Color Atlas of Ear, Nose, and Throat, 268
Color Atlas of General Surgical Diagnosis, 247
Color Atlas of Gynecological Surgery, 279
Color Atlas of Histological Staining Techniques, 263
Color Atlas of Histopathology, 271
The Color Atlas of Intestinal Parasites, 257
Color Atlas of Laparoscopy, 279
Color Atlas of Medical Mycology, 263
Color Atlas of Microbiology, 263
Color Atlas of Neoplasia in the Cat, Dog and Horse, 280
Color Atlas of Oral Pathology, 253
Color Atlas of Pathology, 271
Color Atlas of Pediatric Dermatology, 255
Color Atlas of Renal Diseases, 279
Color Atlas of Rheumatology, 278
Color Atlas of Surgery, 247
A Colour Atlas of Forensic Pathology, 271
A Colour Atlas of Histology, 271

TITLE INDEX

A Colour Atlas of Human Anatomy, 244
A Colour Atlas of Liver Disease, 257
A Colour Atlas of Neuropathology, 250
A Colour Atlas of Tropical Medicine and Parasitology, 263
Common Environmental Terms: A Glossary, 91
Communicable and Infectious Diseases: Diagnosis, Prevention, Treatment, 110
Communicating in Spanish for Medical Personnel, 71
Communicating Nursing Research, 441, 551
Community, Culture, and Care: A Cross-Culture Guide for Health Workers, 235
Community Health Nursing Practice, 441
Community Mental Health: A General Introduction, 339
A Companion to Medical Studies, 193
Comparative & Veterinary Medicine, A Guide to the Resource Literature, 17
Comparative Animal Nutrition, 372
Comparative National Policies on Health Care, 427
COMPENDEX, 626
Compendium of Pharmaceuticals and Specialties, 301
The Compleat Herbal: Being a Description of the Origins, the Lore the Characteristics, the Types, and the Prescribed Uses of Medicinal Herbs, Including an Alphabetical Guide to All Common Medicinal Plants, 123
Complete Dental Assistant's, Secretary's, and Hygienist's Handbook, 103
Complete Desk Reference to Veterinary Pharmaceuticals and Biologicals 78/79, 138
The Complete Handbook for Medical Secretaries and Assistants, 94
Compilation of OTC Drug Regulations, 575
Complications of Diabetes, 418
Composite Index for CRC Handbooks, 94
Composition of Foods, 141
Comprehensive Bibliography of Existing Literature on Tobacco: 1969–1974, 47
Comprehensive Bibliography on Health Maintenance Organizations: 1970–1973, 27
Comprehensive Biochemistry, 374
Comprehensive Cardiac Care: A Text for Nurses and Other Health Professionals, 115
A Comprehensive Dictionary of Audiology, 88
COMPREHENSIVE DISSERTATION ABSTRACTS CDI, 626
Comprehensive Dissertation Index, 1861–1972, 556
Comprehensive Dissertation Index: Five Year Cumulation, 1973–1977, 556
Comprehensive Dissertation Index. 1978 Supplement, 556
Comprehensive Endocrinology, 382
A Comprehensive Guide to the Cannabis Literature, 15, 38
Comprehensive Immunology, 375
Comprehensive Management of Epilepsy in Infancy, Childhood, and Adolescence, 160
Comprehensive Management of Hemophilia, 429
Comprehensive Manuals in Radiology, 392
The Comprehensive Nursing Audiovisual Resource List: 1979, 597
Comprehensive Pediatric Nursing, 441
Comprehensive Textbook of Psychiatry, 479
Comprehensive Virology, 383
Computed Brain and Orbital Tomography: Technique and Interpretation, 277
Computer Glossary for Medical and Health Sciences, 78
Computer-Readable Data Bases: A Directory and Data Sourcebook, 1979 ed., 614

Computers in Biomedical Research, 374
Computers in Chemical and Biochemical Research, 346
Computers in Medicine Abstracts, 507
Computext Book Guides: Conference Publications, 545
Computext Book Guides: Medicine, 18
The Concept of a Blood-Brain Barrier, 404
Concepts and Practices of Intensive Care for Nurse Specialists, 441
Conceptual Index to Psychoanalytic Technique and Training, 42
A Concise Dictionary of Medicine, 78
Concise Dictionary of Soviet Terminology, Institutions, and Abbreviations, 63
A Concise Encyclopedia of Psychiatry, 59
Concise Guide to Biomedical Polymers; Their Design, Fabrication and Molding, 214
A Concise Handbook of Respiratory Diseases, 137
CONFERENCE PAPERS INDEX, 626
Congenital Deformities of the Head and Forearm, 493
Congenital Malformations of the Heart, 380
Consent Handbook, 107
Consolidated Index of Translations Into English, 553
Construction and Utilization of Visual Aids in Dental Health Education, 163
Consultants and Consulting Organizations Directory, 282
Consultations in Dermatology II, 416
Consumer Health and Produce Hazards, 391
Consumer Health Information: A Guide to Sources, 12
Consumer Protection Directory: A Comprehensive Guide to Environmental Organizations in the United States and Canada, 304
Consumer Sourcebook: A Directory and Guide to Government Organizations, Associations, Centers, and Institutes; Media Services; Company and Trademark Information; and Bibliographic Material Relating to Consumer Topics, Sources of Recourse, and Advisory Information, 282
Contact Lens Practice, 456
Contemporary Endocrinology, 311
Contemporary Metabolism, 311
Contemporary Neurology Series, 350, 378
Contemporary Nursing Series, 563
Contemporary Pharmacy Practice, 533
Contemporary Topics in Immunobiology, 347
Contemporary Topics in Molecular Immunology, 347
Contemporary Vocational Rehabilitation, 477
Continuing Medical Education: Perspectives, Problems, Prognosis, 395
Continuing Pharmaceutical Education, Approved Providers, 301
Contraceptive Technology: 1978-1979, 185
Contributions to Epidemiology and Biostatistics, 369
Contributions to Gynecology and Obstetrics, 371
Contributions to Nephrology, 371
Control of Communicable Diseases in Man, 167, 482
Control of Hospital Infection: A Practical Handbook, 107
Conversion Tables for SI Metrication, 140
Cooper and Gun's Dispensing for Pharmaceutical Students, 474
Cooperative Studies in Mental Health and Behavioral Sciences: An Annotated Bibliography Summarizing Two Decades of Cooperation in Mental Health and Behavioral Sciences 1956-1975, 42
Copeman's Textbook of the Rheumatic Diseases, 491
Cope's Early Diagnosis of the Acute Abdomen, 420
Coronary Heart Disease: Clinical Angiographic, and Pathologic Profiles, 252

Corpuscles: Atlas of Red Blood Cell Shapes, 261
Correlation Index: Document Series and PB Reports, 537
Corscaden's Gynecologic Cancer, 493
Cosmetic Surgery: A Consumer's Guide, 208
Cost and Benefit of Fluoride in the Prevention of Dental Caries, 414
Countdown. Canadian Nursing Statistics, 151
A Coursebook in Health Care Delivery, 165
Cowan and Steel's Manual for the Identification of Medical Bacteria, 190
Cowdry's Care of the Geriatric Patient, 426
Craig and Faust's Clinical Parasitology, 110, 433
Cranio-Facial-Cleft Palate Bibliography, 25, 505
The Cranium of the Newborn Infant: An Atlas of Tomography and Anatomical Sections, 273
CRC Critical Reviews in Biochemistry, 373
CRC Critical Reviews in Bioengineering, 373
CRC Critical Reviews in Clinical Laboratory Sciences, 373
CRC Critical Reviews in Clinical Radiology, 373
CRC Critical Reviews in Diagnostic Imaging, 373
CRC Critical Reviews in Microbiology, 373, 530
CRC Critical Reviews in Toxicology, 373
CRC Handbook of Food Additives, 116
CRC Handbook of Radioactive Nuclides, 136
CRC Handbook Series in Clinical Laboratory Science, 112
Creative Teaching in Clinical Nursing, 441
Crisis Center/Hotline: A Guidebook to Beginning and Operating, 107
Critical Care Medicine, 530

Critical Care Medicine Handbook, 112
Critical Care Nursing, 441
A Critical Dictionary of Psychoanalysis, 90
Cross-Sectional Anatomy: An Atlas for Computerized Tomography, 244
CTFA Cosmetic Ingredient Dictionary, 66
Cumulative Index of Hospital Literature, 511
Cumulative Index to English Translations 1948–68, 554
Cumulative Index to Nursing Literature, 513
Cumulative Index to Nursing Literature: Nursing Subject Headings, 513
Cumulative Subject Index to the Monthly Catalog of US Government Publications, 1900–1971, 540
Cunningham's Manual of Practical Anatomy, 157
Current Advances in Oral Surgery, 353
Current Audiovisuals for Mental Health Education, 598
Current Bibliography of Epidemiology: A Guide to the Literature of Epidemiology, Preventive Medicine and Public Health, 47
Current Bibliography of Plastic and Reconstructive Surgery, 23, 505
Current Book Review Citations, 1
Current Cardiovascular Topics, 352
Current Catalog Proof Sheets, 6
Current Citations on Strabismus, Amblyopia, and Other Diseases of Ocular Motility, 506, 515
Current Clinical Dental Terminology: A Glossary of Accepted Terms in All Disciplines of Dentistry, 84
Current Concepts in Nutrition, 385
Current Concepts in Ophthalmology, 361
Current Concepts in Radiology, 370
Current Concepts in the Management of Skin Cancer, 212
Current Contents, 522
Current Controversies in Neurosurgery, 404

Current Dermatologic Management, 163
Current Developments in Psychopharmacology, 366
Current Diagnosis, 346
Current Diagnostic Pediatrics, 389
Current Haematology, 109
Current Index to Conference Papers in Engineering, 545
Current Index to Conference Papers; Science and Technology, 545
Current Literature on Aging, 14
Current Medical Diagnosis and Treatment, 311, 436
Current Medical Information and Technology, 78
Current Medical References, 12
Current Neurology, 350
Current Pediatric Diagnosis and Treatment, 467
Current Pediatric Therapy, 121, 467
Current Practice in Orthopaedic Surgery, 362
Current Problems in Dermatology, 353
Current Problems in Diagnostic Radiology, 370
Current Problems in Surgery, 528
Current Programs, 546
Current Psychiatric Therapies, 368
CURRENT RESEARCH INFORMATION SYSTEM, 627
Current Surgical Practice, 348
Current Therapy, 169
Current Therapy in Dentistry, 353
Current Topics in Biochemistry, 346
Current Topics in Comparative Pathobiology, 363
Current Topics in Developmental Biology, 348
Current Topics in Experimental Endocrinology, 354
Current Topics in Eye Research, 362
Current Topics in Haematology, Immunology and Blood Transfusion, 430
Current Topics in Immunology, 376
Current Topics in Membranes and Transport, 346
Current Topics in Mental Health, 391
Current Topics in Microbiology and Immunology, 357
Current Topics in Radiation Research, 370
Current Topics in Surgical Research, 348
Current Work in the History of Medicine: An International Bibliography, 323
Currents in Alcoholism, 369
Curriculum Building in Nursing: A Process, 441
Cutter Laboratories Annual Report, 585
Cutting's Handbook of Pharmacology: The Actions and Uses of Drugs, 123
Cystic Fibrosis: Manual of Diagnosis and Management, 184
The Cytologic Diagnosis of Cancer, 225
Cytology of the Female Genital Tract: International Histological Classification of Tumours No. 8, 566

d'Abreu's Practice of Cardiothoracic Surgery, 410
Dangerous Plants, Snakes, Arthropods and Marine Life. Toxicity and Treatment, 483
Dangerous Properties of Industrial Materials, 132
Data for Biochemical Research, 142
Data for Protection Against Ionizing Radiation From External Sources: Supplement to ICRP Publication 15, 146
DATRIX (Direct Access to Reference Information, a Xerox Service), 556
Davidson's Biochemistry of the Nucleic Acids, 423
Davis and Geck Surgical Film Catalog, 1969–1970, 595
Davison's Compleat Pediatrician, 467
Dealing with Dilemma: A Manual for Genetic Counselors, 165
Death: A Bibliographical Guide, 42
Death, Grief and Bereavement: A Bibliography 1845–1975, 42
Definition and Measurement of Mental Health, 567
Demographic Yearbook, 149
Dental Abstracts, 509

Dental Abstracts: A Selection of World Dental Literature, 509
The Dental Assistant, 415
Dental Education in the United States and Canada. A Report to the Carnegie Foundation, 331
Dental Practioner Handbooks, 103
Dental Research in the United States, Canada, and Great Britain, 561
Dental-Worterbuch. Dictionary of Dental Practice, 69
Dental X-ray Protection, 415
Dentist's Manual of Emergency Medical Treatment, 163
The Dentists Register, 295
Depression: Clinical, Biological, and Psychological Perspectives, 479
Depression: Theory and Research, 479
Dermatoglyphics in Medical Disorders, 416
Dermatology, 381
Dermatology: An Illustrated Guide, 212
Derwent Publications Ltd. Documentation Services, 581
Design and Analysis in the Animal and Medical Sciences, 393
The Design of a Health Maintenance Organization: A Handbook for Practitioners, 107
Desk Reference for Neuroanatomy: A Guide to Essential Terms, 83
Detection, Prevention and Management of Urinary Tract Infections: A Manual for the Physician, Nurse and Allied Health Worker, 185
Developing Policies and Procedures for Long-Term Care Institutions, 215
Development and Use of Patent Classification Systems, 579
Development of Angiography and Cardiovascular Catheterization, 410
Development of Biochemical Concepts from Ancient to Modern Times, 324
The Development of Medical Bibliography, 324
The Development of Medicine as a Profession, 324

Development of the Human Dentition: An Atlas, 253
The Development of Traditional Psychopathology: A Sourcebook, 203
Developmental and Cell Biology Series, 388
Developmental Disabilities Abstracts, 518
Developmental Neuropathology, 404
Developmental Physiology and Aging, 427
Developments in Biological Standardization, 571
Developments in Medical Microbiology and Infectious Diseases, 357
Diabetes, 529
Diabetes and its Management, 212
Diabetes Guidebook, Diet Section, 213
Diabetes: Its Physiological and Biochemical Basis, 213
Diabetes Literature Index: By Authors, Hierarchy, and By Keywords in the Title, 510
Diabetes Mellitus: Diagnosis and Treatment, 354
The Diabetic Foot, 418
Diagnosis and Early Management of Trauma Emergencies: A Manual for the Emergency Service, 169
The Diagnosis and Treatment of Diseases of the Nervous System, 160
Diagnosis and Treatment of Hemophilia: A Practical Guide, 217
Diagnosis of Diseases of the Chest, 411
Diagnositic and Statistical Manual Mental Disorders, DSM-III, 64
Diagnostic Endocrinology, 104
Diagnostic Methods in Cardiology, 411
Diagnostic Methods in Clinical Virology, 217
Diagnostic Neuroradiology, 99
Diagnostic Parasitology: Clinical Laboratory Manual, 190
Diagnostic Procedures: A Reference for Health Practitioners and a Guide for Patient Counseling, 218
Diagnostic Ultrasound, 485
Diagnostic Ultrasound: Text and Cases, 485

Dictionaries of English and Foreign Languages: A Bibliographical Guide to Both General and Technical Dictionaries with Historical and Explanatory Notes and References, 69
Dictionary Catalog on Deafness and the Deaf, 8
Dictionary of Abbreviations in Medicine and the Health Sciences, 64
Dictionary of American Medical Biography, 319
Dictionary of Bacteriological Equivalents: French-English, German-English, Italian-English, Spanish-English, 71
Dictionary of Behavioral Science, 90
Dictionary of Biochemistry, 75
Dictionary of Biological Terms, 75
A Dictionary of Biology, 75
A Dictionary of Dermatological Words, Terms and Phrases, 84
Dictionary of Epilepsy, 83
A Dictionary of Genetics, 84
A Dictionary of Immunology, 83
Dictionary of Medical Ethics, 78
The Dictionary of Medical Folklore, 78
Dictionary of Medical Syndromes, 78
A Dictionary of Microbial Taxonomy, 85
Dictionary of Microbiology, 86
A Dictionary of Midwifery and Public Health, 91
Dictionary of Nutrition and Food Technology, 87
Dictionary of Radiologic Terminology, 92
Dictionary of Report Series Codes, 537
Dictionary of Scientific Biography, 317
The Dictionary of Sodium, Fats, and Cholesterol, 87
Dictionary of Speech & Hearing, Anatomy & Physiology, 88
Dictionary of the Biological Sciences, 75
Dictionary of the Environmental Sciences, 91
Dictionary/Reference Guide for Respiratory Therapy, 92
Dictionnaire Medical, 69

The Diet Food Finder, 33
Diet Manual, 174
A Diet of Living, 449
Dietary Nutrient Guide, 224
Differential Diagnosis in Dermatology, 416
Differential Diagnosis of Eye Diseases, 265
The Digestive System: An Ultrastructural Atlas and Review, 257
Directory: Departments of Anatomy of the United States and Canada: Schools of Medicine, Dentistry, Osteopathic Medicine, Veterinary Medicine, 294
Directory for Exceptional Children, 300
Directory for the National Clearinghouse Program of the American Association of Blood Banks, 297
Directory of Accredited Allied Medical Educational Programs 1969/70, 292
Directory of Accredited Institutions With Programs in Biocommunications, 292
Directory of Agencies Serving the Visually Handicapped in the United States, 302
Directory of Agencies: U.S. Voluntary, International Voluntary, Intergovernmental, 282
Directory of Approved Internship and Residences, 292
Directory of Architects For Health Facilities, 296
Directory of British Associations, 601
Directory of Canadian Scientific and Technical Periodicals, 524
Directory of Cancer Research Information Resources, 299
Directory of Catholic Special Facilities and Programs in the U.S. for Handicapped Children and Adults, 302
Directory of Certified Nurses, 298
Directory of Contraceptives. Directoire de Contraceptifs. Directorio de Anticonceptivos, 307
Directory of Drug Information and Treatment Organizations, 301

TITLE INDEX

Directory of Engineering, Scientific and Management Document Sources, 563
Directory of Environmental Information Sources, 304
Directory of European Associations, 601
Directory of Federal Health/Medicine Grant and Contract Programs, 283, 288
Directory of Graduate Research: Faculties, Publications, and Doctoral Theses in Departments or Divisions of Chemistry, Chemical Engineering, Biochemistry, and Pharmaceutical and/or Medicinal Chemistry at Universities in the United States and Canada, 292
Directory of Health Sciences Libraries in the United States, 1973, 288
Directory of High-Energy Radiotherapy Centres, 1976 Edition, 307
A Directory of Information Resources in the United States: Biological Sciences, 283
A Directory of Information Resources in the United States: General Toxicology, 304
A Directory of Information Resources in the United States: Physical Sciences, Engineering, 283
Directory of Japanese Scientific Periodicals, 1967, 524
Directory of Medical Specialists, 289
Directory of Medicare Providers and Suppliers of Services, Hospitals Extended Care Facilities, Outpatient Physical Therapy, Independent Laboratories, Portable X-Ray Units, 296
Directory of National Trade and Professional Associations of the United States, and Buyer's Guide, 1972, 601
Directory of On-going Research in Cancer Epidemiology, 1978, 561
Directory of On-going Research in Smoking and Health, 561
The Directory of On-Line Data Bases, 614

Directory of Osteopathic Specialists, 297
Directory of Outpatient Psychiatric Clinics and Other Mental Health Resources in the United States, 303
Directory of Poison Control Centers, 305
Directory of Published Proceedings, Series SEMT—Science/Engineering/Medicine/Technology, 546
Directory of Schools of Nursing in the European Region, 298
Directory of Scientific Directories: A World Guide to Scientific Directories, Including Medicine, Agriculture, Engineering, Manufacturing and Industrial Directories, 281, 283
Directory of Selected Training Facilities in Family Planning and Allied Subjects, 305
Directory of Self-Assessment Programs for Physicians, 289
Directory of Social and Health Agencies of New York City, 303
Directory of Special Libraries and Information Centers, 283
Directory of State and Local Alcoholism Services, 305
Directory of State, Territorial, and Regional Health Authorities, 305
Directory of Technical and Scientific Translators and Services, 554
Directory of United States Standardization Activities, 568
Directory of Universities and Colleges Offering Graduate Programs in the Medical Laboratory Sciences, 293
Directory of Women Physicians in the U.S., 320
A Directory of World Psychiatry, 303
Disability and Rehabilitation: A Selected Bibliography, 40
Disability and Rehabilitation Handbook, 127
Disaster Handbook, 132
Disaster Technology: An Annotated Bibliography, 47
Discharge Planning Handbook, 107

A Discursive Dictionary of Health Care, 85
Disease of Bone and Joints, 459
Diseases of the Breast, 453
Diseases and Destiny: A Bibliography of Medical References to the Famous, 317
Diseases of Muscle: A Study in Pathology, 491
The Diseases of Occupations, 133
Diseases of the Colon and Rectum, 529
Diseases of the Ear, 461
Diseases of the Esophagus, 420
Diseases of the Gallbladder and Biliary System, 420
Diseases of the Heart, 411
Diseases of the Heart and Blood Vessels; Nomenclature and Criteria for Diagnosis, 66
Diseases of the Liver, 421
Diseases of the Liver and Biliary System, 421
Diseases of the Liver and Biliary Tract: Proceedings of the 5th Quadranial Meeting of the International Association for the Study of the Liver, Acapulco 1974, 572
Diseases of the Nervous System, Described for Practitioners and Students, 405
Diseases of the Nervous System in Infancy, Childhood, and Adolescence, 467
Diseases of the Nose, Throat, and Ear, 461
Diseases of the Skin in Children and Adolescents: A Colour Atlas, 255
Diseases Transmitted From Animals to Man, 433
Disorders of the Respiratory Tract in Children, 467
Disorders of the Voluntary Muscle, 492
Dissertation Abstracts International, 557
The Distribution of the Human Blood Groups and Other Polymorphisms, 430
Dm. Disease-A-Month, 530

Doctoral Dissertations in the Health and Behavioral Sciences, 557
Doctoral Programs in Nursing: Nurse Scientist Graduate Training Grants Program, 298
The Doctor's Law Guide: Essentials of Practice Management, 205
Doctors Wanted: No Women Need Apply, 324
Dog Owner's Encyclopedia of Veterinary Medicine, 62
Dorland's Illustrated Medical Dictionary, 78
Dorland's Pocket Medical Dictionary, 79
The Double Contrast Examination of the Colon: Experiences With the Welin Modification, 421
Down-Syndrome: Mongolismus, 26
Down's Syndrome (Mongolism): A Reference Bibliography, 26
Drinking Water and Health, 483
Drug Abuse Current Awareness System (DACAS), 523
Drug Abuse Films, 598
Drug Abuse: A Guide for the Clinician, 235
Drug and Cosmetic Catalog, 301
Drugdex, 592
Drug and Therapeutics Bulletin, 533
Drug Disposition and Pharmacokinetics With a Consideration of Pharmacological and Clinical Relationships, 474
DRUGDOC, 627
Drug Dosage in Laboratory Animals: A Handbook, 112
Drug Effects in Hospitalized Patients, 229
Drug-Induced Ocular Side Effects and Drug Interactions, 474
DRUGINFO, 627
Drug Information for Patients, 230
Drug Information Sources: A Worldwide Annotated Survey, 38
Drug Intelligence and Clinical Pharmacy, 533
Drug Interactions, 124
Drug Interactions: A Handbook of Clinical Use, 124

Drug Interactions Index 1978/79, 124
Drug Literature Index, 516
Drug Metabolism in Man, 474
The Drug, The Nurse, The Patient, 115
Drug Topics Red Book, 584
Drug Use and Abuse Among U.S. Minorities: An Annotated Bibliography, 42
Drugs: An Annotated Bibliography and Guide to the Literature, 38
Drugs and Microbes, 596
Drugs and Nursing Implications, 201
Drugs and the Elderly: Social and Pharmacological Issues, 474
Drugs and the Pharmaceutical Sciences Series, 390
Drugs and Therapy: A Psychotherapist's Handbook of Psychotropic Drugs, 130
Drugs from A to Z: A Dictionary, 89
The Drugs Handbook, 124
Drugs in Current Use and New Drugs, 124
Drugs: International Journal of Current Therapeutics and Applied Pharmacology Reviews, 533
Drugs of Addiction and Non-Addiction; Their Use and Abuse. A Comprehensive Bibliography, 1960–1969, 38
Drugs of Choice, 202
Duncan's Dictionary for Nurses, 86
Duncan's Diseases of Metabolism, 418
DuVries' Surgery of the Foot, 459
Dx and Rx: A Physician's Guide to Medical Writing, 205
Dying and Death: A Clinical Guide for the Caregiver, 235
Dying and Death: An Annotated Bibliography, 43
Dynamics of Law in Nursing and Health Care, 441
Dynamics of Oncology Nursing, 442

Ear, Nose, and Throat Disorders: A Practitioner's Guide, 228
Early American Medical Imprints: A Guide to Works Printed in the United States, 1668–1820, 324
Early Breast Cancer: Its History and Results of Treatment, 453
Early Care of the Injured Patient, 436
Early Childhood Psychosis: Infantile Autism, Childhood Schizophrenia and Related Disorders: An Annotated Bibliography, 1964 to 1969, 43
The Early Diagnosis of the Acute Abdomen, 421
Eater's Digest: The Consumer's Factbook of Food Additives, 144
Eating Disorders: Obesity, Anorexia Nervosa, and the Person Within, 449
Echocardiography, 411
Echocardiography: A Teaching Atlas, 252
Educational Film Locator, 588
Educational Media Catalogs on Microfiche, 588
EEG of Human Sleep, 405
EEG Technology, 405
Effective Psychotherapy: A Handbook of Research, 130
The Effects of Irradiation on the Skeleton, 483
1851 Colney Hatch Asylum: Friern Hospital 1973. A Medical and Social History, 339
The EKG: Basic Techniques for Interpretation, 102
Electricial Activity of the Nervous System, 160, 405
Electrodiagnosis: A Handbook for Neurologists, 99
Electroencephalography and Clinical Neurology: Index to Current Electroencephalographic Literature, 509
An Electron Micrographic Atlas of Viruses, 259
Electronics for Neurobiologists, 99
Elements of Medical Genetics, 424
Elements of Research in Nursing, 442
Elsevier's Dictionary of Pharmaceutical Science and Techniques in Five Languages: English, French, Italian, Spanish, German, 72
Elsevier's Dictionary of Public Health: In Six Languages, English-French-Spanish-Italian-Dutch and German, 72

Elsevier's Medical Dictionary in Five Languages: English/American, French, Italian, Spanish, and German, 72
Emergency Care Handbook: How to Deal With People In Emergencies, 112
Emergency Medical Guide, 218
Emergency Medical Services: Selected Bibliography, 31
Emergency-Room Care, 113
Emergency Treatment and Management, 219
Emmett's Clinical Urography: An Atlas and Textbook of Roentgenologic Diagnosis, 279
Emotions and Bodily Changes: A Survey of Literature on Psychosomatic Interrelationships, 1910–1953, 43
Encyclopaedic Handbook of Medical Psychology, 59
Encyclopedia and Dictionary of Medicine, Nursing, and Allied Health, 86
Encyclopedia of Animal Care, 62
Encyclopedia of Antibiotics, 57
Encyclopedia of Associations, 284, 601
The Encyclopedia of Baby and Child Care, 57
The Encyclopedia of Biochemistry, 52
Encyclopedia of Bioethics, 52
The Encyclopedia of Common Diseases, 55
Encyclopedia of Enzyme Technology, 52
Encyclopedia of Food Science, 56
Encyclopedia of Governmental Advisory Organizations: A Reference Guide to Presidential Advisory Committees, Public Advisory Committees, Interagency Committees and Other Government Related Boards, Panels, Task Forces, Commissions, Conferences, and Other Similar Bodies of Serving in a Consultative, Coordinating, Advisory, Research, or Investigative Capacity, 284
Encyclopedia of Human Behavior: Psychology, Psychiatry, and Mental Health, 59

Encyclopedia of Medical Radiology. Handbuch der Medizinischen Radiologie, 61
Encyclopedia of Medical Sources, 52
Encyclopedia of Mental Health, 59
Encyclopedia of Microscopic Stains, 56
The Encyclopedia of Microscopy and Microtechnique, 57
Encyclopedia of Occupational Health and Safety, 60
The Encyclopedia of Patent Practice and Invention Management, 579
Encyclopedia of Psychoanalysis, 59
Encyclopedia of Psychology, 60
Encyclopedia of Sociology, 52
Encyclopedia of Sport Sciences and Medicine, 59
The Encyclopedia of the Biological Sciences, 52
Encyclopedia of Urology, 61
Encyclopedia Reprints Series, 563
Endocrinology, 104, 529
Endocrinology Index, 505, 510
Endocrinology, Metabolism and Gastroenterology, 418
Endocrinology of Pregnancy, 418
Endoscopy, 421
Endoscopy and Biopsy of the Esophagus and Stomach: A Color Atlas, 257
Energy: A Key-Phrase Dissertation Index, 558
Enfermedades de la Boca: Semiologia, Patologia, Clinica y Terapeutica de la Mucosa Bucal, 380
English-French French-English Dictionary of Medical and Biological Terms, 69
English-Spanish Guide for Medical Personnel, 205
ENVIROLINE, 627
The Environment Film Review: A Critical Guide to Ecology Films, 599
Environment Index: A Guide to the Key Environmental Literature of the Year, 520
Environment Regulation Handbook: Air Pollution, Land Use, Mobile Sources, NEPA, Noise, Pesticides,

Radioactive Materials, Solid Wastes, Water Pollution, 133
Environmental and Industrial Health Hazards, 235
Environmental Biology, 133
Environmental Impact Statements, 627
Environmental Pollution: A Guide to Current Research, 561
Environmental Pollution and Mental Health, 47
Environmental Protection Agency Research Catalog, 562
Environmental Protection Directory: A Comprehensive Guide to Environmental Organizations in the United States and Canada, 305
Environmental Quality—1976, 314
Environmental Radiation Measurements, 133
Environmental Toxicology: A Guide to Information Sources, 16
Enzyme Handbook, 94
Enzyme Handbook Supplement I, 95
The Enzymes, 382
EPB Environmental Periodical Bibliography, 627
Epidemiology and Community Medicine, 483
Epidemiology of Diabetes and Its Vascular Lesions, 418
The Epidemiology of Human Mycotic Diseases, 433
Epilepsy: A Study of the Idiopathic Disease, 405
Epilepsy Bibliography, 1900–1950, 24
Epilepsy Handbook, 99
EPILEPSYLINE, 621
The Esophagus, 421
The Esophagus Handbook and Atlas of Endoscopy, 105
The Essential Guide to Prescription Drugs: What You Need to Know For Safe Drug Use, 230
Essential Immunology, 399
Essentials of Clinical Neuroanatomy and Neurophysiology, 405
The Essentials of Forensic Medicine, 462
Essentials of Geriatric Medicine, 214

Essentials of Human Anatomy, 400
Essentials of Immunology and Microbiology, 433
Essentials of Neuropathology, 405
Essentials of Nursing: A Medical-Surgical Text for Practical Nurses, 442
Essentials of Nursing Research, 442
Essentials of Psychiatric Nursing, 442
The Essentials of Roentgen Interpretation, 486
Ethical Constraints and Imperatives in Medical Research, 395
Ethical Dilemmas and Nursing Practice, 442
Ethics and Health Policy, 428
Ethics in Medicine: Historical Perspectives and Contemporary Concerns, 324
Ethics in Nursing: References and Resources, 32
EUROhealth Handbook, 289
European Research Index, 284
The Euthanasia Controversy 1812–1974: A Bibliography with Select Annotations, 20
The Evaluation of Micropublications; A Handbook for Librarians, 588
Evaluations of Drug Interactions, 202
The Evan Bedford Library of Cardiology, 8
Everyone's Guide to Better Food and Nutrition, 224
Everywoman; A Gynecological Guide for Life, 239
Evolution, 396
The Evolution of Psychoanalytical Technique, 203
EXCEPTIONAL CHILD EDUCATION RESOURCES, 627
Excerpta Medica, 507, 628
Excerpta Medica, International Congress Series, 548
Exercise Manual in Immunology, 187
Exercise Testing and Exercise Training in Coronary Heart Disease, 411
Experimental Models of Epilepsy: A Manual for the Laboratory Worker, 188
Experimental Pharmaceutics, 197

Experimentation with Human Beings: The Authority of the Investigator, Subject, Professions, and State in the Human Experimentations Process, 396
Experiments in Physiology, 158
Explorers of the Body, 325
The Eye, 387
The Eye: Comparative Physiology, 456
Eye Surgery, 226, 456

The Faber Medical Dictionary, 79
The Faber Pocket Medical Dictionary, 79
Facts About Nursing, 151
Facts and Comparisons, 124
Fairbank's Atlas of General Affections of the Skeleton, 267
Familiar Medical Quotations, 79
Family Factbook, 199
Family Health Encyclopedia: An International Reference in the Health Sciences, 53
Family Medicine: Principles and Practice, 437
The Family Prescription and Medication Guide, 230
Family Therapy and Research: An Annotated Bibliography of Articles and Books Published 1950–1970, 20
FASEB Monographs, 374
The Fate of Drugs in the Organism: A Bibliographic Survey, 38
The Father of Child Care—Life of William Cadogan, 1711–1797, 337
FDA Consumer, 523
FDA Drug and Device Product Approvals, 575
FDA Reports, "The Pinksheet," 523
Federal Funds for Research Development and Other Scientific Activities, 558
Federal Information Processing Standards Index, 570
Federal Regulatory Directory 1979–80, 284
Federal Statistical Directory, 148
Federation Proceedings, 548
Feeding, Weight and Obesity Abstracts, 514

Female Reproductive System, 138
Female Sex Anomalies, 493
Female Sterilization: A Handbook for Women, 138
Female Sterilization: Guidelines for the Development of Services, 240
Fertility Modification Thesaurus with Focus on Evaluation of Family Planning Programs, 66
The Fetus and Newly Born Infant: Influences of the Perinatal Environment, 467
Film Guide on Reproduction and Development, 600
Film Reviews in Psychiatry, Psychology and Mental Health: A Descriptive & Evaluative Listing of Educational & Instructional Films, 598
FIND: Financial Information National Directory: Health Careers, 293
Findings of Drug Abuse Research, 16
Fine Structure of Cells and Tissues, 462
First Aid Principles and Procedures, 169
The First Century of Experimental Psychology, 339
The First Three Years of Life, 468
Fitness, Health, and Work Capacity; International Standards for Assessment, 576
Fitting Guide for Hard and Soft Contact Lenses: A Practical Approach, 226
The Flexner Report on Medical Education in the United States and Canada, 325
Flies and Disease, 384
Fluoride Abstracts, 520
Focal Point, 585
Food and Drugs, 575
Food and Nutrition, 531
Food and Nutrition/Alimentation et nutrition/Alimentation y nutricion: Annotated Bibliography, Author, and Subject Index, 33
Food and Nutrition Information and Educational Materials Center Catalog, 34
Food and Nutrition News, 531

Food and Nutrition Terminology: Definitions of Selected Terms and Expressions in Current Use, 87
Food Composition Tables: Updated Annotated Bibliography, 34
Food Consumption Statistics, 1970–1975, 150
Food Ingredients Directory, 299
Food: Multilingual Thesaurus, 67
Food, Nutrition and Diet Therapy, 449
Food Science and Technology Abstracts, 515, 628
Food Science Series, 385
Food: The Gift of Osiris, 336
Foot Disorders: Medical and Surgical Management, 459
Foreign Medical School Catalogue, 293
Foreign Patents: A Guide to Official Patent Literature, 579
Forensic Medicine: A Study in Trauma and Environmental Hazards, 374
Forthcoming International Scientific and Technical Conferences, 544
The Foundation Directory, 284, 628
FOUNDATION GRANTS INDEX, 628
Fractures, 459
Free and Inexpensive Materials, 583
French-English Dictionary of Physical Medicine and Rehabilitation, 69
French's Index of Differential Diagnosis, 513
Freud: The Fusion of Science and Humanism: The Intellectual History of Psychoanalysis, 339
Frontiers in Neuroendocrinology, 354
Frontiers of Biology, 375
Frontiers of Gastrointestinal Research, 550
Frontiers of Hormone Research, 354
Frontiers of Oral Physiology, 381
Frontiers of Radiation Therapy and Oncology, 387
Frozen Blood: A Review of the Literature 1949–1968, 28
Functional Anatomy of the Human Kidney, 585, 600
Functional Neuroanatomy of Man, 406
Functions of the Nervous System, 378

Fundamentals of Clinical Hematology, 430
Fundamentals of Electroencephalography, 406
Fundamentals of Microbiology, 434
Fundamentals of Nursing, 442
Fundamentals of Nursing Practice: Concepts, Roles and Functions, 442
Fundamentals of Operating Roon Nursing, 442
Fundamentals of Public Health Nursing, 115
Fundamentals of Quantity Food Preparation: Desserts and Beverages, 449
Fundamentals of Radiation Therapy and Cancer Chemotherapy, 486
Fundamentals of Radiology, 486
Funk and Scott Index of Corporations and Industries, 285
Funktionelle Dermatologie, 104
The Future of Medical Education, 396

Gaddum's Pharmacology, 474
Gamuts in Radiology: Comprehensive Lists of Roentgen Differential Diagnosis, 146
Gardner's Chemical Synonyms and Trade Names, 76
Gastroenterological Nursing, 222
Gastroenterology, 213, 529
Gastroenterology Abstracts and Citations, 511
Gastroenterology in Clinical Nursing, 442
Gastrointestinal Angiography, 422
Gastrointestinal Disease: Pathophysiology, Diagnosis, Management, 422
Gebbie House Magazine Directory, 583
General Clinical Research Centers: A Research Resources Directory, 289
General Information Concerning Patents: A Brief Introduction to Patent Matters, 580
General Ophthalmology, 456
General Parasitology, 434
General Patents Index—GPI, 582
General Pathology, 462
General Urology, 493
General Veterinary Pathology, 497

Genetic Screening Programs: Principles and Research, 424
Genetical Research, 529
Genetics, 529
Genetics Abstracts, 511
The Genetics of Human Populations, 424
Geochemistry and the Environment, 391
Geriatric Nursing, 222
Geriatric Psychiatry: A Handbook for Psychiatrists and Primary Care Physicians, 106
Geriatrics, 529
Gibbon's Surgery of the Chest, 411
Glaucoma Guidebook, 226
Glossary of Bacteriological Terms, 86
Glossary of Genetics and Cytogenetics, Classical and Molecular, 84
Glossary of Genetics in English, French, Italian, German, and Russian, 72
Glossary of Health Care Terminology, 85
Glossary of Histopathological Terms, 89
Glossary of Immunological Terms, 83
Glossary of Mental Disorders and Guide to Their Classification, 90
Glossary of Molecular Biology, 79
Glossary of Words and Phrases Used in Radiology, Nuclear Medicine, and Ultrasound, 92
Golden's Diagnostic Radiology, 136
Good Health Abroad—A Traveller's Handbook, 133
A Good Idea: The History of the Nutrition Foundation, 336
Goodale's Clinical Interpretation of Laboratory Tests, 396
Gout and Hyperuricemia, 203
Governing Hospitals: Trustees and the New Accountabilities, 215, 428
Government Publications and Their Use, 540
Government Publications Reviews, 540
Government Reference Books 74/75: A Biennial Guide to US Government Publications, 540

Government Reports Announcements and Index, 502, 537, 555
Government Wide Index to Federal Research and Development Reports, 537
Grant and Awards; Fiscal Year 1976, 558
Grant Data Quarterly, 559
GRANTS, 628
Grant's Atlas of Anatomy, 245
Grant's Clinical Electrocardiography, 412
Grant's Dissector, 187
Grassroots, 523
Gray's Anatomy, 207
The Great Medical Bibliographers: A Study in Humanism, 325
Great Teachers of Surgery in the Past, 329
Great Women of Medicine, 317
Greenfield's Neuropathology, 406
Grinker's Neurology, 406
Gross Anatomy Dissector: A Companion for Atlas of Clinical Anatomy, 208
Gross Pathology: A Color Atlas, 271
Group Practice of Dentistry, 212
A Growth Chart for International Use in Maternal and Child Health Care: Guidelines for Primary Health Care Personnel, 142
Growth, Including Reproduction and Morphological Development, 97
Grzimek's Animal Life Encyclopedia, 62
A Guide for Automatic Radiographic Processing and Film Quality Control, 237
A Guide for Beginning Psychotherapists, 232
Guide for Mental Health Workers, 232
A Guide for Nurse Managers, 222
A Guide to Alcohol and Drug Dependence, 233
Guide to American Scientific and Technical Directories, 281
The Guide to Biomedical Standards, 568
A Guide to Canadian Health Science: Information Service and Sources, 12

A Guide to Dental Radiography, 212
A Guide to Dermatohistopathology, 212
Guide to Diagnostic Procedures, 219
A Guide to Dissection in Gross Anatomy, 208
A Guide to Drug Abuse Education and Information Materials, 598
A Guide to Drug Eruptions, 230
Guide to Drug Information, 15
A Guide to Drug Interactions, 230
A Guide to Electrical Hazards and Safety Standards, 576
Guide to Films (16mm) About the Use of Dangerous Drugs, Narcotics, Alcohol and Tobacco (With a Separate Section on Filmstrips), 598
Guide to Films on Mental Handicap: A List of Films on All Aspects of Mental Handicap, Classified by Subject and Suggested Audiences, 599
Guide to Foreign Medical Schools, 293
Guide to House Surgeons in the Surgical Unit, 208
A Guide to International Recommendations on Names and Symbols for Quantities and on Units of Measurement, 565
A Guide to Medical Mathematics, 205
Guide to Medical Writing: A Practical Manual for Physicians, Dentists, Nurses, Pharmacists, 154
A Guide to Microforms and Microform Retrieval Equipment, 591
Guide to Microforms in Print, 588
Guide to Micrographic Equipment, 591
A Guide to Nursing Management of Psychiatric Patients, 194, 222
A Guide to Popular Government Publications: For Libraries and Home Reference, 541
A Guide to Psychiatric Books in English, 15
Guide to Pulmonary Medicine, 239
A Guide to Radiation Protection, 235
Guide to Reference Books, 9
Guide to Reference Material, 9
Guide to Reprints, 563
Guide to Russian Reference Books, 9
Guide to Science and Technology in the USA, 559
Guide to Science and Technology in the USSR; A Reference Guide to Science and Technology in the Soviet Union, 559
A Guide to Scientific and Technical Journals in Translation, 555
Guide to Searching the Biological Literature, 588
Guide to Simple Sanitary Measures for the Control of Enteric Diseases, 236
Guide to Specifications and Standards of the Federal Government, 568
Guide to Surgical Terminology, 83
Guide to the Collection and Transport of Virological Specimens, 218
A Guide to the History of Bacteriology, 333
Guide to the Indexes for Biological Abstracts and Bioresearch Index, 500
Guide to the Literature for the Industrial Microbiologist, 14
Guide to the Literature in Psychiatry, 15
Guide to the Literature of the Life Sciences, 10
Guide to the 1968–1972 International Abortion Research Literature, 17
A Guide to the Use of the Excerpta Medica Abstract Journals: A List of 4,000 Biomedical Terms Most Commonly Used in Search Formulation of Secondary Publications, 4
A Guide to the World's Abstracting and Indexing Services in Science and Technology: National Federation of Indexing and Abstracting Services Report Number 102, 500
Guide to Theses and Dissertations: An Annotated, International Bibliography of Bibliographies, 557
Guide to US Government Publications, 541
Guide to US Government Statistics, 148, 541
Guide to World Science Series, 602
A Guidebook to Microscopial Methods, 205

TITLE INDEX

Guidelines for Format and Production of Scientific and Technical Reports, 537
Guidelines for the Preparation of Radiopharmaceuticals in Hospitals, 230
Guidelines to Metabolic Therapy, 585
Guidelines to Professional Pharmacy, 585
Guides to Scientific Periodicals: An Annotated Bibliography, 524
Gut, 529
Gynaecological Oncology, 453
Gynecologic Cytopathology: A Color Atlas of Differential Diagnosis, 272
Gynecologic Endocrinology, 419
Gynecology: Essentials of Clinical Practice, 493

Haematoloical Aspects of Systemic Disease, 430
Hahnemann Medical College and Hospital of Philadelphia Symposia. Proceedings, 548
Half a Century of Medical Research, 325
A Half-Century of American Medical Education, 325
Hamilton Bailey's Demonstrations of Physical Signs in Clinical Surgery, 402
Hamilton Bailey's Emergency Surgery, 402
Hamilton, Boyd and Mossman's Human Embryology, 400
The Hand Atlas, 245
Handbook for Dental Identification: Techniques in Forensic Dentistry, 103
Handbook for Dental Surgery Assistants and Other Ancillary Workers, 103
Handbook for Differential Diagnosis of Neurological Signs and Symptoms, 100
Handbook for Foreign Medical Graduates, 95
Handbook for Radiologic Technologists and Special Procedures Nurses in Radiology, 115

A Handbook For Specific Learning Disabilities, 130
Handbook for the Differential Diagnosis of Infectious Disease, 110
Handbook for the Medical Secretary, 95
A Handbook for the Study of Suicide, 130
Handbook of Adult Rehabilitative Audiology, 127
Handbook of Aging Series, 106
Handbook of Automated Electronic Clinical Analysis, 113
Handbook of Behavior Modification and Behavior Therapy, 130
Handbook of Biochemistry and Molecular Biology, 95
Handbook of Biological Psychiatry, 131
Handbook of Biomedical Instruments and Measurement, 107
Handbook of Cancer Immunology, 119
Handbook of Cardiology For Nurses: Heart Disease and Its Treatment, the Patient and His Nursing Care, 115
Handbook of Chemical Synonyms and Trade Names, 65
Handbook of Clinical Drug Data, 124
Handbook of Clinical Neurology, 100
Handbook of Clinical Ultrasound, 136
Handbook of Common Poisonings in Children, 121
Handbook of Community Health, 133
A Handbook of Community Medicine, 133
Handbook of Dental Photography, 103
Handbook of Diet Therapy, 116
Handbook of Drug and Chemical Stimulation of the Brain: Behavioural, Pharmacological and Physiological Aspects, 100
Handbook of Drug Interactions [Drug Intelligence Publications], 125
Handbook of Drug Interactions [John Wiley], 125
Handbook of Emergency Toxicology, 134

Handbook of Endocrine Tests in Adults and Children, 104
Handbook of Endocrinology: Diagnosis and Management of Endocrine and Metabolic Disorders, 104
Handbook of Engineering in Medicine and Biology, 95
Handbook of Enzymes Electrophoresis in Human Genetics, 105
Handbook of Epidemiology and Prognosis, 134
Handbook of Experimental Immunology, 97
Handbook of Food Preparation, 117
Handbook of Genetics, 106
Handbook of Hemophilia, 109
Handbook of Histology, 121
Handbook of Human Nutritional Requirements, 117
A Handbook of Human Service Organizations, 108
Handbook of Industrial Toxicology, 134
Handbook of International Documentation and Information, 18
Handbook of Laboratory Animal Science, 139
Handbook of Laboratory Safety, 113
Handbook of Lasers with Selected Data on Optical Technology, 119
Handbook of Lipid Research, 117
Handbook of Medical Emergencies in the Dental Office, 103
Handbook of Medical Library Practice, 95
Handbook of Medical Sociology, 134
Handbook of Medical Treatment, 113
Handbook of Microbiological Investigations for Laboratory Animal Health, 113
Handbook of Microbiology [Van Nostrand Reinhold], 110
Handbook of Microbiology, [Chemical Rubber Company], 110
Handbook of Micromethods for the Biological Sciences, 113
Handbook of Microscopic Anatomy for the Health Sciences, 97
Handbook of Molecular Cytology, 121
Handbook of Mutagenicity Test Procedures, 106
Handbook of Neonatal Respiratory Care, 121
Handbook of Neurochemistry, 101
Handbook of Neurologic Emergencies, 101
Handbook of Nonprescription Drugs, 125
Handbook of Nutrition and Food: Diets, Culture Media and Food Supplements Section, 117
Handbook of Obstetrical and Gynecological Data, 138
Handbook of Orthodontics, 103
Handbook of Pediatric Ophthalmology, 119
Handbook of Pediatrics, 122
Handbook of Perception, 131
Handbook of Physical Medicine and Rehabilitation, 128
Handbook of Physiology, 376
Handbook of Poisoning: Diagnosis and Treatment, 134
Handbook of Practical Pharmacology, 125
Handbook of Psychobiology, 131
Handbook of Psychological Terms, 90
Handbook of Psychopharmacology, 125
Handbook of Sensory Physiology, 101
Handbook of Speech Pathology and Audiology, 128
Handbook of Surgery, 98
Handbook of Teratology, 106
Handbook of the Nutritional Content of Foods, 117
A Handbook of Veterinary Parasitology: Domestic Animals of North America, 139
Handbook of Veterinary Surgical Instruments and Glossary of Surgical Terms, 139
Handbook of Vitamins and Hormones, 117
Handbook on Alcoholism and Its Treatment, 134
A Handbook on Drug and Alcohol Abuse: The Biomedical Aspects, 134

Handbook on Environmental Monitoring, 135
Handbook on Hospital-Associated Infections, 108
Handbook on Human Nutritional Requirements, 117
Handbook on Injectable Drugs, 126
Handbuch der Allgeminen Pathologie, 121
Handbuch der Experimentellen Pharmakologie/Handbook of Experimental Pharmacology, 126
Handbuch der Inneren Medizin, 113
Handbuch der Mikroskopischen Anatomie des Menschen, 97
Handbuch des Diabetes Mellitus, 105
The Handicapped Child: Research Review, 40
Harbeck's Glossary of Medical Terms, 79
The Harriet Lane Handbook: A Manual for Pediatric House Officers, 122
Harrison's Principles of Internal Medicine, 437
The Harvard Guide to Modern Psychiatry, 233
The Harvard List of Books in Psychology, 5
Hastings Center Report, 526
Hayes Druggist Directory, 301
Hazards of Medication: A Manual on Drug Interactions, Incompatibilities, Contraindications, and Adverse Effects, 180
The Healer's Art: The Doctor Through History, 325
The Healers: The Rise of the Medical Establishment, 326
The Healing Hand: Man and Wound in the Ancient World, 437
Health: A Multimedia Source Guide, 289, 593
Health and Crime Abstracts, 1960–1971, 520
Health and Disease of American Indians North of Mexico: A Bibliography, 1800–1969, 48
Health and Medical Economics: A Guide to Information Sources, 14

Health and Safety Guide for Hospitals, 215
Health and Sugar Substitutes, 551
Health Aspects of Pesticides; Abstract Bulletin, 520
Health Care Administration: A Guide to Information Sources, 14
Health Care Administration: A Managerial Perspective, 428
The Health Care Directory, 77–78, 289
Health Care of Women, 442
Health Careers Guidebook, 293
Health Educator's International Guide to Free and Low Cost Audiovisual Teaching/Training Aids, 593
The Health Food Dictionary with Recipes, 88
Health Hazards of the Human Environment, 483
Health Information for International Travel, 182
Health Maintenance Organizations: A Guide to Planning and Development, 215
Health Manpower: An Annotated Bibliography, 27
Health Manpower Source Book, 150
Health/Medicine Legislation in Congress—How It Works, 199
Health Organizations of the United States, Canada and Internationally: A Directory of Voluntary Associations, Professional Societies and Other Groups Concerned With Health and Related Fields, 289, 602
Health Physics Research Abstracts, 31
HEALTH PLANNING & ADMIN (Health Planning and Administration, 621
Health Planning and Manpower Register, 165
Health Policy Cassette Series, 593
Health Project Management: A Manual of Procedures for Formulating and Implementing Health Projects, 166
Health Resources Statistics: Health Manpower and Health Facilities, 1975, 150

Health Sciences and Services: A Guide to Information Sources, 14
Health Sciences Librarianship: A Guide to Information Sources, 12
The Health Sciences Video Directory 1977, 593
Health Service Research, 428
Health Services in the United States, 296
Health. United States 1978, 149
Hearing, Speech, and Communication Disorders: Cumulated Citations 1973, 24
The Heart, 412
Heart and Coronary Arteries: An Anatomical Atlas for Clinical Diagnosis, Radiological Investigation, and Surgical Treatment, 252
Heart and Lung, 528
The Heart Attack Handbook: A Commonsense Guide to Treatment, Recovery, and Prevention, 103
Heart Disease, 412
Heartbook: A Guide to Prevention and Treatment of Cardiovascular Disease, 210
Heinemann Modern Dictionary for Dental Students, 84
The Heinz Handbook of Nutrition, 118
Help for Your Child: A Parent's Guide to Mental Health Services, 233
Helpis-Medical: A Catalogue of Audio-Visual and Other Educational Materials in Medicine and Allied Fields Produced by Institutions of Higher Education in the United Kingdom, 594
Hematology, 430
Hematology of Infancy and Childhood, 468
Hematology: Physiologic, Pathophysiologic, and Clinical Principles, 431
Hepatitis Bibliography, 29, 506
Heredity, 529
Heritable Disorders in Orthopaedic Practice, 460
Hermaphroditism, Genital Anomalies and Related Endocrine Disorders, 493

H-ICDA: Hospital Adaptation of ICDA, 566
The Hip, 552
HISTLINE [History of Medicine Online], 621
Histological Processing for the Neural Sciences, 188
Histological Typing of Skin Tumors, 177
Histopathologic Technic and Practical Histochemistry, 463
Histopathology of the Bone Marrow, 463
Histopathology of the Skin, 416
History and Geography of the Most Important Diseases, 341
The History and Traditions of the Moorfields Eye Hospital, 337
History and Trends of Professional Nursing, 335
The History of Cardiac Surgery 1896–1955, 331
The History of Childhood, 339
The History of Coronary Heart Disease, 331
A History of Dentistry from the Most Ancient Times Until the End of the Eighteenth Century, 331
History of General Physiology 600 B.C. to A.D. 1900, 325
History of Genetics, From Prehistoric Times to the Rediscovery of Mendel's Laws, 332
A History of Immunization, 329
History of Medical Illustration, From Antiquity to 1600 A.D., 326
A History of Medicine, 326
History of Medicine in the United States, 326
The History of Mental Retardation: Collected Papers, 339
A History of Microtechnique, 337
A History of Nursing, 336
A History of Nursing From Ancient to Modern Times, 336
History of Nursing Source Book, 336
The History of Psychiatry: An Evaluation of Psychiatric Thought and Practice from Prehistoric Times to the Present, 340

A History of Public Health, 341
A History of Scientific and Technical Periodicals: The Origins and Development of the Scientific and Technical Press, 1665–1790, 524
The History of the Negro in Medicine, 326
History of the Royal College of Physicians of Edinburgh, 332
The History of Urology, 343
A History of Women in Medicine From Earliest Times to the Beginnings of the Nineteenth Century, 326
HMO Handbook: A Guide for Development of Prepaid Group Practice HMOs, 108
The HMO Sourcebook, 200
Hodgkin's Disease, 453
Homburger and Bonner's Medical Care and Rehabilitation of the Aged and Chronically Ill, 214
Homeopathic Pharmacopeia of the U.S., 575
Homosexuality: A Selective Bibliography of Over Three Thousand Items, 43
Homosexuality: An Annotated Bibliography, 43
Homosexuality Bibliography: Supplement, 1970–1975, 43
Hormone Chemistry, 419
Hormones in Blood, 382
The Hospital: A Social and Architectural History, 332
Hospital Abstracts: A Monthly Survey of World Literature, 511
Hospital Adaptation of ICDA, H-ICDA (International Classification of Diseases, Adapted), 566
Hospital Computer Systems, 428
Hospital Engineering Handbook, 108
Hospital/Health Care Training Media Profiles, Volume One, 596
Hospital Law Manuals, 166
Hospital Literature Index, 506, 512
Hospital Literature Subject Headings, 14
Hospital Literature Subject Headings Transition Guide to Medical Subject Headings, 14
Hospital Management Systems: Multi-unit Organization and Delivery of Health Care, 428
Hospital Medical Records: Guidelines for Their Use and the Release of Medical Information, 572
Hospital Organization Research: Review and Sourcebook, 200
Hospital Pharmacy, 533
Hospital Practice, 529
Hospital Progress, 529
Hospital Purchasing Guide 1978, 301, 584
Hospital Statistics, 152
Hospital Yearbook: An Annual Record of the Hospitals of Great Britain and Ireland Incorporating "Burdett's Hospitals and Charities" Founded 1889, 296
The Hospitalized Adolescent: A Guide to Managing the Ill and Injured Youth, 233
Hospitals, 529
How to Divide Medical Words: Over Twenty-Five Thousand Words in Common Usage Showing Their Spellings and Combinations into Syllables, 73
How to Find Out: A Guide to Sources of Information Arranged by the Dewey Decimal Classification, 10
How to Find Out About Patents, 580
How to Find Out in Psychiatry: A Guide to Sources of Mental Health Information, 16
How to Pay for Your Health Career Education: A Guide for Minority Students, 205
How to Use a Medical Library, 206
How to Write Meaningful Nursing Standards, 573
How to Write Scientific and Technical Papers, 154
The Human Body in Health and Disease, 193
Human Chromosomes, 424
Human Cytogenetics, 383

Human Embryology, 401
Human Endocrinology: A Developmental Approach, 419
Human Experimentation Abstracts, 508
Human Experimentation and the Law, 396
The Human Female Reproductive Tract: A Scanning Electron Microscopic Atlas, 279
Human Haemoglobin Variants and Their Characteristics, 141
Human Health and Disease, 114
Human Larynx-Coronal Section Atlas, 268
Human Multiple Reproduction, 493
Human Neuropsychology, 406
Human Nutrition—A Comprehensive Treatise, 386
Human Sexuality in Physical and Mental Illness and Disabilities: An Annotated Bibliography, 43
Human Viral Hepatitis, 434
Hypersensitivity to Drugs, 58
Hypertension: A Practitioner's Guide to Therapy, 211
Hypertension Manual, 161

IARC Monographs on the Evaluation of Carcinogenic Risk of Chemicals to Humans, 360
IARC Scientific Publications, 552
Identification of Medical Bacteria, 191
IINPADOC (International Patent Documentation Center), 581
Ika, Shika, Waei Hatsuon Buneri Jiten: Japanese-English Medical-Dental Dictionary, 70
Ileostomy: Surgery, Physiology, and Management, 422
Illustrated Dictionary of Eponymic Syndromes and Diseases and Their Synonyms, 89
An Illustrated Guide to Dental Morphology, 212
An Illustrated Guide to Medical Terminology, 79
Illustrated Guide to Orthopedic Nursing, 222

Illustrated Guide to X-Ray Technics, 237
An Illustrated History of Brain Function, 330
Illustrated Manual of Laboratory Diagnosis, 193
Illustrated Manual of Nursing Techniques, 172
Illustrated Medical Dictionary, 80
Illustrated Tumor Nomenclature, 67
Illustration Catalog of the Library of the New York Academy of Medicine, 6
Immediate Care of the Acutely Ill and Injured, 219
The Immune System: A Course on the Molecular and Cellular Basis of Immunity, 399
Immunochemistry of Proteins, 399
Immunologic and Infectious Reactions in the Lung, 488
Immunological Aspects of Allergy and Allergic Diseases, 347, 376
Immunological Diseases, 376
Immunological Reviews, 376
Immunology Abstracts, 508
Immunology: An Introduction to Molecular and Cellular Principles of the Immune Responses, 399
Immunology, Immunopathology, and Immunity, 400
Immunology in Medicine: A Practical Guide to Clinical Immunology, 207
Immunopathology of the Eye, 456
The Impact of Health System Changes on the Nation's Requirements for Registered Nurses in 1985, 143
Implants in Surgery, 402
Improving the Dissemination of Scientific and Technical Information: A Practioner's Guide to Information, 10
Incunabula and Sixteenth Century Printed Books in the National Library of Medicine, Supplement 1, 326
Incunabula Scientifica et Medica: Short Title List, 326
Index Bergeyana, 206

Index Catalogue of the Library of the Surgeon General's Office, United States Army (Army Medical Library), Authors, and Subjects, 326
Index Guide to Drug Information Retrieval, 516
Index-Handbook of Otoxic Agents 1966–1971, 126
Index Medicus, 504, 508, 526, 615
Index Nominum 1978/79, 126
Index of Audiovisual Serials in the Health Sciences, 506, 594
Index of Conference Proceedings Received, 546
Index of Dermatology, 505, 510
Index of Federal Specifications and Standards, 570
Index of Human Ecology, 520
An Index of International Standards, 570
Index of Legal Medicine, 1940–1970: Annotated Bibliography, 20
Index of NLM Serial Titles: A Keyword Listing of Serial Titles Currently Received by the National Library of Medicine, 4
Index of Nutrition Education Materials, 34
Index of Opportunity in the Paramedical Fields: A Directory of Career Opportunities for Mental Health and Social Workers; Public Welfare Workers; Dental, Medical, and Laboratory Technicians; Physical Therapists; and other Allied Paramedical Specialists, 298
Index of Paramaedical Vocabulary: An Index-Indicator Enabling the User Not Versed in Greek and Latin to Locate the Terminology of any Given Subject in a Paramedical, Medical, or Biological Dictionary, 80
Index of Patents, 580
Index of Rheumatology, 504, 521
Index of Suspicion in Treatable Diseases, 147
Index of the Periodical Dental Literature Published in the English Language, 1839–1936/38, 509
Index of Tissue Culture, 506, 513

Index of Trademarks Issued from the United States Patent Office, 580
An Index to Biographical Fragments in Unspecialized Scientific Journals, 500
Index to Book Reviews in the Sciences, 1
Index to Classification, 580
Index to Current Literature, 509
Index to Dental Literature, 504, 509
Index to Dental Literature in the English Language, 510
Index to Producers and Distributors, 592
Index to Public Health Nursing Magazine, 1909–1952, 514
Index to Scientific Reviews, 372
Index to These Accepted for Higher Degrees in the Universities of Great Britain and Ireland, 557
Index Translationum, 554
Index Veterinarius, 522
Indexed Bibliography of Office of Research and Development Reports, Updated to January 1975, 538
Industrial Environmental Health: The Worker and the Community, 183
Industrial Noise: A Selective Bibliography 1963–1973, 48
Infant Nutrition, 450
Infection Control in the Hospital, 108
Infectious Diseases: A Modern Treatise of Infectious Processes, 218
Infectious Diseases of the Fetus and Newborn Infant, 468
Infectious Diseases: Prevention and Treatment in the Nineteenth and Twentieth Centuries, 333
Inflammatory Bowel Disease, 422
Influenza in America, 1918–1976: History, Science, and Politics, 333
Influenza: The Viruses and the Disease, 434
Information Retrieval: On Line, 614
Information Retrieval Systems: Characteristics, Testing, and Evaluation, 614
Information Sources in Science and Technology, 10
Inpharma, 516

Insects and History, 341
Insects and Other Arthropods of Medical Importance, 434
Inservice Education Manual for the Nursing Department, 172
Insta-dex to 140 Medical-Surgical Journals(A Browsing Tool), 523
Instant Spelling Medical Dictionary, 74
Instruments for Measuring Nursing Practice and Other Health Care Variables, 32
Instruments for Use in Nursing Education Research, 33
Insurance Handbook for the Medical Office, 108
Intensive Care Instrumentation, 215
Intensive Care Units: Minimal Criteria and Guidelines, 215
Intensive Coronary Care, 162
Intensive Coronary Care: A Manual for Nurses, 162
Intensive Nursing Care, 443
Interaction of Alcohol and Other Drugs: An Annotated Bibliography of the Scientific Literature on the Interaction of Ethanol and Other Chemical Compounds Normally Absent in Vivo, 38
Interdisciplinary Glossary on Child Abuse and Neglect: Legal, Medical, Social Work Terms, 90
Interdisciplinary Topics in Gerontology, 356
Interferon, 437
Interferon and Antiviral Substances Bibliography, 22, 506
Interferon Bibliography From MEDLARS, September 1973–August 1974, 22
Internal Radiation Dose in Diagnostic Nuclear Medicine, 136
International Abstracts of Biological Sciences, 502
International Academy of Pathology Monographs in Pathology Series, 388
International Advances in Surgical Oncology, 360
International Agency for Research on Cancer: Annual Report, 312

International and Metric Units of Measurement, 140
International Bibliography of Cardiovascular Asculation and Phonocardiography: Journal Articles, 1820–1966; Books, Theses, Dissertations, Phonodiscs, 1819–1968, 25
International Bibliography of Directories of Economics, Science and Technique, 281
International Bibliography of Medicolegal Serials 1736–1967, 524
International Bibliography of Studies on Alcohol, 48
International Bibliography of the History of Legal Medicine, 327
International Bibliography on Burns: Thermal, Electrical, Chemical, Radiation, Cold Injuries, for Better Patient Care, Research, and Teaching, 31
International Classification of Diseases for Oncology, 567
The International Classification of Diseases: 9th Revision, Clinical Modification ICD.9.CM, 565
International Classification of Patents, 580
International Classification of Procedures in Medicine, 565
International Code of Nomenclature of Bacteria: Bacteriological Code, 67
International Congress Calendar, 544
International Critical Tables of Numerical Data, Physics, Chemistry and Technology, 142
International Directory of Genetic Services, 295
International Directory of Mental Retardation Resources, 303
International Directory of Nurses with Doctoral Degrees, 558
International Directory of Occupational Safety and Health Services and Institutions, 306
International Directory of Population Information and Library Resources, 290
International Directory of Research and Development Scientists, 317

International Directory of Specialized Cancer Research and Treatment Establishments, 299
International Directory of Translators and Interpreters, 554
The International Encyclopedia of Pharmacology and Therapeutics, 58
International Encyclopedia of Psychiatry, Psychology, Psychoanalysis, and Neurology, 60
The International File of Micrographics Equipment and Accessories 1979–1980, 592
International Foundation Directory, 285
International Guide to Aids and Appliances for Blind and Visually Impaired Persons, 231
The International Handbook of Medical Science, 114
International Health Regulations, 571
The International Index of Patents, 581
International Index to Film Periodicals, 588
International Index to Multimedia Information, 588
International Journal of Dermatology, 529
International Meeting Reports, 546
International Nursing Index, 504, 514
International Nursing Review, 373
International Pharmaceutical Abstracts, 516, 629
International Review of Connective Tissue Research, 562
International Review of Cytology, 363
International Review of Experimental Pathology, 363
International Review of Neurobiology, 350
International Symposium on Influenza Immunization. Proceedings, 550
Internationales Woerterbuch der Abkuerzungen von Organisationen Pt, 1: A-H. International Dictionary of Abbreviations of Organizations, 63
Interpretation of Diagnostic Tests: A Handbook Synopsis of Laboratory Medicine, 114

Inter-University Electronics Series, 375
Intravenous Medications: A Handbook For Nurses and Other Allied Health Personnel, 115
An Introduction to Clinical Research, 437
Introduction to Food Science and Technology, 450
An Introduction to Human Pharmacology, 474
Introduction to Patient Care: A Comprehensive Approach to Nursing, 443
An Introduction to Radiation Protection, 183
An Introduction to the History of Dentistry in America, 331
An Introduction to the History of Dentistry, With Medical and Dental Chronology and Bibliographic Data, 331
An Introduction to the History of Medicine, 327
An Introduction to the History of Virology, 334
An Introduction to the Literature of the Medical Sciences, 12
An Introduction to the Study of Disease, 437
Introduction to United States Public Documents, 541
Introductory Medical-Surgical Nursing and Student Work Manual, 195
The Inventor's Patent Handbook, 580
The Inverted Medical Dictionary: A Method of Finding Medical Terms Quickly, 80
Investigation of Oncogenic Viruses: I. Recent Articles and Research in Progress, 454
Iowa Drug Information Service, 592
Irregular Serials and Annuals; An International Directory, 344
ISI's Who is Publishing in Science: An International Directory of Research & Development Scientists, 285
Isotope Titles, 502
Issues in Nursing Research, 443

Issues in the Design and Evaluation of Medical Trials, 396
The I.U.D.: A Practical Guide, 240

Jacep, 530
JAMA; Journal of the American Medical Association, 527, 545, 570
JAPTA List 1973; Japanese Drug Directory, 301
JCAH Accreditation Manual for Hospital, 572
The JCAH Standards; A Journal of Nursing Administration Reader, 573
Jewish Physicians: A Biographical Index, 317
The Johns Hopkins Atlas of Human Functional Anatomy, 245
Joslin Diabetes Manual, 164
Joslin's Diabetes Mellitus, 419
Journal of Allergy and Clinical Immunology, 527
Journal of Applied Nutrition, 531
Journal of Applied Physiology, 527
Journal of Bacteriology, 530
Journal of Behavioral Medicine, 526
Journal of Bone and Joint Surgery. American Volume, 532
Journal of Bone and Joint Surgery. British Volume, 532
Journal of Clinical Endocrinology and Metabolism, 529
Journal of Clinical Investigation, 530
Journal of Clinical Pathology, 532
Journal of Clinical Pharmacology, 533
Journal of Family Practice, 530
Journal of General Microbiology, 530
Journal of General Physiology, 527
Journal of Gerontology, 529
Journal of Heredity, 529
Journal of Immunology, 527
Journal of Infectious Disease, 530
Journal of Laboratory and Clinical Medicine, 530
Journal of Laryngology and Otology, 532
Journal of Medical Education, 526
Journal of Nervous and Mental Disease, 534
Journal of Neurosurgery, 528
Journal of Nursing Administration, 531
Journal of Nutrition, 531
Journal of Nutrition Education, 531
Journal of Oral Surgery, 528
Journal of Pediatrics, 532
Journal of Pharmaceutical Sciences, 533
Journal of Pharmacokinetics and Biopharmaceutics, 533
Journal of Pharmacology and Experimental Therapeutics, 533
Journal of Pharmacy and Pharmacology, 533
Journal of Physical and Chemical Reference Data, 142
Journal of Physiology, 527
Journal of Preventive Dentistry, 528
Journal of the American Dietetic Association, 529
Journal of the American Veterinary Medical Association, 535
Journal of the History of Medicine and Allied Sciences, 530
Journal of Thoracic and Cardiovascular Surgery, 528
Journal of Trauma, 530
Journal of Urology, 534
Journal of Veterinary Pharmacology and Therapeutics, 535
Journal of Veterinary Surgery, 535

Karger Highlights, 564
Kazanjian and Converse's Surgical Treatment of Facial Injuries, 402
Key Concepts for the Study and Practice of Nursing, 443
Key Facts on the U.S. Prescription Drug Industry, 152
The Kidney, 392
Kidney Biopsy Interpretation, 240
Kidney Disease and Nephrology Index, 504, 522
Kidney Disease Services, Facilities, and Programs in the United States, 308
Kimber-Gray-Stackpole's Anatomy and Physiology, 98
Kingzett's Chemical Encyclopedia: A Digest of Chemistry and Its Industrial Applications, 53

Kirk-Othmer Encyclopedia of Chemical Technology, 53
Klinik Terminler Lugeti (Ruscha-Latyncha-Azerbaichancha), 70
Kremer's and Urdang's History of Pharmacy, 338

Laboratory and Research Methods in Biology and Medicine, 562
Laboratory Diagnostic Procedures in the Rheumatic Diseases, 198
Laboratory Evaluation of Hemostasis, 189
Laboratory Guide for Biology, 206
Laboratory Guide to Clinical Diagnosis, 219
Laboratory Handbook of Methods of Food Analysis, 118
Laboratory Indices of Nutritional Status in Pregnancy, 144, 574
A Laboratory Manual and Study Guide for Anatomy and Physiology, 187
Laboratory Manual and Study Guide for Clinical Anatomy and Physiology for Allied Health Sciences, 187
Laboratory Manual and Workbook for General Microbiology, 191
Laboratory Manual for Structure and Function in Man, 187
A Laboratory Manual of Blood Coagulation, 189
Laboratory Manual of Cell Biology, 193
Laboratory Manual of Human Anatomy and Physiology, 187
Laboratory Medicine: Hematology, 431
Laboratory Safety Monograph: A Supplement to the NIH Guidelines for Recombinant DNA Research, 397
Laboratory Technique for the Detection of Hereditary Metabolic Disorders, 188
Laboratory Techniques in Brucellosis, 191
Laboratory Techniques in Rabies, 198
Laboratory Training Manual on the Use of Radionuclides and Radiation in Animal Research, 198
Labor-Management Relations in the Health Service Industry, 333

Lancet, 527
Laproscopy in Gynecology, Surgery, and Pediatrics: Textbooks and Atlas, 247
Laser Abstracts for the Medical Profession, 508
Latino Mental Health: Bibliography and Abstracts, 44
Law Every Nurse Should Know, 222
The Law Relating to the Misuse of Drugs, 397
LC Science Tracer Bullet, 10
LC Science Tracer Bullet: Biographical Sources in the Sciences, 318
Legal Accountability in the Nursing Process, 443
Legal Medicine Annual, 308
Leukemia, 454
Leukemia in Childhood, 468
Levels of Health Intervention, 443
Lexicon Medicum: Anglicum, Russicum, Gallicum, Germanicum, Latinum, Polonum, 72
A Lexicon of English Dental Terms With Their Equivalents in Espanol, Deutsch, Francais, Italiano, 72
Library of Congress Catalog. Motion Pictures and Filmstrips, 589
Library Practice in Hospitals: A Basic Guide, 215
Library Resources for Nurses: A Basic Collection for Supporting the Nursing Curriculum, 4
Library Resources for the Blind and Physically Handicapped: A Directory of NLS Network Libraries and Machine-Lending Agencies, 1978, 302
Life Table and Mortality Analysis, 141
Lifting, Moving, Transferring Patients: A Manual, 180
Lilly Digest, 585
The Lippincott Manual of Nursing Practice, 172
LISA, 629
List of Annual Reviews of Progress in Science and Technology; Liste de 'mises au point' annuelles sur les progrès de la science et de la technique, 344
List of Approved Hospitals and Recog-

nized House Officer Posts; England, Wales, Scotland, Northern Ireland, and the Republic of Ireland, 296
List of Journals in Abridged Index Medicus, 4
List of Journals Indexed in Index Medicus, 526
List of Serials with Coden, Title Abbreviations, New, Changed, and Ceased Titles, 526
Lists of International Biological Standards and International Biological Reference Preparations, 1975, 568
Lists of Volatile Compounds in Foods: A Bibliography, 34
The Literature of Science and Technology Approached Historically: A Brief Guide for References, 10
Literature Relating to Neurosurgery and the Neurologic Sciences: A Bibliography From 1945 Through 1968 With A Few Earlier Classics in this Field, 24
The Liver: Normal and Abnormal Functions, 422
Lives of the Fellows of the Royal College of Surgeons of England 1930–1951, 320
Livestock Health Encyclopedia, 62
Living Blood Cells and Their Ultrastructure, 261
Livingstone's Dictionary for Nurses, 86
Livingstone's Pocket Medical Dictionary, 80
Low and Very Low Dose Influences of Ionizing Radiation on Cells and Organisms, Including Man: A Bibliography, 48
LSD: A Total Study, 475
LSD Research: An Annotated Bibliography: 1972–1975, 39
Lung Biology in Health and Disease: Bioengineering Aspects of the Lung, 489
Lung Cancer: Natural History, Prognosis, and Therapy, 489
Lung Function: Assessment and Application in Medicine, 489
Lung Sounds, 489
Lupus Erythematosus: A Review of the Current Status of Discoid and Systemic Lupus Erythematosus and Their Variants, 431
The Lymphatics: Disease, Lymphography and Surgery, 412
Lymphocytes, Isolation, Fractionation and Characterisation, 166
Lysosomes and Storage Diseases, 424

The Macmillan Dictionary for Practical and Vocations Nurses, 87
MacRae's Blue Book, 285
Magazines for Libraries, 583
Mainly on Patents: The Use of Literature of Industrial Property and Its Literature, 578
M&B Pharmaceutical Bulletin, 585
Major Problems in Clinical Pediatrics, 389
Major Problems in Clinical Surgery, 348
Major Problems in Dermatology, 381
Major Problems in Internal Medicine, 358
Major Problems in Neurology, 350, 379
Major Problems in Obstetrics and Gynecology, 393
Major Problems in Ophthalmology, 362
Major Problems in Pathology, 363, 389
Male and Female Homosexuality: A Comprehensive Investigation, 479
The Maltreated Child: The Maltreatment Syndrome in Children—A Medical, Legal, and Social Guide, 233
The Mammalian Myocardium, 412
Mammography: Technique, Diagnosis, Differential Diagnosis, 237
Management by Objectives for Hospitals, 215
The Management of Geriatric Cardiovascular Disease, 106
Management of High-Risk Pregnancy and Intensive Care of the Neonate, 228
Management of Hospitals, 215
The Management of Malignant Disease Series, 454

Management of Neglected Trauma, 219
The Management of Nutritional Emergencies in Large Populations, 224
Management of Ocular Injuries, 119
Management of Surgical Complications, 209
Management of the Patient With Cancer, 225
The Management of 35mm Medical Slides, 594
Managing Contraceptive Pill Patients, 240
Man and the Environment: A Bibliography of Selected Publications of the United Nations System, 1946–1971, 48
A Manpower Policy for Primary Health Care, 428
Man's Haemoglobins, Including the Haemoglobinopathies and Their Investigation, 431
Manson's Tropical Diseases, 435
A Manual for Histologic Technicians, 197
Manual for Nurses in Family and Community Health, 173
Manual for Physical Therapy Technicians, 181
Manual for Staging of Cancer, 1977, 196
Manual for the Organization of Scientific Congresses, 548
Manual of Acute Bacterial Infections: Early Diagnosis and Treatment, 167
Manual of Acute Orthopaedic Therapeutics, 176
A Manual of Adverse Drug Interactions, 170
Manual of Ambulatory Medicine, 170
Manual of Anesthesia, 158
A Manual of Antimicrobial Therapy, 167
Manual of Applied Nutrition, 174
Manual of Basic Neuropathology, 160
A Manual of Basic Virological Techniques, 170, 191
Manual of Classification of Patents, 578

A Manual of Clinical Allergy, 157
Manual of Clinical Biology, 170
Manual of Clinical Dietetics and Physician's Guide, 175
Manual of Clinical Immunology, 157
Manual of Clinical Laboratory Methods, 170, 193
Manual of Clinical Microbiology, 167, 191
Manual of Clinical Mycology, 191
Manual of Clinical Periodontics, 188
Manual of Contact Dermatitis, 164
Manual of Coronary Care, 162
Manual of Critical Care Medicine, 170
Manual of Cyto-Technology, 178
Manual of Dermatologic Syndromes, 164
A Manual of Dissection for Students of Dentistry, 163
Manual of Emergency Medical Therapeutics, 170
Manual of Endocrine Surgery, 165
Manual of Gynecologic and Obstetric Emergencies, 185
A Manual of Head Injuries in General Surgery, 161
Manual of Hematology, 189
Manual of Histopathological Staining Methods, 197
Manual of History Taking, Physical Examination and Record Keeping, 156
Manual of Mechanical Orthopaedics, 177
Manual of Medical Therapeutics, 170
Manual of Mortality Analysis: A Manual on Methods of Analysis of National Mortality Statistics for Public Health Purposes, 182
A Manual of Neurosurgery, 161
A Manual of Newborn Medicine, 178
Manual of Operating Room Technology, 158
Manual of Patent Examining Procedures, 578
Manual of Pediatric Therapeutics, 178
Manual of Practical Entomology in Malaria, 167
A Manual of Practical Orthodontics, 163

Manual of Psychiatric Therapeutics: Practical Psychopharmacology and Psychiatry, 181
A Manual of Radiographic Positioning, 183
Manual of Renal Transplantation, 185
Manual of Respiratory Therapy, 184
Manual of Selected Procedures and Treatment, 185
Manual of Skin Diseases, 164
Manual of Standardized Methods for Veterinary Microbiology, 199
Manual of Surgery of the Gallbladder, Bile Ducts and Exocrine Pancreas, 165
Manual of Surgical Intensive Care, 158
Manual of Surgical Therapeutics, 158
Manual of the International Statistical Classification of Diseases, Injuries, and Causes of Death, 170, 565
Manual of Tropical Medicine, 168
Manual of Tumor Nomenclature and Coding, 176
Manual on Artificial Organs, 185
Manual on Control of Infection in Surgical Patients, 159, 168
A Manual on Drug Dependence, 182
Manual on Larval Control Operations in Malaria Programmes, 168
A Manual on Medical Literature for Law Librarians: A Handbook and Annotated Bibliography, 156
Manual on Radiation Protection in Hospitals and General Practice, 183
Manual on Radiation Sterilization of Medical and Biological Materials, 183
Manual For Health Care Institutions, 166
Marie Curie, 342
Marijuana: A Selective Bibliography, 1924–1979, 49
Marijuana: An Annotated Bibliography, 49
Markets for the Medical Author: A Handbook of Over 500 Journal, Book and Paramedical Publishing Markets for the Medical Writer, 95
Martindale: The Extra Pharmacopeia, 126

Massachusetts General Hospital Handbook of General Hospital Psychiatry, 131
Massachusetts General Hospital Manual of Nursing Procedures, 173
Master Abstracts, 557
Maternal and Infant Drugs and Nursing Intervention, 443
Maternity Nursing: Self Study Guide, 195
Maxcy-Rosenau's Preventive Medicine and Public Health, 483
Mayo Clinic Diet Manual, 175
Mayo Clinic Proceedings, 527
McCance and Widdowson's The Composition of Foods, 144
McGraw-Hill Basic Bibliography of Science and Technology, 20
McGraw-Hill Dictionary of Scientific and Technical Terms, 76
McGraw-Hill Dictionary of the Life Sciences, 76
McGraw-Hill Encyclopedia of Food, Agriculture and Nutrition, 56
McGraw-Hill Encyclopedia of Science and Technology, 53
McGraw-Hill Handbook of Clinical Nursing, 115
McGraw-Hill Modern Men of Science, 318
McGraw-Hill Nursing Dictionary, 87
McGraw-Hill Yearbook of Science and Technology, 308
Measuring Medical Education: The Tests and the Experience of the National Board of Medical Examiners, 206
Mechanisms of Contraction in the Normal and Failing Heart, 412
Medbooks: A Bibliography of New and Forthcoming Books in Human and Dental Medicine, 5
Media Handbook: A Guide to Selecting, Producing, and Using Media for Patient Education, 596
Media: Indexes and Review Sources, 589
Media Review Digest, 589
Medical Abbreviations, 64

Medical Abbreviations and Acronyms, 64
Medical Abbreviations: A Cross Reference Dictionary, 64
Medical and Health Annual, 312
Medical and Health Information Directory: A Guide to State, National and International Organizations, Government Agencies, Educational Institutions, Hospitals, Grant Award Sources, Health Care Delivery Agencies, Journals, Newsletters, Review Serials, Abstracting Services, Publishers, Research Centers, Computerized Data Banks, Audiovisual Services, and Libraries and Information Centers, 290, 602
Medical and Health Related Sciences Thesaurus, 65
The Medical and Health Sciences World Book, 80
The Medical and Healthcare Marketplace Guide, 296
Medical and Surgical Motion Pictures: A Catalog of Selected Films, 595
Medical Assistant's Manual, 171
A Medical Bibliography (Garrison and Morton): An Annotated Check-List of Texts Illustrating the History of Medicine, 327
Medical Books and Serials in Print 1979: An Index to Literature in the Health Sciences, 2
Medical Books for the Layperson: An Annotated Bibliography, 18
Medical Books '79. A Preferred List, 2
Medical Care Chart Book, 142
Medical Clinics of North America, 530
Medical Complications During Pregnancy, 468
Medical Dictionary: Medizinsches Worterbuch: Dictionnaire Medical, 73
Medical Dictionary of the English and German Languages, 69
Medical Disposables: Marketing Guide and Company Directory, 296
Medical Dissertations of Psychiatric Interest (Printed Before 1750), 340
Medical Engineering, 397
Medical Equipment Service Manual: Theory and Maintenance Procedures, 166
Medical Health Film Library, 594
Medical Hieroglyphs: Abbreviations and Symbols, 65
Medical Information Systems: A Resource for Hospitals, 216
Medical Jurisprudence, 397
Medical Legal Dictionary, 81
Medical Letter on Drugs and Therapeutics, 533
Medical Malpractice Law, 397
Medical, Moral and Legal Issues in Mental Health Care, 397
Medical Mycology, 400
Medical Nemesis: The Expropriation of Health, 398
Medical Neurology, 102
Medical Oncology: Medical Aspects of Malignant Disease, 454
Medical Physiology, 401
The Medical Profession in Mid-Victorian London, 327
Medical Radiation Exposure of Pregnant and Potentially Pregnant Women, 136
Medical Readings on Heroin, 30
Medical Records Departments in Hospitals: Guide to Organization, 216
Medical Reference Works, 1679–1966: A Selected Bibliography, 12
Medical Research Index: A Guide to World Medical Research, Including Dentistry, Nursing, Pharmacy, Pschiatry, and Surgery, 559
Medical Risks: Patterns of Mortality and Survival, 152
Medical School Admission Requirements U.S.A. and Canada, 293
Medical School Alumni, 294
Medical Secretary Medi-Speller: A Transcription Aid, 74
Medical Secretary's Manual, 154
Medical Socioeconomic Research Sources, 508
Medical Sociology, 479
Medical Subject Headings, Annotated Alphabetic List, 1979, 623
Medical Subject Headings, Three Structures, 1979, 623

TITLE INDEX

Medical-Surgical Nursing, 443
Medical-Surgical Nursing: A Conceptual Approach, 444
Medical-Surgical Nursing: A Psychophysiologic Approach, 444
Medical Terminology and the Body System, 186
The Medical Transcriptionist Handbook, 96, 208
The Medical Word Book: A Spelling and Vocabulary Guide to Medical Transcription, 74
Medical Writing: The Technic and the Art, 155
Medication Guide for Patient Counseling, 219
Medicinal Chemistry, A Series of Monographs, 390
Medicinal Chemistry Reviews: A Select Bibliography, 39
Medicinal Research: A Series of Monographs, 562
Medicine, 312, 527
Medicine: A Bibliography of Bibliographies, 18
Medicine and Society in America. 1660–1860, 328
Medicine and Sport, 358
The Medicine Show: Physicians and the Perplexities of the Health Revolution in Modern Society, 335
Medicolegal Aspects of Hospital Records, 216
Medicolegal Investigation of Death: Guidelines for the Application to Crime Investigation, 228
Medieval English Medicine, 328
Medi-KWOC Index: An Index to the Published Proceedings of Conferences and Sumposia on Biomedicine, 546
MEDLARS, 615
MEDLARS: The Computerized Literature Retrieval Services of the National Library of Medicine, 614
MEDLINE, 622
MEDOC: A Computerized Index to U.S. Government Publications in the Medical and Health Sciences, 541, 629

Melloni's Illustrated Medical Dictionary, 81
Membership Directory, 307
Mendelian Inheritance in Man, 84
The Menopause: A Guide to Current Research and Practice, 240
Mental Handicap: A Brief Guide, 234
Mental Health Book Review Index: An Annual Bibliography of Book Reviews in the Behavioral Sciences: Cumulative Author-Title Index of Volumes 1–12, 1956–1967, 44
Mental Health Concepts in Medical-Surgical Nursing: A Workbook, 198
Mental Health Digest, 518
Mental Health Directory, 304
Mental Health Emergencies Alert!: An Annotated Bibliography, no. 1, 44
Mental Health Film Guide, 599
Mental Health in the Metropolis: The Midtown Manhattan Study, 480
Mental Health in the United States: A Fifty-Year History, 340
The Mental Health of the Black Community: An Exploratory Bibliography, 44
Mental Illness in Later Life, 480
Mental Institutions in America. Social Policy to 1875, 340
Mental Retardation: An Atlas of Diseases with Associated Physical Abnormalities, 259
The Mental Retardation Dictionary, 91
Mental Retardation Film List, 599
Mercer's Orthopaedic Surgery, 460
The Merck Index: An Encyclopedia of Chemicals and Drugs, 127, 579
The Merck Manual of Diagnosis and Therapy, 171
The Merck Veterinary Manual: A Handbook of Diagnosis and Therapy for the Veterinarian, 186
The Metabolic Basis of Inherited Disease, 424
Metabolic, Degenerative, and Inflammatory Diseases of Bones and Joints, 460
Metabolic, Endocrine and Genetic Disorders of Children, 469
Metabolism, 105

Methadone and Pregnancy: An Annotated Guide to the Literature, 50
Methodology in Evaluating the Quality of Medical Care: An Annotated Selected Bibliography, 1955–1968, 27
Methods and Achievements in Experimental Pathology, 363
Methods for the Analysis of Human Chromosome Aberrations, 189, 213
Methods in Cancer Research, 387
Methods in Cell Biology, 346
Methods in Enzymology: A Multivolume Work, 382
Methods in Human Cytogenetics, 189
Methods in Membrane Biology, 346
Methods in Microbiology, 357
Methods in Pharmacology, 390
Methods of Sampling and Analysis of Contaminants in Food: Report of a Joint FAO/WHO Expert Consultation, 1978, 175
Metric Conversion Tables and Factors, 140
MGH Textbook of Emergency Medicine: Emergency Care As Practiced at the Massachusetts General Hospital, 437
Microanalysis in Medical Biochemistry, 194
Microanatomy of Cell and Tissue Surfaces: An Atlas of Scanning Electron Microscopy, 272
Microbes and Man: A Laboratory Manual for Students in the Health Sciences, 192
Microbiology, 311
Microbiology Abstracts, 512
Microbiology and Pathology, 463
Microbiology Laboratory Manual: A Sequence of Experiments, 192
Microbiology Laboratory Manual and Workbook, 192
Microbiology of Human Skin, 417
Microfilm Source Book, 589
Microform Review, 589
Microforms: The Librarians' View, 1978–79, 589
Microorganisms in Foods, 182
Microsurgery: A Practical Guide for Surgeons, Gynecologists, Urologists, Plastic Surgeons, Neurosurgeons, and Orthopaedists, 209
Microtechniques for the Clinical Laboratory: Concepts and Applications, 219
The Microtomist's Formulary and Guide, 206
Midwives and Medical Men: A History of Inter-Professional Rivalries and Women's Rights, 343
Minorities in Science: The Challenge for Change in Biomedicine, 318
Minority Groups in Medicine: Selected Bibliography, 20
The MMPI: A Practical Guide, 234
Modern Clinical Psychiatry, 480
Modern Concepts of Cerebrovascular Disease, 211
Modern Drug Encyclopedia, 1975–76, 89
Modern Drug Encyclopedia and Therapeutic Index, 89
Modern Food Analysis, 118
Modern Healthcare, 530
Modern Intravenous Therapy Procedures; A Handbook for Nurses and Other Allied Health Personnel, 115
Modern Medical Treatment, 438
Modern Nutrition in Health and Disease Dietotherapy, 450
Modern Pharmacology-Toxicology, 390
Modern Problems in Ophthalmology, 362
Modern Problems in Paediatrics, 552
Modern Problems in Pharmacopsychiatry, 366
Modern Trends in Endocrinology, 354
Modern Trends in Neurology, 350
Modern Trends in Ophthalmology, 362
Modern Trends in Orthopaedics, 362
Molecular Pathology, 463
Monitoring in Anesthesia, 402
Monitoring Quality of Nursing Care, 384
Monograph Series, 587
Monographs in Allergy, 376
Monographs in Clinical Cytology, 363
Monographs in Human Genetics, 383

Monographs in Oral Science, 381
Monographs on Endocrinology, 382
Monthly Bibliography of Medical Reviews, 372
Monthly Catalog, 554
Monthly Catalog of US Government Publications, 541
Monthly Checklist of State Publications, 541
The Morphology of Human Blood Cells, 431
Mosby's Comprehensive Review of Nursing, 444
Mosby's Current Practice and Perspectives in Nursing Series, 359
Mosby's Manual of Critical Care, 173
Mosby's Review of Practical Nursing, 444
Mosquitoes, Malaria and Man: A History of the Hostilities Since 1880, 334
The Mothers' and Fathers' Medical Encyclopedia, 53
Motion Picture Library, 1971–1972, 596
Mountain Medicine: A Clinical Study of Cold and High Altitudes, 438
A Multi-Axial Classification of Child Psychiatric Disorders, 567
A Multidisciplinary Approach to Learning Disability, Handbook for the Classroom Teacher, 131
Multilingual Guide for Medical Personnel, 216
Multilingual Manual for Medical History-Taking, 171
Multilingual Medical Dictionary: Lexicon Medium Polyglottum, 73
Multi-Media Medicine, 594
Multiple Imaging Procedures, 392
Multiple Sclerosis Research, 406
Munro Kerr's Operative Obstetrics, 138
Muscle and Its Innervation: An Atlas of Fine Structure, 267
Muscle Testing: Techniques of Manual Examination, 177
Musculoskeletal Function: An Anatomy and Kinesiology Laboratory Manual, 196

Museum Publications, 21
My Body, My Health: The Concerned Woman's Guide to Gynecology, 240
Myocardial Diseases, 412
Myocardial Infarction, 413

NACDS—Lilly Digest, a Survey of Chain Pharmacy Operations, 585
Nachweise von Vebersetzungen, 554
Names in the History of Psychology: A Biographical Sourcebook, 321
NASA Continuing Bibliography Series, 21
National Atlas of Disease Mortality in the United Kingdom, 274
National Cancer Institute Monograph, 387
National Directory of Mental Health: A Guide to Adult Outpatient Mental Health Facilities and Services Throughout the United States, 304
National Directory of Rehabilitation Facilities, 303
National Directory of State Agencies 1976–77, 285
National Drug Code Directory, 575
National Drug Code Index 1978–79, 575
NATIONAL FOUNDATIONS, 629
A National Guide to Government and Foundation Funding Sources in the Field of Aging, 295
National Health Directory, 1980, 290
National Institute on Drug Abuse Research Monograph Series, 369
National Institutes of Health Publications List, 542
National Institutes of Health Scientific Directory and Annual Bibliography, 291
National Library of Medicine Classification: A Scheme for the Shelf Arrangement of Books in the Field of Medicine and Its Related Sciences, 19
National Library of Medicine Current Catalog, 6
National Library of Medicine Literature Search, 19

National Medical Audiovisual Center Catalog; Audiovisuals for the Health Scientists, 1977, 587
National Medical Audiovisual Center of the National Library of Medicine; Overview, 587
National Patterns of R&D Resources: Funds and Manpower in the United States 1953–1972, 559
The National Survey of Audiovisual Materials for Nursing, 1968–1969, 597
National Trade and Professional Associations of the United States and Canada and Labor Unions, 602
NATO Advanced Study Institutes Series, 546
NATO Conference Series, 547
The National History of Chronic Bronchitis and Emphysema, 342
Nature, 527, 545
Nature of Schizophrenia: New Approaches to Research and Treatment, 480
Neonatal Emergencies and Other Problems, 57
Neonatal Medicine, 460
Neonatology: Pathophysiology and Management of the Newborn, 469
Neurological and Sensory Disease Film Guide, 1966, 596
Neurological Surgery: A Comprehensive Reference Guide to the Diagnosis and Management of Neurosurgical Problems, 209
Neurology, 528
Neurology Series, 350
Neuronal Activity in Sleep: An Annotated Bibliography, 24
Neuropathology of Vision: An Atlas, 250
Neuropsychiatry in World War II, 340
Neuroradiology in Infants and Children, 469
Neurosciences Research, 379
Neurosurgical Biblio-Index, 505, 509
Neurosurgical Management of the Epilepsies, 407
Neurotoxicology, 407

New Concepts in Surgical Pathology of the Skin, 417
New Directions in Public Health Care: An Evaluation of Proposals for National Health Insurance, 428
New England Journal of Medicine, 527, 545
The New Health Professionals: Nurse Practitioners and Physician's Assistants, 201
The New Illustrated Medical Encyclopedia for Home Use: A Practical Guide to Good Health, 53
New Medical Dictionary, 70
The New Nurse in Industry: A Guide for the Newly Employed Occupational Health Nurse, 222
The New Physician Surgical Quiz, 209
New Technical Books: A Selective List with Descriptive Annotations, 2
New Titles in Bioethics, 21
The New York Times Encyclopedia Dictionary of the Environment, 92
The Newborn: A Practical Guide, 228
Newton's Geriatric Nursing, 444
NICEM Index to Health and Safety Education—Multimedia, 594
NICSEM/NIMIS (National Instructional Materials Information System), 629
NIH Almanac 1969, 142
NIH Factbook: Guide to National Institutes of Health Programs and Activities, 291
The N.I.H.—How It Works, 199
NIMH, 629
1980 United States Pharmacopeia XX—National Formulary XV (The United States Pharmacopeia), 576
The 1980–81 International Micrographics Source Book, 589
1980–1981 National Biomedical Research Directory, 559
1980–1981 National Directory of Health/Medicine Organizations, 285
1980–1981 National News Media Directory: Medicine/Health, 285
1970 Film Reference Guide for Medicine and Allied Sciences, 594

1975 Handbook on Women Workers, 96
1971 Drug Abuse Reference: General Terms, Drug Abuse Terms, User Slang, Drugs, Chemicals, Education Source Guide, 91
NLL Announcement Bulletin, 3
NLN Nursing Data Book, 143
Nobel Lectures in Physiology-Medicine, 1901–1970, 335
Nobel Prize Winners in Medicine and Physiology, 1901–1965, 318
Nobel Symposia, 547
Nomenclature and Criteria for Diagnosis and Diseases of the Heart and Great Vessels, 67
Nomenclature Dermatologia, 67
Noninvasive Evaluation of Human Circulation: Clinical, Clinicopharmacological and Data Processing Aspects, 413
Non-Invasive Methods in Cardiology, 413
Noninvasive Techniques in Cardiology for the Nurse and Technician, 211
Nonparametric Methods for Quantitative Analysis, 398
Non-Print Resources; A Union List of Health Science Materials in Connecticut, 595
Nonproprietary Names for Pharmaceutical Substances, 68
Normal Aging I: Reports from the Duke Longitudinal Study 1955–1969, 427
Normal Aging II: Reports from the Duke Longitudinal Study 1970–1973, 427
Normal and Abnormal Development of the Human Nervous System, 407
Normal and Therapeutic Nutrition, 444
Normal Child Development: An Annotated Bibliography of Articles and Books Published 1950–1969, 36
Normal Radiologic Patterns and Variances of the Human Skeleton: An X-Ray Atlas of Adults and Children, 277

Normal Values in Clinical Chemistry: A Guide to Statistical Analysis of Laboratory Data, 220
Notable American Women, 1607–1950: A Biographical Dictionary, 328
Notable Names in Medicine and Surgery, 320
Notes on the History of Nutrition Research, 336
NOVA; Science Adventurers on Television: A Series of Reading Lists, 21
NRC Switchboard: Selected Information Resources on Industrial Safety and Occupational Health, 306
NSF Factbook, 143
NSF Factbook: Guide to National Science Foundation Programs and Activities, 285
NTIS Data Base, 537, 630
Nuclear Air Cleaning Handbook, 135
The Nuclear Fuel Cycle: A Survey of the Public Health, Environmental, and National Security Effects of Nuclear Power, 483
Nuclear Medicine: Clinical and Technological Bases, 454
Nuclear Medicine Science Syllabus, 202
Nuclear Power Reactor Instrumentation Systems Handbook, 135
Nuclear Science Abstracts (NSA), 536, 555
The Nurse Assistant, 195
Nurse Planning Information Series, 384
Nurse Practitioner, 531
The Nurse's Almanac, 143
The Nurse's Drug Handbook, 116
Nurse's Drug Reference, 144, 222
Nurses Guide to Cardiac Monitoring, 222
The Nurse's Guide to Health Services For Patients, 223
A Nurse's Guide to the X-Ray Department, 223
Nurses' Handbook of Fluid Balance, 116
The Nurse's Materia Medica, 116

Nursing Abstracts, 514
Nursing and Medical Terminology: Workbook, 195
Nursing and the Law, 445
Nursing Audit, 445
The Nursing Audit: Self Regulation in Nursing Practice, 445
Nursing Care Evaluation: Concurrent and Retrospective Review Criteria, 573
Nursing Care in Eye, Ear, Nose and Throat Disorders, 445
Nursing Care of Patients with Urologic Diseases, 445
Nursing Care of the Aged: An Annotated Bibliography for Nurses, 32
Nursing Cre of the Alcoholic and Drug Abuser, 445
Nursing Care of the Cancer Patient, 173
Nursing Care of the Growing Family: A Maternal-Newborn Text, 445
Nursing Care of the Labor Patient, 445
Nursing Care of the Patient with Burns, 445
Nursing Care Staffing Requirements in Nursing Homes, 573
Nursing Clinics of North America, 531
Nursing Diagnosis and Intervention in Nursing Practice, 173
Nursing Digest 1975 Review of Medicine and Surgery, 312
Nursing Education Monographs, 384
Nursing Homes: A County and Metropolitan Area Data Book, 144
Nursing in Society: A Historical Perspective, 336
Nursing in the Intensive Respiratory Care Unit, 445
Nursing Job Guide, 298
Nursing Management of Diabetes Mellitus, 446
A Nursing Manual for Care of the Patient with Stroke, 173
Nursing Media Index 16mm Films, 597
Nursing Opportunities, 336
Nursing Outlook, 531

The Nursing Profession: Views Through the Mist, 446
Nursing Research, 531
Nursing Research: A Learning Guide, 223
Nursing Research Conference, 551
Nursing Research: Development, Collaboration and Utilization, 446
Nursing Research: Principles and Practice, 446
Nursing Resources Series, 564
Nursing Skills and Techniques Film Series, 597
Nursing Staffing Methodology: A Review and Critique of Selected Literature, 15
Nursing Standards and Nursing Process, 446
Nursing Studies Index; An Annotated Guide to Reported Studies, Research Methods, and Historical and Biographical Materials in Periodicals, Books and Pamphlets Published in English, 514
Nursing Theory: Analysis, Application, Evaluation, 116
Nursing Theory Conference, 551
Nursing Theses 1932–1961: An Alphabetical Listing and Keyword Index, 558
Nursing Times, 531
Nutrition: A Comprehensive Treatise, 386
Nutrition Abstracts and Reviews, 515
Nutrition Almanac, 144
Nutrition and Aging: A Selected Annotated Bibliography, 1964–1972, 34
Nutrition and Cardiovascular Disease, 450
Nutrition and Diet Therapy: A Learning Guide for Students, 225
Nutrition and Diet Therapy; Reference Dictionary, 88
NUTRITION DATA BANK, 630
Nutrition Education Materials, 34
Nutrition, Immunity and Infection: Mechanisms of Interactions, 450
Nutrition Intervention in Developing Countries, 386
Nutrition News, 531

Nutrition, Nutricion: Index, Indice, 1945–1966, 34
Nutrition Programs for the Elderly—A Guide to Menu Planning, Buying and the Care of Food for Community Programs, 225
Nutrition Reviews, 373
Nutrition Reviews' Present Knowledge in Nutrition, 450
Nutritional Support of Medical Practice, 175
Nutritive Value of American Foods: In Common Units, 144
N. W. Ayer and Sons Directory of Newspapers and Periodicals, 524

Obesity: A Bibliography 1964–1973, 35
Obesity, Anorexia Nervosa, and the Person Within, 225
Obstetric-Gynecologic Terminology with Section on Neonatology and Glossary of Congenital Anomalies, 92
Obstetric Nursing, 446
Obstetrics and Gynecology, 535
Obstetrics and Gynecology Annual, 315
Obtencion Y Manejo De Muestras Para Examenes Microbiologicos De Las Enfermedades Transmisibles, 192
Occupational and Environmental Cancers of the Urinary System, 484
Occupational Diseases: A Guide to Their Recognition, 236
Occupational Diseases: A Syllabus of Signs and Symptoms, 236
Occupational Health and Safety, 60
Occupational Lung Diseases, 484
Occupational Mental Health Notes, 518
Occupational Safety and Health: A Guide to Information Sources, 16, 236, 306
Occupational Safety and Health Abstracts, 521
Occupational Safety and Health Series, 369
Occupational Safety, Health and Fire Index, 577

The Ocular Adnexa, 457
Ocular Differential Diagnosis, 120
Ocular Examination-Basis and Technique, 226
Ocular Pathology: A Text and Atlas, 266
Ocular Syndromes, 457
Ocular Therapeutics and Pharmacology, 457
Official Gazette of the United States Patent Office, 581
Official Methods of Analysis, 236
Oncogenic Viruses, 454
Oncology Abstracts, 515
On Documentation of Scientific Literature, 9
150 Commonly Prescribed Drugs. A Guide to Their Uses and Side Effects, 231
Operative Surgery: Fundamental International Techniques, Colon, Rectum and Anus, 377
Operative Surgery; Fundamental International Techniques: Urology, 280
Ophthalmic Eponyms: An Encyclopedia of Named Signs, Syndromes, and Diseases in Ophthalmology, 88
Ophthalmic Plastic Surgery, 457
Ophthalmology: Principles and Concepts, 457
Ophthalmology Study Guide for Medical Students, 226
The Opium Problem, 480
Opportunistic Pathogens, 192
Optical Society of America Directory, 300
Oral Diagnosis: A Handbook of Modern Diagnostic Techniques Used to Investigate Clinical Problems in Dentistry, 104
Oral Disease, 253
Oral-Facial Genetics, 425
Oral Health Survey, Basic Methods, 163
Oral Maxillo-Facial Surgeons of the World, 319
Oral Pathology, 415
Oral Research Abstracts, 510
Oral Roentgenographic Diagnosis, 253

Oral Surgery, 415
Orban's Oral Histology and Embryology, 253
Organ Preservation for Transplantation, 403
Organization and Administration of Health Care: Theory, Practice, Environment, 428
Organized Medicine in the Progressive Era: The More Toward Monopoly, 328
The Origin and Treatment of Schizophrenic Disorders, 480
The Origin of Medical Terms, 81
Origins of the Healing Art, 328
Orthodontic Directory of the World, 295
Orthodontics: Principles and Practice, 415
Orthopaedic Neurology: A Diagnostic Guide to Neurologic Levels, 227
Orthopaedic Surgery, 120
Orthopaedic Surgery in Infancy and Childhood, 469
Orthopedic Clinics of North America, 532
Orthopedic Diseases: Physiology, Pathology, Radiology, 460
Orthopedic Nursing, 447
OSHA Compliance Guide, 577
An Outline of Dental Materials and Their Selection, 415
An Outline of Food Law: Structure, Principles, Main Provisions, 574
Outline of Orthopaedics, 460

Paediatric Allergy and Clinical Immunology (as Applied to Atopic Disease): A Manual for Students and Practitioners of Medicine, 178
Paediatric Gastroenterology, 469
Paediatric Kidney Disease, 469
Pain: A Sourcebook for Nurses and Other Professionals, 201
PAIS INTERNATIONAL, 630
Paleopathological Diagnosis and Interpretation, Bone Diseases in Ancient Human Populations, 486
PANDEX, 630

Pandex Current Index to Scientific and Technical Literature, 502
Paramedical Dictionary: A Practical Dictionary for the Semi-medical and Ancillary Medical Professions, 81
Parasitology: The Biology of Animal Parasites, 435
Parent-Child Nursing: Psychosocial Aspects, 447
The Parents' Encyclopedia of Infancy, Childhood, and Adolescence, 57
The Parents' Medical Manual, 178
Parkinson's Disease and Related Disorders, Citations from the Literature, 506, 509
Parkinson's Disease and Related Disorders: Cumulative Bibliography: 1800–1970, 25
Parkinson's Disease & Related Disorders: International Directory of Scientists, 1970, 294
Parson's Diseases of the Eye, 227
Patch Testing, 207
Patch Testing Guidelines, 207
A Path to the Double Helix, 332
Pathobiology Annual, 313
Pathologic Basis of Disease, 463
Pathologic Physiology: Mechanisms of Disease, 463
Pathology, 463
Pathology Annual, 313
Pathology of Infancy and Childhood, 470
Pathology of Pulmonary Hypertension, 464
Pathology of the Ear, 461
The Pathology of the Heart, 464
Pathology of the Kidney, 464
Pathology of the Lung (Excluding Pulmonary Tuberculosis), 464
Pathology of the Nervous System, 379
Pathology of Toxaemia of Pregnancy, 138
Pathology of Tumors of the Nervous System, 379
Pathophysiology: Altered Regulatory Mechanisms in Disease, 465
Pathophysiology of Gestation, 393
Patient Assessment Series, 223

The Patient in Surgery: A Guide for Nurses, 223
Patient-Nurse Interaction: A Study of Interaction Patterns in Acute Psychiatric Wards, 447
Patty's Industrial Hygiene and Toxicology, 236, 484
Paul deHaen Information Systems, 592
Pears Medical Encyclopedia, Illustrated, 55
Pediatric and Adolescent Echocardiography: A Handbook, 122
Pediatric and Adolescent Endocrinology, 364
Pediatric Cardiology, 470
Pediatric Clinical Gastroenterology, 470
Pediatric Clinics of North America, 532
Pediatric Dosage Handbook, 122
The Pediatric Examination: Art and Process, 598
Pediatric Nephrology, 470
Pediatric Neurologic Nursing, 447
Pediatric Neurology Handbook, 122
Pediatric Nuclear Medicine, 470
The Pediatric Nurse Practitioner; Guidelines For Practice, 223
The Pediatric Nursing Skills Manual, 173
Pediatric Orthopedics, 470
Pediatric Surgery, 471
Pediatrics, 471, 532
Penguin Library of Nursing, 385
The Penguin Medical Encyclopedia, 56
Perinatal Medicine, 471
Perinatal Nursing: Care of Newborns and Their Families, 447
Periodicals Relevant to Microbiology and Immunology: A World List, 1968, 524
Peripheral Arterial Disease, 413
Peripheral Vascular Surgery, 162
Perspectives in Medicine, 346
Perspectives in Pediatric Pathology, 364
Pesticide Index, 520
Pesticides Abstracts, 521
Peterson's Annual Guides to Graduate Study, 294

Pharmaceutical Directory, 301
Pharmaceutical Handbook, 127
Pharmaceutical Manufacturers of the United States, 301
Pharmaceutical Manufacturing Encyclopedia, 58
Pharmaceutical Marketers Directory, 302
Pharmaceutical News Index, 523, 630
The Pharmacologic Basis of Patient Care, 447
Pharmacological and Biochemical Properties of Drug Substances, 366
Pharmacological and Chemical Synonyms; A Collection of Names of Drugs and Other Compounds Drawn from the Medical Literature of the World, 90
Pharmacological Basis of Patient Care, 116
The Pharmacological Basis of Therapeutics, 475
Pharmacological Reviews, 533
Pharmacology and Therapeutics, 475
Pharmacology, Biochemistry and Behavior, 533
Pharmacology in Nursing, 116, 447
Pharmacology of Steroid Contraceptive Drugs, 475
Pharmacy in History, 533
Pharmacy Law and Ethics, 231
Pharmacy School Admission Requirements, Actual 1977–78, Projected 1978–79, 302
Pharmacy Technicians' Manual, 180
PharmIndex, 231
Photochemical and Photobiological Reviews, 366
Photographic Atlas of Fetal Anatomy, 245
PHRA: Poverty and Human Resources Abstracts, 502
Physical Activities for the Handicapped, 477
Physical Assessment Examinations, 223
The Physical Fitness Encyclopedia, 59
Physical Fitness/Sports Medicine, 31, 505
Physical Therapy, 533

Physical Therapy Procedures: Selected Techniques, 232
Physically Handicapped Children: A Medical Atlas for Teachers, 273
Physicians' Current Procedural Terminology for Naming, Coding, and Reporting Medical Services, 565
Physicians' Desk Reference, 96
Physicians' Desk Reference for Radiology and Nuclear Medicine, 136
Physicians Desk Reference to Pharmaceutical Specialties and Biologicals, 127
Physician's Guide to Negotiations, 216
Physician's Handbook, 114
A Physician's Handbook on Orthomolecular Medicine, 118
Physician's Medical Book Reference, 1978, 294
Physiological Reviews, 373
The Physiology of Physical Stress: A Selective Bibliography, 1500–1964, 31
Physiology, Series One, 377
The Physiopathology of Cancer, 455
A Pictorial History of Medicine, 328
Pilot Study on the Use of Scientific Literature by Scientists, 9
Plague Manual, 183
Plagues and Peoples, 334
Plaster Casting, 227
Plastic and Reconstructive Surgery, 528
Plastic and Reconstructive Surgery of the Breast, 377
Plastic Surgery, 403
The Plastic Surgery Atlas, 247
Platelets: Physiology and Pathology, 431
PMA Annual Report, 586
PMA Bulletin, 586
PMA News Releases, 586
PMA Newsletter, 586
PMD: Pharmaceutical Marketers Directory, 302
PNI [Pharmaceutical News Index], 630
Pocket Atlas of Human Anatomy, 245
Pocketbook of Pediatric Antimicrobial Therapy, 145
Pocket Book of Statistical Tables, 152
Pocket Color Atlas of Dermatology, 255
Pocket Guide to Health Assessment, 220
Poisindex, 592
Poisoning by Drugs and Chemicals, Plant and Animals: An Index of Toxic Effects and Their Treatment, 145
Pollution Abstracts, 521, 630
Pollution Control Companies, U.S.A., 1972, 306
Pollution Research Index: A New Reference Guide, 562
Polyglot Medical Questionnaire in Twenty-Seven Languages with Digital System of Communication, 73
Population Bibliography, 630
Population Sciences: Index of Biomedical Research, 505, 521
Portrait Catalog of the Library of the New York Academy of Medicine, 7
Positioning and Technique Handbook for Radiologic Technologists, 137
Postgraduate Medicine, 527
Potter's New Cyclopedia of Medicinal Herbs and Preparations, 58
A Practical Approach to Pediatric Endocrinology, 228
Practical Clinical Microbiology and Mycology: Techniques and Interpretation, 192
Practical Echocardiography: A Basic Manual, 162
Practical Echocardiology, 413
Practical Electrocardiography, 162
The Practical Encyclopedia of Natural Healing, 54
Practical Guide to Medicine and Veterinarian Mycology, 218, 241
Practical Management of Eye Problems: Glaucoma, Strabismus, Visual Fields, 176
Practical Management of the Elderly, 427
A Practical Manual for Patient Teaching, 173
Practical Manual of Pediatrics: A Pocket Reference for Those Who Treat Children, 178

Practical Medicine: A Guide to Outpatient Management, 216
Practical Neonatal Pediatrics, 471
Practical Nursing Nutrition Education, 174
Practical Nursing Review, 447
Practical Obstetrics and Gynecology: Manual of Selected Procedures and Treatment, 185
Practical Ophthalmic Plastic and Reconstructive Surgery, 457
Practical Paediatric Endocrinology, 179
Practical Pediatric Electrocardiography, 211
Practical Psychiatry for the Primary Physician, 234
Practical Spanish for Medical and Hospital Personnel, 216
Practical Video: The Manager's Guide to Applications, 589
A Practice of Anaesthesia, 159
The Practice of Pediatric Neurology, 471
A Practitioner's Guide to the Diagnostic X-ray Equipment Standard, 577
Pregnancy, Birth and the Newborn Baby: A Complete Guide for Parents and Parents-To-Be, 229
The Prenatal Diagnosis of Hereditary Disorders, 472
Prenatal Intensive Care, 447
Preparing Registered Nurses for Expanded Roles: A Directory of Programs, 298
Prescriber's Guide to Drug Interaction, 127
Prescription Drug Industry Fact Book, 146
Preventive Medicine in the United States, 1900–1975, 341
Previews: Audiovisual Software Reviews, 590
Primary Anatomy, 401
Primary Care Nursing: A Manual of Clinical Skills, 174
Primary Child Care: A Manual for Health Workers, 179
Primary Prevention in Drug Abuse: An Annotated Guide to the Literature, 16
A Primer of Cancer Management, 455

A Primer of Cardiac Diagnosis: The Physical and Technical Study of the Cardiac Patient, 211
A Primer on Chemical Dependency: A Clinical Guide to Alcohol and Drug Problems, 237
Princeton Guide to Microforms: Serials, 590
Princeton Telephone Guide to Microforms, 590
Principles and Practice of Infectious Diseases, 384
Principles and Practice of Nursing, 447
Principles and Practice of Obstetric Anaesthesia, 98
Principles and Practice of Periodontics: With and Atlas of Treatment, 254
Principles and Practices of Medicine, 438
Principles and Techniques of Electron Microscopy: Biological Applications, 389
Principles and Techniques of Scanning Electron Microscopy: Biological Applications, 465
Principles of Anesthesiology, 55
Principles of Biochemical Tests in Diagnostic Microbiology, 192
Principles of Biochemistry, 398
Principles of Clinical Electrocardiography, 188
Principles of Dental Public Health, 415
Principles of Diagnostic Radiology, 486
Principles of Drug Information Services, 180
Principles of Food Science, 451
Principles of Genetics, 425
Principles of Hospital Administration, 429
The Principles of Human Biochemical Genetics, 425
Principles of Immunology, 400
Principles of Medical Statistics, 398
Principles of Modern Immunobiology: Basic and Clinical, 400
Principles of Obstetrics and Gynecology for Nurses, 447
Principles of Successful Radiation Therapy: Introduction to Treatment Planning, 487

Prints Relating to Dentistry, 331
Private Practice: A Handbook for the Independent Mental Health Practitioner, 132
The Problem-Oriented System in Nursing: A Workbook, 195
Problem Pregnancy and Abortion Counseling, 186
Problems of Drug Dependence 1975, 480
Procedures in Vascular Surgery, 261
Proceedings in Print, 547
Proceedings of International Symposium on Infectious Antibiotic Resistance, 551
Proceedings of the Congress of the International Diabetes Federation, 549
The Process of Patient Teaching in Nursing, 448
Professional Nursing: Foundations, Perspectives and Relationships, 224
Progress in Allergy, 347
Progress in Brain Research, 351
Progress in Cancer Research and Therapy, 360
Progress in Cardiac Rehabilitation, 353
Progress in Cardiology, 353
Progress in Cardiovascular Diseases, 528
Progress in Chemical Toxicology, 369
Progress in in Chemotherapy, 552
Progress in Clinical and Biological Research, 358
Progress in Clinical Cancer, 360
Progress in Clinical Immunology, 347
Progress in Clinical Medicine, 438
Progress in Clinical Neurophysiology, 351
Progress in Clinical Pathology, 363
Progress in Drug Metabolism, 366
Progress in Drug Research/Forschritte der Arzneimittelforschung/Progres des Recherches Pharmaceutiques, 366
Progress in Experimental Tumor Research, 360
Progress in Gastroenterology, 355
Progress in Gynecology, 372
Progress in Hematology, 356
Progress in Hemostasis and Thrombosis, 356

Progress in Histochemistry and Cytochemistry, 364
Progress in Immunology, Proceedings, International Congress of Immunology, 549
Progress in Immunology II, 347
Progress in Liver Diseases, 355
Progress in Medical Genetics, 356
Progress in Medical Virology, 358
Progress in Medicinal Chemistry, 366
Progress in Neurobiology, 351
Progress in Neurological Surgery, 351
Progress in Neurology and Psychiatry, An Annual Review, 351
Progress in Neuropathology, 351
Progress in Neurophysiology, 351
Progress in Nuclear Medicine, 361
Progress in Orthopaedic Surgery, 362
Progress in Paediatric Neurosurgery, 472
Progress in Pediatric Radiology, 364
Progress in Pediatric Surgery, 364
Progress in Respiration Research, 371, 562
Progress in Surgery, 349
Progress in Toxicology, 369
Prostaglandin Abstracts. A Guide to the Literature, Volume 1: 1906–1970, 510
The Prostaglandins, 419
Prostheses and Rehabilitation After Arm Amputation, 477
Protection Against Ionizing Radiation from External Sources, 146
The Proteins, 375
Providing Safe Nursing Care for Ethnic People of Color, 448
Psychedelics Encyclopedia, 58
Psychiatric Dictionary, 91
Psychiatric Drugs; A Desk Reference, 146
The Psychiatric Foundations of Medicine, 391
A Psychiatric Glossary, 91
Psychiatric Medicine, 481
Psychiatric Nursing, 448
Psychiatric Nursing: A Basic Manual, 174
Psychiatric Spectator, 586
Psychiatry and the Criminal: A Guide

to Psychiatric Examinations for the Criminal Courts, 234
Psychological Abstracts, 518, 631
Psychological Disorders of Children: A Handbook for Primary Care Physicians, 132
Psychological Index, 1894–1935, 519
The Psychologists, 321
Psychopharmacology, 533
Psychopharmacology: A Generation of Progress, 58
Psychopharmacology Abstracts, 517
Psychopharmacology Bibliography, 39, 505
Psychopharmacology Bulletin, 533
Psychopharmacology: From Theory to Practice, 481
Psychopharmacology of Affective Disorders: A British Association for Psychopharmacology Monograph, 481
Psychosomatic Medicine: Current Trends and Clinical Applications, 481
Psychosources: A Psychology Resource Catalog, 44
Psychotropic Drugs: A Guide for the Practitioner, 234
Psychotropic Drugs: A Manual for Emergency Management of Overdosage, 181
Psychotropic Drugs and Related Compounds, 182
Public Health and the State: Changing Views in Massachusetts, 1842–1936, 342
Public Health Engineering Abstracts, 521
Public Health Law Manual: A Handbook on the Legal Aspects of Public Health Administration and Enforcement, 135
Public Health Reports, 534, 539
Public Welfare Directory, 1940–, 306
Publications: Catalogue 1947–1971, 543
Publications Resulting from National Institute of Mental Health Research Grants, 1947–1961, 44
Publications of the UN Systems: A Reference Guide, 542
Publications of the World Health Organization, 1947–1957: A Bibliography, 543
Pulmonary Diagnostic Techniques, 489
Pulmonary Emboli: A Progress in Cardiovascular Diseases Reprint, 413
Pulmonary Metastasis, 490
Pulmonary Physiology of the Fetus, Newborn and Child, 472

Quality by Objectives: A Practical Method of Care Assessment and Assurance for Ambulatory Health Centers, 217
Quality Control in Blood Banking: Quality Controls in the Clinical Laboratory, 429
Quality of Care Assessment and Assurance An Annotated Bibliography With A Point of View, 31
Quarterly Review of Biology, 373
Quick Reference to Pediatric Emergencies, 123
Quick Reference to Surgical Emergencies, 159

Radiation Dosimetry Data: Catalogue 1976: A Catalogue of Data Sheets Available From the International Atomic Energy Agency, 147
Radiation Oncology: Rationale, Technique, Results, 455
Radiation Protection: A Guide for Scientists and Physicians, 238
Radiation Protection Standards, 577
Radiation Science at the National Physical Laboratory, 1912–1955, 578
A Radiographic Index, 92
Radiologic Anatomy of the Brain, 250
Radiologic Clinics of North America, 534
Radiologic Science: Workbook and Laboratory Manual, 198
Radiologic Transverse Anatomy of the Human Thorax, Abdomen, and Pelvis: An Atlas of Anatomic, Radiologic, Computed Tomography, and Ultrasonic Correlation, 277
Radiological Atlas of Biliary and Pancreatic Disease, 258

Radiological Atlas of Bone Tumours, 264
Radiological Health Training Resources 1975, 50
Radiology, 534
Radiology of Bone Diseases, 487
The Radiology of Skeletal Disorders: Exercise in Diagnosis, 196
Radiology of Syndromes, 238
Radiology of the Abdomen: Anatomic Basis, 258
Radiology of the Gallbladder and Bile Ducts, 423, 487
Radiology of the Newborn and Young Infant, 472
Radiology of the Pancreas and Duodenum, 487
Radiology of the Skull and Brain, 352
Radiology of the Small Intestine, 487
Radiology of Trauma: Textbook and Atlas, 277
Rape and Rape-Related Issues: An Annotated Bibliography, 49
Rape Victimology, 481
Rapid Methods & Automation in Microbiology & Immunology: A Bibliography, 22
Rare Genetic Diseases: A Guidebook, 214
Rational Drug Therapy, 533
Reading Guide to the Cancer-Virology Literature, 35
Readings in Gerontology, 448
Readings on Cancer: An Annotated Bibliography, 36
Realities in Childbearing, 481
Recent Advances in Alcohol and Drug Problems, 369
Recent Advances in Anaesthesia and Analgesia, 403
Recent Advances in Cancer and Radiotherapeutics: Clinical Oncology, 455
Recent Advances in Cardiology, 414
Recent Advances in Clinical Biochemistry, 359
Recent Advances in Clinical Immunology, 347
Recent Advances in Clinical Neurology, 352
Recent Advances in Clinical Nuclear Medicine, 361
Recent Advances in Clinical Pathology, 364
Recent Advances in Clinical Pharmacology, 367
Recent Advances in Clinical Psychiatry, 368
Recent Advances in Clinical Virology, 358
Recent Advances in Dermatology, 417
Recent Advances in Dermato-Pharmacology, 417
Recent Advances in Endocrinology and Metabolism, 354
Recent Advances in Forensic Pathology, 465
Recent Advances in Gastroenterology, 423
Recent Advances in Geriatric Medicine, 356
Recent Advances in Haematology, 356
Recent Advances in Intensive Therapy, 359
Recent Advances in Medicine, 438
Recent Advances in Myology, 371
Recent Advances in in Neuropathology, 364
Recent Advances in Nuclear Medicine, 361
Recent Advances in Obesity Research, 359
Recent Advances in Orthopaedics, 362
Recent Advances in Otolaryngology, 363
Recent Advances in Paediatric Surgery, 365
Recent Advances in Pediatrics, 472
Recent Advances in Plastic Surgery, 349
Recent Advances in Radiology, 370
Recent Advances in Rheumatology, 371
Recent Advances in Studies of Alcoholism, 369
Recent Advances in Surgery, 349
Recent Advances in Thrombosis, 356
Recent Advances in Ultrasound in Biomedicine, 370

Recent Advances on Pain: Pathophysiology and Clinical Aspects, 407
Recent Progress in Hormone Research, 354
Recent Results in Cancer Research, 361
Recent Surveys of Nonmedical Drug Use: A Compendium of Abstracts, 39
Recent Trends in Cardiovascular and Thoracic Surgery, 414
Receptors and Recognition, 391
Recommended Dietary Allowances, 118
Reconstruction Surgery and Traumatology, 377
Recurring Bibliography of Hypertension, 32, 506
Recurring Bibliography on Education in the Allied Health Professions, 21, 506
The Red Blood Cell, 432
Red Cell Manual, 190
Referativnyi Zhurnal, 503
Reference Data on Socioeconomic Issues of Health, 143
Reference Data on the Profile of Medical Practice, 143
Reece-Chamberlain's Manual of Emergency Pediatrics, 179
Reference Encyclopedia of American Psychology and Psychiatry, 60
A Reference Guide to Audiovisual Information, 590
Reflex Testing Methods for Evaluating C.N.S. Development, 161
Regional Differences in the Lung, 490
Registry of Toxic Effects of Chemical Substances, 147
Rehabilitation: A Manual for the Care of the Disabled and the Elderly, 181
Rehabilitation Literature, 517
Rehabilitation Medicine: A Textbook on Physical Medicine and Rehabilitation, 477
Rehabilitation Services in Hospitals and Related Facilities: A Guide to Planning, Organization, and Management, 232
Remington's Pharmaceutical Sciences, 475

Repertorium Commentationum a Societatibus Litterariis Editarum, 503
Report of the Task Group on Reference Man, 571
Research and Clinical Studies in Headache; An International Review, 352
Research and Development in the Federal Budget: FY 1977, 559
Research Centers Directory: A Guide to University-Related and Other Nonprofit Organizations, 286
Research Contracts in the Life Sciences, 559
Research Grant Index, 560
Research in Biological and Medical Sciences; Annual Progress Report, 560
Research in Dental Education: Selected Abstracts, 1933–1968, 25
Research in Nursing Practice, 447
Research in the Service of Mental Health: Report of the Research Task Force of the National Institute of Mental Health, 340
Respiration and Circulation, 137
Respiratory Care, 534
Respiratory Diseases, 490
Respiratory Failure, 490
Respiratory Protection—OSHA and the Small Businessman, 237
Respiratory Research in the People's Republic of China, 490
Respiratory Technology: A Procedure Manual, 184
Respiratory Therapist Manual, 184
The Reston Encyclopedia of Biomedical Engineering Terms, 54
Review of Allied Health Education, 346
A Review of Anatomical Neurology, 407
Review of Gross Anatomy, 246
Review of Medical Pharmacology, 475
Review of Physiological Chemistry, 398
A Review of the US EPA Environmental Research Outlook FY 1976–1980, 562
Review of Urology in Childhood, 472
Reviews of Medical Motion Pictures, 59

Reviews of Physiology, Biochemistry and Pharmacology, 368
Rh: The Intimate History of a Disease and Its Conquest, 332
Rheumatism in Populations, 492
Rheumatology and Rehabilitation, 533
The Rights of Hospital Patients, 217
RINGDOC, 631
The Rise of Surgery: From Empiric Craft to Scientific Discipline, 329
Rites of Passage: Adolescence in America 1790 to the Present, 341
Roentgen Diagnosis of Diseases of Bone, 487
Roentgen Examinations in Acute Abdominal Diseases, 488
Roe's Laboratory Guide to Chemistry, 206
Roget's International Thesaurus, 65
Rohm and Haas Reporter, 586
The Roll of the Royal College of Physicians of London, 320
Royal Society of Medicine International Congress and Symposium Series, 548
RTECS [Registry of Toxic Effects of Chemical Substances], 622
Russian-English Medical Dictionary, 71
Russian-English Translators Dictionary: A Guide to Scientific and Technical Usage, 71
Russian-English Veterinary Dictionary, 71
Rypins' Medical Licensure Examinations, 220

SABIR, 631
Safe Handling of Radiation Sources, 137
Safety Guide for Health Care Institutions, 217
Safety Science Abstracts, 631
Sandoz Atlas of Haematology, 261
Saunders Review for Practical Nurses, 448
Scabies and Pediculosis, 435
Scanning Electron Microscopy, 389, 465
Schistosomiasis: A Bibliography of the World's Literature From 1852–1962, 29
Schistosomiasis: The Evolution of a Medical Literature: Selected Abstracts and Citations, 1852–1972, 29
Schistosomiasis III: Abstracts of the Complete Literature 1963–1974, 29
School Health: A Guide for Health Professionals, 220
School Health Practice, 484
Science, 527, 545
Science Abstracts, 503
The Science and Practice of Clinical Medicine, 359
Science and Technology Research in Progress 1972–1973, 560
Science Books: A Quarterly Review, 3
Science Books and Films, 3, 590
Science Citation Index, 503
Science Fiction Book Review Index, 1923–1973, 1
Science: Guide to Scientific Instruments, 206
Science News Yearbook, 309
Science Research Abstracts, 503
Science Research in Progress, 560
Science, Technology, and Public Policy: A Selected and Annotated Bibliography, 21
Science Year; the World Book Science Annual, 309
Scientific American, 527
Scientific American Medicine, 438
Scientific American Resource Library, 21
Scientific and Technical Aerospace Abstracts, 555
Scientific and Technical Aerospace Reports [STAR], 536
Scientific and Technical Books in Print, 3
Scientific and Technical Information Sources, 11
Scientific and Technical Series, 344
The Scientific Background of the International Sanitary Conferences 1851–1938, 342
Scientific Contributions from the Laboratories 1866–1966, 338, 585

Scientific Directory and Annual Bibliography, 286
Scientific, Engineering and Medical Societies Publications in Prints, 1978–79, 603
Scientific Foundations of Urology, 393
The Scientific Journal: Editorial Policies and Practices; Guidelines for Editors, Reviewers, and Authors, 155, 525
Scientific, Medical, and Technical Book Published in the United States of America: A Selected List of Titles in Print with Annotations, 5
Scientific Meetings, 544
Scientific Periodicals: Their Historical Development, Characteristics and Control, 525
Scientific Principles in Nursing, 448
Scientific Research in British Universities and Colleges, 560
The Scientific Revolution in Victorian Medicine, 330
Scientific, Technical, and Related Societies of the United States, 603
SCISEARCH, 631
Scope and Coverage Manual of the National Library of Medicine, 156
Scope Monographs, 586
Scott-Brown's Disease of the Ear, Nose, and Throat, 388
The Searle Review of Obstetric & Gynecologic Literature, 522
A Select Bibliogaphy of Medical Biography: With an Introductory Essay on Medical Biography, 318
Selected Abstracts on Animal Models for Biomedical Research, 22
Selected Bibliography of Nutrition Materials, 35
Selected Bibliography on Detection of Dependence-Producing Drugs in Body Fluids, 39
Selected Bibliography on Lead Poisoning in Children, 49
A Selected Guide to Audiovisual Materials on Alcohol and Alcoholism, 599
Selected Guide to Food, Dieting, and Beverage Books, 225

Selected Mental Health Audiovisuals, 599
Selected Publications of the Division of Nursing, 543
Selected References on Cereal Grains in Protein Nutrition: Human and Experimental Animal Studies of Major and Minor Cereals, 1910–1966, 35
Selected References on Environment Quality as It Relates to Health, 49
Selected Studies in Building Research, Applicable to the Design and Construction of Health Facilities, 27
Selected Studies in Medical Care and Medical Economics: Annual Report, 311
A Selective Guide to Materials for Mental Health and Family Life Education, 45, 234
Seminars in Arthritis and Rheumatism, 534
Seminars in Hematology, 530
Seminars in Nuclear Medicine, 531
Seminars in Oncology, 531
Seminars in Perinatology, 532
Seminars in Roentgenology, 534
Serial Handbook of Modern Psychiatry, 132
The Series in Clinical and Community Psychology, 368
SERLINE [Serials Online], 622
Services & Organization Guide, 286
Serving Physically Disabled People, 96
Sex and Sex Education: A Bibliography, 51
Sex and the Handicapped: A Selected Bibliography (1927–1975), 41
Sex Education Books for Young Adults 1892–1979, 51
Sexual Options for Paraplegics and Quadriplegics, 128
Sexually Transmitted Diseases, 535
Shands' Handbook of Orthopaedic Surgery, 120
Shelf List Catalog, 8
Shock Trauma Manual, 171
A Short History of Medicine, 328
SI Units, 140

SI Units and Nomenclature in Soil Science, 140
Sicle Cell Disease: Diagnosis Management, Education and Research, 425
The Sickle Cell Hemoglobinopathies: A Comprehensive Bibliography 1910–1972, 28
Side Effects of Drugs, 367, 517
Sights and Sounds in Ophthalmology, 597
Simplified Medical Records System: A Directory of Medical Terminology, 85
Skeletal Research: An Experimental Approach, 562
Skin Signs of Systemic Disease, 417
Skin Surgery, 417
Sleep, 549
Slovar-minimum Po Angliiskomu Iazyku Dlia Studentov Meditisinskikh Vuzov, 71
Slow Transmissible Diseases of the Nervous System, 379
Smith's Blood Diseases of Infancy and Childhood, 472
Smoking and Health Bulletin, 49
Social and Psychological Aspects of Applied Human Genetics: A Bibliography, 26
A Social History of Medicine, 342
Socioeconomic Issues of Health, 152
Sociological Abstracts, 504, 631
The Sociology of Medicine and Health Care: Research Bibliography, 28
Sociology: Nurses and Their Patients in a Modern Society, 448
Source Book for Food Scientists, 201
A Source Book in the History of Psychology, 341
Source Book, Nursing Personnel: Health Manpower References, 201
Sourcebook of Audiology: Speech and Language Terminology, 202
A Source-Book of Biological Names and Terms, 76
A Source Book of Nursing Research, 201
The Source Book of Plastic Surgery, 199, 330
Sourcebook on Aging, 200
Sourcebook on Food and Nutrition, 201
Sourcebook on Health Sciences Librarianship, 13
Source Index Quarterly, 526
Sources of Medical Motion Pictures, 595
Sources of Serials: An International Publisher and Corporate Author Directory, 5
Southern Medical Journal, 527
Southwestern Medical Dictionary: Spanish/English, English/Spanish, 71
Speakers and Lecturers: How to Find Them, 328
Speaking at Medical Meetings, 206
Speciality Board Review: Obstetrics and Gynecology, 199
Specifications and Criteria for Biochemical Compounds, 576
Specifications for the Identity and Purity of Some Food Colors, Flavour Enhancers, Thickening Agents, and Certain Food Additives, 574
Specifications for the Quality Control of Pharmaceutical Preparations: Second Edition of the International Pharmacopoeia, 576
Speech Pathology and Audiology in Medical Settings, 477
Speed: The Current Index to the Drug Abuse Literature, 521
Spina Bifida–Problems and Management, 210
The Spinal Cord: Basic Aspects and Surgical Considerations, 407
Spinal Cord Injuries: Comprehensive Management and Research, 407
Spinal Injury, 477
The Spine, 408
The Spine: A Radiological Text and Atlas, 250
Sports Medicine, 438
Springer Series on the Teaching of Nursing, 385
Sprowl's American Pharmacy: An Introduction to Pharmaceutical Techniques and Dosage Forms, 476
SSIE Current Research, 631
SSIE Science Newsletter, 560

Staff Development in Geriatric Institutions: A Manual for the Trainer, 166
Staffing for Patient Care; A Guide for Nursing Service, Based on A Research Report, 224
Staining Procedures Used by the Biological Stain Commission, 197
Standard Medical Almanac, 143
Standard Nomenclature of Diseases and Operations, 98
Standard Orthopaedic Operations: A Guide for the Junior Surgeon, 227
Standards and Planning Guide for Pharmacy Library Service, 576
Standards and Specifications Information Sources, 569
Standards for Accreditation of Extended Care Facilities, Nursing Care Facilities and Resident Care Facilities, 573
Standards for Cardiopulmonary Resuscitation and Emergency Cardiac Care, 572
Standards for Library Services in Health Care Institutions, 572
Standards of Nursing Practice, 573
State and Local Environmental Libraries: A Directory, 306
State-Approved Schools of Nursing—L.P.N./L.V.N. State Approved Schools of Nursing—R.N., 299
State Government Reference Publications: An Annotated Bibliography, 542
Statistical Indices of Family Health, 149
Statistical Tables of Biological, Agricultural, and Medical Research, 152
Statistics: A Biomedical Introduction, 398
Statistics on Narcotic Drugs for 1976 Furnished by Goverments in Accordance with the International Treaties and Maximum Levels of Opium Stocks, 149
Statistics Sources, 148
Stedman's Medical Dictionary: A Vocabulary of Medicine and Its Allied Sciences, With Pronunciations and Derivations, 81

The Stein and Day International Medical Encyclopedia, 56
Steinbichler's Lexikon fur die Apothedenpraxis in Sieben Sprachen, 73
Stereoscopic Atlas of Human Anatomy, 595
Stereotaxic Atlas of the Human Brainstem and Cerebellar Nuclei: A Variability Study, 251
Strategy of Drug Design: A Molecular Guide to Biological Activity, 231
Strauss and Welt's Diseases of the Kidney, 423
Stress in Health and Disease, 419
Stress Testing: Principles and Practice, 220
The Striated Muscle, 492
Strike Back at Cancer: What You Can Do and Where You Can Go for the Best Medical Care, 299
Stroke and Its Rehabilitation, 478
Structural Units of Medical and Biological Terms, 81
The Structure and Function of Muscle, 392
Structure and Function of the Circulation, 383
Structure of the Human Body, 401
Structure of the Human Brain, 251
Student Manual of Physical Examination, 172
Student Work Manual for Introductory Medical-Surgical Nursing, 195
Studies of Brain Function, 379
Study Guide and Review Manual of Basic Anatomy and Physiology, 208
A Study Guide and Workbook for First Aid and Safety, 194
Study of Nursing Care: Research Project Series, 385
Stylebook/Editorial Manual, 155
Subject Catalog of the Department Library, 7
Subject Catalog of the Library of the New York Academy of Medicine, 7
Subject Directory of Special Libraries and Information Centers, 286
Subject Guide to Government Reference Books, 542

Sudden Infant Death Syndrome: An Annotated Bibliography for the Layman, 37
Sudden Infant Death Syndrome: Selected Annotated Bibliography, 1960–1971, 37
Summary of Grants and Contracts Administered by the National Center for Health Services Research and Development, 287
Supervision in Social Work, 484
Surgery, 528
Surgery Annual, 309
Surgery, Gynecology and Obstetrics, 528
Surgery of the Eyelids and Lacrimal System, 458
Surgery of the Neonate, 273
Surgical Clinics of North America, 528
Surgical Diseases of the Chest, 414
Surgical Gynecological Techniques, 186
Surgical Nutrition, 175
Surgical Pathology, 465
Surgical Treatment of Congenital Heart Disease, 414
Survey of Abstracting Services and Current Bibliographical Tools in Agriculture, Forestry, Fisheries, Nutrition, Veterinary Medicine, and Related Subjects, 500
Swenson's Complete Dentures, 104
The Swine 'Flu Affair, 334
A Syllabus of Medical History, 329
The Symbolic Life: Miscellaneous Writings: The Collected Works of C. G. Jung, 341
Symposia of the Society for Experimental Biology, 548
Symposia on Fundamental Cancer Research. Proceedings, 552
Symposium on Basic Science in Plastic Surgery, 549
Symptoms: The Complete Home Medical Encyclopedia, 54
A Synopsis of Anaesthesia, 403
Synposis of Gynecology, 496
Synopsis of Obstetrics, 496
Synopsis of Surgery, 159
System of Ophthalmology, 56

System of Opthalmology Series, 388
A Systematic Guide to Medical Terminology, 83
Systemic Pathology, 389

Taber's Cyclopedic Medical Dictionary, 82
Take Care of Yourself: A Consumer's Guide to Medical Care, 221
Taking Care of Your Children—A Parent's Guide to Medical Care, 229
TDB [Toxicology Data Bank], 622
Te Linde's Operative Gynecology, 280
The Teaching of Human Sexuality in Schools for Health Professionals, 240
Technical Abstract Bulletin, 537
Technical Aspects of Tomography, 184
Technical Book Review Index, 1
Technical Books in Print: A Reference Catalogue of Books in Print and on Sale in Great Britain, 3
Technical Information Sources: A Guide to Patent Specifications, Standards, and Technical Reports Literature, 569, 579
Technical Literature Search and the Written Report, 155
The Technique of Psychoanalytic Psychotherapy, 482
Techniques in Clinical Immunology, 187
Techniques of Clinical Gastroenterology, 213
Techniques of Medication: A Manual on the Administration of Drug Products, 180
Techniques of Patient Care: A Manual of Bedside Procedures, 174
Technologist Guide to Mammography, 238
A Technology of Health Manpower Utilization: Uniform Measurement and Evaluation, 28
Television and Management: The Manager's Guide to Video, 590
Ten-State Nutrition Survey, 1968–1970, 145

Teratology and Congenital Malformations: A Comprehensive Guide to the Literature, 13
Terminology and Communication Skills in the Health Sciences, 186
Terminology of Communication Disorders: Speech, Language, and Hearing, 88
Text-Atlas of Hematology, 262
A Textbook for Nursing Assistants, 448
Textbook of Endocrinology, 420
Textbook of Geriatric Medicine and Gerontology, 427
Textbook of Medical Physiology, 401
Textbook of Medical-Surgical Nursing, 449
Textbook of Microbiology, 435
A Textbook of Neurology, 408
Textbook of Ophthalmology, 458
Textbook of Orthopaedic Medicine, 461
Textbook of Pediatric Nursing, 449
Textbook of Pediatrics, 472
Textbook of Pulmonary Diseases, 490
Textbook of Radiotherapy, 488
The Thalassaemia Syndromes, 425
Theory and Practice of Histological Techniques, 197
The Theory and Practice of Industrial Pharmacy, 476
Theory of Pharmaceutical Systems, 476
Therapeutic Drug Monitoring, 533
Therapeutics From the Primitives to the 20th Century, 338
Therapeutics in Neurology, 408
Thomas' Register of American Manufacturers and Thomas' Register Catalog File, 287, 583
Three Centuries of Microbiology, 334
Tile and Till, 586
Tissue Culture Abstracts, 513
Tissues and Organs: A Text-Atlas of Scanning Electron Microscopy, 246
TNM Classification of Malignant Tumours, 567
Todd-Sanford Clinical Diagnosis by Laboratory Methods, 221
Topics in Clinical Microbiology, 596

Topics in Hematology, 357
Topics in Therapeutics, 553
Topics on Tropical Neurology, 380
Topley and Wilson's Principles of Bacteriology, Virology and Immunity, 435
Total Management of the Arthritic Patient, 492
Toxic and Hallucinogenic Mushroom Poisoning: A Handbook for Physicians and Mushroom Hunters, 110
Toxic Substances Control Sourcebook, 203
Toxic Substances Sourcebook: The Professional's Guide to the Information Sources, Key Literature and Laws of a Critical New Field, 203
Toxicity Bibliography: A Bibliography Covering Reports of Toxicity Studies, Adverse Drug Reactions, and Poisoning in Man and Animals, 40
Toxicologic Emergencies: A Handbook in Problem Solving, 135
Toxicology Abstracts, 521
Toxicology and Applied Pharmacology, 53
Toxicology Annual, 314
Toxicology of Drugs and Chemicals, 127
Toxicology of the Eye, 458
Toxicology Research Projects Directory, 562
Toxicology: The Basic Science of Poisons, 476
TOXITAPES, 632
TOXLINE [Toxicology Information Online], 622
Tox-tips: Notices of Research Projects, 562
Trace Elements and Iron in Human Metabolism, 451
Traction and Orthopaedic Appliances, 177
Trade Name Dictionary, 76
Trademarks Listed with the Pharmaceutical Manufacturers Association, 68
Traditional Medicine, 22
Training of Medical Laboratory Technicians: A Handbook for Tutors, 96

Transdex/Bibliography and Index to the US Joint Publications Research Services Translations, 554
Translations Register-Index, 554
Translators and Translations; Services and Sources in Science and Technology, 555
Transplantation Proceedings, 549
Trauma in Pregnancy, 496
Trauma Management, 439
Trauma Surgery, 99
Travel Medicine: A Handbook for Practitioners, 114
Travelbee's Intervention in Psychiatric Nursing, 449
Travelers' Guide to U.S.-Certified Doctors Abroad, 207
Travelers to the Tropics—Guidelines for Physicians, 218
The Treatment and Control of Infectious Diseases in Man, 435
Treatment of Cardiac Emergencies, 162
Treatment of Hand Injuries: Preservation and Restoration of Function, 403
Treatment of Heart Disease in the Adult, 211
Treatment of Injuries to Athletes, 478
Treatment of Shock: Principles and Practice, 221
Tredgold's Mental Retardation, 482
Triangle, 586
Triumphs of Medicine, 329
Tropical Diseases: A Handbook for Practitioners, 110
Tropical Diseases Bulletin, 512
Tropical Medicine, 435
Tuberculosis, 490
Tumors in Domestic Animals, 567
Tumors of the Eye, 458
Tumors of the Head and Neck, 455
Tumors of the Kidney, Renal Pelvis, and Ureter, 496
Tumors of the Ovary, 496
Tumours of Childhood: A Clinical Treatise, 473
20,000 Medical Words, 82
Two Centuries of American Medicine 1776–1976, 329

The UFAW Handbook on the Care and Management of Laboratory Animals, 97
Ulrich's International Periodicals Directory, 524
Ulrich's International Periodicals Directory 1977–1978, 525
Ultrasonography of the Eye and Orbit, 458
Ultrasonoscopic Differential Diagnosis in Obstetrics and Gynecology, 280
Ultrastructure of Haemic Cells: A Cytological Atlas of Normal and Leukaemic Blood and Bone Marrow, 262
Understanding Aphasia: A Guide for Medical and Paramedical Professionals, 210
Understanding Arthritis and Rheumatism: A Complete Guide to the Problems and Treatment, 239
Understanding Chemical Patents, 580
Understanding Inherited Disorders, 426
Understanding Medical Terminology, 82
Understanding Piaget, 234
Understanding Research in Nursing, 224
Understanding Scientific Literature: A Bibliometric Approach, 9
The Underwater Handbook: A Guide to Physiology and Performance for the Engineer, 221
Underwater Medicine and Related Sciences: A Guide to the Literature: An Annotated Bibliography, Key Word Index, and Microthesaurus, 32
Undersirable Drug Interactions, 1974–1975, 146
Union Catalog of Medical Periodicals, 632
Union Internationale Centre le Cancer (UICC) Technical Report Series, 539
Union List of Scientific Serials in Canadian Libraries. Catalogue collectif des publications scientifiques dans les bibliothecheques canadiennes, 5
Unique 3-in-1 Research and Development Directory, 561

United Nations Documents Index, 542
The United States Dispensatory, 127
United States Government Manual, 287, 542
Units of Weight and Measure, International (Metric), and US Customary, 140
University College Hospital and Its Medical School: A History, 333
University of London Theses and Dissertations Accepted for Higher Degrees, 557
Unlisted Drugs, 231
The Unseen Minority: A Social History of Blindness in the United States, 337
Upper Extremities Orthotics, 232
Uranium, Plutonium, Transplutonic Elements: Handbook of Experimental Pharmacology, 137
Urban Environments and Human Behavior: An Annotated Bibliography, 45
Urinalysis in Clinical Laboratory Practice, 439
Urologic Clinics of North America, 535
Urologic Surgery: Diagnosis, Techniques and Postoperative Treatment, 280
US Government Research and Development Reports, 538
U.S. Medical Directory, 291
U.S. Nutrition Policies in the Seventies, 451
US Patent Previews, 581
USAN and the USP Dictionary of Drug Names, 68
The Use of Antibiotics: A Comprehensive Review With Clinical Emphasis, 476
The Use of Biological Literature, 11
The Use of Drugs in Psychiatry, 482
Use of Medical Literature: Information Sources for Research and Development, 13
Use of Reports Literature, 538
The User's Guide to Standard Microfiche Formats, 590
The Uterus, 496

The Utilization of Health Services: Indices and Correlates: A Research Bibliography, 1972, 28
Utilization Review: A Selected Bibliography, 1933–1967, 28

Van Nostrand's Scientific Encyclopedia, 54
Vascular Disorders of the Extremities, 56
Vascular Surgery, 403
VD: A Guide for Nurses and Counselors, 224
Venereal Disease Bibliography, 1966–1970, 29
Venom Diseases, 484
Vertical File Index: A Subject and Title Index to Selected Pamphlet Material, 584
VETDOC, 632
The Veterinarian in America 1625–1975, 343
Veterinarians' Product and Therapeutic Reference, 241
The Veterinary Annual, 315
Veterinary Applied Pharmacology and Therapeutics, 497
Veterinary Clinical Parasitology, 186
Veterinary Gastroenterology, 498
Veterinary Multilingual Thesaurus, 67
Veterinary Pathology, 498
Veterinary Pharmacology and Therapeutics, 498
Veterinary Reproduction and Obstetrics, 498
Video in Libraries: A Status Report, 1979–80, 590
The Video Programs Index, 590
The Video Register, 1979–80, 591
The Video Source Book, 591
Videolog: Programs for the Health Sciences, 595
Viewpoints in Biology, 373
Viral and Mycoplasmal Infection of the Respiratory Tract, 491
Viral Infections of Humans, 436
Virology Abstracts, 512
Visible and Palpable Lesions in Children, 229
Vision Index, 515

Visual Aids for Paramedical Vocabulary, 82
Visual Aids Index, 598
Visual Science Information Center Thesaurus, 67
Vital Health Statistics Monographs, 152
Vitamins and Hormones: Advances in Research and Applications, 354
Vitroretinal Disorders: Diagnosis and Management, 458
Vocabulary of Medicine and Related Sciences Principally Containing Terms Not Found in Bilingual and Multilingual Dictionaries, and Terms that May Present Special Problems of Translation: English-French, French-English, 69
Voluntary Social Services: A Handbook of Information and Directory of Organizations, 287
The Volunteer Services Department in a Health Care Institution, 166
Volunteer Services in Mental Health: An Annotated Bibliography, 1955–1969, 45
Volunteers Who Produce Books; Braille, Large Type, Tape, 303
The Vulva, 497

Walter Reed Army Medical Center Television Videotape Catalog, 595
Washington Information Directory, 287
Washington Information Workbook, 291
Washington University Department of Surgery Manual on Techniques of Emergency and Outpatient Surgery, 159
We Call It Bibliotherapy: An Annotated Bibliography on Bibliotherapy and the Adult Hospitalized Patient, 1900–1966, 45
We Want You to Know About Labels on Food, 225
Webster's Medical Speller, 74
Webster's New Collegiate Dictionary, 77

Weekly Government Abstracts, 522, 538
Wellcome Trends in Pharmacy, 586
White Cell Manual, 190
White Sheet; Hospital Pharmacy, 586
WHO Expert Committee on Biological Standardization Report, 571
WHO Handbook for Standardized Cancer Registries, 119
The Whole Pediatrician Catalog, 179
Who's Who in Health Care, 318
Why Not Say It Clearly? A Guide to Scientific Writing, 155
Willard and Spackman's Occupational Therapy, 478
Williams Obstetrics, 497
Wine and the Digestive System; The Effects of Wine and Its Constituents on the Organs and Functions of the Gastrointestinal Tract, 550
Women and Drugs: An Annotated Bibliography, 45
Women and Mental Health: Selected Annotated References 1970–1973, 45
Women in Medicine: A Bibliography of the Literature on Women Physicians, 318
Women in Stress: A Nursing Perspective, 449
A Word-Part Book for Medical Terminology, 82
Words on Aging: A Bibliography of Selected Annotated References Compiled for the Administration on Aging by the Department Library, 26
Work Done in India on Viral and Rickettsial Infections of Vertebrates: A Bibliography, 30
Work Manual For Critical Care Nursing, 196
Workbook for Introductory Medical-Surgical Nursing, 195
Workbook for Pediatric Nurses, 195
Workbook for the Human Body in Health and Disease, 194
Workbook for the Nurses' Aide, 195
A Workbook in Auditory Training for Adults, 197

Workbook in Basic Medical-Surgical Nursing, 196
Workbook in Bedside Maternity Nursing and Answer Key, 196
Workbook of Solutions and Dosage of Drugs: Including Arithmetic, 196
Workbook to Accompany Medicine for the Paramedical Professions, 194
Working with the Elderly: A Training Manual, 165
A World Bibliography of Bibliographies and of Bibliographic Catalogues, Calendars, Abstracts, Digests, Indexes, and the Like, 500
The World Book Illustrated Home Medical Encyclopedia, 54
World Congress of Neurology, Proceedings, 549
World Directory of Collections of Cultures of Microorganisms, 297
World Directory of Environmental Research Centers, 307
World Directory of Schools of Public Health 1971, 307
World Environmental Directory, Volume 2, 1975, 307
World Food and Nutrition Study, 386
The World Food Situation: Problems and Prospects to 1985, 451
A World Geography of Human Diseases, 485
World Guide to Abbreviations of Organizations, 287
World Guide to Scientific Associations/Vernande und Gesellschaften der Wisenschaft: Ein internationales Verzeichnis, 603
World Guide to Technical Information and Documentation Services: Guide Mondial Des Centres de Documentation et d'Information Techniques, 287
World Guide to Trade Associations, 603
World Health, 534
World Health Environmental Surveys, 147
World Health Organization Eighth Revision International Classification of Diseases, Adapted for Use in the United States, 565
World Health Statistics Annual, 149
World Index of Scientific Translations, 555
World List of Forensic Science Laboratories, 300
World List of Scientific Periodicals Published in the Years 1900–1960, 525
World Meetings Outside USA and Canada, 545
World Meetings: United States and Canada, 545
World Patents Index, 582
World Pharmaceutical Directory, 302
World Review of Nutrition and Dietetics, 359
The Worldwide Guide to Medical Electronics Marketing Representation, 297
Wörterbuch der Medizin, 70
Wörterbuch der Neurphysiologie, 70
Wörterbuch der Psychiatrie und Medizinischen Psychologie, 70
WPI, 632
Writer's Guide to Medical Journals, 155
Writing For Nursing Publications, 156
Writing Scientific Papers in English: An ELSE-Ciba Foundation Guide for Authors, 156

Yearbook—American College of Surgeons, 319
Year Book of Anesthesia, 309
Year Book of Cancer, 312
Year Book of Cardiology, 310
Year Book of Cardiovascular Medicine and Surgery, 310
Yearbook of Dentistry, 310
Year Book of Dermatology, 310
Yearbook of Diagnostic Radiology, 315
Year Book of Drug Therapy, 314
Year Book of Endocrinology, 311
Yearbook of Family Practice, 309
Yearbook of International Congress Proceedings: Bibliography of Reports Arising Out of Meetings Held By International Organizations During the Year, 1960–67–, 547
Year Book of Medicine, 312

Yearbook of Neurology and Neurosurgery, 310
Yearbook of Nuclear Medicine, 312
Year Book of Obstetrics and Gynecology, 315
Year Book of Ophthamology, 313
Year Book of Orthopedics and Traumatic Surgery, 313
Year Book of Otolaryngology, 313
Year Book of Pathology and Clinical Pathology, 314
Year Book of Pediatrics, 314
Year Book of Plastic and Reconstructive Surgery, 309
Year Book of Psychiatry and Applied Mental Health, 314
Year Book of Surgery, 310
Yearbook of the American Occupational Therapy Association, 320
Yearbook of Urology, 315
The Year in Hematology, 311

Zinsser Microbiology, 111, 436

AUTHOR INDEX

(Names of individual authors, editors, compilers, translators, etc., and corporate authors)

Abel, Ernest L., 15, 38
Abells, Linda F., 173
Abercrombie, Michael, 75
Abouna, George J. M., 403
Abrahams, Peter, 275
Abrams, Susan, 42
Abramson, David I., 56
Abramson, Harole, 425
Ackerknecht, Erwin H., 328, 338, 341
Ackerman, Lauren V., 465
Ackerman, P., 131
Ackroyd, Ted J., 14
Acri, Michael J., 42
Adams, Catherine F., 145
Adams, George, 214
Adams, J. Crawford, 460
Adams, John C., 227
Adams, Raymond D., 491
Adams, R. L. P., 423
Adamson, Katherine K., 130
Adamson, William C., 130
Aday, Lu Ann, 28
Adler, Gerhard, 339
Adrich, Marian K., 597
Aegerter, Ernest E., 460
Aerospace Medical Association, 613
Affonso, Dyanne D., 440
af Geijerstam, Gunnar, 50
Afifi, Adel K., 269
Afshar, F., 251
Aguilera, Donna, 448
Ahmed, Ali, 270
Ainsworth, Geoffrey C., 85
Ajami, Alfred M. Jr., 38
Akademiia nauk Azerbaidzhanskoi SSR, 70
Akey, Denise, 284
Aladjem, Silvio, 447, 467
Albert, Daniel M., 458
Albert, Joseph S., 103
Albert, Martin L., 406
Al-Doory, Yousef, 433

Alerting Service, Viral Oncology Branch, US National Cancer Institute, 35
Alexander, Franz G., 340
Alexander, Stewart F., 181
Alfaro, Julian H., 216
Allen, Howard N., 251
Allen, Hugh D., 122
Allen, Marshall B., 161
Alpert, Joseph S., 162
Alpiner, Jerome G., 127
Alsever, Robert N., 104
Alter, M., 416
Altman, Isidore, 27
Altman, N. H., 139
Altman, Philip L., 97, 105, 114, 120, 133, 137, 141
Alton, G. G., 191
Altschul, Annie T., 447
Altschule, Mark D., 203
Ambrose, E. J., 451
American Academy for Cerebral Palsy, 611
American Academy of Allergy, 605
American Academy of Dermatology, 606
American Academy of Facial Plastic and Reconstructive Surgery, 605
American Academy of Family Physicians, 603
American Academy of Neurology, 606
American Academy of Nursing, 608
American Academy of Ophthalmology and Otolaryngology, 610
American Academy of Orthopaedic Surgeons, 267, 598
American Academy of Pediatrics, 610
American Association for the Advancement of Science, 590, 604
American Association of Anatomists, 294
American Association of Blood Banks, 608
American Association of Critical Care Nurses, 608
American Association of Dental Colleges, 587

American Association of Medical Assistants, 604
American Association of Neurological Surgeons, 509
American Association of Occupational Health Nursing, 608
American Association on Mental Deficiency, 611
American Burn Association, 608
American Cancer Society, 609
American Chemical Society, 154, 292, 366, 502, 604
American Chiropractic Association, 613
American Cleft Palate Association, 25
American College of Cardiology, 606
American College of Hospital Administration, 607
American College of Obstetricians and Gynecologists, 613
American College of Physicians, 297, 594
American College of Radiology, 307, 612
American College of Surgeons, 596, 605
American Council of Otolaryngology, 010
American Dental Association, 211, 294, 509, 596, 606
American Diabetes Association, 606
American Dietetic Association, 609
America Digestive Disease Society, 607
American Foundation for the Blind, 232, 302, 611
American Gastroenterological Association, 607
American Geriatrics Society, 607
American Heart Association, 32, 210, 572, 606
American Hospital Association, 6, 152, 166, 215, 216, 217, 232, 512, 538, 570, 596, 607
American Institute of Biological Sciences (AIBS), 604
American Joint Committee for Cancer Staging and End-Results Reporting, 196
American Journal of Nursing, 223, 514, 563
American Journal of Nursing Company, 7, 597
American Lung Association, 612
American Medical Association, 78, 155, 179, 288, 292, 293, 294, 320, 508, 594, 595, 604
American Medical Students Association, 604
American National Red Cross, 111
American National Standards Institute, 537, 568
American Nurses Association, 298, 551, 597, 609
American Occupational Medical Association, 612
American Optometric Association, 610
American Osteopathic Association, 613
American Pharmaceutical Association, 68, 202, 301, 610
American Physical Therapy Association, 611
American Physiological Society, 104, 348, 376
American Psychiatric Association, 64, 611
American Psychological Association, 320
American Public Health Association, 47, 152, 612
American Rheumatism Association, 612
American Rheumatism Association Section of the Arthritis Foundation, 521
American Society for Laboratory Animal Care, 613
American Society for Surgery of the Hand, 23
American Society for Testing and Materials, 525, 568, 570
American Society of Abdominal Surgery, 605
American Society of Anesthesiologists, 22, 605
American Society of Clinical Pathologists, 610
American Society of Clinical Pathology, 178
American Society of Cytology, 609
American Society of Electroencephalographic Technologists, 606

AUTHOR INDEX

American Society of Hospital Pharmacists, 610
American Society of Nurse Anesthetists, 609
American Society of Plastic and Reconstructive Surgeons, 23, 605
American Type Culture Collection, 147
American Veterinary Medical Association, 613
Amerine, M. A., 450
Ames, Sue A., 198
Anderson, Alice J., 27
Anderson, Carl E., 175
Anderson, Charles B., 159
Anderson, C. L., 484
Anderson, Charlotte M., 184, 469
Anderson, Ellen M., 196
Anderson, Ferguson, 427
Anderson, Helen C., 444
Anderson, I. G., 601
Anderson, James E., 245
Anderson, Maja C., 439
Anderson, Marilyn J., 22
Anderson, Miles H., 232
Anderson, Neil V., 498
Anderson, Norma J., 195
Anderson, Paul D., 187
Anderson, Philip O., 124
Anderson, Ronald G., 143
Anderson, William A. D., 463
Andrade, Rafael, 254, 416
Andreoli, Kathleen, 115
Andrews, J. T., 454
Andrews, Peter M., 272
Andrews, Theodora, 27, 41
Andriot, John, 148, 540, 541
Andrulis, Richard S., 128
Angell, Marcia, 462
Anlyan, William G., 396
Annan, Gertrude L., 95
Annas, George J., 217
Appelbe, G. E., 231
Aranda, Paul, 44
Archer, W. Harry, 319
Archuleta, Alyce J., 37
Archuleta, Michael J., 37
Arena, Jay M., 467
Arieti, Silvano, 128
Armed Forces Institute of Pathology, 264

Armengol, Joseph, 205
Armstrong, Margaret E., 115
Armstrong, Marsha F., 124
Aronson, Carl E., 138
Aroskar, Mila A., 442
Arthur, Geoffrey H., 498
Artz, Curtis P., 209
Asbell, M. B., 331
Ash, Joan, 289, 593
Ash, Lawrence R., 190
Asimov, Issac, 316
Asperheim, Mary K., 116, 447
Assali, Nicholas S., 393
Association for Education of the Visually Handicapped, 611
Association for the Advancement of Medical Instrumentation, 604
Association of American Medical Colleges, 19, 292, 293, 587
Association of University Professors of Ophthalmology, 226
Atassi, M. Z., 399
Atkinson, R. S., 403
Audio-Visual Association, 588
Auger, Charles P., 538
Aurelia, Joseph C., 160
Ausband, John R., 228
Austen, D. E. G., 189
Austin, Anne L., 336
Austin, George, 407
Austin, Glenn, 178
Austin, Robert B., 324
Austin, Winifred K., 47
Avery, Gordon B., 469
Axelrod, S. J., 142
Ayala, Luis A., 165
Ayd, Frank J., Jr., 397
Aydelotte, Myrtle K., 15
Ayers, Donald M., 74

Babson, S. Gorham, 228
Babyak, Mary A., 48
Bach, Fritz H., 375
Bacon, George E., 228
Baddely, Hiram, 258
Bagshawe, K. D., 454
Bahmanyar, M., 183
Bahn, Anita K., 395
Bahr, Alice H., 589, 590
Baikie, Albert G., 454

Bailey, David, 194
Bailey, Hamilton, 320
Bailey, J. D., 228
Bainbridge, J., 166
Bakalar, James B., 473
Baker, A. B., 378
Balis, George U., 391
Ballabriga, Angel, 270
Ballantyne, John, 388
Ballenger, John J., 461
Ballinger, Walter F., 401
Balows, A., 432
Bancroft, John D., 197
Bander, Edward J., 81
Bandmann, H. J., 207
Banes, Daniel, 229
Banner, E. A., 522
Bannerman, R. H. O., 240
Bannister, Roger, 404
Barabas, Andras, 206
Baranski, Stanislaw, 47
Barchas, Jack D., 481
Bargmann, W., 97
Barker, Kathleen, 27
Barker, W. F., 413
Barman, Thomas E., 94, 95
Barnard, Robin O., 249
Barnes, C. D., 112
Barnes, I. J., 192
Baro, F., 23
Barraclough, Brian, 482
Barratt, T. Martin, 470
Barron, D. N., 438
Barrow, Mark V., 48
Bart, Robert S., 254
Barton, David, 235
Barton, Roger E., 415
Barton, Walter E., 338
Basler, Beatrice K., 12
Basler, Thomas G., 12
Basmajian, John V., 99, 401
Bass, G. E., 231
Bassett, David L., 595
Bate, John, 79
Batey, Marjorie V., 441, 551
Batsakis, John G., 455
Battifora, Hector, 455
Baum, Gerald L., 490
Baumel, Howard, 323
Beacham, Daniel W., 496

Beacham, Woodard D., 496
Beard, Crowell, 176
Beard, Robert J., 240
Beaton, George H., 386
Beaver, Paul C., 497
Beck, K., 279
Beck, William S., 430
Becker, Frederick F., 386, 422
Becker, Joseph, 479
Becker, R. P., 389
Beckett, A. H., 474
Beckwith, J., 412
Beckwith, J. Bruce, 496
Becler, R. D., 233
Beeson, Paul B., 436
Begleiter, Henri, 391
Behnke, J. A., 426
Behrmann, Elmer H., 302
Beland, Irene L., 440
Bell, Alan P., 43
Bell, Ann, 431
Bell, Eleanor J., 217
Bell, Gwen, 45
Bell, J. M., 163
Bell, Whitfield J., Jr., 335
Bellack, Leopold, 106
Bellet, Samuel, 410
Belsjoe, Edith H., 195
Benchimol, A., 211
Bender, Arnold E., 87
Bender, Leonard F., 477
Beneson, Abram S., 482
Benirschke, Kurt, 258
Bennett, A. M. Hastin, 55, 56
Bennett, Donald R., 248
Bennett, Richard G., 212
Bennington, James L., 496
Bennion, Elisabeth, 334
Benson, Douglas C., 312
Berci, George, 421
Berendes, H. W., 475
Berger, Karen J., 220
Bergerson, Betty S., 116, 447
Bergleiter, Rudolf, 277
Bergman, Ronald A., 269
Bergmann, Martin S., 203
Bergsma, Daniel, 259, 295
Berk, Robert N., 423
Berkovitz, B. K. B., 253
Berkow, Robert, 171

AUTHOR INDEX

Berlin, Irving N., 41
Bernat, I., 430
Berner, P., 553
Bernero, Jacqueline R., 148, 328
Bernstein, Theodore M., 154
Bertles, John F., 425
Besch, P. K., 193
Besharov, Douglas J., 233
Bessis, Marcel, 261
Besterman, Theodore, 18
Beswick, T. S. L., 432
Bettman, Otto L., 328
Bevis, Olivia E., 441
Beyer, Charles K., 458
Bhasker, S. N., 253
Bhat, Pachalla K., 274
Biass-Ducroux, Francoise, 72
Bibliographic Retrieval Service (BRS), 623
Bick, Edgar M., 459
Bigler, Helen F., 448
Bikales, N. M., 563
Biloon, Frank, 166
Bineen, J. J., 437
The Bio-Energy Council, 288
Birkner, Rudolf, 277
Birnbaum, Roger W., 215
Birnstingl, Martin, 162
Birren, James E., 106
Birzle, Hermann, 277
Bishop, W. J., 320
Bittar, E. Edward, 390
Bittar, Neville, 390
Black, John, 57
Blackwood, W., 406
Blades, Brian, 414
Blake, John B., 12
Blazevic, Donna J., 192
Bleck, Eugene E., 273
Bleier, Inge J., 196
Blessum, William T., 78
Bliss, Ann A., 201
Bliss, Virginia J., 195
Block, Matthew H., 262
Bloom, Barbara I., 27
Bloom, Bernard L., 339
Bloom, H. J. G., 466
Bloomquist, Harold, 215
Bockus, Henry L., 213
Bodmer, W. F., 424

Boggs, Dane R., 190
Bolander, Donald O., 74
Bolding, A. M., 192
Bomse, Marguerite D., 216
Bondy, Philip K., 418
Bonica, John J., 407
Bonner, Charles D., 214
Bonneville, Mary A., 462
Boomer, Donald S., 340
Boone, Donna C., 429
Boorer, D. R., 36
Bordley, James III, 329
Boretos, John W., 214
Borgaonkar, D. S., 550
Borgstrom, George, 451
Boring, Edwin G., 341
Borman, Joseph B., 414
Boshes, Louis D., 99
Bosma, James F., 273
Bossart, Jane K., 290, 602
Bostock, D. E., 280
The Boston Children's Medical Center, 57
Bottle, R. T., 11
Bouchard, Rosemary E., 173
Boucher, Carl O., 84, 104
Bouchier, Ian A., 423
Bourne, Geoffrey H., 388, 392
Bourne, Peter G., 168
Bouthilet, Lorraine, 340
Bower, E. Olivia, 442
Bower, Fay L., 442
Bowlby, John, 390
Boyce, Henry W., Jr., 213
Boyd, J. D., 400, 401
Boyd, R. J., 439
Boyd, William, 437
Boyer, Paul, 382
Boyle, A. C., 278
Bracegirdle, Brian, 268, 337
Bradbury, M., 404
Brady, Allen J., 412
Branca, Patricia, 335
Branch, Marie F., 448
Brand, William N., 455
Brander, G. C., 497
Branson, Roy, 428
Brashear, H. Robert, 120
Braun, Robert J., 163
Braunwald, Eugene, 412

Braverman, Irwin M., 417
Brazier, Mary A. B., 160, 405
Breathnach, A. S., 254
Bredow, Miriam, 95
Breen, James L., 278
Brehm, Sharon S., 233
Brenner, Barry M., 392
Bricklin, Mark, 54
Brink, Pamela J., 221
Brinkhous, K. M., 109
Brinkman, Charles R., 393
British Institute of Radiology, 230
British Journal of Surgery, 329
Brobeck, John R., 436
Brociner, Grace E., 555
Brocklehurst, John C., 427
Brodman, Estelle, 324
Brodsky, Isadore, 452
Brook, C. G. D., 179
Brookes, Brian, 295
Brooks, Shirley M., 442
Brooks, Stewart M., 144, 222
Brown, Audrey K., 447, 467
Brown Barbara B., 23, 129
Brown, B. W., 398
Brown, J. A. C., 55, 56
Brown, Joseph F., 88
Brown, Marie S., 172
Brown, Mollie, 448
Brown, Montague, 428
Brown, Myra G., 162
Brown, Myrtle I., 32
Brown, Paul B., 99
Brown, R. J. K., 471
Brownlee, Ann T., 235
Bruch, Hilde, 225, 449
Bruinsma, W., 230
Brunner, Lillian S., 158, 172, 449
Bruton, J. W., 263
Bruyn, G. W., 23, 100
Bruyn, Henry B., 122
Bryson, Carolyn Q., 43
Buchanan, Barbara B., 174
Buchanan, F. H., 132
Buchanan, Robert E., 190, 206
Buchanan, William W., 540
Buchsbaum, Herbert J., 496
Buckerly, James, 135
Bucksch, Herbert, 69
Buckton, K. E., 189, 213

Bujdoso, E., 140
Bull, T. R., 268
Bullough, Bonnie, 335
Bullough, Vern W., 324, 335
Bunce, Donald F. M. II, 268
Bunyan, John A., 589, 590
Burchsted, C. A., 135
Burgen, A. S. V., 474
Burgess, Ann Wobert, 443
Burghardt, Erich, 393
Burhenne, H. Joachim, 485
Burian, Frantisek, 247
Burke, Carroll N., 170, 191
Burke, J. F., 439
Burke, Valerie, 469
Burkhalter, Pamela K., 442, 445
Burkhardt, Dietrich, 70
Burkhardt, Rolf, 260
Burnstock, G., 267
Burrage, Walter L., 319
Burrell, Lenette O., 443
Burrell, Zeb L., Jr., 443
Burrow, Gerard N., 468
Burrows, S. J., 216
Burrows, William, 435
Burton, Benjamin T., 118
Burton, J,. 240
Busch, Harris, 387
Bushe, K. A. 472
Bushong, S. C., 198
Busse, Ewald W., 478, 480
Butler, Robert N., 478
Butt, W. R., 419
Butterworth, Thomas, 164
Buttress, F. A., 287
Byrne, Marjorie, 443

Cady, Blake, 175
Caen, J. P., 431
Cahill, Kevin M., 110
Cain, H. D., 219
Caldwell, Eva Wilson, 444
Caldwell, Linton K., 21
Calman, Carl H., 260
Calnan, C. D., 255
Calnan, James, 206
Calne, Donald B., 408
Calvert, Robert Peyton, 579
Cameron, D. C., 182
Camp, J., 325

Campbell, A. C., 163
Campbell, Claire 173
Campbell, E. J. M., 490
Campbell, G. R., 267
Campbell, Patty, 51
Campbell, Robert J., 91
Camps, F. E., 465
Canada, National Science Library, Ottawa 5, 524
Cantlin, Vernita, 158
Cantor, Marjorie M., 573
Cape, Barbara F., 86
Capell, Peter T., 172
Capital Systems Group for the Office of Science Information Service, 10
Caplan, Ronald M., 492
Capron, Alexander M., 396
Carden, Terence S., Jr., 209
Carlin, Harriette L., 74
Carnegie Library of Pittsburgh and Maurice and Laura Falk Library of the Health Professions, University of Pittsburgh, 1
Carr, K. E., 257
Carroll, Anstice, 88
Carstensen, J. Thuro, 476
Carter, G. B., 91
Carter, S. J., 474
Carterette, Edward C., 131
Cartwright, Frederick F., 342
Casale, Joan T., 33
Casarett, Louis J., 476
Case, David B., 172
Case Western Reserve University, 597
Cash, Joan E., 409
Cassan, Stanley M., 239
Cassem, Ned H., 131
Castiglioni, Arturo, 326
Catholic Hospital Association, 607
Catholic University of America, 558
Catron, Donald G., 98
Cavalli-Sforza, L. L., 424
Cavanaugh, D. C., 183
Cave, E. F., 439
Cawley, J. C., 262
Cazalas, Mary W., 445
Center for Disease Control, 145
Central Office Library, US Veterans Administration, 3
Chaff, Sandra L., 318

Chahinian, A. Philippe, 489
Chait, Arnold, 488
Chamberlain, Amparo, 181
Chance, Graham W., 471
Chandler, G., 10
Chandra, R. K., 450
Chapchal, G. Luzern, 377
Chapiro, A., 485
Chapman, Carleton B., 31
Chase, Robert A., 266
Chaskar, Norma L., 446
Chasler, Charles N., 272
Chater, Shirley, 224
Chatoff, Benjamin, 49
Chatterjee, S. N., 185
Chatton, Milton J., 12, 113, 436
Chen, Ching-chih, 1, 11, 13
Cheng, Thomas C., 434
Chereseavich, Gertrude D., 448
Chernick, Victor, 467
Cherubin, Charles E., 235
Chiang, Chin L., 141
Chicago Dietetic Association and South Suburban Dietetic Association of Chicago, 175
Chicago Institute for Psychoanalysis, 314
The Children's Hospital Medical Center, 229
Chilgren, Richard A., 128
Chinn, Peggy I., 440
Chisholm, Geoffrey D., 393
Chisholm, Margaret, 589
Chiswell, B., 140
Chiu, Lee C., 274
Chou, Te-Chuan, 410
Chrispin, A., 389
Christoffersen, Per, 257
Christopherson, W. M., 566
Chrusciel, M., 40
Chrusciel, T. L., 40
Churchill-Davidson, H. C., 159
Ciancutti, Arthur R., 112
Cibis, Gerhard W., 265
City University of New York, Herbert H. Lehman College, Department of Nursing, 223
Ciufo, Sandra, 42
Clain, Allan, 402
Clapp, Jane, 21

Clark, Ann, 440
Clark, A. W. 20
Clark, Gerald R., 339
Clark, George, 197
Clark, Randolph L., 52, 312
Clark, Richard R., 596
Clark, Ronald G., 405
Clarke, D. B., 410
Clarke, Edwin, 330
Classen, M., 256
Claudio, Virginia S., 88
Clawson, D. Kay, 176
Clayton, Bruce D., 125
Clayton, Florence E., 236, 484
Clayton, George D., 236, 484
Clayton, J. M., 231
Clegg, J. B., 425
Clemente, Carmine D., 242
Clemett, Arthur R., 423
Clemmens, Raymond L., 129
Cline, Martin J., 452
Cloudsley-Thompson, J. L., 341
Cluff, Leighton E., 433
Clyde, David F., 435
Clynes, Manfred, 375
Cnumas, Sophie, 570
Cobb, Marguerite, 115
Cockburn, Forrester, 409
Cohen, Alan S., 198
Cohen, Annabelle, 97
Cohen, Eva D., 201
Cohen, Jack S., 332
Cohen, Lilly, 295
Cohen, Myles J., 245
Cohen, Stanley N., 124
Cohn, Helen, 173
Colby, Robert A., 253
Cole, Theodore M., 128
Cole, Warren H., 453
Coleman, D. Jackson, 458
Coleman, Frances, 83
Colgate, Craig, Jr., 602
Colitz, Karen, 34
Collen, M. F., 428
Collin, Mary A., 186, 208
Collins, R. Douglas, 193
Collins, Vincent J., 55
Collis, J. Leigh, 410
Collison, Robert L., 69
Collocott, Thomas C., 75

Colowick, Sidney P., 382
Colwill, John C., 267
Commission of the European Communities Directorate-General for Research, Science and Education, 67
Commission on Professional and Hospital Activities, 565, 566
Committee for the Study of Inborn Errors of Metabolism, US National Research Council, 424
Committee on Control of Surgical Infections and the Committee on Pre- and Postoperative Care, American College of Surgeons, 159, 168
Committee on International Relations, National Research Council, 386
Committee on Maternal Nutrition, US Maternal and Child Health Service, National Research Council, 33
Committee on Nutrition of the Mother and Preschool Child, Food and Nutrition Board, US National Research Council, 144, 574
Committee on Pre- and Post-operative Care, American College of Surgeons, 175
Committee on Professional Education, 176
Committee on School Health, American Academy of Pediatrics, 220
Committee on Trauma, American College of Surgeons, 436
Commonwealth Bureau of Animal Nutrition, 515
Compere, Edward L., 120
Compston, N., 438
Concordia, Sister Mary, OSF, 3
Condon, Robert E., 158
Cone, Thomas E., Jr., 178
Conn, Hadley L., Jr., 409
Conn, Howard F., 169
Conner, Christopher S., 180
Considine, Douglas M., 54
The Consortium of University Film Centers, 588
Constant, Jules, 161
Constantine, Larry L., 130
Conte, Sylvester B., 137
Converse, John M., 402
Conway, Barbara L., 440, 447

Conway, Neville, 251
Cooke, Edward I., 65, 76
Cooke, Richard W. I., 65, 76
Cooke, Robert E., 470
Cooley, Denton A., 414
Coombs, R. R, 399
Coons, Callie M., 35
Cooper, George E., 143
Cooper, Peter, 145
Cooper, R., 405
Cooper, Steven J., 183
Cooper, W. Conrad, 7
Copass, Michael K., 170
Cope, David, 92
Cope, Zachary, 421
Copeland, Keith, 231
Copenhaver, W. M., 462
Copley, M. A. H., 103
Coppen, A., 481
Coran, Arnold C., 273
Corcoran, John W., 390
Corday, Eliot, 413
Coresellis, J. A. N., 406
Corney, Gerald, 493
Cosgriff, James H., Jr., 274
Cosminsky, Sheila, 22
Costrini, Nicholas V., 170
Cotes, J. E., 489
Cotran, Ramzi S., 463
Cottral, George E., 199
Council of Biology Editors, Committee on Form and Style, 154
Council of Europe, 580
Council on Medical Education, American Medical Association, 291, 292
Council on Medical Education and Hospitals, 292
Council on Research and Bibliography, 44
Council on Voluntary Health Agencies, American Medical Association, 288
Coursin, David B., 175
Courtial, Donald, 180
Cowan, S. T., 85, 190
Cozzetto, Frank J., 470
Craig, W. S., 332
Craigmyle, M. B. L., 271
Cralley, Lester V., 483
Crammer, John, 482

Crane, Chilton, 261
Cranley, Mecca S., 446
Crawford, Annie L., 174
Crawford, G. N. C., 66
Crawford, J. Selwyn, 98
Crawford, Susan, 288
Creighton, Helen, 222
Creswell, William H., 484
Crimmins, James C., 589, 590
Critchley, Macdonald, 77
Crofton, John, 490
Cromwell, Leslie, 395
Cromwell, Phyllis E., 45
Cromwell, R., 480
Cronberg, S., 431
Cross, Frank L., Jr., 135
Crowder, Anne S., 218
Crowe, Barry, 63
Crowley, Ellen T., 63, 76
Cruickshank, Bruce, 260
Cryer, Philip E., 104
Csaky, T. Z., 123
Cullinan, John E., 237
Cumley, Russell W., 52, 312
Cunningham, P. J., 79
Cunningham, Robert M., Jr., 215, 428
Curran, R. C., 271
Curran, William J., 324
Curry, Stephen H., 474
Curth, Helen O., 255
Curth, William 255
Custer, R. Philip, 260
Cryiax, J., 461
Czerski, Przemyslaw, 47

da Luz, P. L., 170
Daggett, P. R., 216
The Dahlgren Memorial Library, Georgetown University, 32
Dale, J. R., 231
Dandurand, Gary, 288
Daniel, William A., Jr., 465
Daniels, Lucille, 177
Daniels, Troy E., 103
Darby, W. J., 336
D'Arcy, P. F., 170
Davenport, H. W., 394
Davidorf, Frederick H., 265
Davidsohn, Israel, 221
Davidson, Henry A., 154

Davidson, John K., 213
Davies, G. N., 414
Davis, Anne J., 442
Davis, Lenwood G., 44
Davison, A. N., 406
Davson, Hugh, 387, 456
Dawson, A. M., 438
Dawson, David M. 350
Dawson, R. M. C., 142
Day, Stacy B., 375
Dayhoff, M. O., 259
DeAngelis, Catherine, 466
DeArmond, Stephen J., 251
Dearth, Florean, 163
Deason, Hilary J., 3
Deaton, John G., 95
DeBakey, Lois, 155, 525
Deblock, Nic J. I., 72
DeCastro, Fernando, 223
DeCoursey, Russell M., 187
Deegan, Arthur X., 215
DeGowin, Elmer L., 169
de Goyet, C. de Ville, 225
DeGroot, Leslie J., 418
DeGrouchy, Jean, 259
Deichman, C. S., 165
Deichmann, William B., 127
Delacretaz, Jean, 263
Delagi, E. F., 227
Delamore, I. W., 430
de la Motte, Ingrid, 70
Del Guercio, Louis R. M., 171
Delk, James H., 88
Deloughery, Grace L., 335
DeLuca, H. F., 117
del Regato, J. A., 452
del Signore, Giovanni, 88
Delworth, Ursula, 107
DeMause, Lloyd, 339
Demis, D. Joseph, 381
Demling, L., 256, 257
Demone, Harold W., Jr., 108
D'Encarnacao, Pat, 37
D'Encarnacao, Paul, 37
Denk, R., 416
Dennis, Robert L., 94
Denny-Brown, Derek, 330
Department for Nursing Education, 384
Department of Baccalaureate and Higher Degree Programs, National League for Nursing, 298
Deskins, Barbara B., 224
Desnos, Ernest, 343
DeSola, Ralph, 63
Deson, Norma, 172
Deutsch, Albert, 59
de Vlieger, M., 136
deVryer, F., 34
Dewey, Maynard M., 251
Dewhurst, Kenneth, 330
Diamanti, Joyce, 235
Diaz, Julio, 380
Dibos, Pablo E., 264
Dickason, Elizabeth J., 443
Dickerson, Robert C., 267
Dickey, Richard P., 240
Diers, Donna, 447
Dietary Allowances Committee & Nutrition Board, US National Academy of Sciences, 118
Dietary Staff of Vanderbilt University Hospital, 174
Diethelm, Oskar, 340
di Fiore, Mariano S. H., 269
Diggs, L. W., 431
Dillon, Daniel C., 195
Dillon, Richard S., 101
DiMascio, Albert, 123
DiMascio, Alberto, 58
Dinnage, Rosemary, 40
Dirckx, John H., 205
Dittert, Lewis W., 476
Dittmer, Dorothy S., 97, 105, 109, 133, 137, 141
Division for the Blind and Physically Handicapped, US Library of Congress, 303
Division of Air Pollution, US Public Health Service, 46
Division of Medical Sciences, US National Research Council, 480
Dixon, Allan S. J., 239
Doby, T., 410
Dobzhansky, T., 396
doCarmo, Pamela B., 169
Dock, Lavinia L., 336
Documentation Center, Food and Agriculture Organization of the United Nations, 34

AUTHOR INDEX

Dodds, T. C. 260, 263
Doerr, Wilheim, 270
Doig, Alison G. 148
Dolan, A. M. 215
Dolan, Josephine A., 336
Dolan, Rosemary, 45
Dolyak, Frank, 188
Domaniewska-Sobczak, Kazimiera, 430
Donabedian, A., 142
Donaldson, David D., 265
Donath, Tibor, 66
Donnison, Jean, 343
Donohue, Joseph, 9
Donovan Joan E., 195
Doona, Mary E., 449
Dorland, William A. N., 80
Doucet, Wills, 194
Dougherty, Cary M., 493
Doughty, Dorothy B., 445
Douglas, Andrew, 490
Doull, John, 476
Down, Morgan D., 307
Downer, Ann H., 232
Downer, G. C., 212
Downey, John A., 476
Downs, Florence S., 201, 443
Doyle, Jean M., 94
Doyle, Timothy C., 143
Drakontides, Anna B., 98, 187
Dreisback, Robert H., 134
Drew, L. R. H., 132
Dreyer, Sharon O., 194
Drillien, Cecil M., 469
Droz, R., 235
Drummond, Constance, 102
Duane, Thomas, 387
Dubiny, Mary J., 87
Dubois, Edmund L., 431
Dubos, Rene J., 432
Ducel, Georges, 263
Dudley, H. A. F., 208, 402
Duffy, John, 326
Du Gas, Beverly W., 443
Duker, P., 376
Duke-Elder, Sir Stewart, 56, 388, 457
Dunbar, Claire F., 444
Dunbar, Helen F., 43
Duncan, A. S., 78
Duncan, Helen A., 86
Dunham, Charles S., 127

Dunham, Jerome R., 127
Dunkerley, Gary B., 249
Dunlap, Alice, 14
Dunning, James M., 415
Dunstan, G. R., 78
Duplan, J. F., 485
Dupuis, R., 218
Duranteau, Andre, 69
Durbin, Richard L., 429
Durgin, Jane M., 180
Durizch, M. L., 184
Durling, Richard J., 323
Durrenberger, Robert W., 91
Duterloo, Herman S., 253
Duthie, Robert B., 460
Dybwad, Rosemary F., 303
Dyck, Arthur J., 324
Dyer, Marilyn, 172

Eales, Nellie B., 323
Early, Lawrence E., 423
Eastham, R. D., 55, 109, 219
Eastin, Roy B., 540
Easton, Allan, 107
Eaton, S. Boyd, Jr., 487
Ebert, Myrl, 12
Eck, R. V., 259
Eckenhoff, James E., 309
Eckert, Charles, 113
Eckert, William G., 374
Edeiken, Jack, 487
Edelmann, C. M., Jr., 469
Ederer, Grace M., 192
Edgar, Irving I., 328
Edis, Anthony Jr., 165
Editorial Operations Branch, US National Institutes of Health, 542
Editors of Communications Research Machines, Inc., 44
Education Council for Foreign Medical Graduates, 95
Efron, Daniel H., 182
Egan, Robert L., 238
Egdahl, Richard H., 165
Ehrlich, Ann, 80
Ehrlich, George E., 492
Eichhorn, Robert, 28
Eide, Imogene, 107
Eidelberg, Lawrence, 593, 595
Eidelberg, Ludwig, 59

Eisen, Herman N., 399
Eisenberg, Mickey S., 170
Eisenhauer, Laurel A., 116, 447
Eisner, Gilbert M., 81
Elhart, Dorothy, 448
Eli Lilly & Company, 583
Eliseenkov, U. B., 71
Ellestad, Myrvin H., 220
Elliot, Alfred M., 206
Ellis, Albert, 51
Ellis, Gwynn P., 39
Ellis, Michael D., 483
Ellis, Phillip P., 457
Elster, K., 258
Eltherington, L. G., 112
Emery, Alan E. H., 424
Emmanouilides, George C., 211
Emmett, John L., 279
Emmons, Chester W., 400
Eng, Evelyn, 132
Ennis, Bernice, 15
Ensminger, M. Eugene, 497
Entomological Society of America, 520
Environmental Mutagen Information Center, 16
Epstein, Bernard S., 250
Epstein, E., 417
Epstein, E., Jr., 417
Epstein, M. A., 363
Epstein, Samuel S., 391
Ernest, J. T., 457
Esch, Dortha, 196
Escourolle, Raymond, 160
Eshom, Myreta, 154
Estrin, Norman F., 66
Etter, Lewis E., 92
Evans, Alfred S., 436
Evans, Anthony, 79
Evans, H. J., 189, 213
Even-Odem, Joseph, 70
Ewe, Klaus, 256
Excerpta Medica Foundation, 4
Executive Office of the President, Office of Management and Budget, 148
Eyanson, Paul F., 59
Eyseneck, Hans J., 60

Fahlberg, Willson J., 108
Fairbank, T. J., 267
Falconer, Mary W., 115
Falkner, F., 552
Fanger, Herbert, 220
Farberow, Norman L., 41
Farrell, Jane, 222
Farrer-Brown, Geoffrey, 252
Farzan, Sattar, 137
Fasman, Gerald D., 95
Faust, Ernest C., 110, 433, 497
Favazzo, A. R., 232
Fazzini, E. P., 177
Federal Advisory Council on Medical Training Aids. US National Library of Medicine, 595
Federation of American Societies for Experimental Biology, 548, 604
Federman, D. D., 438
Feher, I., 140
Feigenbaum, Harvey, 411
Feinberg, Barry N., 95
Feinbloom, Richard I., 57
Feiring, Emanuel H., 404
Feldman, Elaine B., 450
Feller, Irving, 31
Felner, Joel M., 252
Felson, Benjamin, 488
Felter, Jacqueline W., 95
Felter, Mark E., 33
Feman, Stephen S., 119
Feneis, Heinz, 245
Fenner, F., 66
Ferguson, Albert B., Jr., 460, 469
Fermaglich, Joseph L., 101
Fernback, Donald J., 466
Ferris, Thomas F., 468
Ferrucci, Joseph T., 487
Fields, Willa L., 220
Figge, Frank H. J., 243
Finch, Bernard E., 216
Finch, Caleb E., 426
Finch, Clement A., 190
Fine, Ben S., 266
Fine, Stuart, 597
Fineberg, H. V., 334
Finegold, Sidney M., 432
Finegold, Wilfred J., 492
Finkelstein, Jerry A., 122
Finnegan, Janet A., 223
Fiorentino, Mary R., 161
Fishbein, Morris, 155

AUTHOR INDEX

Fisher, Alexander A., 254
Fisher, Harold W., 259
Fisher, Harry J., 118
Fisher, Ronald Aylmer, 152
Fisher, Russell S., 229
Fitch, Grace E., 87, 172
Fitz, Charles R., 469
Fleming, David G., 95
Fleming, Juanita W., 443
Fletcher, Charles, 342
Fletcher, Gilbert H., 488
Flexner, Abraham, 325
Flint, T. J., 219
Florey, Lord, 462
Florkin, Marcel, 374
Floyd, Mary K., 46, 50
Fogle, C., 290
Folgueras, Luis E., 597
Fomon, Samuel J., 450
Fontana, Vincent J., 233
Food and Agriculture Organization of the United Nations, 33, 34, 175, 315
Food and Nutrition Information and Educational Materials Center, National Agricultural Library, 34
Ford, Donald H., 99
Ford, Frank R., 467
Fordham, Michael, 339
Fordney, Marilyn T., 108
Fordtran, John S., 422
Forensic Science Society, 300
Forgacs, Paul, 489
Forman, Robert A., 64
Fortuine, Robert, 48
Foster, J. B., 438
Foucault, Michael, 334
Fowler, Jenifer E. H., 84
Fowler, Maureen J. 524
Fowler, Noble O., 409, 411, 412
Fox, H., 496
Fox, John L., 24
Fox, Sidney A., 457
Fraenkel, G. J., 208
Fraenkel-Conrat, Heinz, 383
Frame, Florence K., 25
Francis, Gary S., 162
Francone, Clarice A., 187
Frangenheim, Hans G., 247
Frank, Charles B., 22
Franklin, D. A., 205

Fraser, F. Clarke, 106
Fraser, Robert G., 411
Fraunfelder, F. T., 474
Fredrickson, Donald S., 424
Frederickson, D. T., 210
Free, Alfred H., 439
Free, Helen M., 439
Freedman, Alfred M., 479
Freeman, Howard, 134
Freeman, H. Mackenzie, 458
Freeman, Leonard M., 453
Freeman, Ruth B., 441
Freeman, W. H., 268
Fregert, Sigfrid, 164, 207
Frei, Emil III, 452
Freidman, Herman, 157
Frenay, Agnes C., 82
French, Ruth M., 219
Freud, Anna, 479
Frick, H. C., 493
Friedberg, Charles K., 411
Friede, Reinhard L., 404
Friedman, E. A., 278
Friedman, H., 192
Friedman, Morton P., 131
Friedmann, I., 461
Fries, James F., 221, 229, 239
Frimann-Dahl, J., 488
Frobischer, Martin, 434
Froelich, Robert E., 598
Frohlich, Edward D., 465
Frost, Philip, 417
Fruhmorgen, P., 256
Fry, Lionel, 212
Fuchs, Fritz, 418
Fudenberg, H. H., 399
Fuerst, Elinor V., 442
Fujita, Tsuneo, 270
Fukushima, Hiroyuki, 516
Fuller, A. B., 135
Fullmer, Harold M., 463
Fulton, John F., 325
Fulton, Robert, 42
Furia, Thomas E., 116
Fusco, Madeline M., 251
Futrell, May D., 223
Fyler, Donald C., 470

Gabriel, E., 553
Gabriel, H. Paul, 233

Gahart, Betty L., 115
Gallaudet College, 8
Gallo, Barbara M., 196, 441
Garattini, S., 475
Garb, Solomon, 63, 132, 146, 229
Garcia, Lynne S., 190
Gardner, E. J., 425
Gardner, Pierce, 167
Gardner, William, 65, 75
Gardner, W. D., 401
Garner, A., 456
Garnett, E. R., 68
Garoogian, Andrew, 15
Garoogian, Rhoda, 15
Garrison, Fielding H., 327
Garrison, Young J., 94
Gasser, Raymond F., 243
Gastaut, Henri, 83
Gates, Gary F., 272
Gath, Ann, 132
Gazzaniga, Michael, 131
Gebbie, Kristine M., 441
Gebhardt, Louis P., 192
Geddes, D. M., 216
Gedo, John E., 339
Gee, D. J., 462
Geeraets, Walter J., 457
Geijer, U., 225
Gelbier, S., 103
Gell, P. G. H., 399
Gellis, Sydney S., 121, 467
General Dental Council, 295
Gentry, D. W., 142
Georgopoulos, Basil S., 200
Gerard, Alain, 574
Gerarde, Horace W., 127
Germain, Carol P., 440
Gerstein, Maurice J., 110
Ghalioungui, P., 336
Giannestras, Nicholas J., 459
Gibbons, J. D., 398
Gibbons, Norman E., 190
Gibbs, C. E., 239
Gibbs, Frederic A., 99
Gibbs, R. S., 239
Gibson, John, 116
Gibson, M. H. L., 208
Gies, William J., 331
Gilbert, Harvey A., 451, 490
Gilbert, Judson B., 317

Gilbilisco, J. A., 253
Gill, John L., 393
Gill, William, 171
Gilles, Herbert M., 263
Gillespie, Charles C., 317
Gillies, R. R., 263
Gilman, Alfred, 475
Gilroy, John, 102
Ginsberg, Frances, 158
Girdwood, R. H., 109
Given, Barbara A., 442
Gladstone, William J., 69
Glasby, John S., 57
Glass, Albert J., 340
Glass, Eleanor S., 396
Gleiter, K., 290
Glenn, William A., 39
Glick, Ira D., 20
Gliskstein, Mitchell, 188
Gloeckner, Sallie L., 265
Gmelich, John T., 488
Godden, John O., 471
Godfrey, Lois E., 537
Goeminne, Luc, 26
Gold, Jay J., 419
Gold, Robert S., 47
Goldberg, Morton F., 119
Goldberg, Stanley J., 122
Goldberger, Emanuel, 162
Goldenson, Robert M., 59, 127
Goldfien, Alan, 475
Goldfrank, Lewis R., 135
Goldin, Grace, 332
Goldman, Henry, 415
Goldman, Mervin J., 188
Goldman, Myer, 92, 223
Goldschmidt, Herbert, 255
Goldsmith, Mary, 213
Goldstein, Gerald, 499, 519
Goldstein, Joseph, 479
Goldstein, Lewis P., 120
Goldstein, Louis A., 267
Goldwyn, Robert M., 377
Gomez, Edward C., 417
Gompel, Claude, 269
Gonzalez, Carlos F., 277
Good, R. A., 375
Good, Robert A., 375, 400, 463
Goodchild, Mary C., 184
Goode, Stephen H., 29

AUTHOR INDEX

Goodgold, J., 242
Goodhart, Robert S., 450
Goodlin, Robert C., 138
Goodman, Lawrence R., 277
Goodman, Louis S., 475
Goodman, Richard M., 259
Goodwin, James W., 471
Gordon, Burgess L., 85, 565
Gorlin, Robert, 259, 415
Gorrod, J. W., 474
Goss, Charles M., 207
Gosselin, Robert E., 180, 182
Gosser, Leo G., 82
Gotlin, Ronald W., 104
Gottschalk, Carl W., 423
Gould, Marjorie, 447
Govoni, Laura E., 201
Grabb, William C., 414
Graber, Touro M., 415
Grad, Frank P., 135
Graef, John W., 178
Graf, Rudolf F., 54
Graham, J. D. P., 473, 474
Graham, John R., 234
Graham, L. T., Jr., 456
Graham, Ruth M., 225
Grainger, Ronald G., 161
Grainger, Thomas H., 333
Grant, Julius, 75
Grant, Murray, 133
Grant, W. Morton, 458
Grawunder, Sister Mary Redempta, 447
Gray, G. H., 382
Gray, Peter, 52, 57, 75, 206
Grcevic, Nenad, 407
Great Britain Department of Education and Science, 560
Great Britain General Medical Council, 296
Great Britain General Registry Office, 149
Great Britain: The Patent Office, Department of Trade and Industry, 579
Greeley, A. V., 522
Green, David P., 459
Green, M. M., 84
Green, Marvin H., 140
Green, Thomas H., Jr., 493

Greenberg, Bernard, 384
Greenberg, Bette, 16
Greenberg, Bonita R., 210
Greenblatt, David J., 473
Greenblatt, D. L., 229
Greenfield, George B., 183, 487
Greenwald, Edward S., 452
Greep, R. O., 138
Greer, Melvin, 100
Gresham, Geoffrey A., 271
Gressler, Ion, 437
Grewe, Horst-Eberhard, 246
Gribble, Helen E., 222
Griffen, Ward O., Jr., 99
Griffin, J. P., 170
Griffith, H. Winter, 230
Griffiths, Henry J., 139
Grigoriu, Dodé, 263
Grimstone, A. V., 205
Grinspoon, Lester, 473
Grist, N. R., 217
Grivetti, L., 336
Grob, Gerald N., 340
Grollman, Arthur, 475
Grollman, Evelyn, 475
Groschel, Dieter, 108
Gross, Ludwik, 454
Gross, Robert E., 272
Grossman, Charles B., 277
Grossman, Moses, 123
Grossman, William, 409
Groves, John, 388
Gruendemann, Barbara J., 401
Grundy, Richard D., 391
Grupenhoff, John T., 290
Grzimek, Bernhard, 62
Gudzinowicz, Benjamin J., 220
Guerini, Vincenzo, 331
Guerra, Francisco, 322
Guggenheim, B., 551
Gunn, Alexander, 114
Gunn, John, 303
Gunz, Frederick, 454
Gurman, Alan S., 130
Gurr, Eduard, 56
Gusberg, S. B., 493
Gutgesell, Howard P., 272
Guthrie, D. W., 446
Guthrie, R., 446
Gutman, E., 491

Guttman, Ludwig, 407
Guyton, Arthur C., 377, 380, 401, 409

Haagensen, C. D., 453
Hackett, Thomas P., 131
Hadlow, William J., 379
Hague, Howard, 4
Hahn, Fred E., 390
Hahn, Peter A., 14
Hale, Leslie J., 141
Haley, Jay, 20
Hall, David A., 491
Hall, David C., 193
Hall, H. W., 1
Hall, Reginald, 438
Hall, Thomas S., 325
Haller, Raphael M., 477
Halliday, W. J., 83
Hallman, Grady L., 414
Halnan, K. E., 455
Hamburg, Joseph, 346
Hamerton, John L., 383
Hamilton, W. J., 400, 401
Hamperl, H., 67
Hanan, Zachary I., 180
Hanaway, Joseph, 276
Hanchey, Marguerite M., 499
Hanik, Michael J., 23
Hansell, Peter, 265
Hansten, Philip D., 124
Hanzlikova, V., 491
Harbison, Samuel A., 183
Hardwick, Geraline B., 449
Hardy, James D., 209
Hardy, N., 308
Hardy, R. H., 111
Harmer, M. H., 567
Harper, Harold A., 398
Harrer, Joseph M., 135
Harriman, Philip L., 90
Harris, Ben C., 123
Harris, Harry, 105, 445
Harris, Raymond, 106
Harrison, Gordon, 334
Harrison, Ira E., 22
Harryman, Elizabeth, 89, 202
Harshbarger, Dwight, 108
Hart, Allan H., 62
Hart, F. Dudley, 513
Hart, Frank Leslie, 118

Hart, Henry H., 42
Hartley, H. O., 151
Hartman, Frank R., 203
Hartshorn, Edward A., 125
Harvard Institute for International Development, 386
Harvard University, 5
Harvey, A. McGehee, 322, 329, 438
Harvey, Anthony P., 281, 283
Harvey, W. P., 310
Harwood-Nash, Derek C., 469
Haskell, Charles M., 452
Hatcher, R. A., 185
Hatfield, Philip M., 487
Hauserman, Norma M., 232
Havener, William H., 265
Hawkins, Denis, 240
Hawkins, Reginald Robert, 5
Hawkins, S. E., 193
Hayat, M. A., 389, 465
Hayden, Adaline C., 98
Hayes, Janice E., 201
Hayhoe, F. G. J., 262
Haymaker, Webb D., 403
Haynes, William O., 210
Hayt, Emanuel, 216
Hazlett, Clarke B., 174
Health Law Center, 200
Health Physics Society, 612
Health Resources Administration, Public Health Service, US Department of Health, Education, and Welfare, 539
Health Services Administration, US Department of Health, Education, and Welfare, 27
Hearst, E. S., 339
Hecaen, Henri, 406
Hedley-Whyte, John, 238
Heftmann, Erich, 94
Hegener, Karen C., 294
Heilman, Kenneth M., 100
Heine, Bernard, 482
Heitzman, E. Robert, 243
Held, Bruce J., 237
Helfer, Ray E., 478
Hellemans, J., 420
Hellerstein, Herman K., 411
Helwig, E. B., 177
Hemelt, Mary D., 441

Hemker, H. C., 109
Henderson, Betty, 195
Henderson, G. P., 601
Henderson, Isabella Ferguson, 75
Henderson, John, 218
Henderson, S. P. A., 601
Henderson, Virginia, 447
Henderson, W. D., 75
Henry, John B., 221
Hepler, Opal E., 170, 193
Heptinstall, Robert H., 464
Herbert, W. J., 83
Hermann, R. E., 165
Herrlinger, Robert, 326
Herrmann, Donald E., 59
Herrnstein, Richard J., 341
Hers, H. G., 424
Hershey, Falls B., 260
Hershey, Nathan, 396
Hertig, Arthur T., 496
HeSCA Committee on Education, 292
Hesse, P. R., 140
Hetherington, John, 456
Heumann, Karl F., 374
Hewer, C. L., 403
Hey, D., 53
Hickman, C. J., 75
Higher Education Learning Programmes Information Service, 594
Hild, Walther J., 243
Hill, Austin B., 398
Hill, D. W., 215
Hill, Graham L., 422
Hill, L. R., 85
Hill, Robert L., 375
Hillman, Robert S., 190
Hills, A. Gorman, 394
Himmelsbach, Carl J., 555
Hine, Gerald J., 136
Hingtgen, Joseph N., 43
Hinselmann, M., 280
Hinsie, Leland E., 91
The Hip Society, 552
Hirano, Asao, 249
Hirsch, H. J., 246
Hirsch, James G., 432
Hirschberg, Gerald G., 181
Hirschhorn, Norbert, 31, 217
Hirtz, J., 38
Hobart, M. J., 399

Hobson, J. Allan, 24
Hodes, Philip J., 276, 487
Hodge, H. D., 137
Hodge, James R., 234
Hodge, Melville H., 216
Hodges, Robert E., 386
Hodgman, Eileen C., 312
Hodson, H. V., 285
Hoeffken, Walther, 237
Hoeprich, Paul D., 218
Hoerlein, B. F., 497
Hofer, Doris J., 73
Hoffer, Richard E., 280
Hoffman, Donald B., Jr., 29
Hofmann, Adele, 233
Hofmann, Frederick G., 134
Hogarth, James, 85
Holborow, E. J., 207
Holder, Angela R., 397
Hollaender, A., 383
Holland, James F., 452
Holland, Jennie M., 440
Hollander, M., 398
Holman, H. H., 241
Holmes, Lewis B., 259
Homburg, Roy, 185
Homburger, F., 455
Honigfeld, Gilbert, 146
Hopkins, Helen L., 478
Hopkins, Jenny, 37
Hopkinson, D. A., 105
Hoppenfeld, Stanley, 227
Hopper, John E., 398
Horler, A. R., 438
Hornabrook, R. W., 380
Horrobin, David, 114
Horting-Hansen, E., 253
Horwitz, Orville, 147, 409
Horwitz, William, 236
Hospital Institution and Educational Food Service Society, 607
Hospital Library Standards Committee, Association of Hospital and Institution Libraries, 572
The Hospital Physicists' Association, 576
Houghton, Bernard, 525, 569, 579
House, Earl L., 246
Howard, Alfreda, 146
Howard-Jones, Norman, 342

Howe, G. Melvyn, 274, 485
Howkings, John, 493
Hsu, T. C., 258
Huang, H. K., 244
Huang, Yun Peng, 250
Hubbard, John P., 206
Hubbert, William T., 433
Hubner, P. J. B., 222
Hudak, Carolyn M., 196, 441
Hudson, Helen H., 201
Hueper, Wilhelm C., 484
Hughes, Edward C., 92
Hughes, Harold K., 64
Hughes, William F., 299, 313
Hull, D., 472
Hume, Ruth F., 317
Humphries, Arthur L., Jr., 403
Hungler, Bernadette, 446
Hunsinger, Doris L., 137, 184
Hunt, Ronald D., 498
Hunter, Donald, 133
Hunter, George W., 168, 435
Hunter, Richard, 339
Huntsman, R. G., 431
Hurley, Harry J., Jr., 381
Hurov, Leonard, 139
Hursch, C., 405
Hursh, J. B., 137
Hurst, J. Willis, 412
Hutchings, R. T., 244
Hutchinson, James C., 211
Hyman, Albert S., 59

Illich, Ivan, 398
Imperato, P. J., 435
Inbau, Fred E., 397
Information Center for Hearing, Speech and Disorders of Human Communication, 24
Ingram, Walter R., 407
Inman, Verne T., 459
Insler, Vaclav, 185
Institute for Laboratory Animal Resources, US National Research Council, 308
Institute of Medicine, 395, 428, 465
International Agency for Research on Cancer, 312, 542
International Anesthesia Research Society, 605

International Association of Biological Standardization, 550, 568, 571
International Atomic Energy Agency, 31, 147, 183, 307
International Childbirth Education Association, 613
International College of Surgeons, 605
International Commission on Microbiological Specifications for Foods of the International Association of Microbiological Societies, 182
The International Commission on Radiological Protection, 146, 147
International Commission on Radiological Protection, Task Group of Committee 2, 571
International Dental Federation, 72
International Federation for Documentation, 499
International Federation of Sportive Medicine, 608
International Labour Office, 60, 306
International Labour Organization, 183
International Narcotics Control Board, 149
International Organization for Standardization, 568
International Planned Parenthood Federation, 305
International Reference Center for Abortion Research, 17
International Society of Hematology, 608
International Strabismological Association, 515
International Union Against Cancer, 176
International Union Against Cancer/Union Internationale Centre le Cancer, 299, 539
International Union of Biological Sciences, 604
Iorio, Josephine, 447
Iselin, Marc, 267
Isler, Charlotte, 195
Israel, Lucien, 489
Israels, M. C. G., 430
Iverson, Larry D., 176

Iverson, Leslie L., 125
Iverson, Susan D., 125

Jablonski, Stanley, 89
Jabour, J. T., 122
Jaciow, Douglas, 191
Jack, Robert L., 458
Jackson, Herbert L., 92
Jackson, L. G., 200
Jacob, Alphons, 92
Jacob, Stanley W., 187
Jacobs, Morris B., 110
Jacobs, Philip, 266
Jacobson, Harold G., 197, 392
Jacobson, Michael F., 144
Jacoby, Florence G., 445
Jacox, Ada K., 201
Jaeger, Edmund C., 76
Jaffe, Henry L., 460
Jaffe, Norman S., 456
Jaffurs, William J., 278
James, A. Everette, Jr., 470
James, Edward T., 328
James, Janet W., 328
James, John D., 230
James, V. H. T., 382
Janner, Michel, 255
Jaques Cattell Press, 316, 319, 321
Jarrett, J., 329
Jarrett, John, 418
Jawetz, Ernest, 475
Jayson, M. D., 239
Jeansonne, Louis O., 178
Jefferson, Keith, 485
Jeffrey, Charles, 65
Jeffrey, H. C., 262
Jenkins, Richard J., 466
Jenis, Edwin H., 240
Jirovac, Mary M., 444
Joffe, C. David, 162
Johari, O., 389
Johnson, Alton C., 215
Johnson, Arnold H., 56
Johnson, Joseph E. III, 433
Johnson, M. L., 75
Johnson, Moulton K., 245
Johnson, Philip M., 453
Johnson, Stephen L., 331
Joint Commission on Accreditation Hospitals, 572, 573

Joint Committee on Library Service in Hospitals, Council of National Library Associations, 3
Joint Formulary Committee, 574
Jokl, E., 358
Joklik, Wolfgang K., 111, 436
Jones, C. E., 409
Jones, Dorothy A., 444
Jones, Elizabeth A., 520
Jones, E. L., 271
Jones, Howard W., Jr., 493
Jones, John E., 129
Jones, L. Meyer, 498
Jones, Lester T., 458
Jones, Lois M., 191
Jones, Peter G., 466
Jones, Stacy V., 580
Jones, Thomas C., 498
Jopling, W. H., 133
Journal of Bone and Joint Surgery, 36
Juhl, John H., 486
Julian, Desmond G., 162, 408
Jung, C. G., 341
Jung, Rodney C., 433, 497
Justice, Carson, 63

Kadushin, Alfred, 484
Kagan, Benjamin M., 121, 467
Kahn, Guinter, 254
Kahn, J. E., 135
Kahn, S. B., 452
Kaiser, F. E., 555
Kalbus, Barbara, 187
Kalish, Beatrice J., 335
Kalish, Philip A., 335
Kalita, Dwight K., 118
Kamenetz, G., 69
Kamenetz, H., 69
Kammerer, Kathryn L., 155
Kanely, Edna M., 540
Kanig, Joseph L., 476
Kao, Frederick S., 490
Kaplan, Doris Flax, 35
Kaplan, Harold I., 479
Kaplan, Henry S., 453
Kaplan, Martin M., 198
Kaplan, Nathan O., 382
Karacan, I., 405
Karasu, Toksoz B., 106
Kardon, Randy H., 246

Kardos, G., 140
Kark, Sidney L., 483
Karow, Armand M., Jr., 403
Karp, Adrienne, 197
Kaschak, Marianne C., 48
Kase, Francis J., 579
Kass, Lawrence, 261
Katz, Bill, 583
Katz, Dorothy D., 114, 120
Katz, Jay, 396
Katz, Louis N., 412
Katz, Myron, 277
Kaufman, Martin, 322
Kaufmann, H. J., 277
Kaul, Alexander, 136
Kawamura, Y., 381
Kay, Margarita A., 71
Kaye, Sidney, 134
Keane, Claire Brackman, 86, 442, 448
Keats, Theodore E., 275
Keen, G., 238
Keen, H., 329
Keen, Harry, 418
Keeney, Arthur H., 226
Kelch, Robert P., 228
Kelen, Eva M. A., 51
Keleti, Georg, 113
Kelikian, H., 423
Keller, Donald A., 265
Keller, Mark, 48
Kelleher, Marie J., 223
Kelley, Vincent C., 469
Kelley, William N., 203
Kelly, D. E., 462
Kelly, Emerson C., 52
Kelly, Howard A., 319
Kelly, Patricia T., 165
Kelly, S., 105
Kemme, Douglas H., 137
Kemmer, Elizabeth J., 49
Kemp, R. L., 186
Kempe, C. Henry, 122, 467, 478
Kendall, Maurice G., 148
Kendig, Edwin L., Jr., 467
Kennedy, Dorothy A., 439
Kennedy, Robert L., 449
Kenny, Thomas J., 129
Kepler, Judith A., 179
Kerker, Ann E., 11, 17
Kerr, Avice, 65

Kerr, Donald A., 253
Kessel, Richard G., 246
Kessler, M. M., 304
Kestelman, P., 308
Kett, Joseph F., 341
Key, Jack D., 12
Key, Marcus M., 236
Keys, John D., 180
Keys, Thomas E., 12
Kidney Disease Control Program, 308
Kieffer, Stephen A., 243
Kilbey, B., 106
Killam, Keith F., 58
Kimmig, Joseph, 255
King, Charles G., 336
King, Donald L., 485
King, Eunice M., 172
King, Felicity, 178
King, Lester S., 155
King, Linda S., 588
King, Maurice, 179
King, Michael M., 588
King, Robert C., 84, 106
Kinmonth, John B., 412
Kinney, John M., 158
Kinney, M. B., 166
Kintzel, Kay C., 439
Kirby, Cynthia C., 237
Kirk, Raymond Eller, 53
Kirklin, John W., 408
Kirkpatrick, Charles H., 488
Kirkpatrick, John A., Jr., 460
Kirman, Brian, 234
Kirschman, J. D., 144
Kirsner, Joseph B., 422
Kirstein, Robert, 135
Kissane, John M., 463, 470
Kissin, Benjamin, 391
Kistner, Robert W., 278
Kitchell, J. R., 162
Kivitz, Marvin S., 339
Kjervik, Diane, 449
Klebs, Arnold C., 326
Klein, B., 281
Klein, Barry T., 60
Klein, Jerome O., 468
Klein, Lawrence, 30
Kligman, Albert M., 416
Kline, Nathan S., 181
Klippel, Allen P., 159

AUTHOR INDEX

Kloff, W. J., 436
Klopper, A., 418
Klug, Jay W., 23
Knapp, Rebecca G., 439
Kneisl, Carol R., 198
Knight, Vernon, 491
Knoben, James E., 124
Koch, Gerhard, 26
Koch, Michael S., 65
Koehler, P. Ruben, 486
Koestler, Frances A., 337
Kohnke, Mary F., 440
Kolb, Lawrence C., 480
Kolker, Allan E., 456
Kolmel, Hans Wolfgang, 248
Kolstad, Per, 256
Koneman, Elmer W., 263
Kooi, Kenneth A., 406
Koop, C. Everett, 229
Kopec, Ada C., 430
Kopf, Alfred W., 254
Kopicky, Joyce, 487
Koprowski, Hilary, 198
Koren, Nathan, 317
Korossy, S., 376
Korting, G. W., 255, 416
Kos, L., 278
Kostic, Aleksandar D., 73
Kourany, Miguel, 192
Kowitz, Aletha, 13
Krakauer, Eleanor, 63
Krall, Leo P., 164
Kramer, J. F., 182
Krampitz, Sydney D., 448
Krasowski, J. Owen, 92
Kraus, Barbara, 87
Kraus, Robert, 251
Krause, Marie V., 449
Krause, Urban, 437
Krauss, Stephen, 59
Krawiec, T. S., 321
Kremer, Karl, 246
Kreschek, Janet, 89, 202
Kress, John R., 108
Kretchmer, N., 552
Kreuger, Janelle, 446
Krizek, Thomas J., 169
Kronick, David A., 156, 524
Krugman, Saul, 434
Krupp, Marcus A., 114, 436

Krusen, Frank H., 128
Kruzas, Anthony P., 284, 290, 602
Kubisz, P., 431
Kucers, A., 476
Kuhlenbeck, Hartwig, 378
Kuner, Eugen H., 277
Kunin, Arthur S., 562
Kunin, Calvin M., 185
Kuntzleman, Charles T., 59
Kurdi, William J., 116
Kurylowicz, W., 473
Kutscher, Austin H., 41
Kutscher, Austin H., Jr., 41
Kutsky, R., 117
Kuzemko, Jan A., 207
Kyed, James M., 603
Kynoch, P. A. M., 141

La Beau, Dennis, 316
LaBossiere, Eileen, 188
Lachman, Leon, 476
Lachmann, P. J., 399
Lagua, Rosalinda T., 88
Lajtha, Abel, 101
Lancaster, F. Wilfrid, 614
Lancaster, Henry Oliver, 148
Landsmeer, Johan M. F., 242
Lane, Marc J., 205
Lane, Nancy D., 155
Lange, Crystal M., 597
Langer, Glenn A., 412
Langley, F. A., 496
Langman, Jan, 243
Langs, Robert J., 482
Lanyi, Marton, 237
Lapage, S. P., 67
Lapedes, Daniel N., 56
Laragh, John H., 161
Larson, Carroll B., 447
Larson, Leonard A., 59, 576
Larson, Margaret A., 172
Lascari, Andre D., 468
Laskin, Allen I., 110
Lasky, Paul C., 166
Lassow, Walter J., 187
Laughlin, Alice, 206
Lavin, Paul J., 232
Law, Frank W., 337
Law, John W., 89
Lawler, Marilyn R., 444

Lawrence, J. S., 492
Lawson, Thomas L., 277
Lea, G., 134
Lea, James, 186
Leach, R. M., 262
Leahy, Kathleen M., 115
Leavell, Byrd S., 430
Leavell, Lutie C., 98, 187
Lebowitz, Philip W., 158
Lechevalier, Hubert A., 100, 334
Lederer, William H., 113
Ledley, Robert S., 244
Lee, Jane A., 222
Lee, Richard V., 73
Lees, David H., 279
Lees, Frederick, 160
Lees, R., 118
Leeson, C. Roland, 244, 270
Leeson, Thomas S., 244, 270
Leevy, C. M., 572
Le Fanu, William Richard, 320
Lehmann, H., 141, 431
Lehninger, Albert L., 395
Lehrer, Steven, 325
Leibowitz, J. O., 331
Leicester, Henry M., 324
Leider, Morris, 84, 255
Leigh, Denis, 59
Leitenberg, Harold, 130
LeMaitre, George D., 223
Lemire, Ronald J., 407
Lemp, Helena B., 548
Lennette, Edwin H., 167, 191
Lentz, Thomas L., 270
Lepine, P., 69
Lepley, Marvin, 196
Lequeene, Suzanne E., 22
Lerch, Constance, 195
Lesch, Michael, 413
Levene, G. M., 255
Lever, Walter F., 416
Levey, Samuel, 428
Levin, Marvin E., 418
Levine, Herbert J., 410
Levine, Milton E., 57
Levine, Sol, 134
Levinson, Louis, 152
Lewis, David O., 486
Lewis, Howard L., 428
Lewis, John R., Jr., 246
Lewis, Leon, 181
Lewis, LuVerne W., 195
Lewis, Marianna O., 284
Lewis, Myrna I., 478
Liao, Allen Y., 30
Library Systems Branch, US Environmental Protection Agency, 306
Licht, S. H., 478
Lichtenstein, Louis, 451, 459
Lick, Rainer F., 247
Lidz, Theodore, 480
Liebel, Steve, 487
Lieberman, Herbert A., 476
Liebesny, Felix, 578
Liechty, Richard D., 159
Lillie, R. D., 463
Lima-de-faria, A., 121
Limbacher, James, 590
Limper, Hilda K., 129
Lincoff, Gary, 110
Lindenberg, Richard, 250
Lindner, Arthur E., 487
Lindsay, Cotton M., 428
Lin-Fu, Jane S., 49
Lingeman, Richard R., 89
Linman, James W., 431
Linton, Robert R., 260
Lipkin, Gladys B., 447
Lipman, B. S., 410
Lipowski, Z. J., 481
Lippard, Vernon W., 325
Lipsitt, Don R., 481
Lipton, Morris A., 58
Litman, Theodore J., 28
Livingston, Samuel, 160
Lizzi, Frederic L., 458
Llewellyn-Jones, D., 239
Lockard, Isabel, 83
Lockheed Information Systems (Lockheed), 623
Loebl, Suzanne, 116
Logue, Valentine, 249
Lohr, Thelma, 196, 441
Lokich, Jacob J., 453, 455
Long, James W., 230
Long, William B., 171
Loomba, Narendra P., 428
Loosjes, T. P., 9
Lore, John M., Jr., 246
Losher, Susan, 51

Louttit, Richard T., 23
Low, Neils L., 476
Lowbury, E. J. L., 107
Lowe, D. Armstrong, 565
Lowenthal, David T., 240
Lowry, Sidney, 486
Lucia, Salvatore P., 550
Luckmann, Joan, 444
Ludbrook, J., 208
Ludwig, H., 279
Luisada, Aldo A., 211, 274
Lukert, Barbara, 449
Luna, Lee G., 268
Lunin, Lois F., 14
Luntz, Lester L., 103
Luntz, Phyllys, 103
Lusted, Lee B., 275
Lydiate, P. W. H., 397
Lynch, H. T., 295
Lynch, J. B., 138
Lynch, Malcolm A., 414
Lyon, Leonard J., 102

Macalpine, Ida, 339
Macdonald, John M., 234
MacDonald, Paul C., 497
Mace, D. R., 240
MacFaul, Peter A., 56, 457
MacGillivray, Ian, 493
Mack, Roy, 71
Mackert, Mary E., 441
Madden, John L., 247
Madden, J. S., 233
Maddin, Stuart, 163
Madeley, C. R., 218
Maegraith, Brian, 217
Magalini, Sergio, 78
Magee, Joseph H., 147
Mahan, L. Kathleen, 449
Maichel, Karol, 9
Mainen, Michael W., 273
Maingot, Rodney, 255
Maizell, Robert E., 499
Majno, Guido, 437
Major, Ralph H., 326
Major Scientific Books, Inc., 2
Makino, S., 424
Malamed, Stanley F., 103
Malamud, Nathan, 249
Malcolm, I. V., 239

Malikin, David, 477
Malinowski, Janet S., 445
Malten, K. E., 207
Maltha, D. J., 155
Mandell, G. L., 384
Manfreda, Marguerite L., 448
Mangrum, Robert E., 189
Manning, D., 47
Manpower Resources Staff, US Public Health Service, 150
Manseau, Anna T., 144
Mansfield, Carl M., 453
Manson-Bahr, P. E. C., 435
Marble, Alexander, 419
Margulis, Alexander R., 485
Marien, Daniel, 293
Marks, John, 59
Marler, E. E. J., 90
Marlow, Dorothy R., 449
Marriott, H. J. L., 162
Marshak, Richard H., 487
Marshall, Robert E., 406
Martin, Alan, 183
Martin, Eric W., 124, 180
Martin, Graham, 161
Martin, Horace F., 220
Martin, Leonide L., 442
Martin, M. W., 78
Martin, S. M., 297
Martin, William J., 432
Martinson, Ida, 449
Mash, Norma J., 445
Maslova, Alevtina M., 71
Mason, E. J., 573
Mason, Mildred A., 194, 196
Mason, Rita A., 212
Mason, Thomas J., 264
Massachusetts General Hospital Department of Nursing, 173
Massachusetts General Hospital. Dietary Department, 174
Matarazzo, James M., 603
Matsui, Takayoshi, 276
Matthews, Ruth H., 94
Matthysse, S., 480
Mattingly, Richard F., 280
Maull, Kimball I., 99
Mawson, Stuart, 461
Maxfield, Bruce W., 99
Mayer, Jean, 449

Maynard, John T., 580
Mayo Clinic, 175
Mayor, Georges, 280
Mazziotta, John C., 244
McAlpine, Wallace A., 252
McCarley, Robert W., 24
McCarthy, Daniel J., 431
McCarthy, Margaret D., 201
McCarty, Daniel J., Jr., 239
McCay, Clive M., 336
McClelland, Robert N., 595
McConnell, I., 399
McConnico, Charles T., 96
McCormick, William F., 248, 405
McCulloch, William F., 433
McDermott, Walsh, 436
McDonald, George A., 260
McDowell, Frank, 199, 330
McFarlane, J., 173
McGibony, John R., 429
McGraw-Hill Encyclopedia of Science and Technology, Staff of, 308
McHenry, Earle W., 386
McIntyre, M., 290
McKay, M., 591
McKendry, J. B. J., 228
McKinney, William E. J., 237
McKusick, V. A., 84
McLean, Janice, 282
McMillan, Julia A., 179
McMinn, Alex, 96
McMinn, R. M. H., 244
McNab, Ian, 459
McNeill, William H., 334
McNicol, M. W., 490
McRae, Alexander, 203
M. D. Anderson Hospital and Tumor Institute, 551
Mead, Kate C. H., 326
Mechanic, David, 479
Medical Library Association, 594
Mehregan, Amir H., 212
Meili, W. A. R., 60
Melby, Edward C., Jr., 139
Mello, Nancy K., 369
Melloni, Biagio J., 81
Melloni, Ida D., 81
Melnick and Hamilton, 318
Meltzer, Lawrence E., 162, 441
Meltzer, Yale, 52

Memmler, Ruth L., 193, 194
Mendelson, Jack, 370
Menditto, Joseph, 38
Menninger, Karl A., 15
Mental Health Materials Center, 45, 234, 598
Mereness, Dorothy A., 442
Merriam-Webster Editorial Staff, 74, 77
Merrill, Vinita, 275
Merrington, W. R., 333
Merritt, Houston, 408
Mersky, Roy M., 156
Meschan, Isadore, 242, 485
Metheny, Norma, 116
Metzger, H., 279
Metzger, Norman, 333
Meyer, John S., 102, 211
Meyer, Sharon, 30
Meyers, Frederick H., 475
Miale, John B., 431
Michaelis, A., 84
Michigan Bureau of Health Facilities, 215
Miles, Ashley, 435
Miles, M. A., 29
Milgram, Gail G., 41
Milgrom, Felix, 400
Millard, Patricia, 554
Miller, Albert J., 42
Miller, Benjamin F., 86
Miller, David E., 577
Miller, Denis R., 472
Miller, G., 105
Miller, Genevieve, 323
Miller, Glenn E., 518
Miller, Henry, 438
Miller, M., 194
Miller, Marjorie A., 98, 187
Miller, Michael H., 448
Miller, Robert D., 396
Miller, R. R., 229
Miller, Sigmund S., 54
Miller, S. J. H., 227
Miller, William C., 93
Milne, M. Jean, 454
Milsum, John H., 375
Milunsky, Aubrey, 472
Minckler, Jeff, 379
Minton, Sherman A., Jr., 484

Mirsky, Israel, 409
Mitchel, D. H., 110
Mitchell, J. F., 474
Mitchell, Ross G., 129
Modell, Walter, 115, 124, 202
Moerman, Daniel E., 66
Moffet, Hugh L., 433
Mohan, Surendar, 30
Mohler, Irvin C., 25
Mohr, James C., 343
Moll, Ann D., 302
Mollendorf, W. V., 97
Moment, G. B., 426
Monahan, Robert, 583
Moncure, A. C., 437
Monnier, Marcel, 378
Monroe, Lee S., 257
Moody, Mildred T., 129
Moon, J. R., 132
Mooney, Marion P., 172
Mooney, Thomas O., 128
Moore, Gary S., 191
Moore, Guy W., 199
Moore, M. L., 20
Moore, Mary Lou, 481
Moore, Matthew T., 330
Moraff, Howard, 99
Moragas, Augusto, 270
Morais, Herbert M., 326
Morehead, Joe, 541
Morel, Alice, 445
Morgan, William K. C., 484
Morley, T. P., 404
Morris, Dwight A., 14
Morris, Elaine M., 443
Morris, Lynne D., 14
Morris, R. J., 333
Morton, Barbara M., 224
Morton, Leslie T., 4, 13, 206, 327
Moschella, Samuel L., 381
Moses, Robert A., 455
Moss, Arthur J., 211
Moss, William T., 455
Mossberg, Howard E., 394
Mossman, H. W., 400, 401
Mostofi, F. K., 492
Motta, Pietro, 272
Moulton, Jack E., 567
Mountcastle, Vernon B., 401
Mourant, A. E., 430

Moyers, Robert E., 103
Mueller, Beatriz V., 71
Muench, Eugene V., 11
Muir, C. S., 561
Mullen, Kenneth, 151
Mullins, William S., 340
Munk, William, 320
Murchison, Irene, 443
Murgatroyd, S. J., 36
Murphy, Frank D., 166
Murphy, Henry T., 11
Murphy, Leonard J. T., 343
Murray, Ronald O., 197
Mustard, W. T., 471
Myers, George H., 279
Myers, R. D., 100
Myerscough, P. R., 138
Myrianthopoulos, N. C., 23

Nadas, Alexandar S., 470
Nagel, Donald A., 273
Nagi, Saad Z., 40
Nagler, Willibald, 181
Nakayama, Komei, 256
Nardi, George, 255
Nater, J. P., 207
Nathan, David G., 468
National Association for the Deaf, 611
National Association of Social Workers, 282, 517
National Cancer Institute, US Department of Health, Education, and Welfare, 36, 299, 387, 538
National Clearing House Program, American Association of Blood Banks, 297
National Committee for Careers in the Medical Laboratory, 178, 293
National Coordinating Council on Drug Education, 598
National Council of Social Service, 287
National Environmental Health Association, 612
National Federation of Licensed Practical Nurses, 609
National Federation of the Blind, 611
National Foundation for Cancer Research, 609
National Foundation-March of Dimes, 382, 611

National Geriatrics Society, 573
National Health Federation, 604
National Hemophilia Foundation, 608
National Information Center for Educational Media, 592, 594
National League for Nursing, 609
National Microfilm Association, 588, 590, 591
National Registry of Emergency Medical Technicians, 607
National Resident Matching Program, 604
National Society for Autistic Children, 612
National Translations Center, The John Crerar Library, 553
Natvig, J. B., 166
Naughton, John P., 411
Neal, Kenneth G., 187
Neal-Schuman Publishers, Inc., 304
Nealon, Thomas F., Jr., 225
Needham, J. R., 113
Neiger, Alexander, 257
Nelson, A. M., 133
Nelson, Benjamin, 146
Nelson, James H., Jr., 246
Nelson, John D, 145
Nelson, M. J., 440
Nelson, Waldo E., 472
Nemec, Jaroslav, 327, 524
Netherlands Committee on Bone Tumors, 264
Neu, John, 337
Neudt, R. O., 280
Neuhauser, Duncan, 296
Neurath, Hans, 375
Neustadt, R. E., 334
New York Academy of Medicine, 6, 7
New York Academy of Medicine Library, 317
New York Heart Association, 66
New York Heart Association Criteria Committee, 67
Newberne, P. M., 450
Newby, Frank, 580
Newall, Frank W., 457
Newill, Vaun A., 29
Newman, G. B., 205
Newman, Margaret A., 201
Newton, Thomas H., 392

Nice, Charles, 277
Nicholes, Paul S., 192
Nicholi, Armand M., Jr., 233
Nicholls, Marion E., 446
Nick, William V., 20
Nocolosi, Lucille, 89, 202
Nieburg, Phillip I., 179
Nisonoff, Alfred, 398
Niswander, Jerry D., 48
Nite, Gladys, 447
Nobel, Albert, 73
Noble, Elmer R., 435
Noble, Glenn A., 435
Noble, John H., Jr., 31
Noble, W. C., 417
Noguchi, Michiko, 516
Nolan, Daniel J., 258
Noling, A. W., 33
Norback, Craig T., 289
Norback, Peter G., 289
Norris, Henry J., 496
Nose, Yukihiko, 185
Noshpitz, Joseph, 129
Notter, Lucille E., 224, 442
Novak, F., 186
Nowak, Geraldine D., 50
Noyek, Arnold M., 268
Noyes Data Corporation, 306, 582
Nuclear Medicine Science Syllabus Subcommittee of the Education and Training Committee, Society of Nuclear Medicine, 202
Nueckel, Susan, 225
Nutrition Department, Johns Hopkins Hospital, 174
The Nutrition Foundation, 34
Nutting, Adelaide M., 336
Nyhus, Lloyd M., 158, 221, 309
Nylander, P. S. S. 493

Oakley, W. G., 212
Oberembt, Colette M., 165
Oberhofer, Martin, 137
O'Brien, Donough, 467
O'Brien, Mary, 173
O'Brien, William J., 415
Occupational Safety and Health Information Center, 66
Ockerman, H. W., 201
O'Connor, Andrea, 156

O'Connor, Maeve, 156
Ocran, E. B., 344
Odeh, Robert E., 152
O'Doherty, Desmond S., 101
O'Doherty, Neil, 273
O'Donoghue, Don H., 478
Office of Human Development Services, Administration for Children, Youth, and Families, Children's Bureau, US National Center on Child Abuse and Neglect, 90
Office of Management and Budget Documents, 288
Ogden, Sheila, 195
O'Kane, C. P., 165
Okazaki, Toshiro, 516
Olby, Robert, 332
Olds, R. J., 263
Oliven, John F., 185
Oliver, H. John, 89
Oliver, Michael F., 162
Oliver, William H., 295
Olsen, Arthur M., 421
Olsen, E. G. J., 464
Olson, Arne L., 59
Olsson, O., 61
O'Neal, Lawrence W., 418
Oppedisano-Reich, Marie, 295
Optical Society of America, 300
O'Rahilly, Ronan, 244
Order, Stanley E., 487
Organization for Economic Cooperation and Development, 150
Orkin, Milton, 435
Orth, David, 597
Osberg, Sally, 304, 305
Osborn, June, 333
Osburn, W. A., 401
Oski, Frank A., 179, 468
Osol, Arthur, 77, 127
Osselton, J. W., 405
O'Sullivan, Ward D., 256
Othmer, Donald F., 53
Ottenjann, R., 258
Otto, Peter, 256
Overton, Meredith, 449
Owen, Dolores B., 499
Owen, J., 520
Owen, L. N., 280
Owens, Norma F., 173

Pacela, Allan F., 568
Packard, Francis R., 326
Padilla, Amado M., 44
Palacios, Enrique, 277
Pallett, Phyllis, 173
Palmer, Archie M., 286
Palmer, Eddy D., 213
Palmer, Wendy J., 22
Palmore, Erdman, 427
Pan American Medical Association, 605
Pankey, George A., 167
Pansky, Ben, 246
Pantell, R. H., 229
Paquet, Marc, 272
Pare, C. M. B., 59
Pare, J. A. Peter, 411
Parish, David, 542
Parish, Henry J., 329
Park, Byung H., 400
Parke, Wesley, W., 245
Parker, C. C., 10
Parker, C. W., 58
Parker, William, 43
Parkhouse, J., 402
Parkinson Information Center, US National Institute of Neurological Diseases and Stroke, 25, 294
Parrott, Eugene L., 197
Parry, Shedden C., 73
Partridge, W., 71
Pascoe, Delmer J., 123
Passman, Jerome, 102
Passmore, R., 117
Passmore, Reginald, 193
Passos, Joyce Y., 440
Pasztor, Magda, 37
Paton, David, 119
Patterson, Angelo T., 169
Patton, Grant W., Jr., 278
Patz, Arnall, 597
Pau, Hans, 265
Paul, A. A., 144
Paul, Lester W., 486
Pavlovich, Natalie, 223
Pawlina, Albert, 230
Paxton, Phyllis P., 448
Paykel, E. S., 481
Payne, Barbara P., 474
Payne, W. Spencer, 421

Peacock, P. R., 69
Pearson, C. M., 492
Pearson, E. S., 151
Pearson, Howard A., 472
Peck, Theodore P., 16, 236, 306
Peins, Maryann, 26
Pellens, Mildred, 480
Pemberton, John E., 540
Pennington, Jean A., 224
Perez, Gloria L., 274
Perkins, E. S., 265
Perlin, Seymour, 130
Perlmann, P., 166
Perry, J. F., 20
Personnel Department, American Medical Association, 286
Peters, Uwe H., 70
Peters, Wallace, 263
Petersen, David M., 474
Peterson, M. Jeanne, 327
Peterson, Martin S., 56
Petty, Thomas L., 489
Pfeiffer, Eric, 478, 480
Pfeiffer, Ernst F., 105
Pfeiffer, J. William, 129
Phaneuf, Maria C., 445
Pharmaceutical Manufacturers Association, 68
Pharmaceutical Society of Great Britain, 575
Philbrook, Marilyn M., 18
Phillips, Joel L., 37
Phillips, Mary L., 137
Phillips, Raymond E., 210
Pierce, Robert H., 273
Pietz, D. E., 191
Pilkington, Thomas A., 599
Pilling, Doria, 36
Pillitteri, Adele, 445
Pillsbury, Donald M., 381
Pincus, Stanley, 184
Pindborg, Jens J., 253
Pinkus, Hermann, 212
Pinneo, Rose, 162
Piper, Douglas W., 194
Pleuvry, B. J., 402
Plewig, Gerd, 416
Plomley, N. J. B., 163
Plum, Fred, 209
Plunkett, E. R., 236

Plunkett, Edmond R., 134
Pohle, Linda C., 541
Pointer, Dennis D., 333
Poirier, Jacques, 160
Polacsek, E., 39
Poleman, Charlotte L., 174
Poley, W., 134
Polit, Denise, 446
Pollock, George H., 339
Polson, Cyril J., 462
Pomeranz, Virginia E., 53
Pond, B., 554
Popesko, Peter, 280
Porter, Keith R., 272, 462
Porter Sargent Staff, 300
Portney, G. L., 226
Portugal, Franklin H., 332
Posner, Jerome, 451
Potchen, E. James, 486
Poulson, Hemming, 257
Powell, Nieta W., 115
Power, Sir D'Arcy, 320
Powsner, Henry J., 237, 577
Prall, Robert C., 37
Prasad, Ananda S., 451
Preece, Ann, 197
Prescod, Stephen V., 120
Prescott, G. H., 425
Pressley, Robert J., 119
Pressman, R. M., 132
Prevention Branch, US National Institute on Drug Abuse, 16
Prevention Magazine, Staff of, 55
Price, Elmina M., 224
Prichard, Robert W., 82
Prier, J. E., 192
Principe, William, 144
Pritchard, Jack A., 497
Probst, Calvin, 301
Project Head Start, US Office of Child Development, 36
Pronin, Monica, 203
Provine, Harriet T., 167
Prusiner, Stanley B., 379
Pugh, D. M., 497
Purcell, W. P., 231
Puri, Subhash C., 151
Purpura, Dominick P., 188, 407
Putt, F. A., 197
Pyke, D. A., 212

AUTHOR INDEX

Quickert, Marvin H., 176

Rabello, F. E., 67
Race, R. R., 429
Radcliff, Ruth K., 195
Rahi, A. H. S., 456
Rahmy, M., 235
Rajagopalan, S., 236
Rajka, E., 376
Ramwell, Peter W., 419
Randall, Edwina, 45
Rantz, Marilyn J., 180
Rapaport, Stepehen A., 299
Rassner, Gernot, 254
Raus, Elmer E., 156
Raus, Madonna M., 156
Ravin, Abe, 25
Ray, Charles D., 397
Raybould, Elizabeth, 222
Razin, Andrew M., 130
Read, Herbert, 339
Reagan, T. J., 177
Reap, Charles A., Jr., 103
Reaves, Patterson S., 249
Rechcigl, Miloslav, Jr., 117
Rechenbach, C. W., 68
Rector, Floyd C., 392
Redman, Barbara K., 448
Redman, H. C., 422
Redman, Helen F., 537
Redo, S. Frank, 273
Reece, Robert M., 179
Reed, Richard J., 417
Reeder, Leo G., 134
Reeder, Maurice M., 146
Reeh, Merrill J., 457
Rees, Alan M., 12
Rees, J. M. H., 402
Rees, Simon, 485
Reese, Algernon B., 458
Reeves, W. G., 207
Regional Office for Europe, World Health Organization, 298
Reich, Warren T., 52
Reichel, W., 426
Reid, Robert, 342
Reid, W. Malcolm, 10
Reidel, Donald C., 28
Reilly, Mary J., 179
Reinmiller, Elinor C., 31

Reiser, Stanley, J., 324
Rembolt, Raymond R., 40
Remington, Jack S., 468
Rendel-Short, John, 337
Renetzky, Alvin, 281
Renson, C. E., 253
Research Documentation Section, US National Institutes of Health, 65
The Research Libraries of the New York Public Library and the US Library of Congress, 18, 539, 540, 545
Research Resources Information Center, 289
Reuss, Jeremias D., 503
Reuter, S. R., 422
Revill, J. P., 38
Revolutionary Health Committee of Hunan Province, 169
Reynolds, Herbert Y., 488
Reynolds, James E. F., 126
Reynolds, Michael M., 557
Rhodes, Marie, 401
Rhodin, Johannes A. G., 269
Rhymes, I. L., 189
Richards, Louise G., 39
Richards, Robert K., 395
Richardson, Richard E., 415
Richter, G. W., 363
Rickles, William H., Jr., 49
Ridenour, Nina, 340
Ridley, Constance M., 497
Rieger, R., 84
Rigal, Waldo A., 80
Riley, Lawrence E., 40
Riley, Patrick A., 79
Rimer, Evelyn Harbeck, 79
Rinzler, Carol Ann, 78
Riotton, G., 566
Ritts, Roy E., Jr., 488
Roaf, Robert, 402
Rob, Charles, 55
Robbins, Alan S., 170
Robbins, Perry, 212
Robbins, Stanley L., 462, 463
Roberts, Florence B., 447
Roberts, Mary M., 335
Robertson, J. Craig, 235
Robins, E., 479
Robinson, Corinne H., 444
Robinson, Hamilton B. G., 253

Robinson, Robert E., 82
Robson, J. S., 193
Rockwood, Charles A., Jr., 459
Roe, F. J. C., 451
Roeder, Judith E. R., 45
Roedler, Hans D., 136
Roelandt, J., 413
Roemer, Milton I., 427
Roger, Fred B., 329
Rogers, David E., 312
Rogers, Senta S., 25
Roget, Peter M., 65
Roitt, Ivan M., 399
Roizin, Leon, 407
Roland, Jean-Claude, 268
Romanes, G. J., 157
Ronchi, Lucia, 88
Roody, Peter, 64
Rook, Arthur, 417
Roos, Charles, 12
Roper, Nancy, 80, 86
Rosai, Juan, 465
Rose, Augustus S., 330
Rose, Noel R., 157, 400
Rosen, George, 341
Rosen, Marvin, 339
Rosenberg, Jack M., 127
Rosenberg, Leon E., 418
Rosenblum, Morris, 84
Rosenfeld, Gastao, 51
Rosenkrantz, Barbara G., 342
Rosenthal, S., 208
Ross, Constance A. C., 217
Ross, E. M., 465
Ross, Steven, 203
Rosser, James M., 394
Rossi, E., 552
Rossini, F. P., 256
Rossman, Isadore, 426
Rotem, Yaacov, 70
Roth, Beth, 40
Rothenberg, Robert E., 54
Rothgeb, Carrie L., 338
Rothman, Richard H., 408
Rothstein, William G., 322
Rouse, Jean E., 29
Rovozzo, Grace C., 170, 191
Rowland, Beatrice L., 143
Rowland, Howard S., 143
Roy, Claude C., 470

Roy, Frederick H., 120, 176
Royal College of Surgeons, 8
Ruben, Montague, 456
Rubin, Ira L., 211
Rubin, Mitchell I., 470
Rubin, Stanley, 328
Rubinstein, E., 438
Rubinstein, Lucien J., 160, 379
Ruch, Walter E., 237
Rudd, Robert L., 16
Rudolph, Abraham M., 471
Rudow, Edward H., 107
Rusalem, Herbert, 477
Rushmer, R. F., 102
Rusk, Howard A., 477
Russe, Otto, 266
Russell, B., 192
Russell, Dorothy S., 379
Russell, Gillean, 461
Russell, Graham J., 96
Russell, Paul F., 433
Russell, Phyllis J., 12
Russell, R. W. Ross, 409
Rutherford, Robert B., 403
Rutledge, Felix, 453
Rutstein, David D., 214
Rutter, Michael, 567
Ryan, Sheila A., 125
Rycroft, Charles, 90
Ryge, Gunnar, 415
Rywlin, Arkadi M., 463

Sabiston, David C., 411
Sacks, Joel G., 250
Sadock, Benjamin J., 479
Saffady, William, 592
Saghir, M. T., 479
Sahn, David J., 122
Sahs, Adolph L., 330
Saidie, M. H., 138
Saidman, Lawrence J., 402
Sainani, Gurmukh S., 211
Sainsbury, D., 86
St. al Zaro, Joan, 232
Salamon, George, 250
Salamon, Georges, 249
Salcedo, Ernesto E., 252
Salib, Philip I., 227
Salloway, Jeffrey C., 165
Salmon, Paul R., 258

Salmon, Shirley, 120
Sample, W. Frederick, 485
Sampson, P., 86
Samter, Max, 58, 376
Samuel, Eric, 462
Sanazaro, Paul J., 12
Sanborn, Charlotte J., 338
Sandberg, Eugene, 496
Sandritter, C. Thomas, 270
Sandritter, Walter, 270
Sanger, Ruth, 429
Sani, G., 278
Sankar, D. Siva, 475
Sapira, Joseph D., 235
Sapirie, S., 166
Sarnoff, Paul, 92
Sarti, Dennis A., 485
Sartwell, Philip E., 483
Sasahara, Arthur A., 413
Saski, Witold, 197
Sather, Mike R., 118
Sauer, Gordon C., 164
Sauerland, E. K., 187
Saunders, Cicely M., 454
Saunders, William, 445
Savary, M., 105
Sax, N. Irving, 132
Saxton, Dolores F., 444
Scarpelli, Emile M., 472
Schaefer, H., 104
Schandelmeier, Nancy R., 221
Schapiro, Rolf L., 274
Schaumann, B., 416
Schaumburg-Lever, Gundula, 416
Scheie, Harold G., 458
Schepens, Charles L., 458
Scherer, Jeanne C., 195
Schertel, Albrecht, 64
Schettler, G., 161
Schiff, Leon, 421
Schild, Geoffrey C., 434
Schimke, R. N., 200
Schlant, Robert C., 252
Schlessinger, David, 311
Schmeckebier, Laurence F., 540
Schmidt, Jacob E., 73, 80, 81, 82
Schmitt, Barton D., 130
Schneider, Howard A., 175
Schneider, Marie Louise, 272
Schneider, Volker, 272

Schneierson, S. Stanley, 262
Schnurrenberger, Paul R., 433
Schochet, Sydney S., Jr., 248, 405
Schockmel, Curtis C., 194
Schoenfield, Leslie J., 420
School of Allied Medical Professions, 21
Schottenfeld, David, 452
Schubert, Paul B., 140
Schuknecht, Harold F., 461
Schulman, Janice B., 37
Schult, Martha O., 443
Schultz, Dodi, 53
Schultz, Leroy G., 481
Schulz, Rockwell, 215
Schumann, Gerhild, 270
Schumer, William, 221
Schwartz, Lazar M., 187
Schwartz, Paula, 187
Schwartz, Seymour I., 310
Schwarz, Gerhart S., 237, 577
Schwarzacher, H. G., 189
Schweer, Jean E., 441
Schweitzer, Howard B., 64
Science and Health Publications, 593
Science Service, 309
Scientific Committee, British Herbal Medicine Association, 574
Scientific Publications Section, National Institute of Child Health and Human Development, US Department of Health, Education, and Welfare, 37
Scipien, Gladys M., 441
Scott, Elvyn G., 432
Scott, J. T., 491
Scott, William R., 276
Scott, William W., 493
Seaman, J., 225
Searle, Charles E., 452
Seaton, Anthony, 484
Seeley, H. W., Jr., 192
Segal, Julius, 340
Segal, Maurice S., 61
Seidon, Rudolph, 62
Sela, M., 375
Selesnick, Sheldon T., 340
Seligmann, Jean H., 57
Selikoff, Irving J., 482
Sell, Irene L., 43

Sell, Stewart, 400
Sells, Saul B., 567
Seltz-Petrash, Ann, 593
Selye, Hans, 419
Semioli, William J., 140
Sequin, Marilynne, 597
Seruya, Flora C., 51
Seventh Day Adventist Hospital Association, 513
Seward, Charles, 169
Sewell, Winifred, 15
Seydel, H. Gunter, 488
Shackleton, Alberta D., 174
Shader, R. I., 123
Shader, Richard I., 181, 473
Shafer, Kathleen N., 443
Shaffer, Dale E., 4
Shaffer, David, 567
Shaftan, Gerald W., 159
Sha'ked, Ami, 43
Shanks, Mary D., 439
Shannon, Gerard M., 458
Shapiro, Jacob, 238
Shapiro, Lewis, 255
Shapley, Willis N., 559
Sharma, A., 383, 423
Sharma, A. K., 383, 423
Shaw, J., 472
Shaw, J. C., 405
Shaw, Ralph R., 9
Sheehan, Harold L., 138
Sheehy, Eugene P., 9
Sheldon, Huntington, 437
Sheldon, John M., 157
Sheldon, Neil, 477
Sheldon, William H., 258
Shelley, Walter B., 416
Shepard, Thomas H., 105, 145
Shepherd, Michael, 567
Sheridan, Leslie W., 156
Sherlock, Dame S., 257
Sherlock, Sheila, 421
Sherrill, Claude A., 103
Shields, Thomas W., 488
Shiffman, M. A., 236
Shih, Vivian E., 188
Shilling, Charles W., 30, 32, 221
Shils, Maurice E., 450
Shimoda, A., 192

Shindell, Sidney, 165
Shipps, Fred C., 242
Shiraki, Hirotsugu, 407
Shirkey, Harry C., 122
Sholtys, Phyllis, 307
Shopland, Donald R., 46, 49
Shorter, Ray G., 422
Shrock, John G., 25
Shryock, Richard H., 328
Shubin, H., 112
Shulman, Jonas A., 110
Sicher, Harry, 253
Siegmund, O. H., 186
Siggaard-Andersen, Ole, 429
Silber, Earl N., 412
Silber, Sherman J., 209
Silen, William, 420
Silva, J. Francis, 219
Silver, Henry K., 122, 467
Silverman, Arnold, 470
Silverstein, Martin E., 111
Silverstone, Trevor, 35
Simeone, Frederick A., 408
Simko, Margaret D., 34
Simmons, David J., 562
Simmons, Sandra A., 412
Simonton, D., 563
Simonyi, J., 413
Simring, Marvin R., 188
Singer, Albert, 279
Singer, Charles, 328
Singer, James, 108
Singer, Richard B., 152
Singer, T. E. R., 499
Singleton, P., 86
Sippl, Charles J., 78
Sirridge, Marjorie S., 189
Sitting, Marshall, 58
Skaer, R. J., 205
Skerman, V. B. D., 512
Skinner, Henry A., 81
Skoog, Tord, 403
Skydell, Barbara, 218
Slatt, Bernard J., 226
Sleisenger, Marvin H., 422
Sliosberg A., 72
Sloane, Sheila B., 74
Sloss, Margaret W., 186
Small, W. P., 437

Smith, R. Abbey, 410
Smith, Alice L., 192, 463
Smith, A. N., 462
Smith, Arthur, 263
Smith, Carl H., 472
Smith, Clarissa R., 197
Smith, Donald R., 493
Smith, Dorothy L., 219, 231
Smith, Dorothy W., 440
Smith, E. E., 578
Smith, Helen D., 478
Smith, Hilton A., 498
Smith, Julian F., 499
Smith, Kenneth G. V., 434
Smith, Lendon H., 57
Smith, Margaret G., 470
Smith, Rodney, 55
Smith, Roger C., 10
Smithcors, J. F., 343
Smola, Bonnie K., 196
Smorto, Mario P., 99
Snell, Richard S., 208, 243
Snively, William D., 116
Snow, John C., 158
Snowden, Robert, 240
Snyder, Solomon H., 125
Sobey, Francine, 45
Sobin, L. H., 566
Soccolich, G. V., 304
Social Securities Administration, US Department of Health, Education, and Welfare, 296
Society for Epidemiological Research, 608
Society for Experimental Biology and Medicine, 605
Society of Nuclear Medicine, 609
Soddy, Kenneth, 482
Sodeman, W. A., 463
Sodeman, W. A., Jr., 463
Sollitto, Sharmon, 19
Solnit, Albert J., 479
Solomon, Gail E., 209
Solotorovsky, Morris, 334
Somerville, Dorothy A., 417
Sommers, Sheldon C., 313
Sonnedecker, Glenn, 338
Sonnenblick, Edmund H., 413
Soper, Robert T., 159

Sorensen, Karen, 444
Sorenson, James R., 26
Sourkes, Theodore L., 318
Southgate, D. A. T., 144
Spalding, Eugenia K., 224
Sparks, Richard M., 510
Spaulding, Earle H., 191
Special Libraries Council of Philadelphia and Vicinity, 537
Special Studies Committee of the Michigan Occupational Therapy Association, 64
Speert, Kathryn H., 66
Spencer, Donald D., 63
Spencer, Francis M., 257
Spencer, Frank C., 411
Spencer, H., 464
Spencer, Martha L., 228
Spencer, Rowena, 493
Sperryn, P. N., 438
Spillane, John D., 248
Spillner, P., 63
Spink, Wesley W., 333
Spiro, Howard M., 420
Spitz, Werner U., 228
Spjut, H. J., 452
Spock, Benjamin, 229
Spoerri, O., 472
Sprecher, Daniel, 598
Spreitzer, Elmer A., 40
Spring, Susan B., 398
Springall, W. Herbert, 429
Squire, Lucy F., 486
Srinivasan, T. R., 30
Srole, Leo, 480
Stacy, Ralph W., 374
Staehler, W., 279
Staemmler, Hans-Joachim, 272
Staff of McGraw-Hill Encyclopedia of Science and Technology, 308
Staff of Prevention Magazine, 55
Stafford, Peter, 58
Stafl, Adolf, 256
Stafne, Edward C., 253
Stahr, H. M., 198
Stallard, H. B., 226, 456
Stallworthy, John, 493
Stanbury, John B., 424
Stange, E., 161

Stanley, H. Eugene, 395
Stannard, J. N., 137
Stark, G. T., 210
Statistics and Analysis Branch, Division of Research Grants, US National Institutes of Health, 561
Steen, Edwin B., 64
Steere, Norman V., 113
Steere, William C., 323
Steffl, Bernita M., 107
Stein, Harold A., 226
Steinberg, Franz U., 426
Steinbichler, Eveline, 73
Steinbock, R. T., 486
Stenesh, J., 75
Stephenson, Hugh E., Jr., 200, 219
Stevens, Alan, 197
Stevens, Barbara J., 446
Stevenson, Michael, 289
Stevenson, Roger E., 467
Stewart, Felicia H., 240
Stewart, F. S., 432
Stewart, G. F., 450
Stewart, Isabel M., 336
Stewart, John D. M., 177
Stewart, Mark A., 132
Stewart, R. E., 125
Stewart, William D. P., 147
Stiles, Karl A., 121
Storrs, Alison, 222
Stotz, Elmer H., 374
Strand, Helen R., 79
Strand, Marcella M., 194
Stratford, B. C., 262
Strauss, Herbert S., 217
Strauss, Maurice B., 79
Strohlein, Alfred, 594
Strother, Charles M., 276
Struglia, Erasmus J., 569
Stryker, Ruth P., 221
Stuart, Angus E., 462
Stuart-Harris, Charles H., 434
Stubbe, Hans, 332
Studdard, Gloria J., 91
Student Association for the Study of Hallucinogens (STASH), 301
Sturkie, P. D., 497
Sturm, Dorothy, 431
Sturwold, Virginia G., 25
Stuttgen, G., 104

Subcommittee on Health and the Environment of the Committee on Interstate and Foreign Commerce, US House of Representatives, 85
Subcommittee on Orthopedic Information Services of the Committee on the Skeletal System of the National Research Council, 516
Suddarth, Doris S., 172
Sullivan, Linda E., 284
Summerfield, John A., 257
Surgenor, Douglas M., 432
Sutow, Wataru W., 466
Swaiman, Kenneth F., 471
Swan, H. J. C., 413
Swartzwelder, J. Clyde, 435
Swatek, Frank E., 191
Sweeney, William J., 492
Sweetwood, Hannelore, 445
Swidler, Gerald, 125
Swindler, Daris R., 244
Swishchuh, Leonard E., 472
Swiss Pharmaceutical Society, 126
Swonger, Alvin K., 130
Sykes, M. K., 490
Symmers, William St. C., 389
System Development Corporation (SDC), 623
Szollosi, Annette, 268
Szollosi, Daniel, 268

Taber, Ben-Zion, 185
Tabery, Julia J., 71
Tachdjian, Mihran O., 470
Takahashi, Mutsumasa, 251
Talbott, John H., 316
Tam, Billy K. S., 30
Tam, Miriam S. L., 30
Tamkin, James A., 170
Tashkin, Donald P., 239
Taub, Janet, 107
Taussig, Helen B., 380
Taveras, Juan M., 99
Taybi, Hooshang, 238
Taylor, Cecelia M., 442
Taylor, Clara Mae, 33
Taylor, Joan P., 184
Taylor, K. W., 212
Taylor, Kenneth J. W., 274
Taylor, Lauriston S., 577

AUTHOR INDEX

Taylor, Richard M., 110
Taylor, Robert B., 437
Taylor, Stewart, 466
Technomic Research Staff, 295
Tedeschi, C. G., 374
Tedeschi, Luke G., 374
ten Seldam, R. E. J., 177
Terner, Janet, 318
Terry, Charles E., 480
Tews, Eyvind S., 547
Tharp, Gerald D., 158
Thiele, Victoria F., 88
Thoma, Kurt H., 415
Thomas, Clayton L., 82
Thomas, Harry E., 107, 113
Thomas, M. L. Manson, 7
Thomas, William A., 499, 519
Thompson, Alice M. C., 32
Thompson, Edward T., 98
Thompson, John D., 332
Thompson, Lida F., 443, 448
Thompson, R. A., 187
Thompson, Samuel W. II, 268
Thompson, Thomas T., 237
Thomsen, Carol, 595
Thomson, A. Landsborough, 325
Thomson, R. G., 497
Thomson, William A. R., 77
Thomson, William M., 170
Thorn, George W., 437
Thornton, John L., 318
Thornton, Spencer P., 88
Thorup, Oscar A., 430
Thurmon, T. F. III, 214
Timbury, Morag C., 433
Timiras, P. S., 427
T'ing, Wei Sheng, 111
Tingle, Joyce E., 173
Tissue Culture Association, 513
Todd, Ian P., 377, 382
Tohen, Z. Alfonso, 177
Tolentino, Felipe I., 458
Toner, P. G., 257
Top, Franklin H., 110
Topalis, Mary, 448
Touloukian, Robert J., 169
Travel, Morton E., 410
Travis, Lee E., 128
Tredgold, Roger, 482
Treece, Eleanor W., 442

Treece, James W., 442
Treip, C. S., 250
Trelease, Sam F., 154
Trevethick, R. A., 235
Triche, Charles W. III, 20, 28
Triche, Diane S., 20, 28
Trissel, Lawrence A., 126
Truant, Joseph P., 191
Trzyna, Thaddeus C., 304, 305
Tucker, Gabriel F., Jr., 268
Tucker, Richard P., 406
Tuft, Louis, 157
Tulley, W. J., 163
Tunevall, Goesta, 524
Tunnesson, Walter, 598
Turleau, Catherine, 259
Turley, Raymond V., 10
Turnbull, H. Rutherford, 107
Turner, Anthony C., 114
Turner, Arthur R., 28
Turner, Dorothea, 116
Turner, Glenn O., 210
Turner, James E., 137
Turner, Paul, 124
Turner, Renate G., 137
Turner, William A., 405
Tydesley, W. R., 104
Tyler, H. Richard, 350
Tymchuk, Alexander J., 91

Ufhara, Y., 267
Ule, Günter, 270
Underwood, E. A., 328
Undritz, Erik, 261
UNESCO, 287, 344
Union of Concerned Scientists, 484
UN Document Index Unit, 542
United Nations Statistical Office, 149
United Parkinson Foundation, 606
US Administration on Aging, US Department of Health, Education, and Welfare, 26
US Agricultural Research Service, 225
US Bureau of Radiological Health, 48
US Congress, Office of Technology Assessment, 562
US Consumer and Food Economics Institute, Agricultural Research Service, 141

US Council on Environmental Quality, 314
US Defense Documentation Center, 536
US Defense Documentation Center, Defense Supply Agency, 537
US Department of Agriculture, 117
US Department of Health, Education, and Welfare, 7, 206, 212, 288, 384, 536, 539, 543, 562, 575
US Department of Labor, 293
US Department of Labor, Women's Bureau, 96
US Department of the Army, 115
US Directory Service, 291
US Division of Physician and Health Professions Education, 20
US Energy Research and Development Administration, 35, 536, 559
US Environmental Protection Agency, 46, 539, 562
US Food and Drug Administration, 50, 121, 305, 523, 577, 596
US General Services Administration, 287, 568, 570
US Government Printing Office, 543
US Health Facilities Planning and Construction Service, 27
US Library of Congress, 589
US Library of Congress. Science and Technology Division. Reference Section, 10
US National Academy of Sciences, 317, 576
US National Aeronautics and Space Administration, 536
US National Bureau of Standards, 568, 570
US National Center for Health Services Research and Development, Bureau of Health Manpower Education, National Institutes of Health, 28, 287
US National Center for Health Statistics, 144, 150, 565
US National Clearinghouse for Drug Abuse Literature, National Institute on Drug Abuse, Department of Health, Education, and Welfare, 16, 23, 39, 45
US National Clearinghouse for Mental Health, 41
US National Committee for Geochemistry, US National Research Council, 391
US National Council of Radiation Protection and Measurements, 415
US National Council on Radiation Protection, 133, 136
US National Institute for Occupational Safety and Health, 147, 171, 215
US National Institute of Allergy and Infectious Diseases, 22, 29
US National Institute of Arthritis, Metabolism, and Digestive Diseases, 50, 511, 522
US National Institute of Child Health and Human Development, 600
US National Institute of Child Health and Human Development, Center for Population Research, 521
US National Institute of Dental Research, 561
US National Institute of Mental Health, Department of Health, Education, and Welfare, 39, 44, 304, 598, 599
US National Institute of Neurological and Communicative Disorders and Stroke, Department of Health, Education, and Welfare, 24, 509
US National Institute of Neurological Disease and Stroke, 24
US National Institute on Alcohol Abuse and Alcoholism, Department of Health, Education, and Welfare, 305, 599
US National Institute on Drug Abuse, Department of Health, Education, and Welfare 39, 50, 523
US National Institutes of Health, 46, 142, 286, 291, 397, 536, 539, 560
US National Library of Medicine, 4, 6, 18, 19, 40, 49, 322, 323, 326, 331, 372, 504, 505, 506, 507, 508, 526, 539, 543, 614, 615, 616, 619, 620, 623
US National Library of Medicine. Technical Services Division, 156
US National Library Service for the

Blind and Physically Handicapped, Library of Congress 303
US National Medical Audiovisual Center, 587, 599
US National Referral Center, Science and Technology Division, Library of Congress, 283, 304, 306
US National Research Council, 142, 483
US National Safety Council, 182
US National Science Foundation, 143, 285, 558, 559, 560
US National Technical Information Service, 536, 543
US Naval Medical School of the National Naval Medical Center, 271
US Patent Office, 578, 579, 580, 581
US President's Council on Physical Fitness and Sports, 31
US Public Health Service, 305, 521, 596, 597
US Public Health Service. Pesticides Program, 521
US Rehabilitation Services Administration, 303
US Superintendent of Documents, 541, 554
US Veterans Administration Hospital, 41
Universities Federation for Animal Welfare, 97
University of Iowa, College of Pharmacy, 592
University of Kansas Medical Center, Department of Nursing Education, 551
Unseld, Dieter W., 69
Usdin, Earl, 182
Usdin, Gene, 426, 479, 481
Utz, David C., 279

Vaeth, J. M., 387
Vaillancourt, Pauline M., 35
Vainshtein, Zinaida I., 71
Valdoni, Pietro, 225
Valenstein, Elliot S., 330
Vallance-Owen, J., 213
Valman, H. B., 121, 471
Vanbreuseghem, R., 218, 241
VanDemark, P. J., 192

van der Linden, Frans P. G. M., 253
van der Reis, L., 550
Van Hoof, F., 424
van Ketel, W. G., 207
Van Leeuwen, Gerard, 178
Vannier, Maryhelen, 477
van Oss, Carel J., 400
van Praag, Herman M., 131, 234
Van Sell Davidson, Sharon, 573
van Straten, S., 34
Vantrappen, G., 420
Vaughan, Patricia, 181
Vaughan-Wrobel, Beth C., 195
Vaughn, D., 456
Vaughn, Janet M., 483
Veaner, A. B., 588
Veatch, Robert M., 19, 428
Veillon, Emanuel, 73
Velleman, Ruth A., 96
Vellucci, Matthew J., 285
Verel, David, 161
Vervoren, Thora M., 196
Verzar, F., 336
Vibe, G., 134
Vick, Nicholas A., 406
Vickery, Donald M., 221, 229
Vidal, Maria T., 270
Vidic, Branislav, 244
Vietti, Teresa J., 466
Villee, Dorothy B., 419
Villiger, Emil, 248
Vinken, P. J., 100
Visscher, M. B., 395
Vlodaver, Zeev, 252
Vodra, Richard E., 199
Volans, Glyn, 124
Vollman, Rudolf, F., 26
von der Mosel, Hans A., 568
von Frauendorfer, Sigmund, 500
Vona, Embree De-Persiis, 88

Wade, Ainley, 126
Wade, Carol, 563
Wade, Jenny, 4
Wagenvoort, C. A., 464
Wagenvoort, Noeke, 464
Wagner, Henry N., Jr., 264, 470
Wagner, Monica Mary, 172
Wagner, Robert R., 383
Wakeley, Cecil, 79

Walen, Susan R., 232
Walford, Albert J., 9
Walker, William F., 247
Wallach, Jacques B., 114
Wallach, Jeffrey J., 81
Waller, Coy W., 49
Walsh, Frank B., 250
Walsh, Mary Roth, 324
Walsh, Robert J., 152
Walshe, Francis M. R., 405
Walter Reed Army Institute of Research, 560
Walter Reed Army Medical Center, US Department of Defense, 595
Walters, LeRoy, 19
Walton, John N., 404, 492
Waltz, Jon R., 397
Wang, Yen, 136
Wangensteen, Owen H., 329
Wangensteen, Sarah D., 329
Ward, Charles O., 180
Ward, Howard L., 188
Ward, Mary Jane, 33
Ward, Michael, 438
Waring, William W., 178
Warren, Kenneth S., 29
Warren, Richard, 261
Warwick, Roger, 207, 406
Wasserman, Paul, 148, 281, 282, 290, 328, 602
Watanabe, Arthur S., 125, 180
Waterhouse, J. A. H., 118, 134
Waters, Harold, 119
Waters, T. R. W., 332
Waterson, A. P., 334
Watkins, E. S., 251
Watson, Craig, 250
Watson, N. K., 589
Watson, Robert T., 100
Waxman, Bruce D., 374
Weakley, Brenda S., 120
Weast, Robert C., 94
Weatherall, D. J., 425
Weathers, Doris L., 425
Webb, Marion R., 71
Weber, D. L., 177
Weckesser, Elden C., 403
Weed, Robert, 261
Wehrle, Paul F., 110
Weil, M. H., 112, 170

Weinberg, Martin S., 43
Weinberg, Samuel, 255
Weinberger, Bernhard W., 331
Weiner, John M., 396
Weinstein, Lois, 13
Weir, D. M., 97
Weir, Jamie, 275
Weisberg, Leon A., 277
Weiss, Earle B., 61
Weiss, Leonard, 451, 490
Weiss, Nathaniel, 83
Welbourn, R. B., 78
Welin, Grethe, 421
Welin, Solve, 421
Wellcome Historical Medical Library, 323
Wellcome Historical Medical Museum Library, 323
Wells, P. N. T., 485
Wentz, Frank M., 254
Werner, Mario, 219
Werts, Margaret F., 30, 32, 221
Wessells, Virginia G., 446
West, Geoffrey, P., 62, 93
West, John B., 489, 490
West, Kelly M., 418
Westermeyer, Joseph, 237
Western Reserve University, 8
Whalen, George J., 54
Whalen, Joseph P., 258
Whaley, Lucille F., 426
Wheat, Myron W., Jr., 162
Whelen, Hilary, 35
Whipple, Gerald H., 439
Whitaker, Charlotte, 19
White, Abraham, 398
White, Burton L., 468
White, David C., 275
White, M. J. D., 61
White, Robert G., 433
White, Robert P., 272
White, Sarah, 559
Whitson, B. J., 173
Whittington, Frank J., 474
Whybrow, Peter C., 481
Widmann, Frances K., 396
Wieck, Lynn, 172
Wied, G. L., 363
Wigzell, H., 166
Wilcocks, C., 435

AUTHOR INDEX

Wilcox, William H., 499, 519
Wilding, P., 192
Wilkes, I. H., 63
Wilkins, E. W., Jr., 437
Wilkins, Robert H., 378
Wilkinson, Lise, 334
Wilkinson, P. C., 83
Willet, Joseph W., 451
Willett, Hilda P., 111, 436
Williams, Cecil C., 178
Williams, D. F., 402
Williams, D. Innes, 280
Williams, David I., 393
Williams, George, 279
Williams, I. G., 473
Williams, Innes, 472
Williams, J. G. P., 438
Williams, John S., Jr., 47
Williams, Margaret, 240
Williams, Martha E., 614
Williams, P. C., 525
Williams, Peter L., 207, 406
Williams, Preston P., 199
Williams, R. M., 405
Williams, Robert H., 420
Williams, Robley C., 259
Williams, Roger J., 118
Williams, Roger John, 52
Williams, Sue R., 225
Williams, Sylvia, 46
Williams, Thomas J., 121
Williams, Trevor I., 316
Williams, W. J., 430
Williams, Wilbur K., 110
Wilson, Florence A., 296
Wilson, Graham S., 435
Wilson, James G., 106
Wilson, John L., 98
Wilson, Robert R., 186
Wilson, William K., 307
Winchell, Constance M., 9
Windholz, M., 127
Winek, C. L., 314
Winek, Charles L., 91
Wingate, Peter, 56
Winick, Myron, 385
Winkelstein, Alan, 190
Winslow, Ken, 590
Winter, C. C., 445
Winton, Harry N. M., 48, 542

Wintrobe, Maxwell M., 109, 429
Wischnitzer, Saul, 205, 242
Wise, Robert E., 487
Wishik, Samuel M., 66
Wissler, R. W., 161
Witten, David M., 279
Wobig, John L., 458
Woerdeman, M. W., 243
Wolf, P. L., 192
Wolf, U., 189
Wolff, M. E., 473
Wolman, Benjamin B., 60, 90, 130
Wood, Charles D., 244
Wood, Dena L., 193, 194
Wood, Ernest H., 99
Wood, Marilyn J., 221
Wood, R. L., 462
Woodburne, Russell T., 208, 400
Woodford, F. Peter, 156
Wootton, A. C., 338
Wootton, I. D. P., 194
World Federation of Neurological Society, 606
World Health Organization, 90, 119, 142, 149, 167, 168, 171, 183, 240, 307, 483, 536, 539, 542, 543, 565, 566, 567, 568, 569, 571, 574, 576
World Health Organization, Study Group, 149
Worthingham, Catherine, 177
Worthington, E. Louisa, 126
Wren, R. C., 58
Wright, Arthur W., 220
Wright, Francis S., 471
Wright, I. S., 210
Wyatt, G. B., 171
Wyatt, H. V., 11
Wyatt, J. L., 171
Wyburn, G. M., 257
Wyman, Alvin C., 277
Wyngaarden, James B., 203, 424
Wynkoop, Sally, 542
Wynn, Ralph M., 315
Wynne, Lyman C., 480
Wynne, Ronald D., 37
Wynne-Davies, Ruth, 267, 460

Yakes, Nancy, 284
Yale University. School of Nursing. Index Staff, 514

Yamauchi, Ryutaro, 70
Yanoff, Myron, 266
Yap, J. C., 251
Yashon, David, 477
Yates, Frank, 152
Youmans, Guy P., 490
Youmans, Julian R., 209
Young, Harold C., 283, 286
Young, James H., 337
Young, Margaret L., 283, 286
Youngson, A. J., 330

Zachau-Christiansen, B., 465
Zachert, Martha J. K., 576
Zacks, Sumner I., 249
Zahorski, Withold W., 482
Zaias, Nardo, 417
Zainie, Carla M., 138
Zaman, Viqar, 262

Zander, Karen, 173
Zetkin, Maxim, 70
Ziegal, Erna E., 446
Zils, Michael, 603
Zimmerli, William H., 47
Zimmerman, Clarence E., 174
Zimmerman, David R., 332
Zimmerman, Mikhail G., 71
Zingg, Ernst J., 280
Zizmor, Judith, 268
Zollinger, Robert M., 247
Zollinger, Robert M., Jr., 247
Zoneraich, Samuel, 413
Zschoche, Donna A., 444
Zubkoff, Helene, 593
Zuckerman, A. J., 434
Zuidema, George D., 245
Zulch, Klaus J., 269
Zusne, Leonard, 321

Author Index to Reference List

Abrams, F. A., 650
Adams, Scott, 633, 644
Agranovs, A. I., 639
Aitchison, T. M., 636
Algermissen, Virginia L., 647
Allyn, Richard, 640
American Standards Association, 637
Anderson, David C., 637
Armstrong, Robert P., 642
Arndt, K., 648
Ash, J., 651
Asher, Gordon, 648
Ashwroth, W., 633
Auger, C. P., 649

Baer, K. A., 635
Baker, D. B., 633
Bailery, J. L., 650
Baldwin, Carol, 645
Barker, Frances H., 641
Bartlett, Marjorie H., 646
Basile, Victor A., 651
Bastille, J. D., 638
Basu, R. N., 646
Baum, Harry, 639
Bearman, T. C., 650
Beatty, William K., 642
Beauchamp, Sister E. A., 647
Bell, J. A. H., 647
Billings, John Shaw, 643
Birnbaum, H., 645
Bishop, David, 650
Bloomfield, M., 641
Bock, Rochelle, 637
Boston Medical Library, 637
Bottle, R. T., 635
Bourni, C. P., 633
Bowden, Charles L., 651
Bowden, Virginia M., 651
Bower, C. A., 652
Boyer, Calvin James, 642
Brand, R., 650
Brandon, Alfred N., 633, 640
Brantz, Malcolm H., 647
Braude, Robert M., 637, 644
British Standards Institution, 637
Broaduf, H., 645

Broadus, Robert N., 638
Brodman, Estelle, 635, 651
Buckland, M. K., 635
Burke, M. S., 649
Burkett, J., 633
Butkovich, Margaret, 637

Callard, J. C., 642
Cantu, Jane Q., 643
Cermakova, Jirina, 639
Charen, Thelma, 644
Chen, Ching-chih, 636, 638, 651
Chillag, J. P., 650
Clark, C. V., 648
Cobb, Mary M., 642
Cornelius, E. H., 642
Cosma, M., 650
Crane, Diana, 646
Cross, L. C., 648
Cunningham, Eileen R., 637

Damerau, F. J., 636
Dannatt, R. J., 649
Davies, G., 646
Day, Philip E., 633
Dickson, W. M., 642
Doe, Janet, 644
Dolcourt, Joyce L., 644
Dorr, H. A., 633
Drage, J. R., 633
Drott, M. C., 638, 650
Duncan, Howertine Farrell, 640
Dwyer, Thomas F., 647

Elias, A. W., 642
Elliot, C. K., 633
Elliot, M., 634
Elwin, C. E., 646

Flanagan, C., 634
Fleming, Thomas P., 651
Flood, B., 637
Ford, M., 650
Foreman, Gertrude, 645
Foster, Willis R., 646
Fox, Sir Theodor, 646
Fraser, M. D. E., 651

AUTHOR INDEX

Fried, C., 634
Friedlander, J., 646
Fruehauf, E. L., 642

Gaffney, Inez, 641
Gannett, Elwood K., 649
Gardner, A. L., 642
Garfield, Eugene, 633, 636, 639, 642, 648
Garrison, Fielding H., 643
Garvey, W. D., 639, 646
Gee, Helen H., 643
Getchell, Marjorie E., 640
Ginski, J. M., 651
Gnudi, Martha Teach, 643
Goffman, William, 638
Gomes, Stella S., 651
Gordon, B. L., 644
Gould, A. M., 633
Graber, T. M., 640
Graf, F., 649
Gregory, M. W., 646
Griffith, B. C., 638, 646, 650

Haigh, P. A., 639
Hall, A. M., 636
Hathorn, Isabel B., 640
Herschman, A., 648
Hill, Dorothy R., 640
Hines, Lois E., 637
Hitchingham, Eileen E., 645
Hollander, S., 634, 644
Holton, G., 636
Houghton, Bernard, 649
Hudson, S., 649

Ingelfinger, Franz J., 642
International Council of Scientific Unions, 643

Jacobus, David P., 634
Jones, M. Irene, 637

Keenan, Stella, 634
Kennedy, H. E., 634
Kennedy, Jean, 637
Kilgour, Frederick G., 651, 652
Knox, William T., 646
Kochen, M., 642
Korfhage, R. R., 646

Kossmann, Charles B., 637
Kovacs, H., 651
Kraft, M., 639
Kronick, David A., 647
Kuney, J. H., 648

Lakie, M. H., 650
Lancaster, F. W., 634, 645
Lavalle, K. H., 636
Leeds, Alice A., 643
Lehman, L. J., 646
Leiter, J., 645
Lewis, R. F., 639
Library Association, Medical Section, 640
Lloyd, H. A., 651
Lufkin, J. M., 650

Maddox, John, 648
Malcolm, M. E., 648
Mankin, C. J., 638
Manten, A. A., 649
Martyn, J., 636
McCarn, D. B., 645
McMurtray, H. F., 651
Meakin, F. A., 639
Meiboom, Esther R., 647
Messinger, K., 637
Mick, C. K., 651
Miller, J. K., 645
Miller, Lois B., 642
Mills, P. R., 639
Mitchell, P. C., 645
Moll, W., 645
Moore, J. A., 649
Morris, Thomas G., 638
Mountstephens, Brenda, 643

Narin, Francis, 643, 648

Olch, Peter D., 643
Onsager, L. W., 640
Orr, Richard H., 643
Oseasohn, Robert, 652

Parkins, P. V., 634
Parr, T., 635
Peters, B., 640
Pings, Vern M., 644
Pinski, Gabriel, 643

AUTHOR INDEX

Postell, William Dosite, 635
Poynter, F. N. L., 643
Prevel, J. J., 634
Price, D. J. de Solla, 636, 646
Price, K., 635
Pukteris, Sophie, 650

Raisig, L. Miles, 648, 652
Ramsden, M. J., 637
Raskin, Robert B., 640
Ratcliff, Wendy W., 640
Rathbun, Edith N., 642
Raymond, Sue L., 647
Reck, D., 649
Redowska, C. A., 642
Rees, A. M., 652
Richman, J. T., 645
Ring, Malvin E., 634
Ruhl, Mary Jane, 635

Sanders, E., 635
Sanders, T. R. B., 649
Saracevic, T., 637
Sarett, L. H., 643
Schad, Jasper G., 639
Scheerer, George, 637
Schneider, J. H., 642
Schultz, Louise, 634
Schwartz, J. H., 648
Science Information Exchange, 641
Scott, P. H., 650
Sengupta, I. N., 646, 648
Sequin, Marilynne, 647
Seymour, C. A., 639
Sher, I. H., 633
Shilling, C. W., 635
Simon, H. R., 635
Smith, E. B., 650
Smith, Joan M. B., 652
Smith, Reginald W., 651
Sodergren, Linnea, 645
Spiller, David, 639
Staiger, D. L., 648
Stangl, Peter, 652
Stavely, Ronald, 634
Stearns, Norman S., 640
Sutherland, F. M., 634, 635, 649
Swanson, D. R., 638, 645

Tagliacozzo, R., 641
Taine, Seymour I., 644
Tauber, S. J., 642
Temkin, Owsei, 643
Thompson, C. W. N., 634
Tibbetts, Pamela, 652
Timour, John A., 641
Torr, D. V., 634
Tracy, J. M., 636
Truelson, Stanley D., Jr., 634
Tschirgi, Robert D., 647

Urguhart, D. J., 642
US National Academy of Sciences, 647
US National Library of Medicine, 638, 644
US Office of Technical Services, 650
US Veterans Administration, Central Office Library, 641
Utterback, Robert A., 647

Veaner, Allen, 647
Velleman, R. A., 635
Virgo, J. A., 649

Walden, W. E., 645
Weinman, J., 640
Weinstock, M., 636
Wellisch, H., 638
Welt, Isaac D., 644
Wendt, R. E., 643
Wente, Van A., 641
Werner, G., 645
West, K. M., 644
Wilkinson, Doris, 634, 644
Williams, Martha E., 641, 645
Wood, D. N., 652
Wood, G. C., 652
Wood, J. L., 634
Wood, M. S., 646
Woodward, A. M., 649
Wright, Arthuree M., 636
Wright, K. C., 638
Wyatt, H. V., 643

Yast, Helen T., 641
Yokote, Gail, 647
Young, Clifford A., 641

Zeller, Karen, 641

Ref
Z
6658
C44

APR 2 1981